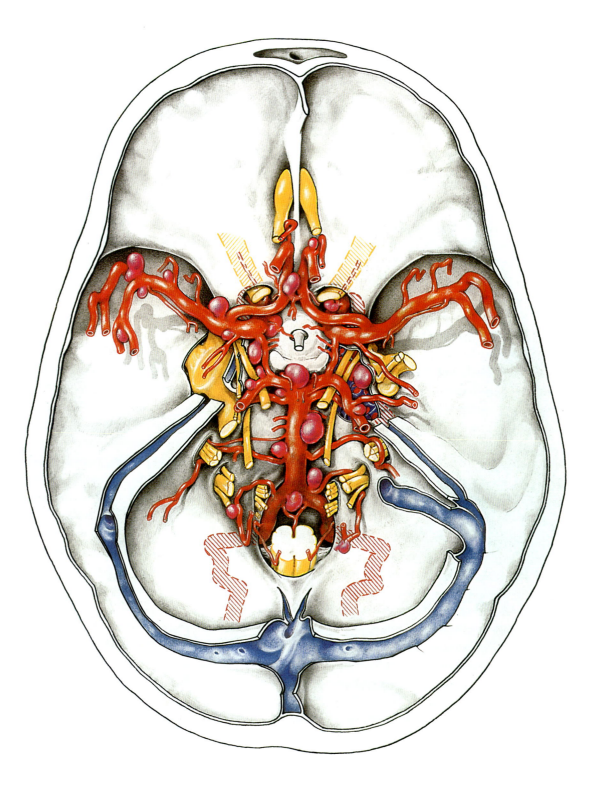

Schematic illustration of aneurysms of the Circle of Willis in relation to the basal cranial nerves.

Microneurosurgery

in 4 Volumes

M. G. Yaşargil

I

Microsurgical Anatomy of the Basal Cisterns and Vessels of the Brain, Diagnostic Studies, General Operative Techniques and Pathological Considerations of the Intracranial Aneurysms

II

Clinical Considerations, Surgery of the Intracranial Aneurysms and Results

III

Clinical Considerations and Microsurgery of the Arteriovenous Racemose Angiomas

IV

Clinical Considerations and Microsurgery of the Tumors

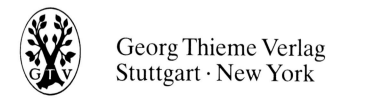

Georg Thieme Verlag
Stuttgart · New York

Thieme Stratton Inc.
New York

II Clinical Considerations, Surgery of the Intracranial Aneurysms and Results

M. G. Yaşargil

Collaborators:
R. D. Smith, P. H. Young and P. J. Teddy

Illustrated by P. Roth

169 Figures in 705 Illustrations
145 Tables

1984
Georg Thieme Verlag
Stuttgart · New York

Thieme Stratton Inc.
New York

Addresses

Yaşargil, M. G., M.D., Professor and Chairman,
Neurosurgical Department
University Hospital, Zurich

Smith, R. D., M.D., Department of Neurosurgery,
Louisiana State University Medical Center
New Orleans, Louisiana

Young, P. H., M.D., Section of Neurological Surgery
St. Louis University Medical Center
St. Louis, Missouri

Teddy, P. J., DPhil, FRCS, Consultant Neurosurgeon
The Department of Neurological Surgery
The Radcliffe Infirmary, Oxford

Roth, P., Scientific artist
Neurosurgical Department
University Hospital, Zurich

Deutsche Bibliothek Cataloguing in Publication Data

Yaşargil, M. Gazi:
Microneurosurgery : in 4 vol. / M. G. Yaşargil.
– Stuttgart ; New York : Thieme; New York :
Thieme Stratton

2. → Yaşargil, M. Gazi: Clinical considerations, surgery of the intracranial aneurysms and results

Yaşargil, M. Gazi:
Clinical considerations, surgery of the intracranial aneurysms and results / M. G. Yaşargil. Collab.: R. D. Smith ... Ill. by P. Roth. – Stuttgart ; New York : Thieme; New York : Thieme Stratton, 1984

(Microneurosurgery / M. G. Yaşargil ; 2)

Important Note: Medicine is an ever-changing science. Research and clinical experience are continually broadening our knowledge, in particular our knowledge of proper treatment and drug therapy. Insofar as this book mentions any dosage or application, readers may rest assured that the authors, editors and publishers have made every effort to ensure that such references are strictly in accordance with the state of knowledge at the time of production of the book. Nevertheless, every user is requested to carefully examine the manufacturers' leaflets accompanying each drug to check on his own responsibility whether the dosage schedules recommended therein or the contraindications stated by the manufacturers differ from the statements made in the present book. Such examination is particularly important with drugs which are either rarely used or have been newly released on the market.

Some of the product names, patents and registered designs referred to in this book are in fact registered trademarks or proprietary names even though specific reference to this fact is not always made in the text. Therefore, the appearance of a name without designation as proprietary is not to be construed as a representation by the publishers that it is in the public domain.

All rights, including the rights of publication, distribution and sales, as well as the right to translation, are reserved. No part of this work covered by the copyrights hereon may be reproduced or copied in any form or by any means – graphic, electronic or mechanical including photocopying, recording, taping, or information and retrieval systems – without written permission of the publisher.

© 1984 Georg Thieme Verlag, Rüdigerstrasse 14,
D-7000 Stuttgart 30, FRG
Typesetting: Printing-House Dörr
D-7140 Ludwigsburg; typeset on System 5 (Linotron 202)
Printed and bound in India by
Replika Press Pvt. Ltd.

ISBN 3-13-644901-0 (Georg Thieme Verlag, Stuttgart)
ISBN 0-86577-142-1 (Thieme-Stratton Inc., New York)
LC 83-051137

Acknowledgements

Although the cases described in this volume constitute a personal series, the clinical work could never have been carried out nor the book completed without the considerable help of very many colleagues and friends.

I should like to acknowledge in particular the excellent work, professional skills and help of our anesthetic team, notably Drs. Marijan Curcic, Mirjana Kis, and Claudia Champion our senior anesthetists past and present, and Dr. Anton Valavanis in the Department of Radiology in Zurich.

The patients whose clinical records form the basis of this book were referred from hospitals and departments not only in Zurich and other cantons but also many different countries outside Switzerland. Several of the radiographs depicted in the text were supplied by neuroradiologists from these other units. I would like to thank all my colleagues – physicians, surgeons and radiologists, who by virtue of referral laid the groundwork both for the surgery and for this publication.

I am greatly indebted to the operating theatre staff whose expertise and quiet efficiency have been a source of unfailing support over the years.

Sophisticated operations can be useful to the patient only if the pre- and postoperative care are of equal sophistication and in this respect I am most grateful for the very high standards set by the nursing and medical staff and the physiotherapists on the intensive care unit and general nursing wards in the University Hospital of Zurich.

I wish again to thank Dr. Gertrud Siegenthaler not only for her help in supervising the medical aspect of the intensive care, but also on this occasion for the contribution to the chapter on complications.

I would particularly like to thank Dr. Peter Teddy for his many contributions to this text and for his general help and advise in preparing and correcting the manuscript.

The draft copies of Volume II have all been corrected and typed by Mrs. Margrit Traber, who also helped to compile the index to Volumes I and II. I am once again most grateful to her.

Preface

Publication of the first two volumes of this series on Microneurosurgery was originally scheduled for 1980. The intention was to describe the results achieved and experience gained by the senior author from the 1,012 cases of intracranial aneurysm operated upon in the Neurosurgical Department in the University Hospital, Zurich between January 1967 and July 31, 1979.

For several reasons publication had to be delayed for four years and in the interim a further 355 cases had been operated upon between August 1, 1979 and December 31, 1983. It seemed reasonable to include these additional cases in the present text as it provided an opportunity to compare at least the early results from this group with the other larger series all operated upon by a single surgeon using microtechniques. Chapter 10 deals with this second series as an addendum.

We hoped to establish whether or not improved neurosurgical nursing and anesthetic methods and above all, experience of the individual surgeon in dealing with ruptured aneurysms had significantly improved outcome in the latter group. My own opinion regarding surgical expertise is that for the first one or two hundred cases results will improve as experience is gained in dealing with these lesions. Beyond this level I doubt that increased dexterity leads to significant reduction in morbidity and mortality. What is probably more important is that the greater the surgical experience the better one becomes at selecting patients for surgery and at timing radiological and operative intervention.

This must lead me once more to emphasize the overriding necessity always to consider the overall management of subarachnoid hemorrhage and the need to find ways of bringing more patients presenting in poorer clinical condition to safe and effective surgery.

The first nine chapters of this present volume are devoted to a comprehensive analysis of the 1,012 aneurysm cases treated between 1967 and 1979. The first chapter deals with general considerations, chapters 2–5 with operative results in relation to the site of various aneurysms, chapters 6 and 7 with giant multiple aneurysms respectively, and chapter 8 with those cases not treated surgically. Chapter 9 deals with operative complications and chapter 11 is reserved for general comments and conclusions.

I hope that this publication which makes no attempt to camouflage the uncertainties and difficulties we have experienced in over 16 years of aneurysm surgery will help others to overcome similar problems as they encounter them, and thereby help to reduce just a little the still appallingly high mortality and morbidity from subarachnoid hemorrhage.

M. G. Yaşargil

Contents

1 Clinical Considerations 1

Clinical Presentation 1
Ruptured Cerebral Aneurysm with
Symptoms of Meningeal Irritation 1
Unruptured Cerebral Aneurysm 2
   Symptomatic 2
   Asymptomatic 2
Timing of Operation 7
   Relationship to Clinical Condition 7
   General Medical Condition 16
   Relationship to Angiographically
   Demonstrated Vasospasm 17
   Relationship to Intracranial Pressure ... 25
   Relationship to Cerebral Blood Flow ... 26

Reducing Preoperative Rebleeding Risk ... 26
   General Medical Care 26
   Hypotension 27
   Antifibrinolytic Agents 27
   Partial Cervical Carotid Artery Occlusion . 28

Special Clinical Presentations 28
Unruptured Asymptomatic Aneurysms ... 28
Pregnancy 29
Age 29
Children 30
Laterality 32

2 Internal Carotid Artery Aneurysms 33

Introduction 33

Infraclinoid Internal Carotid Artery Aneurysms 33
Anatomical Relationships 33
   Aneurysms of the Cervical ICA 33
   Aneurysms in the Petrous Portion of ICA . 37
   Intracavernous Aneurysms 37
Operative Technique 38
   Cervical Carotid Ligation 38
Clinical Presentation and Operative Results . 39
Summary 41

Carotid-Ophthalmic Aneurysms 43
Anatomical Relationships 43
   Laterality and Multiplicity of Aneurysms . 43
   Projection of Aneurysm Fundus 44
   Relationship to Ophthalmic Artery 44
   Relationship to Anterior Clinoid Process . 44
Operative Technique 44
   Initial Approach and Proximal Control .. 44
   Gaining Distal Control 45

Exposure of the Ophthalmic Artery 45
The Carotid and Chiasmatic Cisterns ... 46
Elevation of a Suprachiasmatic
Aneurysm 46
Clip Application 46
Multiple and Bilateral Aneurysms 46
Unclipped Aneurysms 47
Summary 48
Clinical Presentation and Operative Results . 48
   Timing and Results 54
Summary 55

Distal Medial Wall Aneurysms 58
Anatomical Relationships 58
Operative Technique 58
Clinical Presentation and Operative Results . 58

Aneurysms of Superior Wall of Internal Carotid Artery 59
Anatomical Relationships 59
Operative Technique 59
Clinical Presentation and Operative Results . 59

Inferior Wall Aneurysms of the Internal Carotid Artery ... 60
Anatomical Relationships ... 60
  Multiplicity ... 60
Operative Technique ... 60
Clinical Presentation and Operative Results ... 68
  Timing and Results ... 70
Summary ... 70

Carotid-Posterior Communicating Aneurysms ... 71
Anatomical Relationships ... 71
  Laterality and Multiplicity ... 71
  General Remarks ... 71
  Direction of Fundus ... 72
  Relationship to the Subarachnoid Cisterns ... 74
  Relationship to Posterior Communicating Artery ... 76
  Relationship to Anterior Thalamoperforating (Diencephalic or Central) Arteries ... 77
  Relationship to the Anterior Choroidal Artery ... 77
  Relationship to the Oculomotor Nerve ... 77
  Relationship to the Tentorium Cerebelli ... 78
  Relationship to Clinoid Processes ... 78
  Relationship to the Mesial Temporal Lobe ... 78
  Epidural Extension ... 78
Operative Technique ... 78
  Identification of the Posterior Communicating Artery ... 78
  Identification of the Anterior Choroidal Artery ... 82
  Identification of the Oculomotor Nerve ... 82
  Dissection of Aneurysm Neck ... 83
  Coagulation ... 84
  Clip Application ... 85
  Fundus Resection and Closure ... 85
  Intraoperative Rupture of the Aneurysm ... 85
  Ligated Aneurysms ... 85
  Bilateral Aneurysms ... 85
  Summary ... 88
Clinical Presentation and Operative Results ... 88
  Background ... 88
  Presenting Features ... 88
  Outcome of Oculomotor Palsy ... 90
  Operative Results ... 90
  Mortality and Morbidity Analysis ... 92

Anterior Choroidal Artery Aneurysms ... 99
Anatomical Relationships ... 99
  Incidence ... 99
  Relationship to the Anterior Choroidal Artery ... 99
  Relationship to the Uncus and Tentorium ... 100
  Multiple and Bilateral Aneurysms ... 100
Operative Technique ... 102
  Initial Exposure ... 102
  Dissection of the Carotid Cistern ... 102
  Dissection of the Aneurysm Neck ... 102
  Clip Application ... 102
  Summary ... 103
Clinical Presentation and Operative Results ... 103
  Background ... 103
  Presenting Features ... 103
  Operative Results ... 104
  Operative Timing ... 106
Summary ... 106

Aneurysms of the Internal Carotid Artery Bifurcation (ICBi-Aneurysms) ... 109
Anatomical Relationships ... 109
  Incidence, Laterality ... 109
  Size and Direction of Fundus ... 109
  Relationship to Subarachnoid Cisterns ... 109
  Arterial Relationships ... 109
  Venous Relationships ... 113
Operative Technique ... 113
  Initial Exposure ... 113
  Dissection of the Sylvian Fissure ... 113
  Dissection of the Lamina Terminalis Cistern ... 113
  Dissection Beneath the Bifurcation ... 114
  Ligature and Clip Application ... 114
  Fundus Resection and Closure ... 115
  Summary ... 115
Bilateral and Multiple Aneurysms ... 116
Clinical Presentation and Operative Results ... 118
  Background ... 118
  Presenting Features ... 118
  Operative Results ... 118
  Timing and Results ... 120
Summary of Internal Carotid Artery Aneurysms ... 122

3 Middle Cerebral Artery Aneurysms ... 124

Anatomical Relationships ... 124
  Incidence, Laterality, Multiplicity ... 124
  Size and Morphology ... 125
  Relationship to the Subarachnoid Cisterns ... 125
  Relationship to the Middle Cerebral Artery ... 126
Operative Technique ... 132
  Initial Exposure ... 132
  Dissection of the Aneurysm ... 134

Contents IX

Clip Application	136	Background	149
Closure	139	Presenting Features	150
Summary of Operative Technique	139	Operative Results	150
Bilateral and Multiple Aneurysms	140	Complications	159
Giant Aneurysms	146	Analysis of Results	160
Clinical Presentation and Operative Results	149	Conclusion	164

4 Anterior Cerebral and Anterior Communicating Artery Aneurysms 165

Introduction	165	Initial Approach	185
		Dissection of the Aneurysm	186
Proximal Anterior Cerebral Artery		Clip Application	193
Aneurysms	165	Fundus Resection	199
Anatomical Relationships	165	Hemostasis and Closure	199
Operative Technique	167	Summary of Operative Technique	199
Initial Approach	167	Clinical Presentation and Operative Results	200
Cisternal Dissection	167	Presenting Features	200
Aneurysm Dissection	167	Operative Results	200
Aneurysm Clipping	167	Analysis of Results	206
Clinical Presentation and Operative Results	168	Summary	221
		Distal Anterior Cerebral Artery Aneurysms	
Anterior Communicating Artery Aneurysms	169	**(pericallosal artery aneurysms)**	224
Background	169	Anatomical Relationships	224
Anatomical Relationships	169	Operative Technique	226
Incidence	169	Initial Approach	226
Multiplicity	170	Removal of Hematoma	228
Location	173	Identification of Parent Arteries	228
Arterial Relationships	178	Aneurysm Dissection	228
Direction of Fundus	180	Aneurysm Clipping	228
Venous Relationships	184	Fundus Resection	228
Relationship to the Subarachnoid		Summary	228
Cisterns	184	Clinical Presentation and Operative Results	229
Operative Technique	185	Timing and Results	229

5 Vertebrobasilar Aneurysms 232

Background	232	Dissection of the Posterior Cerebral	
		Arteries	240
Basilar Artery Bifurcation Aneurysms	233	Dividing the Circle of Willis	240
Anatomical Relationships	233	Removal of the Posterior Clinoid Process	242
Incidence and Multiplicity	233	Dissection of Aneurysm Neck	242
Projection of Fundus	233	Clip Application	242
Size of Aneurysm	236	Closure	246
Relation to Posterior Communicating and		Summary of Operative Technique	246
Posterior Cerebral Arteries	236	Clinical Presentation and Operative Results	247
Relationship to the Dorsum Sellae	236	Presenting Features	247
Operative Technique	237	Operative Results	247
Initial Approach	237	Outcome of Oculomotor Paralysis	252
Entering the Interpeduncular Cistern	237	Analysis of Operative Results	252
Dissection of the Posterior Communi-		Operative Problems	254
cating Arteries	240	Summary	255

Upper Basilar Artery Trunk Aneurysms ... 257
Anatomical Relationships ... 257
Operative Technique ... 257
Clinical Presentation and Operative Results . 259

Posterior Cerebral Artery Aneurysms (P₁ Segment) ... 260
Anatomical Relationships ... 260
Operative Technique ... 260
Clinical Presentation and Operative Results . 264

Posterior Cerebral Artery Aneurysms (P₁/P₂ Junction) ... 265
Anatomical Relationships ... 265
Operative Technique ... 266
Clinical Presentation and Operative Results . 266

Posterior Cerebral Artery Aneurysms (P₂ Segment) ... 266
Anatomical Relationships ... 266
Operative Technique ... 266
Clinical Presentation and Operative Results . 267

Posterior Cerebral Artery Aneurysms (P₃ Segment) ... 268
Anatomical Relationships ... 268
Operative Technique ... 268
Clinical Presentation and Operative Results . 268

Saccular Aneurysms of the Lower Basilar Artery ... 270
Anatomical Relationships ... 270
Operative Technique ... 270
Clinical Presentation and Operative Results . 271

Fusiform Aneurysms of the Lower Basilar Artery ... 272
Anatomical Relationships ... 272
Operative Technique and Results ... 272

Distal Superior Cerebellar Artery Aneurysms ... 279
Anatomical Relationships ... 279
Operative Technique and Results ... 279

Saccular Aneurysms of the Vertebral Artery ... 281
Anatomical Relationships ... 281
Operative Technique ... 281
Clinical Presentation and Operative Results . 284

Fusiform Aneurysms of the Vertebral Artery ... 286
Anatomical Relationships ... 286
Operative Technique and Surgical Results . 286

Distal Posterior Inferior Cerebrellar Artery Aneurysms ... 290
Anatomical Relationships ... 290
Operative Technique ... 290
Clinical Presentation and Operative Results . 290
Summary ... 294

6 Giant Intracranial Aneurysms ... 296

7 Multiple Aneurysms ... 305

8 Unoperated Cases ... 329

9 Complications of Aneurysm Surgery ... 331

Introduction ... 331
Classification ... 331
Central Nervous System Complications ... 333
   Intracranial Hematoma ... 333
   Infection ... 333
   Ischemia ... 333
   Alterations of CSF Circulation ... 336
General Medical Complications ... 338
Conclusions ... 338

10 Addendum ... 340

11 Final Comments ... 346

References ... 349

Index ... 385

1 Clinical Considerations

Clinical Presentation

Ruptured Cerebral Aneurysm with Symptoms of Meningeal Irritation

The most common presentation of cerebral aneurysm is that of subarachnoid hemorrhage. This syndrome is classically characterized by explosive onset of severe headache, decreased level of consciousness, nuchal rigidity, and vomiting. Symptoms range from rather mild and transient headache and neck stiffness to deep coma with failing vital signs and little residual neurological function. Subarachnoid hemorrhage can mimic meningitis. Papilledema and retinal hemorrhages may be present. Symptoms of nausea, vomiting and headache may mimic systemic disease. Rarely a patient suffering a subarachnoid hemorrhage may present with hysterical, delusional, or psychotic behavior (with signs similar to those seen with hallucinatory drug ingestion such as LSD) or even as a forensic case.

Of particular importance is the recognition of patients suffering a mild, so-called "warning" hemorrhage. These patients may present with a variety of headache complaints and their differentiation from the more common headache syndromes may be difficult. A high index of suspicion should be aroused by complaints of new onset of worsening headache, by descriptions of "the worst headache I ever had", and by headache associated with signs of meningeal irritation.

Focal deficits accompany the presenting symptoms when there is hemorrhage into the brain substance or occasionally into the cranial nerves, or when regional blood flow to important areas of the brain is diminished. Patients presenting with focal neurological signs may incorrectly be considered to have sustained a thrombotic or hemorrhagic stroke on the basis of hypertension or

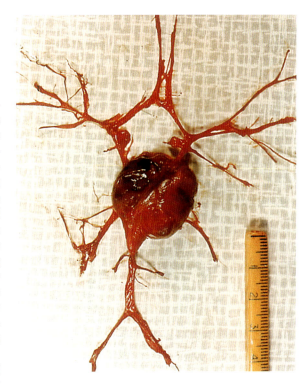

Fig 1 Autopsy specimen of an unrecognized basilar bifurcation aneurysm in a 2½ year old infant.

atherosclerotic cerebrovascular disease, or they may be thought to have a brain tumor:

B. F., a 2 year old male was in good health until 2 August, 1972, when he suddenly began crying and then lost consciousness. He exhibited a right hemiparesis when first examined. He was febrile with a leukocytosis, and lumbar puncture was xanthochromic. Bilateral carotid angiography did not reveal any pathological structures. He was returned to his local hospital where he made some recovery. On 9 September, 1972, he suddenly had a respiratory arrest and died. Autopsy revealed a ruptured 3 cm aneurysm of the basilar artery bifurcation (Fig **1**). Diagnostic failures such as this are now avoidable through the use of CT scanning.

Sometimes patients who have lost consciousness following subarachnoid hemorrhage are involved in automobile accidents or sustain falls, and their clinical condition is considered due to the secondary event. Psychiatric, behavioral, and even criminal changes have been seen following aneurysm rupture.

Unruptured Cerebral Aneurysm

Symptomatic

A second group of cerebral aneurysms present because of mass effect or their involvement of adjacent structures. Aneurysms of the intracavernous portion of the internal carotid artery generally present with cranial nerve deficits. Aneurysms of the internal carotid-ophthalmic arteries, the inferior wall of the internal carotid artery, and of the anterior communicating artery, may present as chiasmatic lesions with visual field deficits and pituitary dysfunction. Oculomotor palsies are common with aneurysms of the internal carotid-posterior communicating arteries and the basilar artery bifurcation area. Large aneurysms of the middle cerebral artery and internal carotid artery bifurcation have presented as hemisphere tumors, with hemiparesis and speech deficits, and large aneurysms of the anterior communicating and upper basilar arteries have presented as psychoorganic syndromes. A large basilar artery bifurcation aneurysm was discovered because of Parkinsonian complaints. Another presented with a pseudobulbar syndrome. Similarly aneurysms of the vertebrobasilar circulation have been misdiagnosed as posterior fossa tumors or as multiple sclerosis because of their involvement with brain stem structures (see pages 272, 286).

Asymptomatic

A third and increasingly common group are those aneurysms which are found incidentally during evaluation for headache, dizziness, or other neurological complaints. The common use of angiography in evaluation of neurological problems has brought many asymptomatic aneurysms to light, and the widespread use of computerized tomography for relatively benign problems promises to increase the discovery of asymptomatic aneurysms. The handling of such lesions is considered below (Figs **2A–D, 3A–C, 4A–H, 5A–D**).

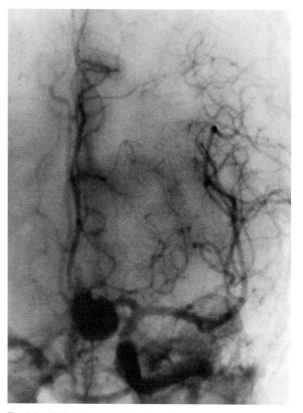

Fig **2A** This 54 year old patient had noticed visual blurring but this could not be objectively documented. The CT scan appearance was suggestive of a frontobasal tumor. Carotid angiography showed a large aneurysm at the left corner of the anterior communicating artery (**A**).

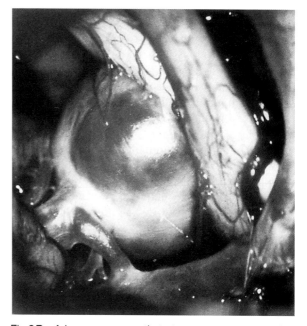

Fig **2B** A large aneurysm that at surgery was seen to be arising from the left A_1 segment and projecting into the left optic nerve (**B**). Operative photographs show the aneurysm bulging into the nerve.

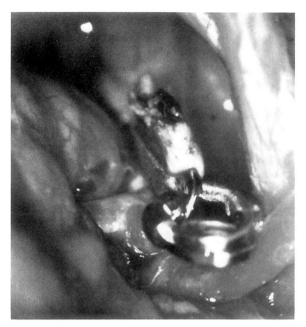
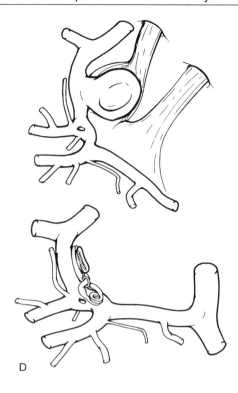

Fig 2C Clipped aneurysm and the compressed optic nerve.

2D Schematical drawing of operative findings and the aneurysmal neck after clipping and resection of the aneurysm.

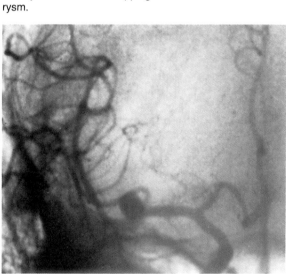
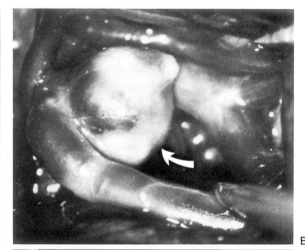
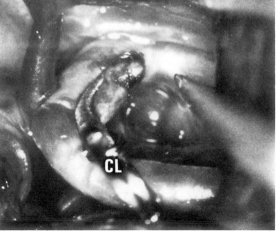

Fig 3A–C To evaluate a right sided Horner's syndrome a medical doctor underwent vertebral angiography that led to spontaneous filling of the right middle cerebral artery and branches and showed surprisingly an unruptured aneurysm at the right middle cerebral artery bifurcation. Right carotid angiography confirmed the presence of this aneurysm better (**A**). The patient insisted on the elimination of this asymptomatic aneurysm. At surgery the aneurysm (arrow) presented as a thin walled sac with lobulations (**B**). Dissection and clipping of the large based aneurysm was successfully carried out (**C**).

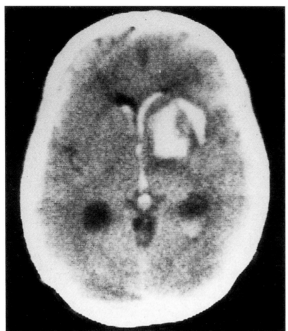

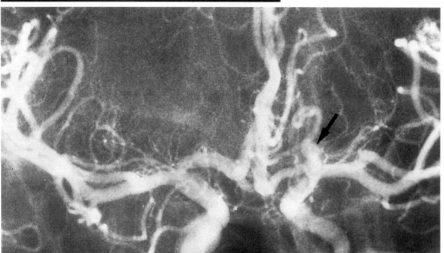

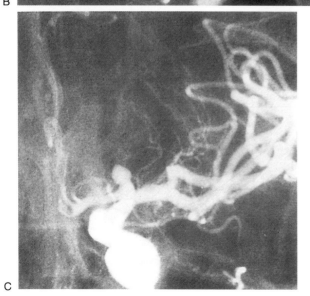

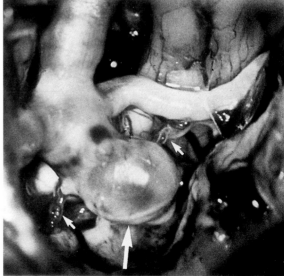

Fig 4 A–H A 41 year old patient suffered a subarachnoid hemorrhage with a left hemisyndrome. CT scan showed a deep right frontal hematoma (**A**). Right carotid angiography with cross compression revealed surprisingly no aneurysm on the right but an aneurysm (arrow) at the left carotid bifurcation (**B**). The left carotid angiogram confirmed this (**C**). Operative photograph shows the posteriorly directed fundus of the aneurysm within the trigonum olfactorium (large arrow) hiding behind the Heubner artery (small arrows, **D**).

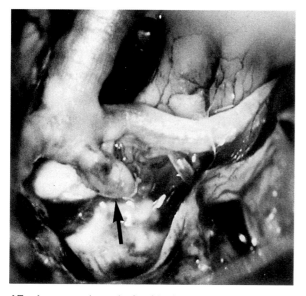

4E Aneurysm (arrow) after bipolar coagulation.

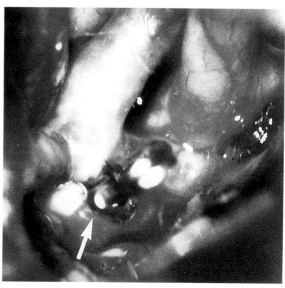

4F Clipped aneurysm (arrow).

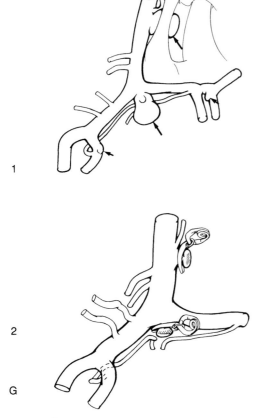

4G Schematical drawing of the operative findings. An incidental aneurysm of the left ophthalmic artery was also clipped. Baby aneurysms on M_2 and AcoA (small arrows).

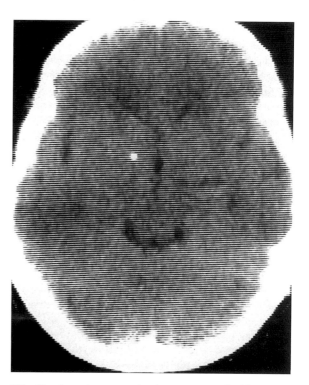

4H The hematoma resolved spontaneously (Case 54, Table **45**).

6   1 Clinical Considerations

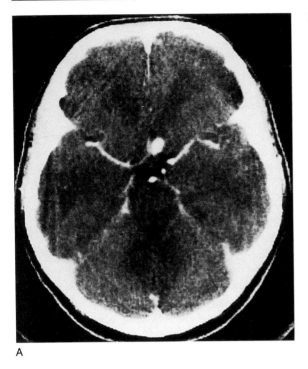

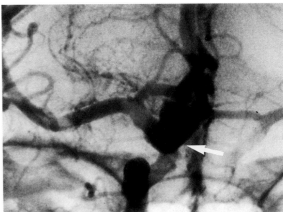

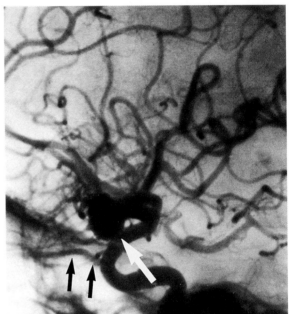

Fig 5A–D This 45 year old female patient with migraine showed on CT scan, surprisingly, an aneurysm of the right A₁ segment (**A**). The right carotid angiogram demonstrated an aneurysm (white arrow) of the internal carotid artery, about 6 mm distal to the origin of the ophthalmic artery (black arrows) (**B** and **C**). Operative exploration confirmed the site of the aneurysm, it compressed and displaced the right optic nerve.

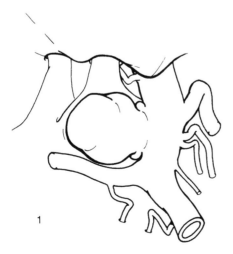
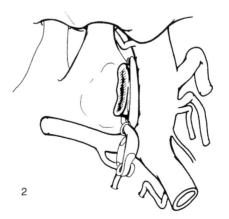

5D Schematic drawing of operative findings and procedures.

Timing of Operation

In 1953, Norlén and Olivecrona published a series of cerebral aneurysm patients, showing that excellent results could be expected in grade I and II patients if operations were performed 2 to 3 weeks after subarachnoid hemorrhage. In the same surgeons' series morbidity and mortality remained high when similar patients underwent operation within the first 2 weeks. Other surgeons reported similar experiences, so that the timing of operation and other associated factors that affected the outcome began to receive increasing attention.

It is unlikely that the factors which increase the risk of operation also significantly protect the patient from rerupture during the waiting period. Elevated intracranial pressure has been suggested by Nornes (1973) to give increased support to the aneurysm wall, but it remains unproven whether patients with increased intracranial pressure, in fact, have a lower incidence of rebleeding. Suzuki (1979), using CSF drainage is convinced of the benefit of decreased intracranial pressure. Nibbelink et al (1975) found the incidence of rerupture higher in the presence of vasospasm.

The natural history of rerupture, perhaps modified by various therapeutic techniques discussed below, must be weighed against the risk of operation in the early posthemorrhage period in determining the optimal time for operative intervention. Risk factors include:

1) *Clinical condition,*
2) *Angiographically demonstrated severe generalized vasospasm,*
3) *Increased intracranial pressure,*
4) *Cerebral blood flow alterations (ischemia, e.g. infarct on CT scan).*

Relationship to Clinical Condition

By the middle 1950's, several substantial series of operated cerebral aneurysms had been reported (Hamby 1952; Norlén and Olivecrona 1953; Steelman et al. 1953). A significant mortality and morbidity in both operated and unoperated cases was discouraging, and neurosurgeons and neurologists tended to become polarized in their positions as to the proper method of handling ruptured cerebral aneurysms. Neurosurgeons drew attention to the rapidly improving techniques and presented reports of successfully handled cases. They were in turn criticized for case selection, a fundamental precept of successful surgical care. Reports generally included consecutive cases without attempting to separate various risk factors.

Graf (1955) presented a series of patients and called attention to the fact that reports on aneurysm surgery usually placed all patients together without considering the multiple variables present. He was especially impressed by the added risk of intracerebral hematoma. Botterell and associates (1956) picked up this theme and devised a scheme of preoperative grading, assigning patients a number graded from I to V, depending on clinical condition. This system emphasized level of consciousness and focal deficits, again relating as a major factor to the patient's condition the presence of intracerebral hematoma. Hunt and Hess (1968) presented a grading system which combined level of consciousness, meningeal signs, and neurological deficits, and placed patients in a higher grade if systemic disease or angiographic spasm was present.

Previous publications concerning the present series of patients have generally employed the Botterell system of grading as revised by Lougheed and Marshall (1973). The system emphasizes level of consciousness, and disregards focal neurological deficit in determining preoperative grade. Review of over 1012 patients undergoing operation in the present series showed that this concept remains valid when preoperative grade is used as a prognostic indicator of mortality. On the other hand, morbidity rates, as might be expected, are much higher in the group of patients which have a preoperative neurological deficit which may or may not resolve. It was, therefore, decided that a more complete picture of preoperative status could be given by adding "a" and "b" categories to each of the Roman numeral grades to indicate those patients with (b) and without (a) focal neurological deficits in the preoperative period. The grading system used throughout this book will be as follows:

Grade 0a	– Unruptured aneurysm, no neurological deficit.
Grade 0b	– Unruptured aneurysm associated with neurological deficit. Deficits such as III nerve palsy or progressive hemisyndrome may be severe in these patients, especially in the case of giant aneurysm (chiasmatic, mesodiencephalic, pontobulbar syndrome).
Grade Ia	– Asymptomatic following subarachnoid hemorrhage.
Grade Ib	– Alert and oriented, no meningism, but with focal pronounced neurological deficit following subarachnoid hemorrhage. Deficits include hemiparesis, paraparesis, asphasia, sensory deficits, visual field losses (due to lesions of temporal or occipital lobes), but not simple lesions of cranial nerves such as chiasmatic visual field losses, or III–IV nerve palsies.
Grade IIa	– Alert, but with headache and meningism following subarachnoid hemorrhage.
Grade IIb	– Same, with focal neurological deficit.
Grade IIIa	– Lethargic, confused, disoriented, combative following subarachnoid hemorrhage.
Grade IIIb	– Same, with focal neurological deficit.
Grade IV	– Semicomatose, responding to pain but not to voice following subarachnoid hemorrhage. Pupils are reactive to light but patient may show extensor posturing. Although it may be possible in most cases to lateralize neurological deficits there was no prognostic benefit to assigning "a" and "b" categories to these patients.
Grade V	– Comatose following subarachnoid hemorrhage. Pupils not reactive to light, extensor posturing or no reaction to pain, failing vital signs.

Systemic disease is an important part of the preoperative evaluation, but is considered independently of patient grade. Angiographically demonstrated vasospasm is not a part of the grading system. Grading is of course not a static designation, but depends on the patient's course. Preoperative grades given in the various tables describe the patient's neurological condition at the time he was taken to the operating room.

Any grading system, however, presents certain difficulties. Each proposed grade includes a spectrum of patients – for instance, drowsy patients (grade III) are grouped together regardless of age, general medical state, and basic physical condition. Some patients have only minimal signs or deficits, while others fall just short of being placed in the next higher grade. While this particular grading system used in this series of patients has proved useful in analyzing operative results, and in establishing general guidelines as to the timing and need for operation, it should be kept in mind that judgement is required for each case. Hopefully, in the future advanced scanning techniques and neurophysiological examinations will provide a better appraisal of brain damage following ruptured cerebral aneurysm, but for this series of patients, neurological examination provided the most consistent operative and prognostic indicator.

Grade 0a

Asymptomatic unruptured aneurysms comprise a group of clinically silent lesions generally discovered incidentally during various neuroradiologic procedures. Under these fortunate circumstances, such aneurysms should be surgically corrected before a catastrophic rupture occurs. In the present series, there were 12 such patients and good operative results were obtained in 11 (Table **1a**). These results suggest that in the vast majority of grade 0a patients, good results can be assured, thereby demanding that once a silent aneurysm is identified, operative intervention should be undertaken without unnecessary delay. Occasionally, associated medical disabilities may hinder good operative results, but long delays during medical evaluation and treatment must be prudently weighed against the threat of rupture. Patient No. 14 (Table **40**) had an unruptured aneurysm of the anterior choroidal artery but a hypertensive intracerebral hematoma.

Grade 0b

Symptomatic unruptured aneurysms (mostly large or giant) generally produce focal, or generalized perifocal neurological deficits due to their size and inherent mass effect. These patients present like those in grade 0a without hemorrhage-associated neurological dysfunction, although localized neurovascular compression places them in a less satisfactory category. Postoperative results would be expected to reflect this difference. In the current series of 59 such patients, good results were obtained in 45, while 3 suffered poor results and 5 died (Table **1a**). The less favorable outcome achieved in this group thus reflects both persisting preoperative deficits as well as additional neurological disability related to the more difficult correction of larger aneurysms. Despite these slightly less favorable results, operative intervention in this group should commence as expeditiously as for the previous group (0a), especially in the face of progressing symptomatology. In addition to the real danger of rupture, the consequences of untreated, persistent neurovascular compression must be considered before delaying operation for any length of time.

Grades Ia and IIa

With experience gained during the past 30 years, many neurosurgeons prefer to delay operation with the most optimal clinical grade patients until 1 or 2 weeks after hemorrhage, thereby avoiding an unacceptable increase in the operative morbidity and mortality (Drake 1971; Mullan 1975; Gillingham et al. 1976). Recent reports (Sano and Saito 1978; Samson et al. 1979; Suzuki 1979) suggest that more favorable outcomes are achieved by earlier surgical intervention within the first 48 hours following hemorrhage, than later during the first week. Since the application of microtechniques to the treatment of intracranial aneurysms our policy has been to perform surgery as soon as possible if the patient belongs to groups I or II (1967). As most of the cases, especially the patients in condition I and II have been delayed in their admission to our clinic from other hospitals, the policy of "as soon as possible" could not be applied in a large number of patients. As Table **2** shows, only 7 patients (1.3%) in the groups Ia–IIa could be operated on within 3 days. However, in these patients there was no morbidity and no mortality.

In the present series, 556 aneurysm patients underwent an intracranial procedure while in a good clinical state (orientated and alert) and without focal neurological deficits (I–IIa). In this group the time of operation was within the first 2 weeks following hemorrhage in 227 (40.8%), between the 2nd and 4th week in 183 (32.9%), and after 4 weeks in 146 (26.3%). Unlike previous series, the results show no difference in postoperative states between these time intervals. Patients undergoing operation during the first 2 weeks fared just as well as those during the subsequent 2 weeks, with a good outcome in the majority (Table 2). Similarly, no difference in mortality rates was revealed, with very low mortality occurring in each time period.

This experience suggests that good operative results can be obtained in the vast majority (95%) of good grade patients regardless of timing. It would therefore seem that random or arbitrary waiting periods before operating on these patients are not justified. The increased risk of rebleeding while delaying surgery for several weeks must be plotted against the good surgical results obtainable during this period. Our results justify early operation for this group of patients.

Grades Ib and IIb

Alert patients with pronounced focal neurological impairment form a distinct group. While the general state of consciousness in this group is similar to the previous group (Ia and IIa), localized posthemorrhagic neurological dysfunction is characteristic and often manifests underlying vascular spasm, infarct or hematoma. The frequent irreversible sequelae of these pathological processes are reflected in fewer good operative results and more numerous fair results in these patients (Table 1a and 1b).

In the current series, 156 patients underwent operation for aneurysm in this group; neurologically alert, but with some focal impairment (i.e. hemisyndrome or paraparesis). This group of patients was nearly equally divided as to the operative timing between the initial 2 weeks (60 = 38.5%), the following 2 weeks (51 = 32.7%), and thereafter (45 = 28.8%). As in the previous groups, no additional operative morbidity or mortality was seen in those patients undergoing a procedure during the first 2 weeks when compared with subsequent time periods.

The timing of surgery in this group should be based upon the underlying cause of the focal neurological deficit. The presence of mass effect due to intracranial hematoma demands early operative intervention in most instances. When the CT scan shows ischemia in relation to the focal deficit and angiography shows severe vasospasm or a vascular occlusion it is generally better to wait until the patient's condition has stabilized. Experience has shown that surgery in the face of progressive cerebral ischemia generally leads to a poor result, so, for the most part, patients in the present series with CT suggesting impending cerebral infarction were allowed time to recover before operation.

In contrast, younger patients (under 50 years) with internal carotid artery, middle and anterior cerebral artery aneurysms underwent early operation in the face of local unilateral mild or severe vasospasm. In these patients it was rewarding to open the basal cisterns and remove the blood clot bathing the affected vessels, relieving the vasospasm with local papaverine application and stripping the network of nervous tissue from the vessel wall. It might even seem reasonable as a general rule to clip the aneurysm early despite evidence of progressive spasm, in order to allow safer and more vigorous pharmacological control of the blood pressure and intraventricular volume.

Grades IIIa and IIIb

Patients with significantly altered states of consciousness following aneurysmal hemorrhage comprise a rather different category. Compared with the previous groups (I and II), the diminished state of consciousness in these patients implies widespread cerebral dysfunction. Therefore, regardless of associated focal neurological deficits, the overall clinical condition of these patients is much less favorable. This is reflected in dramatically fewer good operative results and a many fold increase in operative mortality (Table 1a and 1b). The generalized nature of hemorrhagic brain injury overshadows the effects of associated localized cerebral dysfunction on operative results, although the sequelae of focal preoperative deficits can be recognized in fewer good results and more numerous fair results (Table 3). Japanese colleagues (Sano and Saito 1979) recently reported good results in patients who were operated upon in condition III–IV within 1–3 days. Further experience with "emergency surgery" of aneurysms will prove the benefit of this policy. It is to be noted, however, that some patients who are initially categorized in level III–IV would spontaneously improve to a better condition within hours or 1–3 days. The patients who are still in condition III–IV after 3 days or specially after 1–2 weeks are a special group, usually with a poor prognosis. As there is no objective method available to measure brain metabolism and predict the prognosis, one must not perform "emergency surgery" in every case.

In the present series, 175 lethargic or confused but rousable patients underwent aneurysm surgery. The majority (100) were operated upon during the first 2 weeks with nearly 69.0% achieving a good result. The operative mortality in this group was over 14.0% (Table 2). In the remaining 75 patients (42.8%) surgery was delayed until sometime after the first 2 weeks, being performed usually during the third week (44 cases). Of these patients (66.7%) had a good clinical result, while 6.6% died (Table 2). This experience indicates that delaying operative intervention in this group of patients for at least 2 weeks following hemorrhage results in fewer operative deaths but also culminates in fewer good results. This is in most cases due to the preoperative existing lesions occurring at the time of hemorrhage.

From our experience these patients, in general, should be given time to recover to better grades (I or II) before proceeding with an operation with the exception of those cases who have subdural or intracerebral hematomas with mass effect. At present this group of aneurysm patients requires the greatest clinical judgement in timing operative intervention.

Although confirmatory statistical data have not yet been fully analyzed, there is a definite impression that among those cases treated in Zurich in the past few years there is a group of younger patients who are admitted in good general condition and in grade IIb who develop a moderate hemiparesis without change in conscious level over the course of a few days following a subarachnoid hemorrhage. There is usually no evidence clinically, on CT scan or at angiography of a rebleed, of significant vasospasm or of hydrocephalus although some show CT evidence of hemisphere low density.

What has been established is that early surgery in such cases, and particularly in those with a CT scan suggesting changes of early infarction, uniformly results in a poor outcome. For this reason, surgery in this special group is always delayed until significant clinical and/or CT scan improvement is demonstrated.

Consequently few precise guidelines can be given for planning a surgical procedure in these patients. If a patient is young and otherwise healthy with no infarcts on CT scan, surgery is generally performed earlier, usually within the first 2 weeks. In older patients, on the other hand, especially those with associated medical problems such as hypertension, heart disease and those showing wide swings in blood pressure, surgery is delayed. Patients with ruptured middle cerebral artery aneurysms are generally taken to the operating room earlier so that the subarachnoid cisterns can be opened and surrounding hematoma evacuated in the hope of relieving vasospasm and preventing chronic arterial changes. Patients with space-occupying hematomas, especially when associated with middle cerebral artery aneurysms usually come to early operation. Other patients might undergo operation earlier so as to avoid long weekend or holiday delays.

It is generally suggested that patients who deteriorate rapidly from good to poor grades whilst awaiting surgery should have their operation further postponed to await possible improvement. Such improvement may never occur in many instances and it has become the practice of the senior surgeon to operate as an emergency on those patients who present initially in grade Ia or IIa and in good general condition but who subsequently show sudden deterioration due to rebleeding.

This approach is based on the premise that rapid deterioration due to spasm is generally progressive and largely irreversible while that due to recurrent hemorrhage or to intracerebral hematoma with mass effect is potentially treatable. These patients usually undergo emergency angiography with surgery following on under the same anesthetic. On rare occasions surgery has even been undertaken without angiography when the CT scan has provided good localizing evidence for the site of the aneurysm rupture.

The problem of preventing rupture while awaiting neurological improvement often influences the surgeon to proceed with earlier operation. The selection of which patients in this group will be benefited by early surgery must be guided by sound clinical judgement in the absence of other objective measurement concerning brain metabolism. It is in this area of quantifying cerebral metabolism that the PET scan may offer new insights in the future.

Grades IV and V

Semiconscious, comatose, and moribund patients following aneurysmal hemorrhage comprise the least favorable group. Diffuse irreversible brain injury often occurs as is demonstrated on CT scan at the time of hemorrhage in these patients accounting for their poor presenting neurological state. Operative results in this worst group mirror this pessimism. In our experience good operative results can be expected in less than 20% of patients undergoing surgery while semiconscious, and only poor results or death obtain in comatose or moribund patients.

However, of all patients (41 cases) presenting in a semicomatose state following hemorrhage, nearly 21.9% eventually will make a good recovery, while another 14.6% will be at least self-sufficient.

This suggests that these patients fare much better with delayed surgical intervention (allowing their clinical status to improve to a better grade: I, II, or III). Based on this conclusion, early operation in these patients should be abandoned except in the presence of a space-occupying intracranial hematoma. Frequently, patients presenting with large intracerebral or subdural hematomas may go on to make reasonably good recoveries once the clot has been evacuated and the brain decompressed. The patient's presenting grade in these cases is a combination of mass effect from hematoma and hemorrhagic brain injury. The relative importance of each component has great bearing on the final outcome and thus on the decision to intervene operatively. It is in this context that new diagnostic techniques to ascertain the integrity of deep brain structures would be most valuable.

Comatose and moribund patients have little chance of survival and early operative intervention is generally abandoned. Most of these patients will succumb to their ruptured aneurysm, and ethical considerations preclude surgical intervention at this stage to prolong a vegetative existence. In this series, some young patients with large hematomas underwent operation when the time interval between diagnosis and clinical deterioration was short and some hope for restoring brain function was felt to remain. The results were generally futile with 14 out of 15 patients dying and one remaining in extremely poor condition.

Table 1a Preoperative condition and surgical results

	Total No.	Good	Fair	Poor	Death
Non ruptured (71 cases)					
0a	12 (1.2%)	11 (91.7%)	–	–	1 (8.3%)
0b	59 (5.8%)	45 (76.3%)	6	3	5 (8.4%)
	71 (7.0%)	56 (78.9%)	6	3	6
Ruptured (941 cases)					
Ia	242 (23.9%)	241 (99.6%)	1	–	– (0.0%)
Ib	9 (0.9%)	8 (88.9%)	–	–	1 (11.1%)
IIa	314 (31.0%)	301 (95.9%)	7	–	6 (1.9%)
IIb	147 (14.5%)	132 (89.8%)	11	2	2 (1.4%)
IIIa	75 (7.4%)	63 (84.0%)	2	1	9 (12.0%)
IIIb	100 (9.9%)	56 (56.0%)	24	10	10 (10.0%)
IV	41 (4.1%)	9 (21.9%)	6	13	13 (31.7%)
V	13 (1.3%)	–	–	2	11 (84.6%)
	941	810 (86.1%)	51 (5.4%)	28 (3.0%)	52 (5.5%)
Total	1012	866 (85.6%)	57 (5.6%)	31 (3.1%)	58 (5.7%)

Timing of Operation   13

Table 1b Surgical results and preoperative condition of patients with ruptured aneurysms

		Total No.	Good	Fair	Poor	Death
Ruptured Cases (941 patients)						
Without neurologic lesion	Ia	242	241	1	–	–
	IIa	314	301	7	–	6
	IIIa	75	63	2	1	9
		631 (67.1%)	605 (95.9%)	10 (1.6%)	1 (0.2%)	15 (2.4%)
With neurologic lesion	Ib	9	8	–	–	1
	IIb	147	130	13	2	2
	IIIb	100	56	24	10	10
	IV	41	9	6	13	13
	V	13	–	–	2	11
		310 (32.9%)	203 (66.1%)	43 (13.8%)	27 (8.7%)	37 (11.9%)
	Total	941				

Table 2 Timing, preoperative condition, and operative results in 941 patients with subarachnoid hemorrhage

	Total	Good							Fair						Poor					Death						
		Ia	Ib	IIa	IIb	IIIa	IIIb	IV	Ia	IIa	IIb	IIIa	IIIb	IV	IIb	IIIa	IIIb	IV	V	Ib	IIa	IIb	IIIa	IIIb	IV	V
1–3 d	42 4.5%	–	–	7	4	5	2	3	–	–	–	–	1	1	–	–	–	2	2	–	–	–	–	–	6	9
4–7 d	129 13.7%	12	–	62	16	8	9	3	–	2	–	–	3	3	1	–	–	4	–	–	–	–	1	1	3	1
1–2 w	259 27.5%	32	–	110	34	30	15	2	1	–	4	2	7	–	–	–	4	1	–	–	1	1	7	5	2	1
2–4 w	285 30.3%	85	3	91	46	14	17	1	–	3	–	–	4	1	1	1	5	3	–	–	4	1	–	3	2	–
1–3 m	152 16.2%	69	2	19	23	6	13	–	–	2	3	–	7	1	–	–	1	2	–	1	1	–	1	1	–	–
> 3 m	74 7.9%	43	3	12	7	–	–	–	–	–	6	–	2	–	–	–	–	1	–	–	–	–	–	–	–	–
	941	241	8	301	130	63	56	9	1	7	13	2	24	6	2	1	10	13	2	1	6	2	9	10	13	11

Table 3 Clinical condition, site of aneurysm, and outcome

		Total No.	Good	Fair	Poor	Death	
0a	Ophth.	2	2	–	–	–	
	inf.	1	1	–	–	–	
	sup.	1	1	–	–	–	
	P co A	2	2	–	–	–	
	A cho A	1	–	–	–	1	(ICH)
	med.	3	3	–	–	–	
	A co A	2	2	–	–	–	
		12	11	–	–	1	
0b	C c	11	10	1	–	–	
	Ophth.	8	7	–	–	1	(EIA)
	inf.	3	2	–	1	–	
	P co A	10	10	–	–	–	
	Ic Bi.	4	2	2	–	–	
	MCA	11	8	2	1	–	
	A co A	2	–	1	–	1	(accident)
	Ba Bi.	2	1	–	–	1	(m)
	Ba Br.	3	2	–	1	–	
	Ba Tr.	2	1	–	–	1	
	Vertebr.	3	2	–	–	1	(m)
		59	45	6	3	5	
Ia	C c	2	2	–	–	–	
	Ophth.	8	8	–	–	–	
	med.	1	1	–	–	–	
	inf.	6	6	–	–	–	
	P co A	45	45	–	–	–	
	A cho A	6	6	–	–	–	
	Ic Bi.	24	24	–	–	–	
	MCA	42	41	1	–	–	
	A_1	5	5	–	–	–	
	A co A	82	82	–	–	–	
	Pe A	5	5	–	–	–	
	Ba Bi.	12	12	–	–	–	
	Ba Br.	3	3	–	–	–	
	Ba Tr.	–	–	–	–	–	
	Vertebr.	1	1	–	–	–	
		242	241	1	–	–	

ICH = intracerebral hematoma
EIA = extra-intracranial anastomosis
m = muscle wrapping
RR = rupture of aneurysm after clipping

Table 3
(Continuation)

			Total No.	Good	Fair	Poor	Death	
IIa	Ophth.		8	8	–	–	–	
	med.		1	1	–	–	–	
	inf.		6	6	–	–	–	
	P co A		56	51	5	–	–	
	A cho A		8	8	–	–	–	
	Ic Bi.		13	13	–	–	–	
	MCA		29	29	–	–	–	
	A_1		5	5	–	–	–	
	A co A		150	146	1	–	3	
	Pe A		6	6	–	–	–	
	Ba Bi.		16	15	1	–	–	
	Ba Br.		5	4	–	–	1	(RR)
	Ba Tr.		3	1	–	–	2	
	Vertebr.		8	8	–	–	–	
			314	301	7	–	6	
Ib	Ophth.		1	1	–	–	–	
	MCA		2	2	–	–	–	
	Ba Bi.		2	1	–	–	1	(m)
	Ba Br.		4	4	–	–	–	
			9	8	–	–	1	
IIb	Ophth.		1	1	–	–	–	
	inf.		2	2	–	–	–	
	P co A		18	16	2	–	–	
	A cho A		1	–	1	–	–	
	Ic Bi.		3	3	–	–	–	
	MCA		40	36	4	–	–	
	A_1		1	1	–	–	–	
	A co A		66	60	3	1	2	
	Pe A		2	2	–	–	–	
	Ba Bi.		7	5	1	1	–	
	Ba Br.		4	3	1	–	–	
	Vertebr.		2	1	1	–	–	
			147	130	13	2	2	
IIIa	Ophth.		3	3	–	–	–	
	inf.		1	–	–	–	1	
	P co A		14	12	–	–	2	
	A cho A		2	2	–	–	–	
	Ic Bi.		5	5	–	–	–	
	MCA		7	6	1	–	–	
	A_1		1	1	–	–	–	
	A co A		28	21	1	1	5	
	Pe A		5	5	–	–	–	
	Ba Bi.		4	3	–	–	1	
	Ba Br.		1	1	–	–	–	
	Ba Tr.		1	1	–	–	–	
	Vertebr.		3	3	–	–	–	
			75	63	2	1	9	

16   1 Clinical Considerations

Table 3
(Continuation)

			Total No.	Good	Fair	Poor	Death	
IIIb		Ophth.	1	1	–	–	–	
		inf.	2	1	–	–	1	
		P co A	16	6	6	1	3	
		A cho A	2	–	1	1	–	
		Ic Bi.	3	–	2	–	1	
		MCA	32	25	6	–	1	
		A_1	2	–	2	–	–	
		A co A	27	18	5	2	2	
		Pe A	4	2	–	2	–	
		Ba Bi.	7	–	2	4	1	
		Ba Br.	1	1	–	–	–	
		Ba Tr.	2	1	–	–	1	(m)
		Vertebr.	1	1	–	–	–	
			100	56	24	10	10	
IV		Ophth.	1	1	–	–	–	
		P co A	10	2	4	1	3	
		A cho A	1	–	–	–	1	
		Ic Bi.	2	2	–	–	–	
		MCA	9	4	1	3	1	
		A co A	17	–	–	9	8	
		Pe A	1	–	1	–	–	
			41	9	6	13	13	
V		P co A	2	–	–	–	2	
		Ic Bi.	1	–	–	–	1	
		MCA	9	–	–	2	7	
		A co A	1	–	–	–	1	
			13	–	–	2	11	

General Medical Condition

In addition to neurological grade, each patient will have individual risk factors that must be taken into account when determining the appropriate time for operative intervention. In the present series the following medical conditions influenced timing or even need for operation.

Age: Patients over 60 years old carry a somewhat higher risk from both angiography and surgery and this increases with advancing age. Many medical advances have helped diminish the risk associated with age, and older patients in good medical condition are generally acceptable operative candidates. The disparity between chronological and biological age is often apparent, however.

Hypertension. Preexisting hypertension which has been adequately controlled with medication seems to present less of a hazard to the patient than the labile hypertension associated with subarachnoid hemorrhage. Marked swings in blood pressure in the preoperative period should delay operation until well controlled. However, there are cases in which the blood pressure cannot be controlled with any medical treatment and these patients usually died before surgery. The combination of a clear state of consciousness and stabilized high blood pressure is not a difficult problem, while a decreased level of consciousness and labile, uncontrollable high blood pressure presents real difficulty.

Diabetes mellitus. Diabetes and its associated coronary artery disease, renal disease, and generalized atherosclerosis adds risk to any major operation. Diabetes should be under control prior to operation, and this may be difficult with the stress of subarachnoid hemorrhage and corticosteroid treatment.

Renal insufficiency. Hypertension, diabetes mellitus and occasionally polycystic kidney disease may cause a patient to present with electrolyte imbalance and/or azotemia. This should delay operation until corrected.

Heart disease. Patients with cardiac ischemia or congestive heart failure may not be suitable operative candidates.

Obstructive pulmonary disease. Poor ventilation will require preoperative therapy and perhaps endotracheal intubation or tracheostomy prior to considering an operative procedure.

Other. Obesity, blood coagulopathy, thrombophlebitis, and other medical problems may cause an intended operative procedure to be postponed or abandoned.

Relationship to Angiographically Demonstrated Vasospasm

One of the most debated topics among neurosurgeons has been the relevance of vasospasm demonstrated by angiography to the timing of operative intervention and to the ultimate operative result. Several neurosurgeons have recommended that surgery be delayed until vasospasm has disappeared on repeat angiography (Drake 1971; Hunt and Kosnik 1974). Other studies have failed to substantiate a relationship between the presence of preoperative vasospasm and a poor operative result (Graf and Nibbelink 1974; Millikan 1975).

Allcock and Drake (1965) reported on 83 ruptured aneurysm patients undergoing pre- and postoperative angiography. In this series 31 patients had some degree of preoperative vasospasm, with postoperative spasm still present in 48%. By contrast of 52 patients with no preoperative vasospasm, spasm was demonstrated postoperatively in only 38%. The average preoperative clinical grade was comparable in the two groups, although large intracranial hematomas were present in more patients with preoperative spasm (17%) than without (12%). Including this variable, satisfactory results were obtained in only 45% of patients with preoperative vasospasm, while 60% of those without spasm before surgery had a comparable result. Although these findings suggest that the presence of preoperative vasospasm hinders a good operative result, certainly the effects of associated factors (such as large hematomas) must be accounted for.

Graf and Nibbelink (1974), reporting results of the Cooperative Aneurysm Study, found a different relationship between the presence of preoperative vasospasm and operative results. In this series, while 39% of patients without preoperative spasm and 37% of patients with localized spasm succumbed postoperatively, only 29% of patients with diffuse spasm suffered a fatal result. Obviously factors other than preoperative vasospasm contributed to the high mortality figures in this study. In another report, Millikan (1975) found a 19% mortality in patients both with and without vasospasm, again suggesting the limited effect of spasm on operative results. During a period of over 7 years Flamm and Ransohoff (1979) observed spasm in 35 per cent of the patients with SAH from aneurysms. This is in agreement with other reports in the literature (Perret and Nishioka 1966; Wilkins et al. 1968).

In the 30 years since Ecker and Riemenschneider (1951) first reported an association between vasospasm and ruptured cerebral aneurysm, there have been repeated attempts in centers around the world to piece together a general hypothesis for the phenomenon of vasospasm. In 1972, 18 investigators from the United States and Canada met in Jackson, Mississippi, for a workshop on cerebrovascular spasm, the proceedings of which were published in 1975 by Smith and Robertson. In 1979, 77 senior authors from nine countries presented 119 papers at the 2nd International Workshop held in Amsterdam. The proceedings of that meeting were published in 1980 by Wilkins. In 1980 the monograph of Boullin was published presenting the historical, clinical, radiographic and pathological aspects of vasospasm including experimental work. Unfortunately in most published reports, variations in the timing of angiography as related to the hemorrhage and to the time of operation, variations in technical factors related to obtaining adequate angiography, variations in the degree of spasm and variations in the clinical condition of individual patients have made a convincing comprehensive statement on the pathogenesis and relevance of vasospasm impossible. A study comparing operative results in alert patients (grades I and II) with angiographically demonstrable vasospasm just prior to operation to a similar group of patients without spasm is currently lacking. A prospective series comparing surgical results in alert patients with vasospasm randomly allocated to either immediate or delayed surgery would also be valuable. It must be concluded that at present much remains unknown about vasospasm: exactly when and why it occurs, why there is such marked variation in degree and duration among individual patients, when and how it should be treated, and what relationship it has to cerebral ischemia. There is no adequate explanation regarding the mechanism of the occurrence of vasospasm after SAH. The substance that may trigger the vasoconstriction has also remained obscure. There is currently no established way to prevent vasospasm or to treat patients who suffer from severe cerebral ischemia due to vasospasm (Suzuki 1979). A great many pharmacological agents have been tried without success in this respect but recent preliminary trials using systemically administered calcium antagonists have been viewed optimistically. Further carefully controlled studies with large numbers of patients must be undertaken.

Cerebral vasospasm is only one of several pathophysiological processes affecting cerebral blood flow in any given patient. The arteries visualized on angiography are the conduits through which the blood must pass on its way to the cerebral microcirculation where metabolic exchange occurs. Brain metabolism begins to fail when inadequate blood flow is maintained at the capillary level. Physical principles require a severe decrement in arterial luminal diameter before a significant reduction in flow takes place. The cerebral perfusion pressure and the resistance at the arteriolar and perhaps venous levels are other important factors influencing the flow of blood through the capillaries. Alterations in these factors may be suggested by a slowed circulation time or poor vessel filling on angiography, but cannot be correlated with cerebral vasospasm per se.

Thus marked discrepancies between the angiographic picture of vasospasm and neurological function are observed, bringing the physiological importance of angiographic vasospasm into question. When the cerebral circulation is marginal, a small insult may tip the balance towards cerebral ischemia, and in these cases vasospasm may be playing a role. On the other hand, ischemic deficits are seen in the absence of angiographically observed spasm, so the failure of circulation must be occurring in smaller more distal vessels.

If vasospasm is indeed a cause of cerebral ischemia, one important consideration would be some type of quantification of the degree of vasospasm present. Most earlier reports have only stated whether vasospasm was present or not and have failed to precisely describe the degree of spasm, making comparisons of operative results and recommendations about operative timing generally inconclusive.

A few recent publications (Sano and Saito 1979; Saito et al. 1977, 1979) have begun to differentiate patients on the basis of degree of vasospasm. They have described direct relationship between the degree of angiographically demonstrated vasospasm (diffuse, multisegmental, local) and the patient's outcome. As previously discussed (Vol. I, Chapter 5), vasospasm can be localized, segmental, or diffuse, and it can be unilateral or bilateral. Certainly mild vasospasm localized around the site of aneurysm rupture (which probably occurs in almost every case for some period of time) is less important than severe, diffuse, bilateral vasospasm. On this basis vasospasm should be graded as either mild, moderate, or severe, and each degree as being either localized, segmental, or diffuse. Hopefully in the future on the basis of the categorization of the precise degree of vasospasm in each case, its relationship to the patient's clinical condition, to the timing of angiography and surgery, and to the operative results can be more clearly defined.

Previous publications have suggested that the correlation of vasospasm with clinical condition is poor when vasospasm is mild, but is more useful when vasospasm is severe. Most neurosurgeons would agree that there is a general trend toward increasing impairment in those patients demonstrating increasing degrees of vasospasm, but the question remains whether the presence of angiographically demonstrated mild or moderate, local or segmental vasospasm in a patient who shows no neurological impairment represents a contraindication to operation. The experience with the present series of patients has been that the vasospasm of patients presenting as grade I or II has not correlated well enough with the clinical condition either pre- or postoperatively to be used as a specific contraindication to surgery in the absence of positive neurological findings that would by themselves delay the operation.

Because of the variations in timing of angiography in relation to the subarachnoid hemorrhage and the operative intervention, and the fact that many of the angiographic studies were performed outside the University of Zurich, a meaningful statistical analysis of vasospasm and subsequent operative results is not possible. A few exemplary cases (Figs **6–9**), however, demonstrate our impressions from this large series of cases about the importance of vasospasm on operative timing and results.

During the course of this series, clinical bedside observation of the patient proved a more reliable guide to timing of operation and ultimate prognosis than did the finding of vasospasm on angiography. It was found that careful microscopic operative technique with strict attention to anatomical details, avoidance of brain retraction, and precise dissection of the arachnoid were more important to a patient's postoperative course,

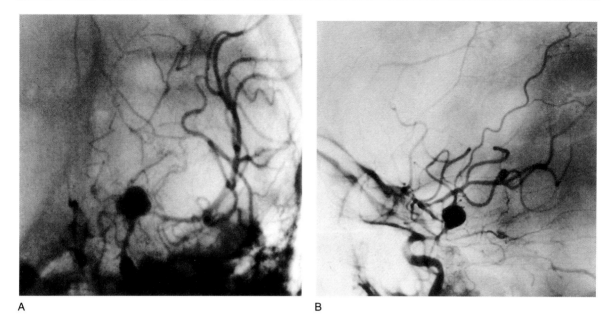

Fig 6 A–B This 17 year old patient with a left carotid bifurcation aneurysm and severe spasm (**A** and **B**) was operated upon in grade Ia. Hematoma was evacuated from the basal cisterns and papaverine applied; the patient made a full recovery (Case 45, Table **45**).

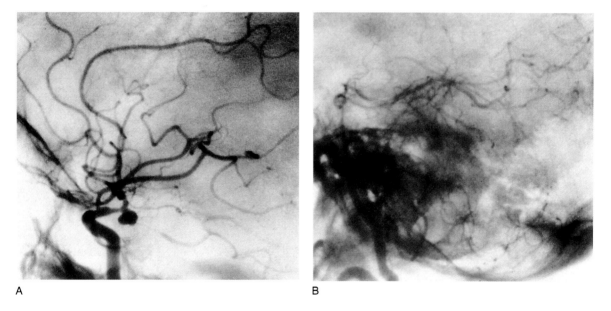

Fig 7 A–B 2 weeks following a subarachnoid hemorrhage, angiography demonstrated a posterior communicating aneurysm with marked spasm of the neighboring vessels (**A**) including the basilar artery (**B**). Despite this the patient underwent surgery (grade IIa) and made an uneventful recovery.

than was the presence of slight or moderate vasospasm preoperatively (Figs **6–11**).

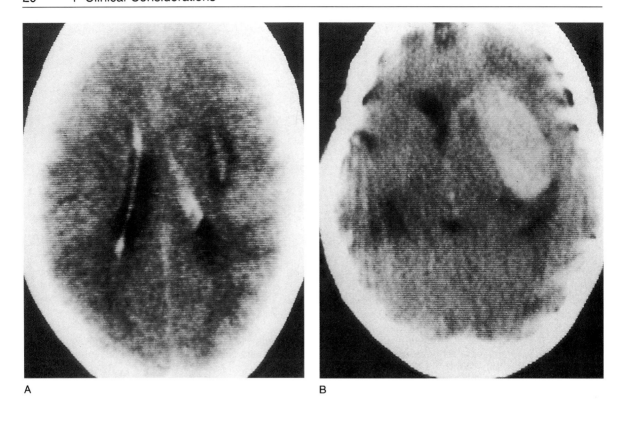
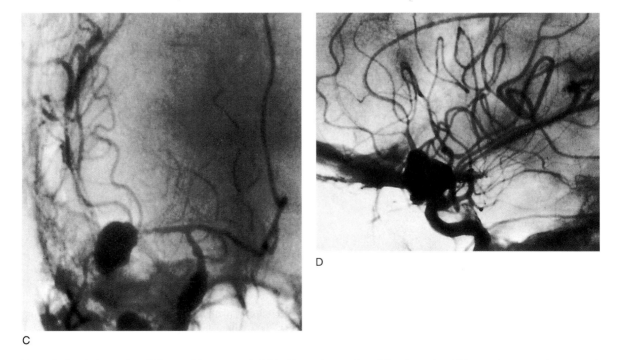

Fig. 8 A–D 2 days after delivery of her second child, this patient suffered 2 subarachnoid hemorrhages within a week with both intraventricular (**A**) and intracerebral (**B**) hematomas evident on CT scan. Angiography showed a large right middle cerebral bifurcation aneurysm (**C** and **D**) with spasm of the neighboring vessels. The aneurysm was explored and clipped successfully on the third day (grade IIIb). The hematoma was also evacuated. The patient made a full recovery.

Timing of Operation

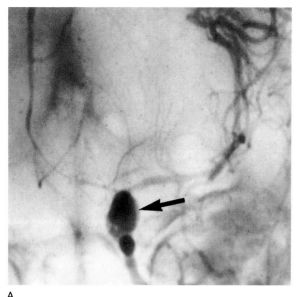
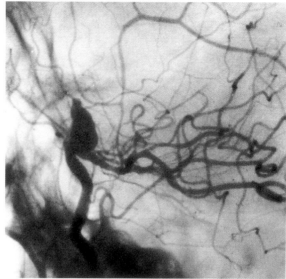
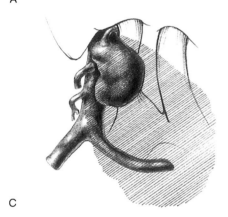
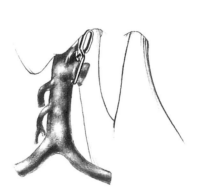

Fig **9 A–C** This 67 year old patient with diabetes and hypertension suffered a severe subarachnoid hemorrhage with drowsiness, a right hemisyndrome, and aphasia. Following angiography (**A** and **B**) which revealed a large left carotid-ophthalmic aneurysm (arrow) with severe spasm and mass effect, she became comatose with a dilated pupil. Surgical evacuation of a large left frontal hematoma and clipping of the aneurysm (**C**) resulted in her full recovery (Case 5, Table **16**).

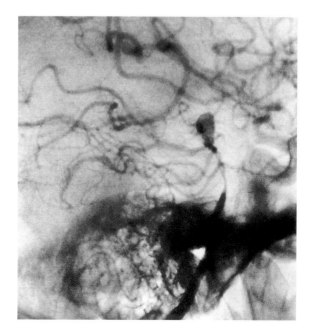

Fig **10** While looking at this angiogram, this 48 year old neurology professor who was in good condition 8 days after his subarachnoid hemorrhage, jokingly wondered whether surgery should be postponed because of the severe basilar artery spasm. He made an uneventful recovery following surgery the next day.

1 Clinical Considerations

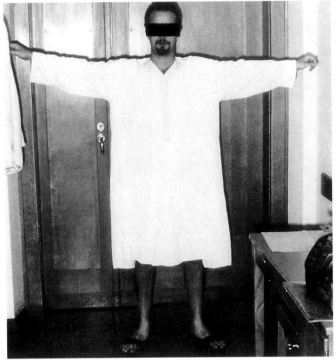

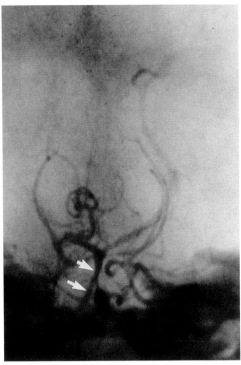

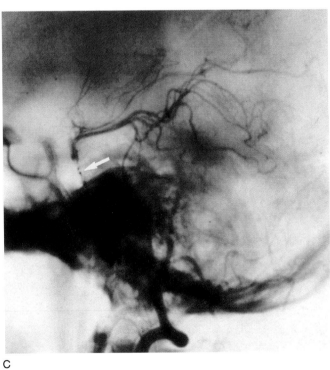

Fig 11 A–C This picture (**A**) was taken one day after the angiogram (B and C) was completed showing no evidence of an aneurysm but remarkable basilar artery vasospasm (arrows). The patient's condition is evident.

Because it was felt that vasospasm might to some degree protect the aneurysm from rerupture, operation was usually undertaken to eliminate the aneurysm before vasospasm had disappeared. At operation, active attempts to relieve spasm were made, – opening the subarachnoid cisterns, removing the hematoma, reestablishing the normal flow of cerebrospinal fluid over the arteries, applying papaverine to the arteries, and removing the periadventitial sympathetic plexus from the arterial wall. The anatomical bounderies of the Sylvian and pericallosal cisterns differ from the other basal cisterns, in that they are tightly confined by the adjacent lobes of the brain. It was therefore considered especially important with aneurysms at these locations to remove hematomas early, even when small, to restore cerebrospinal fluid circulation over the arteries, and establish the proper milieu for arterial metabolism hoping to prevent the chronic constrictive changes in the arteries previously discussed in Vol. I, Chapter 5.

The same principles also apply to the postoperative period. When a patient is doing poorly and vasospasm is present on angiography, there is a tendency to equate the two and perhaps ignore other pathological alterations amenable to treatment. For instance, cases have been seen that demonstrated not only vasospasm, but also hydrocephalus. Shunting completely reversed the decreased level of consciousness and the focal neurological deficits. In the past 6 years, computerized tomography has been used almost exclusively to evaluate postoperative complications, and vasospasm has been rarely classified as an etiology for a poor postoperative course. It is probable that some local vasospasm would be present in most cases if angiography were done in every operated case in the first few days postoperatively, but no consistent relationship between the presence of vasospasm and the patient's clinical condition has been appreciated in those cases which did undergo angiography.

While a final answer to the importance of vasospasm cannot be given, it must be emphasized that angiographically demonstrated vasospasm is only one of many neurological and medical factors that must be considered in the preoperative assessment of a patient. When vasospasm (grade I or II) is present and the patient is in good clinical and medical condition (grade I or II), it does not seem necessary to delay operation. When a patient is a marginal operative risk because of obtundation or medical complications (grade III), vasospasm may support a decision to postpone operation. *Severe and diffuse vasospasm is seen only in semicomatose and comatose patients (grades IV and V) and abandoning early surgery in this group of patients is recommended in general, regardless of the presence of such spasm. From our observations, there has not been a single patient in grades I to III who presented with severe or diffuse spasm.*

The presence of symptomatic postoperative vasospasm is not independent of other factors as proposed by some authors (Artiola i Fortuny and Prieto-Valiente 1981); rather it is primarily related to untimely operative intervention in a poorer grade, deteriorating patient regardless of the presence of vasospasm. It may also be due to prolonged, excessive brain retraction during the procedure, improper application of a clip, or injury to vessels, especially the perforators (Fig **12A–F**).

Recent experience in Zurich has suggested that too rapid postoperative mobilization, particularly in patients undergoing early surgery, may lead to cerebral ischemic deficits (see page 345, Vol. II). Vasospasm seen on postoperative angiography in these cases might represent changes in vessel calibre secondary to orthostatic influence in the face of disturbed autoregulation.

24   1 Clinical Considerations

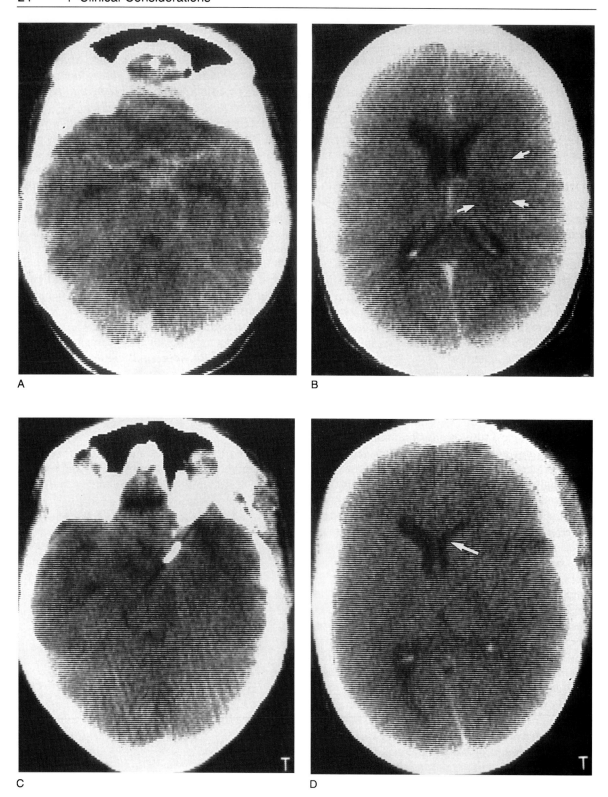

Fig 12 A–F   Angiography in this 24 year old female patient with a subarachnoid hemorrhage showed an aneurysm of the right posterior communicating artery and local spasm. The CT scan (**A–B**) demonstrated slight infarction of the right middle cerebral artery territory (arrows) and compression of the right ventricular system. The patient was drowsy but was operated upon 2 days after subarachnoid hemorrhage and immediately after the angiography. The right internal carotid and middle cerebral arteries showed severe spasm on exploration. The aneurysm could be clipped, but the blood pressure dropped for about 10 minutes. The postoperative condition of the patient was excellent for 6 days. She then developed acute left sided hemiplegia. The CT scan showed edema (arrow) of the right hemisphere (**C–D**).

Fig. **12 E, F** ▶

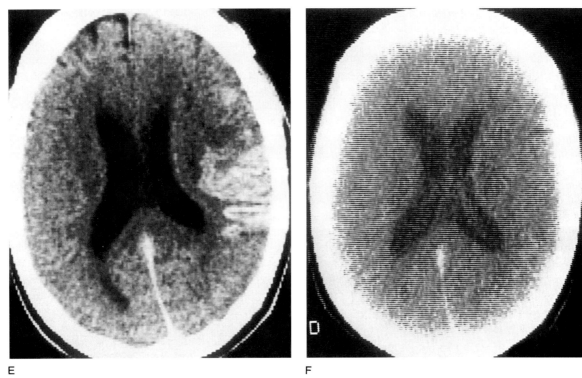

Fig 12E–F Three weeks after surgery the area of infarction could be seen more clearly on the CT scan (**E**). Over the next three months there was a moderate recovery of her clinical state and in the CT scan appearance (**F**).

Relationship to Intracranial Pressure

The importance of intracranial pressure in the timing of operation has not been satisfactorily resolved. Klafta and Hamby (1969) examined intracranial pressure by lumbar puncture in 112 operated cases. They found no difference in mortality in relation to intracranial pressure in grade I and II patients, or in grade IV patients. In 40 grade III patients, however, they found a 17 per cent mortality in patients with lumbar subarachnoid pressure less than 200 mm of water, and a 41 per cent mortality in patients with pressures greater than 200 mm. Since neurological recovery is often seen in grade III patients, they felt that operative intervention might be justified only when intracranial pressure had become normal.

Nornes (1973) suggested that the appropriate time for operative intervention was when the intracranial pressure as measured epidurally fell below 400 mm of water, since the theoretical probability for rupture increased with decreasing intracranial pressure. He did not have a clinical series.

The findings of Klafta and Hamby (1969) suggest that the clinical grade is not directly related to intracranial pressure, but more recent investigators have attempted to show a correlation between these factors. Hayashi et al. (1977) evaluated 26 patients classified between grades III and V and found that increased morbidity was related to elevated intracranial pressure. Hase and associates (1978) followed the development of intracranial pressure patterns in 21 patients with subarachnoid hemorrhage and also found some correlation between increasing pressure and grade, although several patients in poorer grades were shown to have normal intracranial pressure. Hayashi and co-workers (1978) undertook longer periods of pressure recording in 12 patients and found that pressure usually declined at about the 7th posthemorrhage day and this was coincidental with the onset of angiographically recognizable vasospasm. The clinical condition could not be related to the presence of vasospasm. Following this period of lowered intracranial pressure, the pressure again climbed in some patients with diffuse vasospasm and those patients had a less favorable outcome. This secondary increase in intracranial pressure presumably represents cerebral infarction. These studies thus tend to relate clinical condition and intracranial pressure without specifying intracranial pressure as a parameter for the timing of operation.

While intracranial pressure monitoring may be useful for patients in poor condition, it is not likely to be helpful in patients who are alert. Intracranial pressure would thus be relevant to timing of operation in poorer grade patients only, a group where intracranial pressure per se is only one of many factors contributing to the patient's clinical condition.

Sakamoto et al 1979 (in the monograph of Suzuki 1979) performed, in order to improve the patient's condition, continuous ventricular drainage in 25 patients (4 were grade III and 21 were grade IV). The drainage was performed within 1 to 12 days after rupture. Due to the drainage the grade of consciousness improved in 12 cases; i.e. 11 cases improved from grade IV to grade III and 1 case improved from grade III to grade I. Direct surgery was performed at the earliest 1 day and at the latest 10 days following drainage, with an average time span of 2.6 days. 11 patients died, 2 patients remained in fair condition, but 2 patients showed good, and 9 patients excellent results.

In our series preoperative ventricular drainage was performed in only 1 case who was grade IV, 10 days after SAH. The clipping of a ruptured AcoA aneurysm was uneventful, but the patient remained in poor condition.

Relationship to Cerebral Blood Flow

Alterations in cerebral blood flow commonly occur in the presence of subarachnoid hemorrhage. Many reports have been able to relate decreases in regional cerebral blood flow with neurological deficits, and have suggested that such measurements might provide a rational basis for the timing of operation (Zingesser et al. 1968; Symon 1971; Ferguson et al. 1972; Grubb et al. 1975; Kohlmeyer 1979). The relationship between angiographic vasospasm and decreased cerebral blood flow has been variable in these reports. Most of these studies have utilized intraarterial injection of radioisotopes to assess regional cerebral blood flow, although more recently inhalation techniques have become available (Obrist et al. 1975; Meyer et al. 1978, 1979).

Nilsson (1977) measured cerebral blood flow by an intravenous isotope method in 207 patients with ruptured intracranial aneurysms and found a good correlation between patient grade and the level of isotope counts and transit times of the intravenously injected radionuclides. More importantly, however, he found that 21 of 160 patients in grades I or II showed low count rates and/or transit times. There was a 30 per cent incidence of postoperative mortality or serious morbidity in this group of patients, as compared to an 8 per cent incidence in those who demonstrated normal or only slightly abnormal findings on the isotope test. He recommended delaying operation in those patients who showed low values, although values often remained low for several weeks and some patients were lost to rebleeding.

Kelly and associates (1977) conducted a similar study in 44 patients using the standard dynamic brain scan. They used only qualitative measurements as opposed to Nilsson's semiquantitative method. They also found some correlation between brain scan abnormalities and clinical grade, but found that 9 patients in good condition had normal brain scans. While 17 of 19 patients in good condition with normal scans did well after operation, 4 of 8 clinically similar patients with abnormal scans died and 3 were left seriously disabled. They also found that patients with normal scans tended to rebleed at a greater rate, and recommended that a patient in good condition with a normal scan be operated upon as early as possible. They could find no association between angiographic vasospasm and clinical outcome or dynamic brain scan except when vasospasm was especially severe.

These methods have not been tried with the present series of patients, but seem worthy of investigation. Inhalation and intraarterial injection techniques are more precise than intravenous methods in evaluation of cerebral blood flow, but few hospitals are able to conduct such studies on a routine basis. Future developments in PET (single position emission tomography) or NMR (nuclear magnetic resonance) may allow us to follow the local and general metabolic condition of the brain.

Reducing Preoperative Rebleeding Risk

In the absence of intracranial hematoma with mass effect, operation is aimed primarily at eliminating the possibility of aneurysm rerupture. As noted above, outcome is generally more satisfactory when the patient has improved to good condition prior to operation. The following measures have been suggested to reduce the incidence of rebleeding in the preoperative period:

General Medical Care

Patients with ruptured cerebral aneurysm should be placed on bed rest, with sedation and analgesia as required. Stool softeners are given, and in obtunded patients and most women, an urinary catheter is more satisfactory than a bedpan. All patients in this series were placed on anticonvulsants and dexamethasone on admission.

Hypotension

Elevation of blood pressure is common following rupture of a cerebral aneurysm, and may reflect preexisting hypertension, hypothalamic dysfunction, a general reaction to stress, or a systemic response to intracranial hypertension. Slosberg (1956) introduced the concept of titrated hypotension in the treatment of subarachnoid hemorrhage, and has proposed this as a definite form of treatment; this despite a 17 per cent mortality in his hands for all forms of subarachnoid hemorrhage (Slosberg 1973). More recent figures of Nibbelink (1975) with results of the Cooperative Aneurysm Study show a mortality rate of 28.9% when hypotension alone was used as treatment. Many patients following ruptured cerebral aneurysm show increasing obtundation and focal neurological deficits as blood pressure is lowered. The general policy of this department has been to try to bring blood pressure into the normal range and to avoid large swings in blood pressure.

There is some evidence that hypotensive agents may interfere with the action of antifibrinolytic agents as is discussed in the next section.

Antifibrinolytic Agents

The antifibrinolytic agent epsilon aminocaproic acid was introduced by Mullan and Dawley (1968) as a possible means by which clot lysis and thus aneurysm rerupture might be retarded to allow a patient more time for recovery prior to operation. Reports concerning the use of this drug and a similar compound, tranexamic acid have generally shown a favorable effect on the prevention of rebleeding (Tovi et al. 1972). Nibbelink (1975), Post et al. (1977), and Beck (1979) reported results of the Cooperative Aneurysm Study which showed a mortality rate, primarily from rebleeding, of 28.9% with hypotension alone as therapy, 5.8% for antifibrinolytic therapy alone, and 23.8% for combined hypotension and antifibrinolytic therapy. The antagonistic effect of antihypertensive agents on antifibrinolytic therapy could not be explained. Fodstad and associates (1978) conducted a randomized trial of 46 patients of whom 23 received tranexamic acid and 23 served as controls. 1 patient in the treated group rebled while 9 of the controls rebled. 2 recent large randomized series show no benefit from antifibrinolytic therapy (Girvin 1975; Kaste and Ramsay 1979). In both series no difference in rebleeding rate were noted between treated and untreated patients. Differences in dosage, fluid administration, and the use of antihypertensive agents were considered possible factors explaining these results. The Glasgow/Dutch trial on the use of antifibrinolytic agents should provide more definite information as to their effectiveness or otherwise and the results are awaited with great interest.

While antifibrinolytic therapy is seemingly effective in preventing rebleeding from an aneurysm, concern has been expressed about possible complications of these agents:

Cerebral ischemia. Kagström and Palma (1972) reported that although the incidence of rebleeding had been reduced by antifibrinolytic agents, the incidence of ischemic complications in patients so treated seemed to be higher. Sonntag and Stein (1974) described 3 of 7 cases who showed increasing focal ischemic deficits while receiving epsilon aminocaproic acid, and noted arteriographic changes suggestive of cerebral thrombosis or arteritis. Rydin and Lundberg (1976) reported two cases of cerebral artery thrombosis in patients taking tranexamic acid for metrorrhagia. In the series reported by Fodstad and associates (1978) while only 1 patient treated with tranexamic acid rebled, 2 others died of cerebral infarction and 1 of a postangiographic carotid artery occlusion. They noted increased incidence of spasm in treated patients and this tended to correlate with neurological deficit.

Hydrocephalus. Knibestöl and colleagues (1976) evaluated ventricular size by echoencephalography and found a higher incidence of ventricular enlargement in patients treated with tranexamic acid. There was no difference in patients with clinically significant hydrocephalus at late follow-up however. In the series of Fodstad and associates (1978) there was a somewhat higher incidence of third ventricular dilatation in the control group, while neither group showed lateral ventricular dilatation by angiography. A similar study with computerized tomography showed the incidence of hydrocephalus associated with antifibrinolytic agents to be increased.

Venous thrombosis. Because phlebothrombosis and pulmonary embolism are not uncommon following subarachnoid hemorrhage, it is difficult to determine whether antifibrinolytic agents actually increase the incidence of venous thrombosis.

Rebound fibrinolysis. Abrupt discontinuation of antifibrinolytic agents may be associated with rebleeding from an aneurysm. The drugs are rapidly excreted in the urine and require continuous administration. Generally, the drug has not been given during operation, and in the present series of patients, an increased tendency to small vessel oozing from muscle, bone, and brain sur-

face has been noted. As clot lysis times were not performed on these patients, this bleeding tendency can be reported only as an observation.
Difficulty of dissection at operation. Hematoma in patients treated with antifibrinolytic agents is more tenacious and hampers dissection. Extra care must be given to small perforation vessels and to exposure of the aneurysm.
Antifibrinolytic therapy has not been used in Zurich.

Partial Cervical Carotid Artery Occlusion

For many years ligation of the common or internal carotid arteries in the neck was a basic treatment for cerebral aneurysm. This method has now been generally replaced by intracranial procedures. Mullan (1975) has proposed that in the preoperative period, the incidence of rebleeding might be lowered by subtotal carotid artery occlusion, regulating the amount of occlusion by pressure measured in the superficial temporal artery. He has reported success with internal carotid and middle cerebral artery aneurysms, but does not recommend the procedure for anterior communicating or basilar artery aneurysms.

Special Clinical Presentations

Unruptured Asymptomatic Aneurysms

The natural history of unruptured cerebral aneurysms is not clearly defined. Certainly the chance of rupture is increased as the aneurysm enlarges to greater than 5 or 6 mm in diameter, although bleeding from smaller aneurysms does occur. One way of gathering a rough estimate of the likelihood of an aneurysm to bleed is to compare the incidence of ruptured aneurysms in the population with the autopsy incidence. While autopsy figures vary as noted in Chapter 2, it seems that about 1 to 2% of the population has an aneurysm which is greater than 5 mm in diameter, or between 100 and 200 in each 10,000 people. If the annual incidence of ruptured aneurysm is 1 in 10,000 (Pakarinen 1967) and if the number of people remaining in a given 10,000 population declines toward 0 over the 40 years that aneurysm rupture is most likely (between ages 30 and 70), then the number of cases of ruptured aneurysm in this group will be between 20 and 30 depending on the shape of the natural mortality curve. Thus the likelihood of rupture will be 20 to 30 of a possible 100 to 200 people or between 10 and 30%. This figure is in fair agreement with the findings of Heiskanen and Marttila (1970) who found that 8 of 76 (10.5%) patients with multiple aneurysms ruptured a previously unruptured aneurysm over a period of from 4 to 11 years. Moyes (1971) found that of 29 patients with an untreated second aneurysm, 4 reruptured (14%) and another 4 showed angiographic evidence of enlargement.

It is generally conceded that operation on an unruptured aneurysm is far safer than an operation following subarachnoid hemorrhage. In Moyes' series 16 patients were subjected to operation for second unruptured aneurysms. There were no deaths, but 2 patients sustained relatively severe neurological deficits. In 5 cases of purely incidental aneurysms, there was no death or morbidity. Samson and associates (1977) operated on 49 patients for asymptomatic aneurysms. 37 of these patients had had a previous craniotomy – 29 for ruptured cerebral aneurysm, and 8 others for tumor, arteriovenous malformation, or cerebral ischemia. 8 patients had undergone a carotid endarterectomy and 2 a transsphenoidal hypophysectomy. There was no mortality in the 49 patients, and the only morbidity described was frontalis muscle paralysis in 3 patients. Salazar (1980) reported 15 patients who underwent angiography for various nonhemorrhagic disorders in whom a total of 18 asymptomatic aneurysms were found. These patients were operated on with no mortality.

Thus it would seem that most patients in whom an aneurysm is found during evaluation for neurological complaints should be advised to have the aneurysm clipped. Age and coexistent illness may of course weigh against operative therapy. A number of aneurysms which were unruptured and asymptomatic were encountered in the present series. Multiple aneurysms which could not be treated at one operation (Vol. II, Chapter 7), and aneurysms found incidentally with tumors or arteriovenous malformations are discussed in Vol. I, Chapter 5. Only 5 cases underwent operation as a prophylactic procedure for incidentally discovered aneurysms.

Cerebral angiography has been used frequently to evaluate neurological symptoms which are vague or non-localizing and occasionally an aneurysm is found.

Computerized tomography has brought about some decrease in the use of angiography, and with the use of contrast enhancement, CT scanning itself can be expected to turn up unruptured aneurysms in patients complaining of headache, dizziness, fatigue, visual disturbances, depression, forgetfulness, and other rather generalized symptoms. While this can save some patients the tragedy of a subarachnoid hemorrhage, it gives added responsibility to the neurosurgeon to exercise sound clinical judgement in case selection (see Figs 2–4).

Pregnancy

As cerebral aneurysms commonly make their appearance after 35 years of age, and childbearing is far more common under 35 years of age, the incidence of ruptured aneurysms during pregnancy is not high. The frequency has been estimated at about 1 in 10,000 live births (Miller and Hinckley 1970). Nevertheless ruptured aneurysm accounts for about 25% of maternal mortality and therefore represents an important clinicopathological problem.

Pool (1965) collected 37 cases from the medical literature, a questionnaire sent to other neurosurgeons, and personal experience. Subarachnoid hemorrhage was more common in the last half of pregnancy and slightly more common in the last trimester. 26 of the 37 patients were treated by operation – 6 with cervical carotid ligation and 20 with intracranial procedures. 2 patients died (7.7%). Of 11 patients treated with bed rest, 8 died from recurrent hemorrhage (72.7%). It was noted that each of the 8 patients had recovered from the first hemorrhage. Fetal mortality rate was low in both groups. Pool thus concluded that pregnant patients with ruptured aneurysms should be treated as non-pregnant patients, and undergo operation when in good clinical condition.

Hunt and associates (1974) have more recently reviewed the existing literature on this subject and added cases of their own. They are in agreement with Pool that operative treatment of the aneurysm is recommended. Addressing the problem of delivery in a patient with an untreated aneurysm or an aneurysm treated by carotid ligation, they felt that Caesarian section was not indicated and preferred segmental block anesthesia. Robinson and associates (1974) also advised early intracranial operation for ruptured aneurysm in pregnant patients and found this carried no additional hazard to the fetus, although they recommend avoiding hypotension during surgery.

In the present series, 7 patients suffered one or more subarachnoid hemorrhages during pregnancy. Ages ranged from 26 to 39 years old. All subarachnoid hemorrhages occurred between the 5th and 9th month of pregnancy. Details are summarized in Table **4**. Two of these patients had Caesarian section with operation for aneurysm performed afterwards. The other 5 patients had operation for cerebral aneurysm performed within the 5th to 7th months of pregnancy and all had normal subsequent deliveries. This experience would support the opinion of Pool (1965) that the aneurysm be treated as if the patient were not pregnant.

Age

In the present series, the peak age for presentation with ruptured intracranial aneurysm was around 46 years, with 68.2 per cent of the patients under the age of 50 (Tables **16** [p. 286, Vol. I], **19–21** [pp. 300–302, Vol. I]). This is a somewhat younger group than that reported by "Cooperative Study" where the peak age was between 50 and 54. Aneurysms at different locations varied with respect to the most common age of presentation. Aneurysms of the anterior communicating, middle cerebral, and internal carotid-posterior communicating arteries were most frequent between the ages 40 and 60, while 100 per cent of fusiform basilar aneurysms, 59 per cent of internal carotid artery bifurcation aneurysms, and 40 per cent of aneurysms of the posterior cerebral artery were found in patients less than 30 years old.

Jones (1978) reviewed 56 patients over 50 years old with ruptured cerebral aneurysms of whom 37 underwent operation. There was an overall 27 per cent mortality in operated cases, with 17 per cent mortality in grades I and II. He felt that angiography could be more limited in this group if the site of rupture could be documented by computerized tomography. In his series anterior communicating artery aneurysm patients showed a less favorable outcome after operation, although his conclusion that these patients are better treated conservatively would require further documentation.

Amacher and associates (1977) reviewed the

Table 4 Clinical details and outcome in seven patients suffering subarachnoid hemorrhage during pregnancy

	Age					Grade	Date of operation	Site	Surgery	Deficit	Result
O. R.	29	SAH	24 Feb 67 6 Mar 67 8 Mar 67	R. Hpr. + aphasia Sectio Caesarea	9 m. 2nd	Ib mild hpr.	20 Mar 67 14 d.	r.p.c.	Clip	No	Good, Child healthy
K. R.	37	SAH	24 Jan 78	Pregnancy Sectio Caesarea	9 m.	Ia	27 Jun 78 5 m. 8 Nov 78	r.MCA l.MCA	Clip Clip	No	Good, Child healthy
V. D.	29	SAH	8 Oct 75	Pregnant	5 m. 1st	Ia	6 Nov 75 29 d.	r. ophth. 2nd aneur.	Clip Muscle	No	Good, Normal delivery, Child healthy
O. J.	29	SAH	23 Mar 71	Pregnant	5 m. 2nd	IIa	7 Apr 77 11 d.	l.p.c.	Clip	No	Good, Normal delivery, Child healthy
A. A.	34	SAH SAH	1958 ACA operated 25 Oct 79	Pregnant	5 m.	IIa	29 Nov 79 4 w.	l.inf. l.c.A. A.C.A.	Clip Clip (old clip slipped)		Good, Normal delivery, Child healthy
S. M.	39	SAH	Spring 66 13 Nov 66	Pregnant	7 m. 4th	Ia	26 Jan 67 2½ m.	r.l.c.A. bifurc.	Clip	No	Good, Normal delivery, Child healthy
B. C.	26	SAH	16 Oct 73	Pregnant	7 m. 2nd	IIa	28 Oct 73 12 d.	r.A.C.A.	Clip	No	Good, Normal delivery, Child healthy

courses of 93 patients over 60 years old in grades I or II from Drake's large series of patients and found only a mild difference in mortality accounted for primarily by unexpected death from myocardial infarction and pulmonary embolism with no significant difference in morbidity.

Children

Cerebral aneurysms do not occur commonly in childhood, in the Cooperative Study only 2.5 per cent of aneurysms occurred in patients under 20 years old (41 aneurysms in 6343 patients). Matson (1965) reported 14 cases of aneurysms occurring in childhood. In 6 of these cases the aneurysm was found on the anterior communicating artery, in 4 on the internal carotid artery with 1 on the bifurcation, in 2 on the middle cerebral artery, in 1 on the basilar bifurcation, and in 1 on the left posterior inferior cerebellar artery. 3 of his patients had coarctation of the aorta and 1 had endocarditis. He felt the incidences of early rebleeding and ischemia were less in this age group. Patel and Richardson (1971) found 58 cases of childhood aneurysm in 3,000 cases seen at Atkinson-Morley Hospital in London. 7 patients had coarctation of the aorta and 2 polycystic kidney disease. 23 patients had aneurysms of the anterior communicating artery and 20 patients had aneurysms of the internal carotid artery bifurcation. In 3 cases there were multiple aneurysms.

Thompson et al. (1973) reported 22 cases of intracranial aneurysm in children, of which 15 were congenital saccular aneurysms and the others mycotic or traumatic. 6 of the saccular aneurysms were located at the internal carotid artery bifurcation. These authors were impressed by the larger size of aneurysms in childhood – from 10 to 35 mm. They also mentioned that no incidental aneurysms had been seen in this age group in over 1500 angiograms. Grode et al. (1978) reported 2 infant cases (30 weeks and 3 months old) who were successfully operated upon with aneurysms of the left and right middle cerebral artery clipped. Lipper et al. (1978) reported a congenital saccular aneurysm of the left ICA in a 19 day old neonate and found 19 cases in the first year of life that have been reported between 1943 and 1977.

Hungerford et al. (1981) reported a 1 month old infant with an aneurysm and reviewed 17 cases in the literature of aneurysms occurring in infants between the ages of 3 days and 3 months. Becker et al. (1978) reported a case of a 5 year old girl with a large aneurysm on the left MCA and reviewed 15 cases of the literature of early childhood aneurysms diagnosed during life. Richardson (1979) reported 74 cases in 3900 proven aneurysm-bearing patients (1.9%). None of the 74 cases had a family history of ruptured aneurysm and none had clinically obvious atheroma, inflammatory angiopathy, bacterial endocarditis, blood dyscrasia or collagen disease. 7 had coarctation of the aorta, 2 had bilateral polycystic kidney, and 1 patient had ductus arteriosus. The incidence of associated anomalies was, therefore, high but the overall incidence of hypertension was only 15 per cent. Complicating subdural or intracerebral hematomas were present in 15/74 (20%). The "warning bleeds", seemed more common in young patients than in adults. Vascular spasm, however, was only seen at angiography in 9/74 (12%) of cases, although the significance of this finding is doubtful as most cases were admitted very soon after the hemorrhage. Relevant is the observation that at necropsy, pale infarction was not seen even when the premorbid angiogram had shown severe spasm. All the aneurysms fell within the average range of size from 5–30 mm in diameter. The 30 per cent incidence of aneurysm of the carotid termination contrasts remarkably with quoted figures of 3–5% in most adult series. It is also interesting that of 17 cases presenting with hemiplegia or hemiparesis, no less than 12 harbored a contralateral terminal carotid aneurysm.

Interestingly, in the large series of Suzuki (1979) there are no cases below the age of 10 years, and only 5 cases below the age of 20 years (0.5%).

In the present series 41 of 1012 operated cases were under 20 years of age (4.1%), with 4 cases under 10 years of age (0.4%) (Vol. I, Table **21**). Location of aneurysms, age of patients, preoperative condition and results in the first two decades of life are given in Tables **5, 6,** and **7**. It is noted that 16 patients or almost half of these cases had aneurysms of the internal carotid bifurcation. One patient had bilateral aneurysms of the carotid bifurcation. 11 cases had aneurysms of the anterior communicating artery, and 4 cases had aneurysms of the middle cerebral artery. In 9 cases, aneurysms were found on the posterior circulation including 2 fusiform dilatations of the basilar artery. In the youngest case of our series (2½ years old) the diagnosis was made at autopsy

Table 5 Distribution of aneurysms in operated patients under 20 years old

	Under 10 years No. of cases			11 to 20 years No. of cases		
Internal carotid artery	2			16		
Intracavernous	–			1	M	(18 years)
Posterior communicating	–			1	F	(12 years)
Bifurcation	2	1 F 1 M	(9 years) (10 years)	14	5 F 9 M	
Middle cerebral artery	–			4	3 F 1 M	
Anterior communicating artery	1	F	(8 years)	10	3 F 7 M	
Basilar artery and branches	1	F	(5 years)	4	1 F 3 M	(19 years) (13, 18*, 19* years)
Vertebral artery	–			3	1 F 2 M	(15 years) (14 years)
	4			37 = 41		

* died

32   1 Clinical Considerations

Table 6 Outcome in operated juvenile aneurysm cases related to site

Location	Total No.	Good	Fair	Death
Intracavernous	1	1	–	–
PcoA	1	1	–	–
ICA-Bi	16	15	1	–
MCA	4	4	–	–
AcoA	11	11	–	–
VA	3	3	–	–
BA	5	3	–	2*
	41	38	1	2

* later death after muscle wrapping of fusiform aneurysms

Table 7 Patients under 20 years of age

Preoperative condition	Total No.	Good	Fair	Death
0b	4	3	1	–
Ia	15	15	–	–
Ib	2	2	–	–
IIa	12	11	–	1*
IIb	2	2	–	–
IIIa	3	3	–	–
IIIb	3	2	–	1*
	41	38 (92.7%)	1	2 (4.9%)

* muscle wrapping

(p. 1 of this Chapter). In our series of children none of the 41 cases had a family history of ruptured aneurysm and none had clinically obvious associated diseases.

None of the cases had a subdural hematoma, but 8 cases presented with an intracerebral hematoma. In 16 cases the aneurysm was localized at the bifurcation of the internal carotid artery (39%). In all patients the aneurysm was directly explored and clipped. In 1 case bilateral aneurysms of both ICA could be clipped through a one-sided exploration. In 38 patients (92.7%) the operative result was good, in 2 patients large basilar aneurysms could not be clipped but only wrapped with muscle. Both patients died later.

Among 227 patients who died in other hospitals of the Canton Zurich (in the time-period 1967–1979) before surgery, 4 patients were under 20 years old (Table 8).

Table 8 Unoperated cases (died before surgery)

Age	Sex	Location	Condition		
9 y	M	AcoA	V	died within hours	IVH
12 y	M	AcoA	IV	died within hours	IVH + ICH
15 y	F	Ba-Bi	IV	died after shunting	+
9 y	M	MCA (R.)	V	died within hours	IVH + ICH

Laterality

The lateralization of 1012 aneurysms is shown in Table 18, Vol. I, Chapter 5. It is noted that aneurysms of the internal carotid artery are slightly more common on the right side (53.6%), while aneurysms on the anterior communicating artery arise more frequently from the left corner (52.5%) and aneurysms of the middle cerebral artery are equally distributed on both sides.

2 Internal Carotid Artery Aneurysms

Introduction

Aneurysms may arise at any of several locations along the intracranial course of the internal carotid artery. Each of these aneurysm locations is associated with its own local symptomatology, epidemiology, operative problems, and prognostic factors. As increasing numbers of aneurysms of the intracranial internal carotid artery have been treated, it has been recognized that aneurysms should be discussed for each location independently, and many reports of patients with aneurysm at a given site of the internal carotid artery have appeared. It is therefore appropriate that the anatomical relationships, operative techniques, and case presentation and results be presented for each particular location in the present series of aneurysm patients. A general summary of internal carotid artery aneurysms is then given at the end of the chapter.

In dividing aneurysms of the internal carotid artery into various groups by location, however, there arises the problem of terminology. Aneurysms of the internal carotid artery most commonly arise at the origin of a major branch. The aneurysm orifice may be completely situated on the internal carotid artery or may involve the arterial branch to a varying degree. Only uncommonly will the aneurysm be completely situated on the branch, and thus the terms "ophthalmic artery aneurysm" and "posterior communicating artery aneurysm" convey a false anatomical impression of most internal carotid artery aneurysms. The following grouping of aneurysms has been adopted for the present series:

1) Infraclinoid internal carotid artery aneurysms (Intracavernous aneurysms) (Icav An),
2) Medial wall internal carotid artery aneurysms
   a) Proximal (Carotid-ophthalmic aneurysms, ophthalmic artery aneurysms) (Oph An),
   b) Distal (very rare, two cases),
3) Inferior wall internal carotid artery aneurysms (Inf An),
4) Superior wall internal carotid artery aneurysms (one case),
5) Lateral wall internal carotid artery aneurysms
   a) Proximal (Carotid-posterior communicating artery aneurysms PCOA An),
   b) Distal (Carotid-choroidal aneurysms, anterior choroidal artery aneurysms, Ach An),
6) At the bifurcation of ICA; (Bi An).

The location and frequency of these aneurysms is shown diagrammatically in Fig **57 A–B**, p. 122.

Infraclinoid Internal Carotid Artery Aneurysms

Anatomical Relationships

Aneurysms of the Cervical ICA

Aneurysms arising from the cervical portion of the internal carotid artery have been treated by vascular surgeons, otolaryngologists, and occasionally neurosurgeons. Cooper (1836) reported the first successful operation of an aneurysm of the cervical carotid artery. Killian (1951) reported 173 aneurysms of the ICA in the neck out of 787 cases of extracranial carotid aneurysms. Brihaye (1979) reviewed the world literature and found 47 well documented cases between 1931 and 1977. These cases are listed in the publication of Pia (1979), Table I, pages 47–54. Schechter (1979) also reviewed the world literature and found 853 extracranial carotid aneurysms in 830 patients between 1687 and 1977. He noted that the aneurysms were almost equally divided between the common and internal carotid arteries, with traumatic aneurysms affecting primarily the common carotid artery.

The presentation of patients with cervical carotid aneurysms was reviewed by Mokri et al. (1982). Aneurysms in this location usually present as masses protruding into the pharynx or bulging at the angle of the mandible beneath the skin. Pulsation and bruit identify the vascular nature of the lesions. Some patients suffer ischemic neurologic events, while a few may present with bleeding from the pharynx, ear, or nose.

Cervical carotid aneurysms have diverse etiologies, including atherosclerosis, fibromuscular dysplasia, cystic medial necrosis, trauma, and infection. Both primary infectious processes such as syphilis, as well as secondary contiguous infections in the neck or mastoids may result in their production.

Winslow (1926) reported a mortality of 70 per cent in the patients treated conservatively versus a mortality of 30 per cent in those undergoing ligation of the artery. A number of recent reports have outlined a variety of treatment techniques for these aneurysms (Lin et al. 1956; Beall et al. 1962; Raphael et al. 1963; Buxton et al. 1964; Mokri et al. 1982). Pia (1979) reviewed the treatment of these lesions in his series of patients. This consists of ligating the common carotid artery or more frequently the internal carotid artery. In some instances this was accompanied by resection of the lesion and/or an EC–IC bypass procedure. In other cases an end-to-end reconstruction of the artery or an aneurysmorrhaphy was performed. His results were good in 33 cases, fair in 2, poor in 2, and fatal in 6. In 5 patients undergoing conservative treatment, 3 had died and 2 recovered.

Within the time period of 1967–1979, there were no cases in our series of an aneurysm in the cervical portion of the ICA, but in 1980 we observed a unique case of bilateral giant fusiform aneurysms of the ICA in the cervical and petrocavernous portions. These presented with bilateral exophthalmus (right > left) and headache in a 16 year old boy. The patient underwent a right-sided EC–IC anastomosis followed by resection of the accessible parts of the right sided aneurysm by a vascular surgeon. The patient recovered from his headache and bilateral exophthalmus within a few months and the postoperative angiogram showed patency of the anastomosis, and not only diminution of the cavernous portion of the right sided aneurysm but surprisingly also a decreased size of the left cervical carotid aneurysm. The scheduled left sided EC-IC-bypass surgery was therefore postponed (Fig **13A–G**).

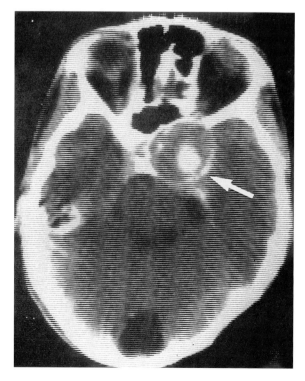

Fig **13A** CT scan of a 16 year old patient with headaches, bilateral exophthalmus, hyperacusis, decreased visual acuity, and a pulsating mass in the neck suggestive of a giant aneurysm (arrow).

Anatomical Relationships

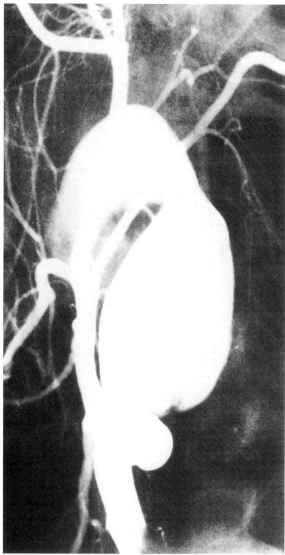

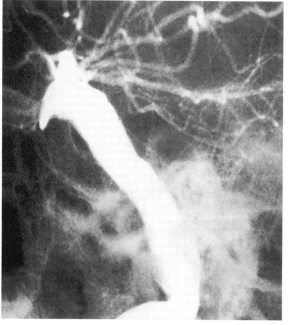

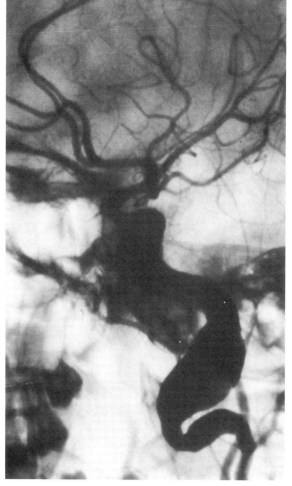

Fig **13B–D** Right cervical (**B**) and intracranial (**C**) angiograms revealed a giant fusiform aneurysm of the entire internal carotid artery. Left carotid angiography (**D**) confirmed the presence of a similar though smaller aneurysm on the left internal carotid artery.

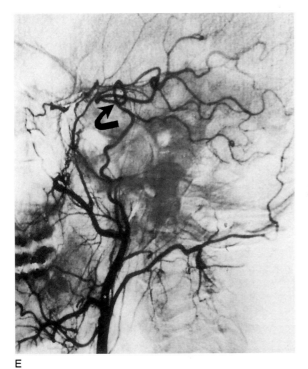

E

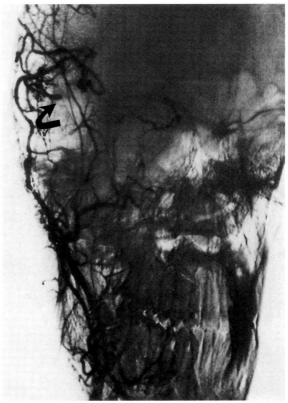

F

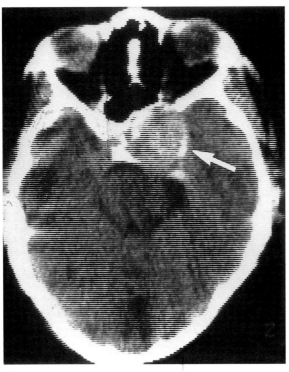

G

Fig 13 E–G The patient underwent a right EC-IC bypass (Dr. Zumstein) followed by resection of the cervical aneurysm and ligation of the right internal carotid artery at its entrance into the carotid canal (Profs. Turina and Schwartz, Zurich). The patient improved and angiography (arrows) (**E** and **F**) showed a patent anastomosis without filling of the aneurysm which was thrombosed on CT scan (arrow) (**G**). The left sided asymptomatic aneurysm is untreated.

Aneurysms in the Petrous Portion of ICA

Brihaye (1979b) found in the literature only 20 cases of these very rare aneurysms (see Table 1, pp. 56–60 in the monograph of Pia). In 11 cases the aneurysm was large and in 8 cases it was small; in 1 case the aneurysm was not visualized. The treatments of choice were ligatures of the CCA or ICA: successfully performed in 12 cases, but ineffective in 2 cases. In these two cases and in another 5 cases, a direct attempt with mastoidectomy was made. This was successful in 5 cases, whereas 2 patients died, 1 due to uncontrollable hemorrhage. Also 1 patient died who was treated with ligature of the ECA.

We observed 2 cases of aneurysms in the petrous portion of the ICA, which have been successfully treated by vascular and neuro-oto-laryngological surgeons with resection of the aneurysm and reconstruction of the ICA.

Intracavernous Aneurysms

Most infraclinoid internal carotid aneurysms arise from the intracavernous portion of the artery. From the clinical history they can be divided into 2 groups, traumatic and spontaneous (Brihaye 1979c). Parkinson (1979), however, distinguished further divisions: "basically there are two types of aneurysms in the region, the saccular and the fistulous. The fistulous type can again be divided into two, the spontaneous and the traumatic."

The incidence of intracavernous carotid aneurysms is approximately 5 per cent of all intracranial aneurysms (Jeanmart et al. 1973). Within the 13 years of the microsurgical era, we have observed 30 fistulous and 13 (1.3%) spontaneous non-traumatic non-fistulous saccular aneurysms, together constituting 4.2% of the series.

In this monograph only the last group of 13 patients will be discussed.

In unusual cases they may be infectious in origin, as the case reported by de Rougemont et al. (1966). A congenital etiology is conjectured in many observations (Brihaye 1979c). Drake (1968) observed 2 aneurysms in a 14 year old girl, one on the intracavernous carotid, the other on the basilar artery. The most frequent association is with those aneurysms which arise from the persistent trigeminal artery itself (Davis et al. 1965; Morrison et al. 1974). Out of 16 cases reported by Djindjian et al. (1965) 4 had such an association. However, this high incidence has not been seen in other series where the frequency is around 15 per cent (Brihaye 1979c). It is assumed that these aneurysms may arise in association with other smaller branches within the cavernous sinus, as do aneurysms at other intracranial locations (Barr et al. 1971).

An atherosclerotic origin is likely in many cases; this etiology could explain the greater incidence in patients who are 50 years old or more (Brihaye 1979c).

There were 13 cases of intracavernous aneurysm in the present series; in 7 cases the lesion was on the right side and in 6 on the left. In 2 cases there were bilateral cavernous aneurysms, larger on the left in one case and on the right in the other. There were no instances of associated intracranial aneurysms. However, in 1 case of ruptured intracranial aneurysm, there was an associated incidental cavernous aneurysm.

These aneurysms may attain a large diameter, and are frequently partially thrombosed. Their intracavernous location may lead to dysfunction of cranial nerves III, IV, and VI, the first and sometimes second divisions of V, and occasionally II. The lesion may erode the sella turcica, although pituitary abnormalities are exceptional. The clinicoanatomical correlations of the various cavernous sinus syndromes that may be associated with aneurysms of this portion of the internal carotid artery were discussed in a classical paper by Jefferson (1938).

If the aneurysm comes into continuity with the carotid cistern, rupture may lead to subarachnoid hemorrhage. On the other hand, if the aneurysm is totally within the cavernous sinus, rupture may lead to internal carotid-cavernous sinus fistula, with exophthalmus, chemosis, and a bruit.

Finally, we observed an unusual case with a left-sided giant cavernous aneurysm which was clearly demonstrated on CT scan, although carotid angiography failed to show any suspicious change along the cavernous portion of the left internal carotid artery. Subsequent subtemporal exploration confirmed a fully thrombosed aneurysm (Fig **14A–B**).

2 Internal Carotid Artery Aneurysms

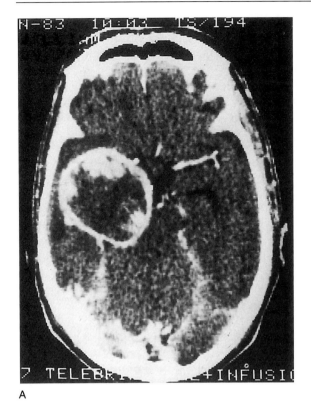
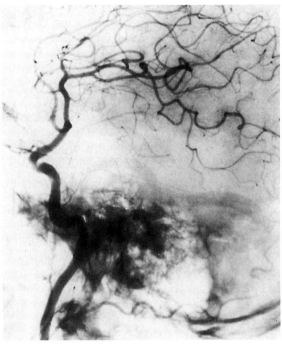

Fig 14A–B   A giant aneurysm on CT scan (**A**), carotid angiography surprisingly failed to demonstrate any part of the aneurysm.

Operative Technique

There are at present several possible methods of treatment available for intracavernous internal carotid artery aneurysm.
1) Cervical, internal, or common carotid artery ligation. 10 of 13 cases in the present series were treated with carotid artery ligation alone.
2) Carotid ligation with preliminary extracranial, intracranial arterial anastomosis procedure. 2 cases in the present series had such a procedure performed.
3) Balloon catheter techniques. No patients in the present series have had an attempt at balloon catheter occlusion of an intracavernous aneurysm. Serbinenko (1974), Debrun et al. (1975, 1978, 1981), Prolo et al. (1977), and Romodanov and Shcheglov (1979) have reported success with this technique.
4) Wire thrombosis techniques. Mullan (1974) and Hosobuchi (1975) have reported success in inducing thrombosis in these aneurysms by the direct introduction of thin gauge wire.
5) Direct clipping of aneurysm. Parkinson (1965, 1979) has described opening of the cavernous sinus under hypothermia and cardiac arrest, and more recently Johnston (1979) has described a case of bilateral intracavernous aneurysms

handled in this way. The generally acceptable results following carotid ligation have tempered enthusiasm for a more radical approach in most cases, but in some situations, such techniques may be required.

Cervical Carotid Ligation

The general concepts of cervical carotid artery ligation were discussed in Chapter 6, and will not be repeated here. Prior to performing cervical carotid artery ligation, the adequacy of cerebral collateral circulation must be carefully evaluated. The following methods have been employed.
1) *Cerebral angiography*. A complete study should include cross-compression of the ipsilateral (aneurysm bearing) carotid artery to evaluate the anterior communicating artery, and compression of the ipsilateral carotid artery during vertebral injection to evaluate the posterior communicating artery.
2) *Matas test*. Digital compression of the ipsilateral carotid artery is monitored by neurological evaluation and by electroencephalography (Matas and Allen 1911).
3) *Wada test*. It will occasionally be necessary to determine cerebral dominance prior to carotid ligation. This is evaluated by intra-arterial injec-

tion of barbiturate at the time of angiography (Wada and Rasmussen 1960).
4) *EEG with compression.* Under local anesthesia, the common carotid artery bifurcation in the neck is exposed. The common carotid artery is compressed for 15 minutes while the neurological condition is continuously checked. If this is well tolerated, a bulldog or Crutchfield clamp is applied to the internal carotid artery, and closed completely again checking the patient's neurological condition. A silk ligature is also loosely placed around the internal carotid artery and the wound is closed. If the patient's neurological condition changes over the next 24 hours, the clamp is immediately re-opened. The wound is then re-opened and the same procedure followed with the clamp now placed on the common carotid artery. In either instance, if the patient's neurological status remains unchanged for 24 hours with the clamp completely closed, then the wound is re-opened under local anesthesia and the previously applied suture firmly fastened to permanently ligate the vessel. During this entire process, the patient's blood pressure must be maintained at normal to high levels.

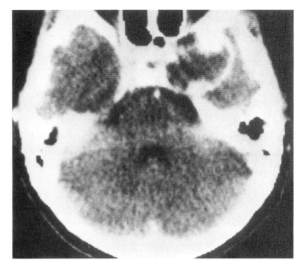

Fig 15A A giant right sided fusiform intracavernous aneurysm as seen on CT scan in a 50 year old woman with ophthalmoparesis. The small left sided intracavernous aneurysm is not demonstrated.

Clinical Presentation and Operative Results

One patient early in the series would not tolerate carotid occlusion and an attempt was made to reinforce the collateral circulation with an extra-intracranial bypass procedure. This case was presented previously (Yaşargil 1969). Despite the failure in this case, the idea of performing an extracranial-intracranial bypass procedure seemed a good one for cases where the collateral circulation was insufficient. In 1979, the following patients (see Table **9**, Nos. 12 and 13) with bilateral cavernous aneurysms came to treatment: (Figs **15** and **16**).

In these 13 cases, straightforward cervical carotid artery ligation was possible in 10 cases with a good result in all. 3 cases required extracranial-intracranial anastomosis however, which was successful in 2 more recent cases but failed in 1 case early in the series. It is recommended that a bypass procedure be considered in the operative therapy of these aneurysms when collateral circulation is insufficient or when bilateral intracavernous carotid artery aneurysms are present.

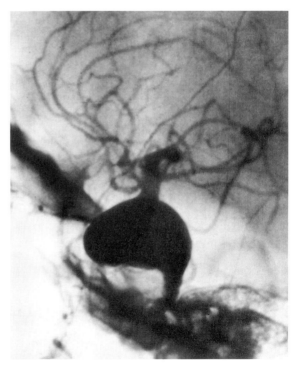

Fig 15B Right carotid angiography confirmed the lesion with subtotal thrombosis of the sac.

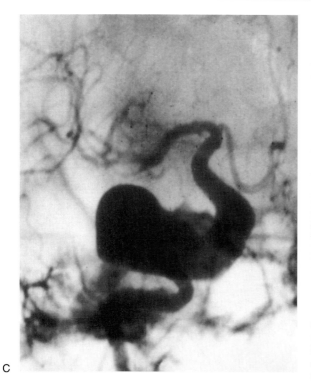

C

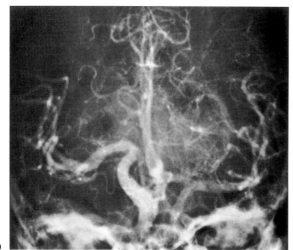

D

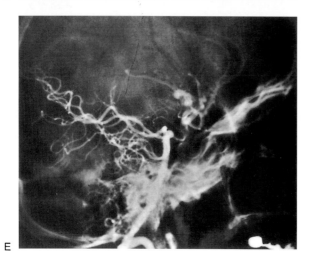

E

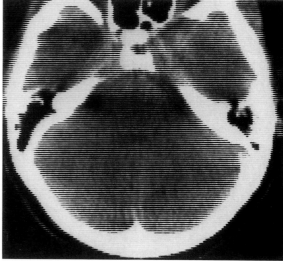

F

Fig 15 C–F The AP view of the right carotid angiogram shows the full extent of this aneurysm (**C**). The right internal carotid artery was ligated in the neck and EC-IC bypass performed. Repeat left carotid (**D**) and vertebral angiograms (**E**) showed good collateral flow with filling of the right internal carotid artery but not the aneurysm which was found to be thrombosed and shrunken on CT (**F**) (Case 13, Table **9**). The patient has had no left sided symptoms over the past four years. If she should develop an enlargement of the aneurysm a left sided EC-IC bypass and left internal carotid artery ligation or intraarterial balloon occlusion may be considered.

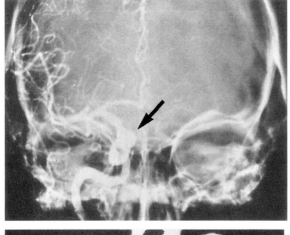
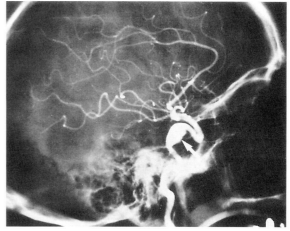
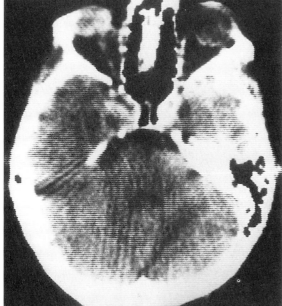
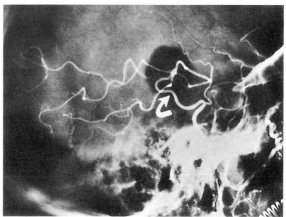
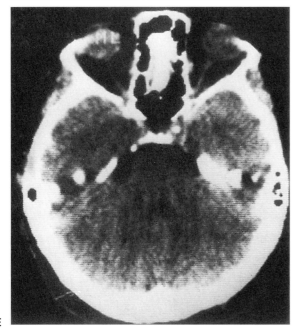

Fig 16A–E Bilateral intracavernous carotid aneurysm (arrow) (**A**-right and **B**-left) with the left larger and symptomatic, partially thrombosed on CT scan (**C**). The patient underwent a left EC-IC bypass (arrow) (**D**) followed by ligation of the left internal carotid artery in the neck with good results as confirmed by postoperative CT scan (**E**) (Case 12, Table **9**). The patient has remained asymptomatic for the past 4 years from the right intracavernous aneurysm. Again, balloon occlusion would be considered should the aneurysm undergo symptomatic enlargement.

Summary

Of 13 patients with cavernous internal carotid artery aneurysms, 5 were men and 8 women. Ages ranged from 18 to 57. In the 21 cases of Brihaye (1979) the ratio of female to male was 14:3, and the patients' ages ranged from 19 to 76 years. 2 patients had bilateral aneurysms at this location. The presenting symptoms are summarized in Table **9**. Nine patients complained of ipsilateral retro-orbital pain. 11 patients had cranial nerve deficits, 2 of these associated with subarachnoid hemorrhage. 9 patients had abducens palsy or paresis, 5 patients had partial oculomotor palsy, 4 patients had sensory changes in the distribution of the trigeminal nerve, 1 patient had visual loss associated with destruction of the sella turcica, and 2 had complete cavernous sinus syndromes with exophthalmos. One patient developed a carotid-cavernous fistula, and 1 patient had only severe headaches with no neurological findings. Several patients gave a history of acute episodes of headache suggesting either sudden enlargement of the aneurysm or a small rupture.

Surgical results are also noted in Table 9. 12 of the 13 patients (92.3%) are in good condition from 1 to 11 years postoperatively. 2 of these cases required a preliminary superficial temporal artery-middle cerebral artery anastomosis, and this has worked well. An earlier attempt to anastomose the two fronto-orbital arteries failed, and this patient remains only in fair condition.

Table 9 Intracavernous internal carotid artery aneurysm patients

Patient	Year	Age	Sex	History	Findings	Site	Size	Procedure	Remarks	Result
1. Wy	1967	57	M	Pain Diplopia 0b	Exophth. III, IV, V, VI palsy	Left	Giant	Frontopolar to frontopolar anast. No ligation	Aplastic AcoA, hypoplastic PcoA, Poor collat. circ., postop. infection	Fair
2. Schi	1967	34	F	SAH Diplopia Ia	Right VI palsy	Right	Large	Right ICA ligation	Improvement	Good
3. Gü	1968	38	F	Diplopia Mild Exoph. 0b	Left VI Partial III paresis	Left	Small	Left ICA ligation	Improvement	Good
4. Sche	1969	42	F	SAH Diplopia Ia	Right VI paresis	Right	Small	Right ICA ligation	Improvement	Good
5. Mu	1969	34	F	Right orbital pain 0b	Right VI paresis	Right	Small	Right ICA ligation	Improvement	Good
6. Os	1969	42	F	Left frontal pain 0b	Left VI paresis Left V_1 hypesth.	Left	Medium	Left ICA clamp (17 Oct 69) Left CCA ligation (11 Nov 69)	Postop. Transient right hemiparesis and aphasia, Fully Recovered	Good
7. Cl	1970	52	M	0b	Exophth.	Right	Medium	Right ICA ligation	Improvement	Good
8. Me	1974	18	M	Pain Diplopia 0b	Left VI paresis	Left	Large	Left ICA ligation	Improvement	Good
9. Wa	1975	57	M	Pain, Decr. Vision 0b	VF Defect Left VI paresis	Left	Giant	Left ICA ligation	Improvement	Good
10. Kl	1976	40	M	Pain 0b	None	Right	Small	Right ICA ligation	Improvement	Good
11. Po	1979	33	F	Pain Diplopia 0b	Exophth. Right III paresis	Right	Large	Right ICA ligation	Improvement	Good
12. Cl	1979	50	F	Pain Diplopia 0b	Left III Left paresis V_{1-3}	Right Left	Small Giant	EIA and Left ICA ligation	Improvement	Good
13. Ne	1979	50	F	Pain Diplopia 0b	Right III, IV, V, VI paresis	Right Left	Large Small	EIA and Right ICA ligation	Improvement	Good

Carotid-Ophthalmic Aneurysms

Anatomical Relationships

Aneurysms arising from the medial or superomedial wall of the internal carotid artery and projecting in a variety of directions are included in this category (Fig 17). These aneurysms usually arise in relation to the ophthalmic artery and classically have been called ophthalmic artery aneurysms. Pool and Potts (1965) reported that these aneurysms comprise about 1.3 per cent of intracranial aneurysms, while Locksley (1966) and Iwabuchi (1978) estimed their occurrence at 5.4 per cent and 3.8 per cent respectively. In the present series a total of 33 patients presented with symptomatic aneurysms in this location, comprising 3.3 per cent of the entire series.

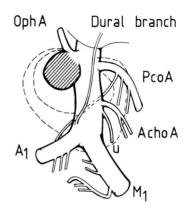

Fig 17 Schematic illustration of proximal medial wall aneurysms (carotid-ophthalmic) that sometimes involve the origin of the ophthalmic artery, showing their growing tendency with involvement of other carotid artery branches.

Laterality and Multiplicity of Aneurysms

In the present series the aneurysm was located on the left side in 14 cases and on the right side in 19. Striking in this group of aneurysms is the incidence of associated aneurysms and especially the occurrence of symmetrical aneurysms on the opposite internal carotid artery. 7 of 33 cases (21.2%) showed bilaterally symmetrical carotid-ophthalmic aneurysms. Aneurysms were present at other locations in 11 patients including 1 at the opposite internal carotid and middle cerebral artery bifurcation, giving a total of 16 patients (48.5%) with multiple aneurysms. There were a total of 55 aneurysms (5 micro) in this group of 33 patients (Table 10). In addition, 11 patients with ruptured aneurysms at other locations had incidental carotid-ophthalmic aneurysms (see Table 11a–b); 7 of these have been clipped, 4 microaneurysms coagulated and wrapped with muscle.

Table 10 Ophthalmic artery aneurysms. Clinical data from various series

	No. of cases	Sex Male	Sex Female	SAH	Side Right	Side Left	Multiple aneurysms	Visual changes
Co-operative study 1966	143	36	107	101	65	78	–	–
Drake et al. 1968b	14	3	11	13	5	9	9	1
Kothandaram et al. 1971	19	4	15	15	7	12	4	4
Thurel et al. 1974	17	6	11	14	6	11	4	3
Almeida et al. 1976	8	3	5	7	4	4	3	1
Guidetti 1977	38	14	24	34	17	21	12	15
Own 1981	33	3	30	23	19	14	16	6
Total	272	69	203	207	123	149	48	30

Projection of Aneurysm Fundus

Aneurysms at this location arise from the medial or superomedial wall of the internal carotid artery at or just beyond the origin of the ophthalmic artery. The position of the fundus is variable, however, and two main varieties and five subdivisions of fundus projection can be recognized:

Suprachiasmatic

1) *Supero-anterior*. In 4 cases the fundus projected anteriorly over the anterior clinoid process or laterally over the internal carotid artery and had no significant relationship to the optic nerves or chiasm. In this instance the neck of the aneurysm and the ophthalmic artery are concealed from the surgeon's view by the fundus of the aneurysm.
2) *Supero-posterior*. 8 aneurysms projected above the optic nerves and chiasm. An aneurysm of this group may extend posteriorly and is often buried in the lateral orbital gyri; a point to remember when traction is applied to the undersurface of the frontal lobe.

Subchiasmatic

3) *Inferomedial*. This is the most common presentation of internal carotid-ophthalmic artery aneurysm, as it was found in 20 of 39 cases (including the 6 bilateral cases). The fundus lies beneath the adjacent optic nerve, often elevating it, and compressing it. The aneurysm is in a close relationship with the pituitary stalk, which may be displaced laterally towards the opposite side or inferiorly. Subchiasmatic aneurysms may be associated with loss of visual acuity and altitudinal visual field defects due to compression of the optic nerves and chiasm. When thrombosed they may be confused with suprasellar tumors (see Vol. I, Fig **254 A–D**). In one case, the fundus of a subchiasmatic aneurysm protruded between the optic nerves and ruptured into the overlying gyrus rectus, imitating an anterior communicating artery aneurysm (see Vol. I, Fig **259 A–B**).
4) Giant *subchiasmal* aneurysms filling the entire suprasellar area have been termed "global" (Thurel et al 1974). The aneurysm may involve both ICA, the PcoA and its branches, the ACA, the AcoA and its branches, both optic nerves, and the chiasm. 4 patients in the present series fell into this category.
5) *Extradural*. Because of their close relationship to the cavernous sinus, and the variable location of the origin of the ophthalmic artery, these aneurysms may be partially extradural. One patient had bilateral aneurysms, both of which were partially extradural and another had one aneurysm which was partially extradural.

Relationship to Ophthalmic Artery

An aneurysm at this location usually arises just distal to the origin of the ophthalmic artery on the superomedial wall of the internal carotid artery. The aneurysm displaces the ophthalmic artery proximally toward the cavernous sinus. The artery is fixed in the optic canal and, therefore, becomes stretched around the proximal neck portion of the aneurysm. The origin of the ophthalmic artery may be just within the cavernous sinus or up to several millimeters along the intraarachnoidal internal carotid artery, making identification of the artery at times quite difficult in the presence of an aneurysm. In most of our cases there was either no segment or a small 1–2 mm segment of the ICA proximal to the ophthalmic artery available for dissection and for the possible placement of a temporary clip. The surgeon should keep this anatomical situation in mind, especially in cases of larger carotid-ophthalmic aneurysms, when it is often necessary to leave the area of the ICA in the neck open for possible compression.

Relationship to Anterior Clinoid Process

The shape and length of the anterior clinoid process and the relationship of the aneurysm and the ophthalmic artery to the body of the sphenoid and to the cavernous sinus, determine whether the proximal side of the aneurysm neck and the ophthalmic artery will be hidden from the surgeon's view. It may be helpful to remove a portion of the anterior clinoid process or to unroof the optic canal to gain a small but appreciable amount of mobilization of the optic nerve, resulting in a better view. This is described under Operative Technique.

Operative Technique

Initial Approach and Proximal Control

Through a standard pterional craniotomy, the dura is retracted and the proximal end of the Sylvian cistern opened to expose the origin of the middle cerebral artery. The arachnoid over the middle cerebral artery is opened across the internal carotid artery bifurcation. The frontal lobe should not be retracted very quickly to expose the internal carotid artery and optic nerve since the fundus of the aneurysm may be adherent to the orbital surface of the frontal lobe and be avulsed with retraction.

The carotid cistern is opened lateral to the internal carotid artery to release cerebrospinal fluid from this cistern and from the interpeduncular cistern. The relationship of the internal carotid artery to the anterior clinoid process is evaluated. The most proximal portion of the internal carotid artery is exposed, so that a temporary clip can be placed across it if necessary to control bleeding. How close the aneurysm is to the dura of the cavernous sinus and how far posteriorly the anterior clinoid process projects will determine whether an opportunity exists for the creation of the necessary space. Proximal control of the internal carotid artery may not be possible intracranially. The anesthesiologist should be advised that it may be necessary to compress the carotid artery in the neck, and he should have prepared himself for this by ascertaining the point on the neck where pressure need be applied. An alternative is to drape the neck into the operative field to allow the surgeon's assistant to perform digital compression. With aneurysms that are especially large or complicated, the surgeon may wish to expose the internal carotid artery in the neck prior to the craniotomy in order to temporarily or permanently ligate it in the face of adversity.

Gaining Distal Control

In those aneurysms that project beneath the optic nerves and chiasm, the anterior cerebral arteries and anterior communicating artery are next inspected by opening the lamina terminalis cistern over the antero-superior aspect of these arteries. The relative sizes of the anterior cerebral arteries and the adequacy of the anterior communicating artery are noted to determine the degree of cross-filling should a temporary clip be applied to the internal carotid artery. Opening this cistern also allows the frontal lobe to fall away a bit more from the optic nerves, giving the surgeon more operating space. When the aneurysm sits above the optic nerves and chiasm, this exposure of the anterior cerebral arteries must be deferred.

Attention is then turned to the lateral aspect of the carotid cistern, where the posterior communicating and anterior choroidal arteries are identified. The first few millimeters of each artery are dissected free of arachnoid, and space created on the internal carotid artery for a temporary clip to be placed just distal to the neck of the aneurysm if required. Ideally the surgeon would like to be able to place a clip proximal to the origin of the posterior communicating artery to maximize collateral filling of the ipsilateral middle cerebral artery. If the aneurysm has involved the internal carotid artery too close to the posterior communicating artery to allow placement of a temporary clip, however, then the proximal portion of the posterior communicating artery must be adequately prepared to permit placement of a temporary clip on it without compromise of the perforating branches. The location and direction of these perforating arteries is noted and their relationship to the aneurysm fundus ascertained.

Exposure of the Ophthalmic Artery

In those cases in which the origin of the ophthalmic artery is visible, a plane is developed between it and the neck of the aneurysm by separating and dividing the arachnoid adhesions holding them together. 2 or 3 millimeters of separation will give enough space to pass the blade of a clip between the two structures. The optic nerve may overlie the origin of the ophthalmic artery, and this can be gently elevated by sliding a small cottonoid sponge between the nerve and carotid artery.

Frequently, however, the origin of the ophthalmic artery will be hidden by the base of the aneurysm or by the anterior clinoid process. In these cases, it is preferable to remove the anterior clinoid process and unroof the posterior end of the optic canal to identify the artery distal to the aneurysm. In addition to aiding in identification of the ophthalmic artery, this maneuver helps mobilize the optic nerve which is often rather tightly stretched over the aneurysm fundus. The dura over the anterior clinoid process is incised from the lateral edge of the process to near the ipsilateral optic canal, and reflected anteriorly over the medial orbit with a periosteal elevator, exposing about 1 cm of bone. A small piece of sterile rubber surgeon's glove is placed over the internal carotid artery and optic nerve to protect them, and the clinoid process is drilled off using a high speed electric drill with a diamond burr. Pneumatization of the sphenoid bone is variable, but may be extensive. The surgeon should avoid drilling too much in a medial direction as he may enter the optic recess of the sphenoid sinus or even the ethmoid air cells. In one case, an air cell was present lateral to the optic nerve within the anterior clinoid process, and this was entered as soon as drilling had begun. This was packed with muscle, but later it gave rise to severe pneumocephalus and required a subsequent formal repair (see Fig **169 A–D**).

As the dura propria follows the optic nerve and ophthalmic artery into the optic canal, a layer of dura propria will be seen to cover these structures after the optic canal has been unroofed. This dura is opened with microscissors far enough anteriorly so that the optic nerve has been relieved of tension and the ophthalmic artery can be identified. The artery is usually on the inferolateral side of the nerve. The artery is followed proximally, and a plane developed between it and the aneurysm wall. The internal carotid artery may be followed a short distance into the cavernous sinus to identify the neck proximally.

The Carotid and Chiasmatic Cisterns

Arteries to the optic chiasm from the internal carotid artery and branches of the PcoA are most often stretched. Where these lie close to the neck of the aneurysm they are dissected free. This will further help to define the neck of aneurysm on its distal side.

Larger aneurysms may extend to the pituitary stalk and hypothalamus. These structures are identified so that they will not be injured during attempts to shrink the neck of the aneurysm with bipolar coagulation or during the dissection and removal of a large sac from the subchiasmatic region.

Elevation of a Suprachiasmatic Aneurysm

For those large suprachiasmatic aneurysms in which the fundus covers the neck of the aneurysm, the aneurysm itself or its arachnoidal fibers must be lifted and a plane developed between it and the internal carotid artery. With all structures in the vicinity of the aneurysm exposed, the fundus of the aneurysm can be separated from the carotid bifurcation area and from the anterior cerebral artery and gently nudged forward with a suction tip over a cottonoid sponge while adhesions are divided until the neck of the aneurysm is exposed. If the dome of the aneurysm is buried in the fronto-orbital gyrus, the pia around the fundus is coagulated and dissected in order that the fundus be mobilized with the adjacent pia.

Clip Application

As with all aneurysms, the size, shape, and physical characteristics of the neck will dictate the preparation of the neck required before a clip can be placed. Bipolar coagulation can help to create a suitable neck. A clip should generally be introduced over the internal carotid artery with the blades pointing medially and inferiorly.

In 1 case a silk ligature placed around the neck of an aneurysm was used to reduce the size of the neck so that a clip could be subsequently applied. 3 cases required temporary clips on the internal carotid artery to allow the removal of thrombus and atheroma before a clip could be satisfactorily applied to the aneurysmal neck. 2 cases required temporary occlusion of the cervical carotid artery to control bleeding.

The fundus of the aneurysm should be resected to decompress the adjacent optic nerve and to assure adequate clip placement. Enough aneurysm wall is left that a second clip can be applied if the first clip requires adjustment. The edges can be sealed with bipolar coagulation to allow additional manipulation of the clip, until the best position of clip is reached. Papaverine is applied to the arteries, and the sympathetic plexus stripped from the internal carotid artery. With good hemostasis and removal of blood from the subarachnoid space, the wound is closed in the usual manner.

Multiple and Bilateral Aneurysms

Of the 33 carotid-ophthalmic aneurysms, 17 had only a single aneurysm (left 7, right 10), whereas 16 (48.5%) had additional aneurysms (left 8, right 8) (Table **11a** and **b**). There were 7 bilateral ophthalmic aneurysms (21.2%) and in 5 of these cases (see Table **16**, Nos. 9, 10, 11, 18, and 22), both aneurysms could be clipped at the same pterional approach. In these cases after clipping the ruptured aneurysm, the contralateral aneurysm could be clipped through a small tunnel extending either under or over the opposite optic nerve. In some cases bipolar coagulation was first used to narrow the neck, but in all cases the opposite ophthalmic artery was preserved. In one case (No. 13) a small contralateral aneurysm was simply covered with muscle, and in another case (No. 12), neither aneurysm could be clipped because of a broad based, partially extradural configuration. In one other case (No. 17), an aneurysm was present on the right internal carotid artery bifurcation together with a symptomatic left internal carotid-ophthalmic artery aneurysm. Both could be clipped through a left pterional approach.

Thus in only 1 of the 33 cases, was it not possible to treat all additional aneurysms at one operation. This patient underwent clipping of a contralateral middle cerebral artery bifurcation aneurysm one year after the first operation (No. 9).

Table 11a Multiplicity of ophthalmic aneurysms

Side	No.	Size	Opp. Ophth.	Post. comm.	Ant. chor.	ICB	MCA	Ant. com.	Bas.	Total
Left	8	Micro	1 (m)	–	1 (m)	–	–	–	–	2
		Macro	4 (c)	2 (c)	–	2 (c)	2 (c)	–	–	10
Right	8	Micro	1 (m)	1 (m)	–	–	1 (m)	–	–	3
		Macro	1 (c)	2 (c)	–	1 (c)	1 (c)	1 (c)	1 (c)	7
	16		7	5	1	3	4	1	1	22

c = clipped, m = muscle wrapped

Unclipped Aneurysms

6 patients did not have their aneurysms clipped. One case, with a flat aneurysm, was treated early in the series with muscle wrapping and cyanoacrylate coating (No. 1). 2 additional cases were also wrapped and coated. One (No. 30) was a single flat aneurysm, and one (No. 12) had bilateral, symmetrical, asymptomatic (discovered during an angiographic investigation for headache), unruptured aneurysms (Fig 18A–B).

The flat configuration of these aneurysms did not allow clipping. These thin walled aneurysms were 2–3 mm wide, 4–6 mm long, but only 1–2 mm high, and partially within the cavernous sinus. Removal of the anterior clinoid process still did not permit the creation of an aneurysmal neck for clipping, without possible strangulation of the ICA. None of these patients subsequently suffered subarachnoid hemorrhage.

One patient (No. 7) was treated by carotid ligation

Table 11b Total numbers of ophthalmic aneurysms

		Total No.
Single aneurysm	17 patients	17
1 additional aneurysm	11 patients	22
2 additional aneurysms	4 patients	12
3 additional aneurysms	1 patient	4
	33	55

55 aneurysms were seen in 33 patients; 50 were clipped (c) 5 wrapped with muscle (m)

at her request, and an elderly lady (No. 29) with a giant, sclerotic, partially calcified and subtotally thrombosed aneurysm with symptoms relating to increased intracranial pressure underwent decompressive craniectomy only. The final patient (No. 33) ruptured her aneurysm following a superficial temporal-middle cerebral artery anastomosis. This case is described in detail on page 54.

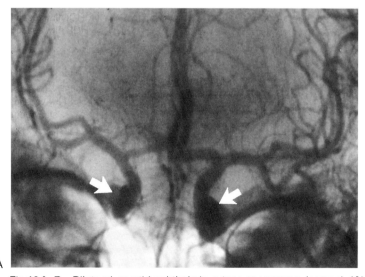
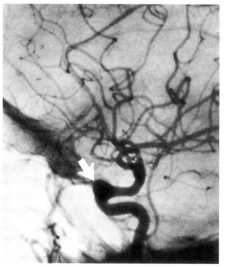

Fig 18A–B Bilateral carotid-ophthalmic artery aneurysms (arrows) (A). Though asymptomatic the family requested exploration which revealed both aneurysms to be partially intracavernous (arrow) as predicted on the right lateral carotid angiogram (B) (Case 12, Table 16).

Summary

In summary, the steps in the operative treatment of these ophthalmic aneurysms include the following:
1) (Pterional) craniotomy,
2) Opening the proximal Sylvian cistern,
3) Minimal retraction of the frontal lobe,
4) Preparation of the proximal internal carotid artery,
5) Identification of the posterior communicating and anterior choroidal arteries and their branches,
6) Inspection of the anterior cerebral-anterior communicating artery complex to evaluate collateral circulation in case of large and giant aneurysms,
7) Exposure of the ophthalmic artery,
8) Mobilization of the optic nerve, if necessary,
9) Identification of the pituitary stalk,
10) Identification of the hypophyseal and optic arteries,
11) Inspection of the opposite internal carotid-ophthalmic artery junction,
12) Clip application,
13) Puncture and collapse of fundus,
14) Fundus resection, sealing of cut edges by bipolar coagulation, staging re-application of the clip if necessary,
15) Final inspection,
16) Papaverine and local sympathectomy,
17) Routine hemostasis and closure.

Clinical Presentation and Operative Results

Several series of carotid-ophthalmic aneurysms have been reported. Mortality has been high with these aneurysms when subjected to intracranial operation. Drake and associates (1968b) reported a 50 per cent mortality in 6 cases, Kothandaram and co-workers (1971) a 20 per cent mortality in 10 cases, Thurel and co-authors (1974) a 50 per cent mortality in 6 cases, and Guidetti and La Torre (1975) a 19 per cent mortality in 32 cases. Kodama et al. (1979) reported a 16.7 per cent mortality in 6 cases and Benedetti et al. (1975) reported 6 cases, Sundt and Murphey (1969) 8 cases, and Almeida and associates (1976) 7 cases with no mortality.

Of the 33 patients undergoing operation for aneurysms of the proximal and medial wall of the internal carotid artery in the present series, 30 were female (90.9%) and only 3 male (Figs 19–23). Drake (1968) has reported that 85 per cent of these lesions occur in females, and overall 70.9 per cent of collected cases in the literature have occurred in women. In the present series, ages ranged from 28 to 71 with an average of 44 (Table 12). Presenting symptomatology is summarized in Table 13. Subarachnoid hemorrhage occurred in 23 of 33 cases (70 per cent), and 6 patients (18 per cent) presented with visual field deficit. One of these had associated pituitary dysfunction (No. 16,

Table 12 Age and sex of 33 ophthalmic artery aneurysm patients

Age	Male	Female	Total
21–30 years	–	3	3
31–40 years	1	7	8
41–50 years	2	8	10
51–60 years	–	7	7
61–70 years	–	4	4
over 70 years	–	1	1
	3	30	33

Table 13 Symptoms in 33 ophthalmic artery aneurysm patients

SAH	23 cases
Visual deficit	5 cases
Visual deficit and pituitary symptoms	1 case
Epileptic seizures	1 case
Papilledema	1 case
Headache	2 cases

Clinical Presentation and Operative Results

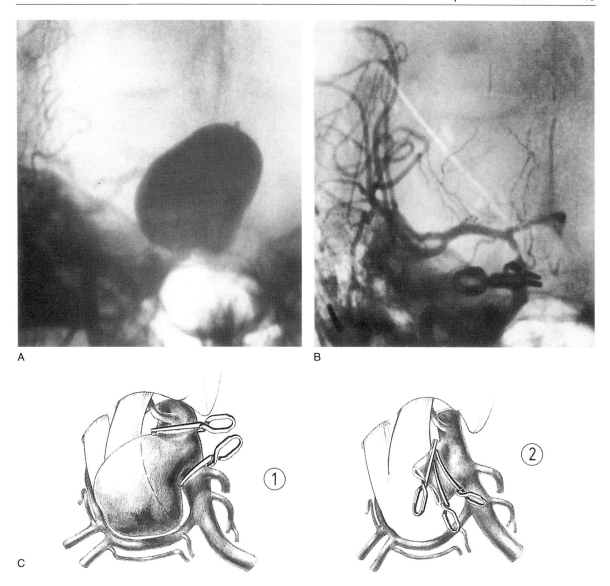

Fig 19 A–C Giant right carotid ophthalmic aneurysm (Case 24, Table 16) whose sclerotic broad base (A) could be clipped and resected after placing temporary clips on right internal carotid artery. The postoperative course was uneventful but angiography (B) was carried out on request of the husband. It showed some spasm, but the patient was asymptomatic and left hospital the same day. Schematic drawing (C) showing operative procedure with temporary clipping of internal carotid artery (1). The broad based sclerotic aneurysm could not be shrunk in order to apply a single clip. Successful occlusion was obtained using 3 clips (2).

Table 16). In the other 4 cases, headache was the chief complaint in 2, a third presented with deteriorating mental function and papilledema from a giant aneurysm (No. 29), and a fourth (No. 21) presented with seizures. This patient was found to have a parasagittal meningioma in conjunction with her aneurysm. 1 of the patients presenting with visual loss had an associated pituitary adenoma. None of the patients who presented with subarachnoid hemorrhage was found to have a visual deficit, although examination was limited in some by drowsiness and lack of cooperation (Table 16).

2 Internal Carotid Artery Aneurysms

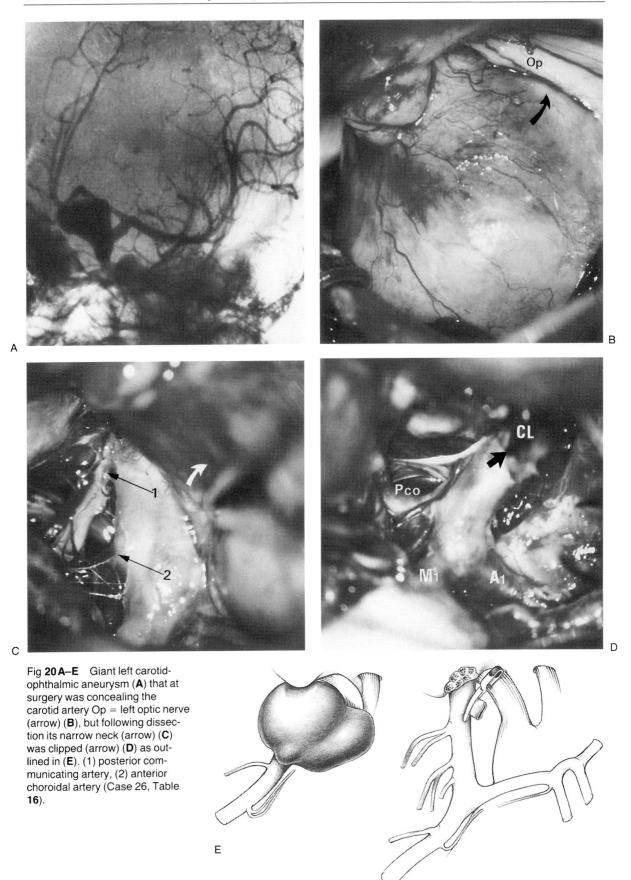

Fig 20 A–E Giant left carotid-ophthalmic aneurysm (A) that at surgery was concealing the carotid artery Op = left optic nerve (arrow) (B), but following dissection its narrow neck (arrow) (C) was clipped (arrow) (D) as outlined in (E). (1) posterior communicating artery, (2) anterior choroidal artery (Case 26, Table 16).

Clinical Presentation and Operative Results 51

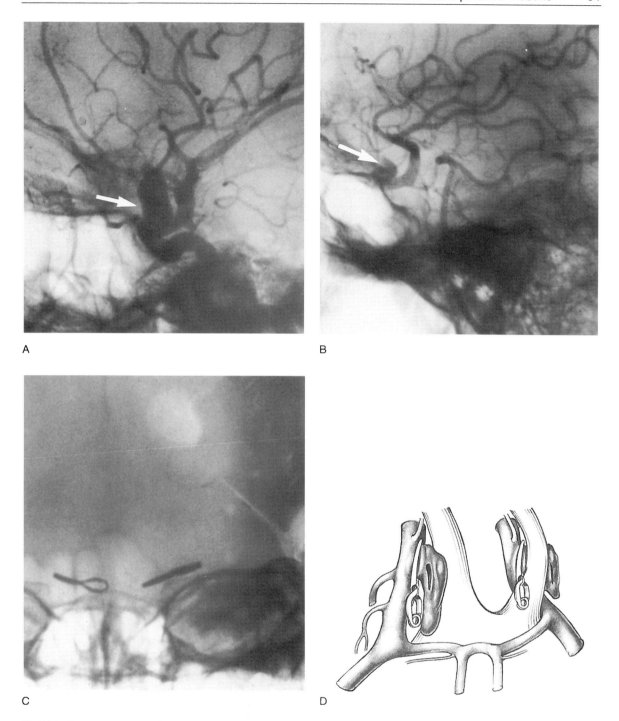

Fig 21 A–D   Larger ruptured left (arrow) (A) and smaller asymptomatic right (arrow) (B) carotid-ophthalmic aneurysms that were both clipped through a single left pterional approach (C) as outlined in (D).

52 2 Internal Carotid Artery Aneurysms

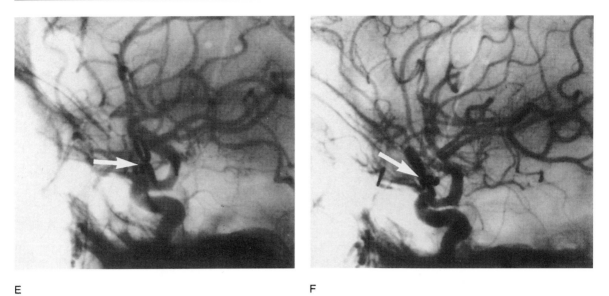

Fig 21 E–F Postoperative angiography confirmed complete obliteration of both aneurysms (arrows) (**E**-left and **F**-right) (Case 11, Table **16**).

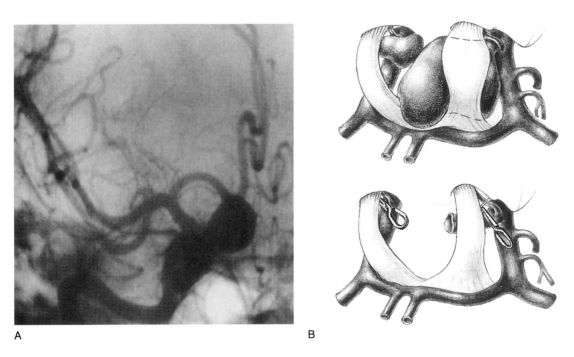

Fig **22 A–B** Large right carotid-ophthalmic aneurysm (**A**) that was clipped. A small hidden left ophthalmic aneurysm was found at surgery (**B**) and also clipped (Case 22, Table **16**).

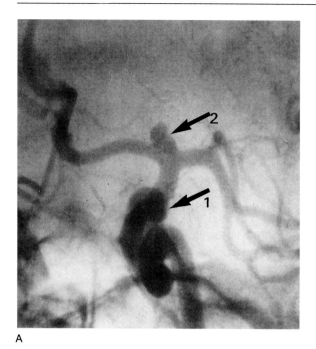
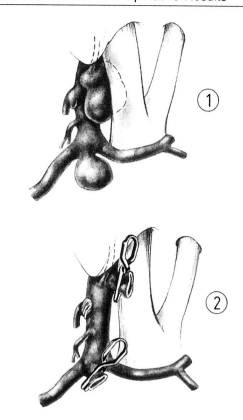

Fig 23A–B Ruptured left carotid-ophthalmic aneurysm (arrow 1) associated with an unruptured carotid bifurcation aneurysm (arrow 2) (**A**). Both were clipped at operation (**B**) (Case 17, Table **16**).

The preoperative condition is related to surgical results for these 33 patients in Table **14**. 18 (54.5%) of these patients were grades 0a, Ia, or IIa at the time of operation. All patients made a good recovery, including a patient in grade IV at the time of operation (Case 5, Table **16**) (see also page 298, Fig **147**).

In 2 patients, however, there was some additional deficit postoperatively. Fortunately, they went on to recover:

Ka., a 41 year old lady, presented in grade 0b with right sided visual loss. There was no history of subarachnoid hemorrhage. Angiography revealed a large subchiasmatic aneurysm on the right internal carotid artery. At operation on 22 April, 1970, the aneurysm could be clipped and excised.

Postoperatively the patient developed diabetes insipidus and amenorrhea, which recovered after several months. It was not clear whether stretching of the

Table 14 Surgical results related to preoperative grade

	Grade	Total	Good	Death
Unruptured	0a	2	2 (1)	–
	0b	8	7 (1)	1*
	Ia	8	8 (1)	–
	Ib	1	1°	–
	IIa	8	8	–
	IIb	1	1	–
	IIIa	3	3 (1)	–
	IIIb	1	1	–
	IV	1	1	–
		33	32 (4)	1

* only EIA, not direct surgical approach to aneurysm
( ) coagulation and muscle wrapping
° extracranial carotid ligature

hypophyseal arterial branches or direct injury to the hypothalamus led to the postoperative hormonal dysfunction. She was later symptom free.

Tu., a 40 year old woman, presented with decreased vision in the right eye and a right homonymous inferior temporal quadranopia, with no history of subarachnoid hemorrhage. Angiography demonstrated a suprachiasmatic carotid-ophthalmic aneurysm which appeared subtotally thrombosed because both A_1 segments were elevated. At operation the aneurysm was found to be associated with a large chromophobe adenoma. While the right optic nerve was compressed between the lesions, the primary injury seemed to be to the right optic tract where a deep groove had been excavated by the anterior cerebral artery crossing over the tumor. Postoperatively, the visual field loss had extended to an almost complete right homonymous hemianopia, but when examined 6 months later, visual fields had returned to their preoperative state. She has returned to her previous profession (see Vol. I, Fig **246A–C**).

There was one death in this series. This patient had an extracranial-intracranial bypass procedure which was uneventful, but in the postoperative period ruptured her aneurysm. No direct attack on the aneurysm had been undertaken:

Ma., a 50 year old woman, noted a progressive loss of vision in the right eye over 18 months prior to admission. Vision had become rapidly impaired in the last four weeks. CT scan in Dec 76 was unremarkable, but angiography at the time of admission showed a giant aneurysm of the right internal carotid-ophthalmic artery, which appeared to extend into the cavernous sinus. The left A_1 segment was hypoplastic, and both A_1's filled only from the right side. The right carotid artery also filled the right posterior cerebral artery. Because collateral circulation was so poor into the right internal carotid system, it was decided to first perform a right superficial temporal-middle cerebral artery anastomosis, in case the right internal carotid artery was lost at operation. This was done without incident on 15 June, 1977, but 24 hours after operation she had a grand mal seizure and lapsed into coma. Reexploration of the anastomosis site showed only edema. At autopsy it was seen that the aneurysm had ruptured. It seems an inescapable conclusion that the operation somehow led to rupture of the aneurysm. With such a case in the future, a clamp should be placed on the internal carotid artery immediately following the extracranial-intracranial anastomosis, or the aneurysm should be clipped at the same sitting.

Timing and Results

23 of the 33 patients in this group of patients presented with subarachnoid hemorrhage. Of these 23, 8 underwent surgical intervention one month or longer after the hemorrhage, while the remaining 14 cases were operated upon during the first month after rupture. Only 1 patient had surgery during the first week. Good results were obtained in all of these patients, irrespective of the surgical timing (Table **15**).

Table 15 Timing of surgery and results in 23 patients with ruptured aneurysm of the ophthalmic artery

	\multicolumn{7}{c	}{Good}	
	Ia	Ib	IIa	IIb	IIIa	IIIb	IV	
1–3 d	–	–	–	–	–	–	–	
4–7 d	–	–	–	–	–	–	1	
1–2 w	–	–	1	–	3	1	–	
2–4 w	5	–	4	–	–	–	–	
1–3 m	2	–	2	1	–	–	–	
> 3 m	1	1	1	–	–	–	–	
	8	1	8	1	3	1	1	= 23

Summary

Of 33 patients, 32 have enjoyed complete recovery, while 1 patient who underwent only a microvascular bypass procedure died before a definitive operation could be carried out. None of the 31 patients living is known to have had a recurrent hemorrhage in a period from 1 to 13 years including 3 cases treated with muscle wrapping only and one patient treated by cervical carotid artery ligation, but the patient (No. 18) with bilateral ophthalmic and second additional aneurysm on the posterior communicating artery suffered a second hemorrhage 4 years later. Further information was not available (see Table **16**).

In 27 of 33 patients the aneurysms were clipped together with 17 additional aneurysms (7 contralateral ophthalmic artery aneurysms). In 4 cases the aneurysm was only wrapped with muscle, in 1 case a ligature was performed and 1 patient underwent an extra-intracranial anastomosis and died before carotid ligation could be performed (Case 33, Table **16**).

2 Internal Carotid Artery Aneurysms

Table 16 Clinical details, operative findings and outcome in ophthalmic artery aneurysm cases

No.	Age	Sex	Signs and symptoms	Aneurysm site	Size	Assoc. aneurysms	Grade	Interval	Surgery	Deficit	Result
1	40	F	SAH	L., supraoptic	Small	R. MCA (small)	IIIa	10 d	Muscle	1967 —	Good
2	53	F	SAH	R., supraoptic	Medium	—	IIa	4 w	Clip	1968 —	Good
3	42	M	SAH	R., supraoptic	Medium	—	Ia	6 w	Clip	1970 —	Good
4	41	F	Headache, right nasal field decrease	R., global	Large	—	0b	—	Clip	1970 Transient diabetes insipidus	Good
5	67	F	SAH, Hpr.r., aphasia i.c.H. l. frontal	L. supraoptic	Giant	—	IV	3 d	Clip	1971 Recovery	Good
6	42	M	SAH	R., suboptic	Medium	—	IIa	6 w	Clip	1971 —	Good
7	52	F	SAH, Hpr. l. mild	R., suboptic	Medium	—	IIa	1 y	Lig. ICA, r.	1972 Recovery	Good
8	43	F	SAH	R., suboptic	Medium	AcoA (medium)	Ia	3 w	Cl/Cl	1973 —	Good
9	39	F	SAH, Hpr.r., aphasia i.c.H. l. frontal	L., supraoptic	Medium (bi)	R. ophth. supraopt. (medium) L. MCA, L.AchoA (micro)	IIIa	11 d	Cl/Cl/Cl/M	1973 Transient III-palsy	Good
10	69	F	SAH	R., suboptic	Medium (bi)	L. ophth. subopt. (medium) R. PcoA (medium)	IIa	3 w	Cl/Cl/Cl	1973 —	Good
11	39	F	SAH 2 ×	L. supraopt.	Medium (bi)	R. ophth. supraopt. (medium)	IIa	4 w	Cl/Cl	1974 —	Good
12	52	F	Headache	R. superior part. intracavern.	Small (bi)	L. ophth. superior (micro)	0a	—	Muscle	1974 —	Good
13	47	F	SAH	L., suboptic	Medium (bi)	R. ophth. superior (micro)	Ia	3 m	Cl/Muscle	1975 —	Good
14	32	F	SAH, frontal hemat.	R., suboptic	Medium	—	IIIa	10 d	Clip	1975 Recovery	Good
15	29	F	SAH, diplopia	R., suboptic	Medium	—	Ia	28 d	Clip	1975 —	Good
16	40	F	Vision decrease r., r. inferior temp. defect	R., supraoptic	Medium	Chromophobe adenoma	0b	—	Cl/removal of tumor	1975 Recovery	Good
17	53	F	SAH	L., supraoptic	Medium	R. IC-Bifurcation	IIa	24 d	Cl/Cl	1976 —	Good
18	35	F	SAH 2 ×	R. supraoptic	Medium (bi)	L. ophth. subopt. (medium) R. PcoA	Ia	6 w	Cl/Cl/M	1976 —	Good Recurrent SAH 1980
19	45	F	SAH 3 ×, l. Hpr. mild right VI-palsy	R., suboptic	Medium	—	IIb	2 w	Clip	1976 Recovery	Good

20	29	F	SAH, 3 ×, right Hpr.	L., suboptic	Medium	–	IIIb	2 w	Clip	1976 Recovery	Good
21	45	F	Epilepsy, r. Hpr.	L., supraoptic	Medium	L. IC-Bifurcation L. frontal meningioma	0b	–	Cl/Cl/removal of tumor	1976 Recovery	Good
22	45	M	SAH	R., suboptic	Medium (bi)	L. ophth. suboptic (medium)	Ia	3 w	Cl/Cl	1976 –	Good
23	52	F	Headache	L., suboptic	Medium	L. IC-Bi, L. PcoA	0a	–	Cl/Cl/Cl	1976 –	Good
24	37	F	R. visual defect (inferior temporal)	R., global	Giant	–	0b	–	Clip	1976 Recovery	Good
25	28	F	SAH	L., supraoptic	Medium	L. MCA R. MCA	IIa	4 w	Cl/Cl 2nd expl. Cl	1976 –	Good
26	65	F	L. amblyopia bitemp. hemianop.	L., global	Giant	–	0b	–	Clip	1976 Recovery	Good
27	62	F	SAH	L., suboptic	Large	L. PcoA	Ia	3 w	Cl/Cl	1977 –	Good
28	60	F	L. visual defect (nasal)	L., global (thrombosed)	Large	–	0b	–	Clip, removal of aneurysm	1977 Recovery	Good
29	71	F	Headache, PE, CT = giant tumor left frontal	L., supraoptic	Giant	–	0b	–	inoperable, de- compr. bone flap, Muscle	1977 Recovery	Good Died 4 years later
30	50	F	SAH	L., superior partially intracav.	Medium	–	Ia	3 w	Muscle	1978 –	Good
31	49	F	SAH	R., suboptic	Medium	R. PcoA	IIa	2 w	Cl/Cl	1978 –	Good
32	55	F	SAH, CT shows 2 aneurysms	R., supraoptic	Medium	Basil.-Bi.	IIa	7 w	Cl/Muscle	1978 –	Good
33	50	F	R. amblyopia, Q.A. nasal right. CT = large aneurysm	R., global no collaterals to the right ICA	Large	–	0b	–	EI anastomosis June 15, 1977 No expl. of aneurysm	June 17, 1977 SAH, i.c.H., coma June 20, 1977	Death

(bi) = bilateral

Distal Medial Wall Aneurysms

Anatomical Relationships

2 patients presented with ruptured aneurysms arising from the medial wall of the internal carotid artery, slightly proximal to the bifurcation. The smaller of these was buried in the optic tract while the larger was subchiasmatic and directed toward the pituitary stalk. Both aneurysms were on the right side and both occurred in women. The anterior cerebral artery, recurrent artery of Heubner, pituitary stalk and optic tract are the principle anatomical structures adjacent to these aneurysms. Aneurysms in such a location have not been previously published to our knowledge.

Operative Technique

Careful dissection should avoid injury especially to the optic tract, pituitary stalk, and recurrent artery of Heubner, which may be concealed by the aneurysm.

Clinical Presentation and Operative Results

As only 2 aneurysms occurred at this location, these cases will be presented:

Le., S., a 64 year old woman, fell striking her head on 6 November 1968. On 12 November, 1968, she suffered a subarachnoid hemorrhage and presented drowsy and disorientated. Visual fields were thought to be intact. Angiography showed an aneurysm of the right internal carotid artery, which was proximal to the bifurcation. At operation on 11 December, 1969, the distal medial wall aneurysm was clipped. The fundus was buried in the right optic tract. She did well postoperatively.

Scha., a 42 year old lady, suffered a subarachnoid hemorrhage on 1 August, 1972, and was somnolent with meningism. Rebleeding occurred on 18 August, 1972, with loss of consciousness, followed by some improvement. Angiography showed an aneurysm of the distal medial wall of the right internal carotid artery. There was poor collateral circulation from the left side. At operation on 23 August, 1972, the aneurysm was identified by opening the Sylvian cistern and following the middle cerebral artery proximal to the internal carotid artery bifurcation. The aneurysm was extremely thin

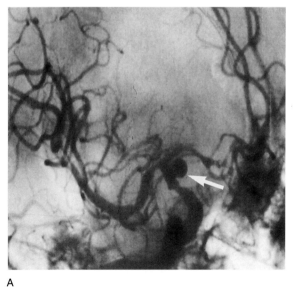

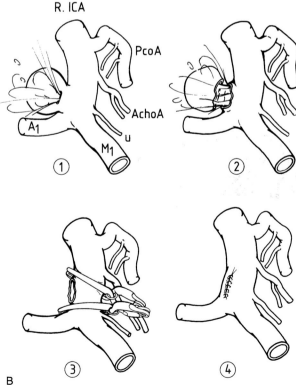

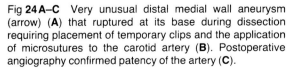

Fig 24 A–C Very unusual distal medial wall aneurysm (arrow) (**A**) that ruptured at its base during dissection requiring placement of temporary clips and the application of microsutures to the carotid artery (**B**). Postoperative angiography confirmed patency of the artery (**C**).

Fig. 24 C ▶

walled, and ruptured at the base during dissection. Temporary clips were applied to the internal carotid artery placing one clip just distal to the origin of the posterior communicating artery and one clip just proximal to the origin of the anterior choroidal artery. The right internal carotid was then repaired with interrupted microsutures, the first case in which this had been done. The patient made a good recovery (Fig **24A–C**). See also Fig **5A–D**, p. 6, Vol. II.

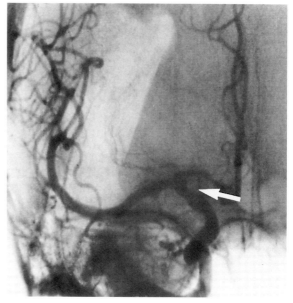

C

Aneurysms of Superior Wall of Internal Carotid Artery

Anatomical Relationships

One patient presented with an unruptured aneurysm arising entirely from the superior wall of the internal carotid artery without relation to any arterial branch.

Operative Technique

Aneurysms in this location project towards the operator as he approaches the carotid artery. This should be remembered when first retracting the frontal lobe to gain access to the artery as the aneurysm may be ruptured inadvertently during this maneuver.

Clinical Presentation and Operative Results

The one patient (29 year old female) in this series presented not only with a large superior wall aneurysm, but also with a basilar bifurcation aneurysm and an occipital arteriovenous malformation. Both aneurysms were clipped through a right sided pterional approach with good results. The AVM will be removed later (see Vol. I, Fig **241A–C**).

Inferior Wall Aneurysms of the Internal Carotid Artery

Anatomical Relationships

A special group of aneurysms include those that arise from the inferior wall of the internal carotid artery and project inferiorly into the carotid and interpeduncular cisterns (see Table **19**). These aneurysms have not been adequately described in the medical literature. The lesions are large, have an ill-defined (7 cases) or absent neck, and may be fusiform, often including more than half the circumference of the internal carotid artery (14 cases). They frequently show significant sclerosis with calcification and are often partially to subtotally thrombosed. It is not clear whether these aneurysms are typical saccular aneurysms, that have become large, or whether they represent a form of arteriosclerotic aneurysm or ectasia of the internal carotid artery, as is occasionally seen in the cervical carotid and basilar arteries (see Fig **57B**).

The origins of the posterior communicating and anterior choroidal arteries may be included within the neck. These arteries usually course laterally over the fundus of the aneurysm and then along its inferior surface although in 2 cases the arteries were displaced medially and in another 2 cases, the posterior communicating artery coursed lateral to the aneurysm with the anterior choroidal artery medial, so that the internal carotid artery was twisted over the aneurysm.

These aneurysms present a typical angiographic picture: In the anteroposterior view they are directed medially and appear to be internal carotid-ophthalmic artery or carotid bifurcation aneurysms, while in the lateral view they are directed posteriorly and appear to arise from the internal carotid-posterior communicating artery.

21 such cases were seen in the present series; 14 arose from the left internal carotid artery and 7 from the right.

Multiplicity

In only 1 case was there an additional aneurysm of the contralateral PcoA. Since concluding this series for publication, 5 additional aneurysms have been seen at this location, 2 associated with unruptured anterior communicating artery aneurysms and 1 with a contralateral anterior choroidal artery aneurysm. In addition, 1 patient with a ruptured aneurysm of the right MCA had co- incidentally a large inferior aneurysm of the right ICA, which was clipped (see Fig **77A–G**, p. 143).

Operative Technique

Because of the variability of presentation of these aneurysms, it is not possible to give a standard approach to operation as has been given for the more frequent internal carotid artery aneurysms. Several methods were used in the 21 cases which can be grouped into 6 basic procedures:

1) *Cervical carotid artery ligation.* 2 patients (Nos. 10 and 11) were treated by ligation of the cervical internal carotid artery, as they refused craniotomy. Carotid ligation was well tolerated by each patient, and as both have remained free of symptoms, no further operations have been undertaken.
2) *Extracranial-intracranial trapping.* One patient (No. 15) was treated by ligation of the internal carotid artery in the neck, and clipping of the intracranial internal carotid artery proximal to the posterior communicating artery.
3) *Intracranial internal carotid artery trapping.* In 1 patient (No. 14), the aneurysm ruptured during craniotomy. Bleeding could only be controlled by placing a clip above and below the aneurysm on the internal carotid artery. In another case in 1981 the intracranial trapping of ICA was achieved without any deficit as in this case the collateral supply had been well developed (see Fig **28**).
4) *Extra-intracranial anastomosis with carotid ligation or clipping.* 2 patients (Nos. 12 and 13) underwent an extracranial-middle cerebral branch anastomosis (one occipital and one superficial temporal artery) before in 1 case definitive attack on the aneurysm.
5) *Muscle wrapping.* 2 aneurysms (Nos. 2 and 6) were covered with muscle. These aneurysms were, in fact, diffuse fusiform dilatations of the entire supraclinoid internal carotid artery. They were sclerotic and involved the origins of the posterior communicating and anterior choroidal arteries. Application of a clip was not possible.
6) *Creation of a neck and clipping of aneurysm.* In 14 of the 21 cases a clip could be applied to the aneurysm although only with considerable difficulty. Following exposure of the aneurysm through a standard pterional craniotomy, the

aneurysm was exposed in the carotid cistern. Dissection of the posterior communicating and anterior choroidal arteries and their branches is extremely tedious and demanding. Perforating branches of the posterior communicating artery are especially likely to be involved with the aneurysm when the fundus extends posteriorly and inferiorly toward the basilar bifurcation.

In 5 cases, the aneurysm could be shrivelled with bipolar coagulation, and a large, curved clip applied. In 2 other cases, the sac of the aneurysm was narrowed with a ligature and then a large clip applied (Nos. 1 and 8). Often there was not a true neck for clipping and the application of a large, curved clip primarily served to fashion an internal carotid artery from the aneurysm sac. In the remaining 5 cases, the aneurysm was too large to be manipulated, and it was necessary to apply temporary clips above and below the aneurysm, aspirate the contents of the aneurysm, and shrink it with bipolar coagulation before a final large, curved clip could be applied and the temporary clips removed. The large size of these aneurysms may make it difficult to include the aneurysm initially within a clip without strangulating the internal carotid artery (Figs **25–29**).

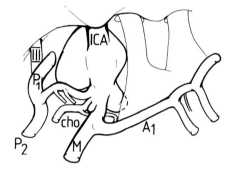

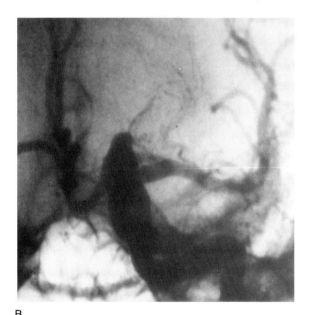

Fig **25A–C** Schematic illustration of an inferior wall aneurysm of the left internal carotid artery (**A**). Aneurysms that on AP angiography (**B**) appear to arise from either the ophthalmic or the carotid bifurcation but on lateral films (**C**) seem to come from the posterior communicating artery (Case 20, Table **19**).

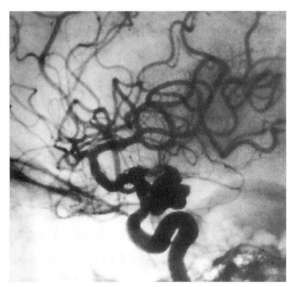

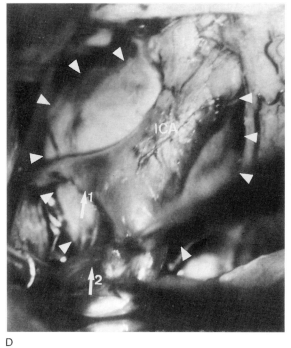
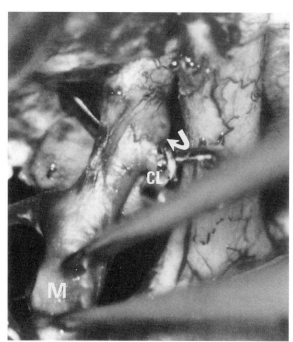

D

E

Fig 25 D–F Exploration showed that the aneurysm actually arose from the inferior wall of the internal carotid artery (arrow heads). Posterior communicating artery (arrow 1), anterior communicating artery (arrow 2) (**D**). Though broad based a neck can occasionally be created (arrow) (**E**) and a clip applied as outlined in (**F**). The left posterior communicating artery and anterior communicating artery could be readily dissected and preserved. The small aneurysm at the origin of the anterior choroidal artery was coagulated and wrapped as shown diagrammatically in (**F**).

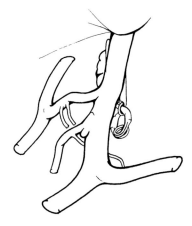

F

Operative Technique 63

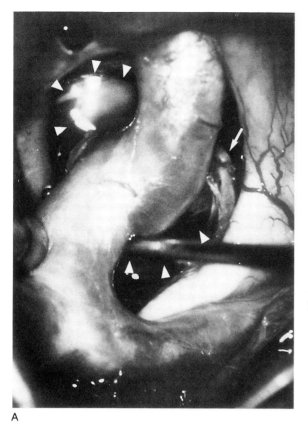

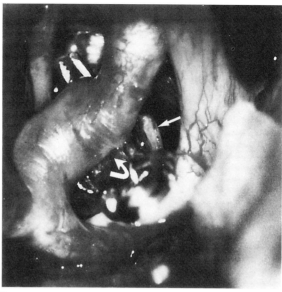

Fig 26 A–C Operative photographs of an inferior wall aneurysm of the left internal carotid artery (arrow heads) that was pushing the posterior communicating artery and its branches medially toward the optic nerve (arrow) as seen before (**A**) and after (**B**) clipping, PcoA (straight arrow), Clip (curved arrow) (Case 14, Table **19**).

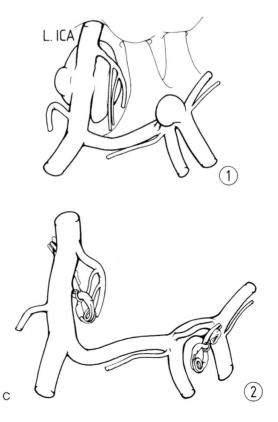

C Schematic illustration with incidental aneurysm of the anterior communicating artery. (1) before, (2) after clipping of both aneurysms.

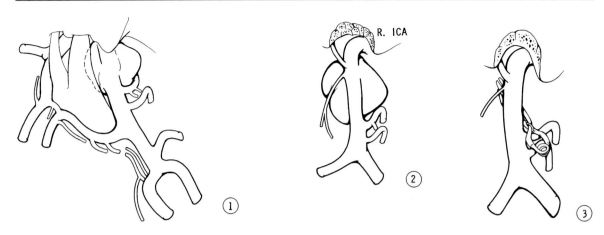

Fig 27A Inferior wall aneurysm of the right internal carotid artery. The posterior communicating artery is displaced medially. The anterior clinoid process had to be drilled away to dissect the proximal part of aneurysm (2). Thereafter a clip could be applied (3) (Case 18, Table **19**).

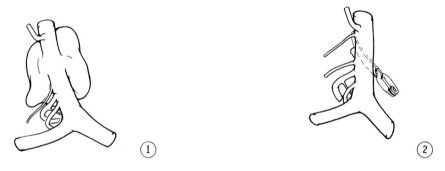

Fig 27B Inferior wall aneurysm of the right internal carotid artery with a well shaped neck, which could be clipped directly (Case 19, Table **19**).

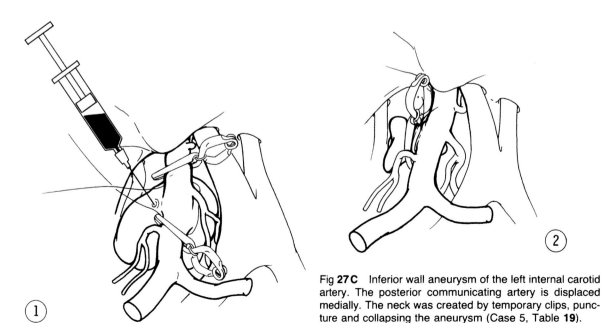

Fig 27C Inferior wall aneurysm of the left internal carotid artery. The posterior communicating artery is displaced medially. The neck was created by temporary clips, puncture and collapsing the aneurysm (Case 5, Table **19**).

Operative Technique 65

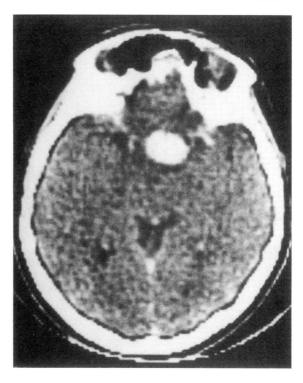

Fig 28A The origin of this large aneurysm could not be defined by CT scan (Case 15, Table 19).

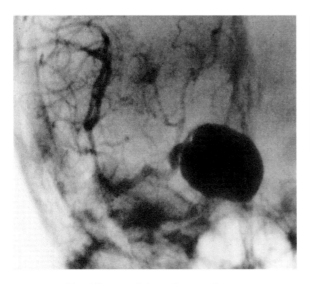

Fig 28B The AP view of the right carotid angiogram was suspicious of an ophthalmic aneurysm.

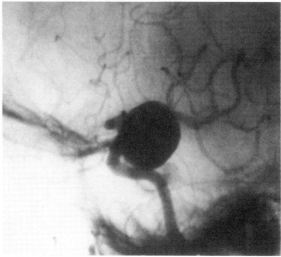

Fig 28C The lateral view, however, was suspicious of an aneurysm of the posterior communicating artery or at the carotid bifurcation.

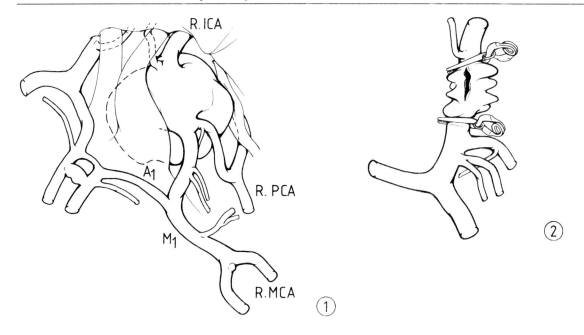

Fig 28 D Exploration showed an inferior wall aneurysm with a broad base (1), which did not allow the creation of a neck by any method. A trapping technique was therefore used, the right ophthalmic and posterior communicating arteries saved, and the internal carotid sacrificed, knowing that there was a sufficient collateral from the left side (2).

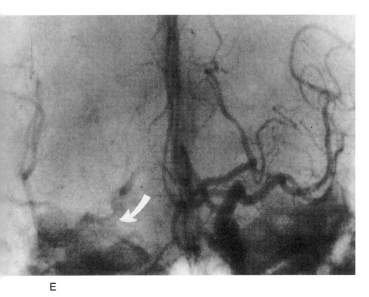

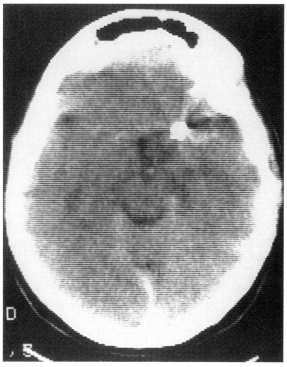

Fig 28 E–F Left sided carotid angiogram shows good filling of the right anterior and middle cerebral arteries (arrow). The postoperative course was uneventful. The postoperative CT does not show any infarction (F).

Operative Technique 67

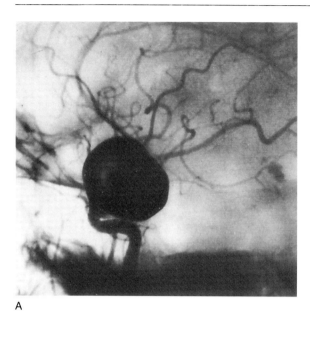

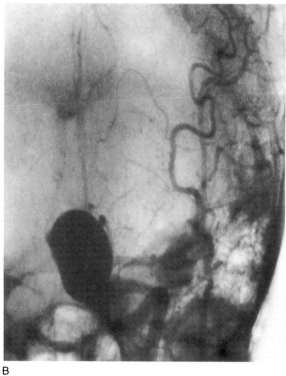

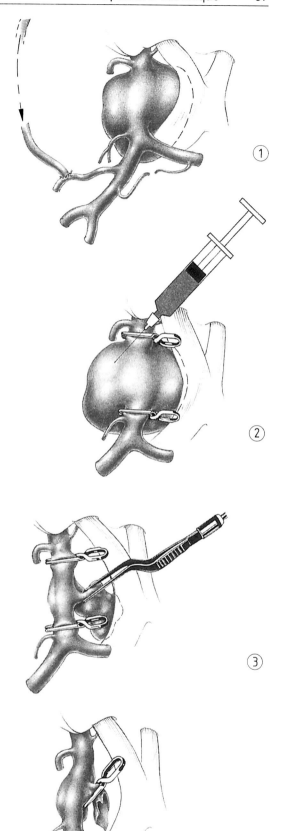

Fig 29 A–C Giant left inferior wall aneurysm of the internal carotid artery (**A** and **B**) presenting with chiasmal compression and pituitary insufficiency in a patient with poor collateral flow from the right. The EC-IC bypass did not succeed (1); the patient became hemiplegic and aphasic following the clipping of the aneurysm (**C**) and remained for years in poor condition (Case 13, Table **19**). During surgery temporary clips had been applied for 2 min while puncturing the aneurysm sac (2). A neck was then created using bipolar coagulation (3) followed by application of a final clip (4).

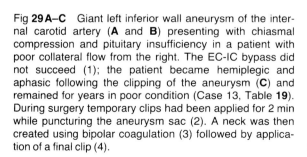

Clinical Presentation and Operative Results

Of the 21 cases with aneurysms at this location, 11 were men and 10 were women. Ages ranged from 41 to 70 (Table **17**). 17 patients (81 per cent) presented with subarachnoid hemorrhage, 1 of these associated with an oculomotor palsy, 1 associated with decreased visual acuity, and 1 associated with both. One patient presented with blindness in the left eye and decreased visual acuity in the right eye from a large left sided aneurysm, and another patient presented with a classical lateral chiasmal syndrome – decreased visual acuity on the right and a left homonymous insufficiency. One patient exhibited rather sudden onset of dementia and a left oculomotor palsy. She was thought to have ruptured her aneurysm with a resultant left frontal intracerebral hematoma, but was found at operation to have a left frontal reticulum cell sarcoma. The aneurysm was incidental in this case. A final case presented with rather bizarre paresthesias which were possibly transient ischemic attacks caused by embolization from her aneurysm (No. 17). These cases are summarized in Table **21**.

Surgical results are related to preoperative grade in Table **18**. A good result was achieved in 18 patients (85.7%). 2 patients were treated by cervical carotid artery ligation only, 2 by wrapping with muscle, and 12 by aneurysm clipping (Table **20**). 2 patients experienced protracted postoperative courses before going on to full recovery (cases Nos. 12 and 15).

There was one poor result (case No. 13). This man had undergone an extracranial-intracranial anastomosis performed prior to his giant aneurysm operation. He was operated on in condition 0b, but unfortunately the aneurysm bled at the beginning of the craniotomy.

At craniotomy the dura was very tense, it was seen that the aneurysm had ruptured and was actively bleeding. The giant aneurysm could not be rapidly dissected free, so clamps were placed on the internal carotid artery above the anterior choroidal artery. The aneurysm was opened and thrombosed hematoma removed. The sac was freed from surrounding structures and shrunk with bipolar coagulation. The neck of the aneurysm could then be clipped with 2 clips and the temporary clips removed. Postoperatively the patient showed a right hemiparesis, aphasia, and a severe psychoorganic syndrome. He remained severely disabled.

2 patients died (9.5 per cent). The first patient (No. 1) died of cerebral infarction and it was felt that the internal carotid, posterior communicating, and anterior choroidal arteries had been compromised by ligating the aneurysm. The second patient sustained rupture of the aneurysm during craniotomy, and trapping of the lesion did not prevent her death (No. 4).

In 2 cases (Nos. 4 and 13), 1 with a poor result and 1 who died, the aneurysm ruptured during or just prior to the craniotomy. In both these cases the cervical carotid arteries had been exposed in the neck and manipulated. Whether this contributed to the rupture of the aneurysms one cannot say, but it seems possible (Table **19**).

Table 17 Age and sex of 21 patients with aneurysms of the inferior wall of the internal carotid artery

Age	Male	Female	Total	
41–50 years	5	1	6	(28.6%)
51–60 years	2	7	9	(42.9%)
61–70 years	4	2	6	(28.6%)
	11 (52.4%)	10 (47.6%)	21	

Table 18 Surgical results related to preoperative grade

Grade	Total No.	Good	Poor	Death
0a	1	1	–	–
0b	3	2	1	–
Ia	6	6 (2 m) (2 lig)	–	–
IIa	6	6	–	–
IIb	2	2	–	–
IIIa	1	–	–	1
IIIb	2	1	–	1
	21	18	1	2

Table 19 Inferior wall internal carotid artery aneurysm patients

Patient	Year	Age	Sex	SAH	Signs	Site	Time	Grade	Operation	Shape	Size	Remarks	Result
1. St	1967	68	F	1	–	Right	2 w	IIIa	Lig. + clip	F	Large	Sclerotic aneurysm, ICA strangulated by ligature	Dead
2. Re	1969	56	F	1	–	Right	3 w	Ia	Muscle	F	Medium	Sclerotic	Good
3. Schü	1969	59	F	1	–	Left	4 m	Ia	Clip	S	Large	Temporary clips, aspiration	Good
4. Yüs	1969	50	F	3	Aphasia Hpl. R.	Left	10d	IIIb	Intracranial trapping	F	Large	Ruptured during craniotomy	Dead
5. Ce	1970	45	M	1	L. CN III palsy	Left	2m	Ia	Clip	S	Medium	Temporary clips, aspiration	Good
6. Te	1971	41	M	1	–	Left	4 w	Ia	Muscle	F	Large		Good
7. Un	1972	64	M	2	R. Hemip. l. CN III palsy	Left	2 w	IIIb	Clip	F	Large	Temporary clips, aspiration, shunt	Good
8. Tü	1972	54	M	2	R. Hemip. L. CN III palsy, POS	Left	5 m	IIb	Lig. + clip	F	Medium	Ruptured during operation	Good
9. Ob	1972	65	M	1	–	Left	7 d	IIa	Clip	S	Medium	Sclerotic, shunt	Good
10. Ka	1972	51	F	1	R. CN III palsy	Right	1 y	Ia	Cerv. r. ICA ligation	S	Medium	Pt. refused craniotomy	Good
11. Bo	1972	66	M	1	–	Left	2 m	Ia	Cerv. l. ICA ligation	S	Medium	Pt. refused craniotomy	Good
12. Bi	1973	50	M	1	Dec. vis. acuity l. l. CN III paresis r. hpr. POS	Left	7 m	IIb	Muscle + EIA + Cerv. l. ICA ligation 1976	F	Giant	90% thrombosed, sclerotic, shunt 1974 – recovery from chiasm sympt.	Good
13. Gu	1973	42	M	–	Blind l. Dec. VA r. Pit. Insuff.	Left	–	Ob	EIA Clip	F	Giant	Sclerotic, temporary clips to ICA, Hemiplegia, Aphasia	Poor
14. Mi	1974	60	F	1	–	Left	2 w	IIa	Clip	S	Medium		Good
15. Pr	1976	56	F	–	Chiasm Syn. Right pit. insuff.	Right	1 y	Ob	Trapping	F	Giant	Part. cavern., subtot. thromb., post-op. transient l. hpr.	Good
16. Al	1976	70	F	–	POS l. CN III palsy	Left	–	Ob	Clip	S	Medium	Reticulum cell sarcoma of left frontal lobe	Good
17. Gi	1977	51	F	–	TIA's *r. PcoA	Left	–	OA	Clip Muscle	F	Medium	Sclerotic aneurysm	Good
18. Yür	1979	54	M	1		Right	3 w	IIa	Clip	F	Large	Sclerotic	Good
19. Schü	1979	52	F	1		Right	2 w	IIa	Clip	F	Medium		Good
20. He	1979	48	M	1		Left	2 w	IIa	Clip	F	Medium	Sclerotic	Good
21. Fr	1979	67	M	1		Right	3 w	IIa	Clip	F	Medium		Good

* = additional aneurysms
F = fusiform
S = saccular
POS = psychoorganic syndrome

Table 20 Type of surgery and results – internal carotid artery aneurysms

	Results				Total
	Good	Fair	Poor	Death	
Extracranial ligature ICA	2	–	–	–	2
Extracranial ligature ICA + EIA + Muscle	1	–	–	–	1
Trapping extra-intracranial	1**	–	–	–	1
Trapping intracranial (also p.co + ant.ch.)	–	–	–	1*	1
Clip + EIA	–	–	1***	–	1
Clip	12	–	–	1****	13
Muscle wrapping	2	–	–	–	2
	18	–	1	2	21

* No. 4
** No. 15
*** No. 13
**** No. 1

Table 21 Timing and results (17 cases with SAH) – internal carotid artery aneurysms

	Good				Death		
	Ia	IIa	IIb	IIIb	IIIa	IIIb	
0–3 d	–	–	–	–	–	–	
3–8 d	–	1	–	–	–	–	
1–2 w	–	1	–	1	1	1	
2–4 w	1	4	–	–	–	–	
1–3 m	3	–	–	–	–	–	
> 3 m	2	–	2	–	–	–	
	6	6	2	1	1	1	= 17

Timing and Results

17 of the 21 patients in this group presented with subarachnoid hemorrhage. Of these 17, seven underwent surgical intervention one month or longer after the hemorrhage, while the remainder were operated upon during the first month (4 cases after 2 weeks, 5 cases after 3 weeks) after rupture. Only 1 patient had surgery during the first week. Good results were not related to timing, but to the preoperative condition of the patient and operative difficulties (Table 21).

Summary

In conclusion, aneurysms arising from the inferior wall of the internal carotid artery present a considerable challenge. In this series only 14 of 21 aneurysms could be properly clipped, and of these there was 1 death and 1 poor result. The aneurysms differ from the typical internal carotid artery aneurysm in being large, sclerotic, and particularly in involving a large portion of the circumference of the artery. Each case must be individually evaluated, and treatment tailored to each particular lesion.

Carotid-Posterior Communicating Aneurysms

Anatomical Relationships

Laterality and Multiplicity

At, or near, the origin of the posterior communicating artery is the most common site of aneurysm formation on the internal carotid artery. There were 173 patients in the present series with aneurysms at this location accounting for 54.2 per cent of aneurysms on the internal carotid artery and (17 per cent) of all aneurysms in the series. Suzuki (1979) showed 213 posterior communicating artery aneurysms in 1000 cases for an incidence of 21.3%. The aneurysms arose from the right internal carotid artery in 100 cases (58%) and from the left in 73 (42%), unlike observations from Suzuki, who saw 52.6% on the left and 47.4% on the right. Only 4 aneurysms in this location were large (15–25 mm) and there were no giant aneurysms (over 25 mm). This suggests that expanding aneurysms at this site generally fail to reach a large size owing to the early appearance of oculomotor symptoms.

Single aneurysms were present in 122 patients while 51 (29.5%) had other additional aneurysms. Of these 97 additional aneurysms, 43 were large enough for clipping, while 54 of the additional aneurysms were too small for clipping and were merely coagulated and covered with muscle. Thus in this group of 173 patients there were a total of 270 aneurysms of which 209 were clipped. The distribution of multiple aneurysms is shown in Table 22a and b.

In addition, 47 patients with ruptured aneurysms at other locations had, in 17 cases, microaneurysms on the PcoA, which have been coagulated and in 30 cases larger asymptomatic aneurysms of the PcoA, which have been clipped (see Table 129).

General Remarks

The dissection and clipping of an aneurysm along the lateral wall of the ICA at the origin of the PcoA and the AchoA can be performed from two very different approaches:

1) *Lateral subtemporal approach.* This was never used by the senior author, as in most of the cases the fundus of the aneurysm is directed laterally and the dome is fixed in arachnoidal adhesions between the temporal pole, the tentorial edge, and the III nerve. Thus in using this approach, the fundus is first faced and the neck is away from the surgeon.

2) *Supero-lateral approach.* Through a pterional craniotomy, the proximal Sylvian fissure is opened. The surgeon is then perpedicular to the axis of the ICA-MCA with optimal visualization

Table **22a** Size and location of multiple aneurysms associated with internal carotid – posterior communicating artery aneurysms

		Ipsilateral P.co.A.	Contra-lat. P. co. A.	Intra-cav.	Oph. A.	A. cho. A.	I. C. B.	M_1	M.C.B.	A. co. A.	Pe. A.	Ba. B.	Total
Left P. co. A.	Micro	–	1	1	1	7	5	2	5	5	–	–	27
	Macro	21	2	–	2	2	3	1	2	6	1	–	40
Right P. co. A.	Micro	–	1	–	1	3	4	1	10	8	–	–	28
	Macro	30	6	–	–	2	–	1	6	6	1	1	53
		51	10	1	4	14	12	5	23	25	2	1	148

Table **22b**

Single	122	patients		122	
1 additional aneurysm	29	patients	=	58	
2 additional aneurysms	8	patients	=	24	
3 additional aneurysms	6	patients	=	24	148
4 additional aneurysms	6	patients	=	30	
5 additional aneurysms	2	patients	=	12	
	173			270	

of the ICA along its whole length. The head position with slight rotation to the opposite side rotates the ICA and brings the origin of the PcoA to the surface. The clipping of an aneurysm in this location may on occasion be one of the easiest, but on other occasions can also turn into one of the most difficult procedures. This depends on the size of the aneurysm, the size of its neck, the thickness of its wall, and its relation to the PcoA, the thalamoperforators, and the AchoA.

Occasionally, a well defined aneurysmal neck with a well defined relationship to the PcoA offers itself to the clip. In such a case the operation can be accomplished within seconds without even opening of the Sylvian fissure. However, if the neck is large, if the PcoA and its branches are covered by the aneurysm, or if the AchoA is adherent to the wall of the neck or fundus of the aneurysm, then the procedure may require all technical refinements. The delicacy of the procedure is highlighted by the smallness of the triangular space between the clinoid – tentorial edge and medio-basal temporal pole, and the importance of structures in the immediate neighbourhood like tie ICA, the PcoA, branches of the PcoA, and III nerve.

A pterional craniotomy with opening of the proximal Sylvian fissure medial to the Sylvian vein and slight retraction of the frontolateral lobe opens the way directly to the ICA and the origin of the aneurysm.

Direction of Fundus

While a wide variety of configurations for the fundus projection of these aneurysms is possible, five general categories can be recognized (Fig 30, 31A–F):

1) *Anterolateral.* Some aneurysms, usually smaller ones, project upwards from the internal carotid artery. When larger, these aneurysms may hide the origin of the posterior communicating artery.

2) *Superolateral.* The fundus of these aneurysms projects upwards between the sphenoid ridge and tentorial edge.

3) *Posterolateral superior* (supratentorial). The fundus is directed into the adjacent temporal lobe. Rupture may lead to intracerebral and intraventricular hematoma, and care must be taken not to avulse the aneurysm by retraction of the frontal or temporal lobe or during the application of a clip to the neck of the aneurysm.

4) *Posterolateral inferior* (infratentorial). A common direction of the fundus is toward the interpeduncular cistern and the oculomotor nerve and this is often associated with an oculomotor palsy.

5) *Posteromedial inferior.* These aneurysms are similar to inferior wall aneurysms.

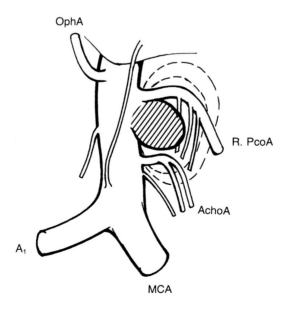

Fig 30 Schematic illustration of the so-called aneurysm of the posterior communicating artery and its tendency to enlarge within the lateral carotid cistern.

Anatomical Relationships 73

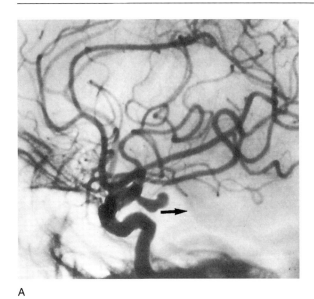

A

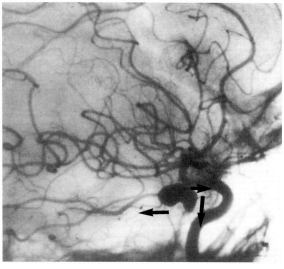

B

Fig 31A–F The radiographic description of aneurysms of the posterior communicating artery as related to the surgeon's view.
A This posteriorly directed aneurysm will project inferiorly at operation (arrow).
B This anterior-inferior-posteriorly directed aneurysm (arrows) will appear superior-anterior-inferior.

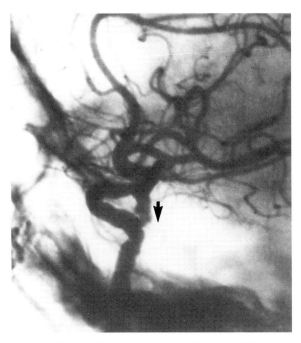

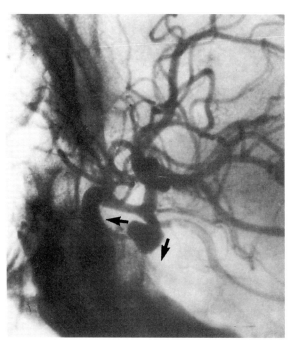

C An inferiorly directed aneurysm (arrow) will be seen anterior.

D Angiographically inferior-anteriorly directed aneurysms (arrows) will become anterior-superior.

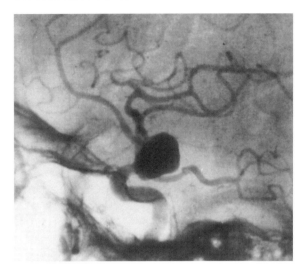
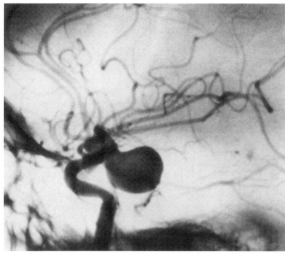

Fig 31 E Superior-posteriorly directed aneurysm will be found posterior-inferior.

F Posterior-inferiorly directed aneurysm will be seen inferior-anterior.

Relationship to the Subarachnoid Cisterns

Relationships of the subarachnoid cisterns to the aneurysm, to normal anatomical structures, and to each other, are of paramount importance for accurate dissection. The posterior communicating artery arises in the carotid cistern. The whole segment of this artery within the carotid cistern carries its own sleeve of arachnoid down to the interpeduncular cistern, where the P_1 segment of the posterior cerebral comes through a window as it exits the interpeduncular cistern to enter the ambient cistern. This occurs just at the medial border of the 3rd nerve. The anterior choroidal artery also carries a sleeve of arachnoid through the carotid cistern, and this arachnoid becomes contiguous with the arachnoid of the crural cistern. Finally, the oculomotor nerve comes out of the interpeduncular cistern by piercing Liliequist's membrane and carries a sleeve of arachnoid into the dural leaflets of the cavernous sinus. Points of arachnoid thickening and fixation that especially apply to aneurysms of the internal carotid-posterior communicating artery are:
1) The corner joining the uncus, tentorium, and oculomotor nerve;
2) The exit of the oculomotor nerve into the cavernous sinus; and
3) The point where the sleeves of arachnoid covering the posterior communicating artery and oculomotor nerve are adjacent to each other over Liliequist's membrane (see Vol I, Figs **10–12**).

The epiarachnoid space anterior to the carotid and the interpeduncular cistern back to the clivus are free. In some cases, however, there will be a rather dense adherence of the arachnoid sheath of the posterior communicating artery to the clinoid, and at times an actual groove or sulcus has been observed in the posterior clinoid process where the posterior communicating artery crosses it. This adherence will hinder mobilization of the posterior communicating artery and retraction of the internal carotid artery (Fig **32A–B**).

An aneurysm arising at the origin of the posterior communicating artery is within the carotid cistern, and as it enlarges it carries with it the arachnoid of this cistern. A potential plane of dissection remains between the arachnoid over the aneurysm and the arachnoid sleeves of the posterior communicating and anterior choroidal arteries (Fig **33A–B**). With further enlargement of the fundus, the arachnoid layer becomes apposed to the arachnoid of the crural and interpeduncular cisterns. Where the arachnoid over the aneurysm becomes attached to the points of arachnoid reinforcement and fixation described above, separation of the layers can be quite difficult and usually requires sharp dissection.

Anatomical Relationships

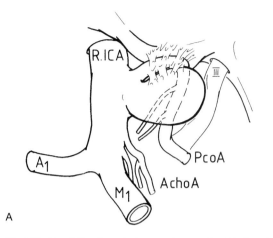

A

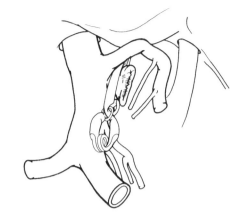

B

Fig 32A–B Adhesions between the arachnoid sheath of the posterior communicating artery and the aneurysm and the dura of the anterior clinoid process.

B After dissection and coagulation of the aneurysm with division of the adhesions between aneurysm and the dura the posterior communicating artery and branches could be clearly demonstrated and the aneurysm clipped.

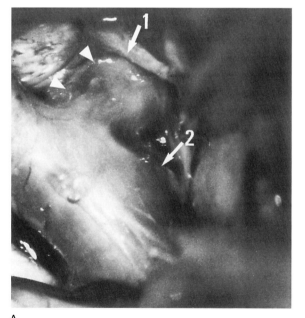

A

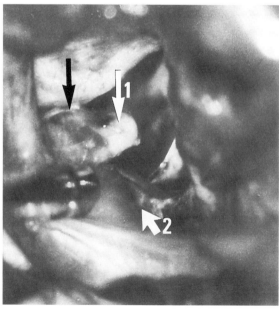

B

Fig 33A–B Operative photographs before dissection (**A**), aneurysm and right posterior communicating artery (arrow 1), anterior choroidal artery (arrow 2). Dissected and coagulated aneurysm (white arrow 1) and posterior communicating artery (black arrow), anterior choroidal artery (white arrow 2) (**B**).

Relationship to Posterior Communicating Artery

The contribution of the posterior communicating artery to the posterior cerebral artery is variable, but may be expected to predominate in about 15 per cent of cases. Von Mitterwallner (1955) found that in only 0.3 per cent of anatomical specimens did the posterior cerebral artery arise exclusively from the internal carotid artery, with absence of the P_1 segment of the posterior cerebral artery. Angiographically, in the present series of patients, the posterior cerebral artery was filled by the internal carotid artery injection on the side of an internal carotid-posterior communicating artery aneurysm in about 60 per cent of cases. In the other 40 per cent of angiograms the posterior communicating artery could not be identified. At operation, however, there were no cases of true aplasia of the posterior communicating artery. The artery may be hypoplastic or it may be compressed by the aneurysm sac, especially as it crosses the posterior clinoid process. Thus, the angiographic assessment of the importance of the posterior communicating artery is not entirely reliable. It was felt that in about 6 per cent of cases at operation, the posterior communicating artery was hyperplastic and appeared to be the primary source of blood supply to the posterior cerebral artery.

In 4 cases (2.3%), there was a second posterior communicating artery (or second PCA) which did not, in fact, communicate with the posterior cerebral artery, but coursed along the tentorium to the mesiobasal temporo-occipital area. This artery, previously described by Windle (1888) and Dandy (1944) may cause confusion during dissection, assuming it is the AchoA. In 3 cases, the aneurysm arose proximal to the posterior communicating artery, and in 1 of these there was also an aneurysm proximal to the anterior choroidal artery on the same side. In 1 case, there was a fenestration in the origin of the posterior communicating artery and an aneurysm was present on the proximal segment of this fenestration (see Fig **43A–C**, p. 65, Vol. I). Microsurgery has enabled us to recognise the relation of these aneurysms to the PcoA and precise dissection and care of this artery and its branches is possible. In only 8 cases in the present series did the aneurysm actually arise from the posterior communicating artery. In the remaining 165 cases, the lesion bore a variable relationship to the internal carotid and posterior communicating arteries (Fig **34**).

Arachnoid adhesions between the aneurysm and the posterior communicating artery may create the impression of more involvement of the posterior communicating artery than is actually present.

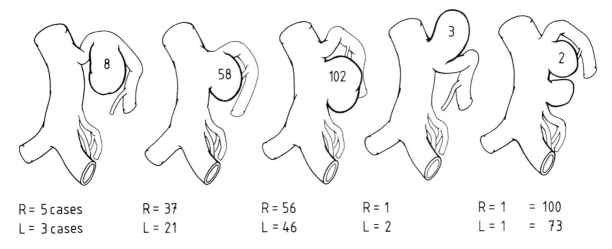

Fig **34** Schematic representation of the variable relationship between the proximal lateral wall of the ICA and true posterior communicating artery in own 173 cases.

The posterior communicating artery courses into the interpeduncular cistern and will be on the proximal inferior side of the aneurysm fundus. The origin of the artery is frequently covered by the aneurysm neck and the arachnoid dissection plane between these must be developed to identify the artery. At times the artery can be identified medial to the internal carotid artery as it courses medio-inferiorly toward the posterior cerebral artery.

Relationship to Anterior Thalamoperforating (Diencephalic or Central) Arteries

The thalamoperforating branches of the posterior communicating artery course medially and are generally displaced posteriorly and medially with growth of the aneurysm. Arachnoid of the interpeduncular and carotid cisterns is interposed between these vessels and the fundus of the aneurysm. Some of these branches, especially the tuberomammillary (premammillary) artery may be quite well developed even in the presence of a hypoplastic posterior communicating artery. The origins of these arteries are somewhat variable, arising between 2–5 mm distal to the carotid artery (most commonly at 2 mm). In one case from the present series the tuberomammillary artery arose directly from the ICA. Despite their differing origins, the entrance sites of these vessels into the diencephalon are surprisingly regular. It is important to determine the location of the thalamoperforate branches so that a clip can be properly placed without any strangulation of these arteries.

Relationship to the Anterior Choroidal Artery

The anterior choroidal artery regularly arises from the internal carotid artery as a single branch or as two or more arteries. When of single origin, the artery may branch very early, or may not give off a branch until well into the crural cistern. The anterior choroidal artery remains separated from an aneurysm at the origin of the posterior communicating artery first by the sleeve of arachnoid enclosing its origin in the carotid cistern and then by the arachnoid of the crural cistern. The anterior choroidal artery is usually displaced posteriorly and medially by a large aneurysm, and may be mistaken for a medial striate artery because of its proximity to the internal carotid artery bifurcation.

Relationship to the Oculomotor Nerve

The oculomotor nerve courses through the interpeduncular cistern in close relationship to the posterior communicating artery, but each structure is invested with its own arachnoid sheath. As these structures leave the interpeduncular cistern through Liliequist's membrane they diverge, with the posterior communicating artery taking its sleeve of arachnoid into the carotid cistern and the oculomotor nerve carrying its arachnoid into the cavernous sinus.

Growth of an aneurysm may injure the nerve by compression, or the aneurysm may rupture into the nerve. Many cases have been seen where the nerve was severely stretched or was hemorrhagic following rupture of an aneurysm, but remained functionally intact, whereas a nerve that seemed anatomically intact was completely non-functional. The exact mechanism of injury is not clear. The aneurysm fundus can become quite densely attached to the oculomotor nerve at its exit point into the cavernous sinus; in these cases the dissection of the fundus is not undertaken. In one case the fundus of the aneurysm was seen to project through a rent in the nerve, but there were no symptoms (Fig **35A–B**).

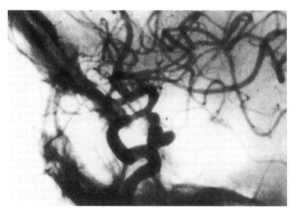

A

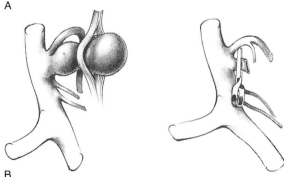

B

Fig **35A–B** Long inferiorly directed posterior communicating artery aneurysm (**A**) that at surgery was projecting anterolaterally through a fenestration in the oculomotor nerve (**B**).

Relationship to the Tentorium Cerebelli

The tentorial edge may be quite close to the internal carotid artery offering little space for dissection or may be far enough removed to allow easy visualization of the oculomotor nerve. The fundus of the aneurysm may project above or below the tentorium or may be firmly attached to it.

Relationship to Clinoid Processes

When the origin of the posterior communicating artery is quite proximal or the anterior clinoid process long, this bony process may cover the proximal portion of the aneurysm neck. The posterior clinoid process may also be quite wide or prominent and have the posterior communicating artery attached to it.

Relationship to the Mesial Temporal Lobe

Aneurysms at this location are generally directed toward the parahippocampal gyrus (uncus) of the temporal lobe, and in some cases will be adherent to or even buried in the temporal lobe. A small subpial resection of the mediobasal pole of the temporal lobe may be necessary to expose the relationship of the aneurysm to the posterior communicating and especially anterior choroidal arteries.

Epidural Extension

No cases were observed where an aneurysm of the PcoA extended along the ICA as far proximally as the cavernous sinus. This occurs commonly with the ophthalmic and inferior wall of ICA aneurysms.

Operative Technique

Through a frontotemporosphenoidal craniotomy, the proximal Sylvian cistern is opened on the frontal side of the superficial middle cerebral veins, and the arachnoid dissected down to the internal carotid artery bifurcation, dividing the thickened bands of arachnoid which cross the origins of the anterior and middle cerebral arteries. Minimal retraction (medially and superiorly) should be applied to the frontal lobe at this point, and the temporal pole should be untouched. The microsurgeon should be able to perform these manipulations in this narrow space without retraction of the temporal lobe.

The carotid and interpeduncular cisterns are opened on their medial sides to allow the release of cerebrospinal fluid and the proximal internal carotid artery beneath the anterior clinoid process is dissected free of arachnoid to allow the placement of a temporary clip if necessary.

The lamina terminalis cistern is next opened over both optic nerves and over both anterior cerebral arteries. This is important for several reasons. First it further mobilizes the frontal lobes to that they will fall away from the basal cisterns without significant retraction. Because the fundus of the aneurysm may be adherent to the temporal lobe, it is important that traction on the laterobasal frontal lobe not be transmitted to the aneurysm. Retraction of the frontal lobe before it has been adequately mobilized by opening the basal cisterns may cause the dome of the aneurysm to be avulsed, leading to hemorrhage before the internal carotid artery has been adequately dissected. Secondly opening of the lamina terminalis cistern allows the surgeon to evaluate cross-circulation through the anterior cerebral arteries should temporary clips be required.

Identification of the Posterior Communicating Artery

The origin and course of the posterior communicating artery may next be determined. It is usually possible to identify the origin of the posterior communicating artery just proximal to the aneurysm on the posterolateral wall of the internal carotid artery. Occasionally however, the aneurysm will overlie the origin of the posterior communicating artery and obscure its course.

Attention should then be directed to the medial side of the internal carotid artery where the carotid and the interpeduncular cistern (Liliequist's membrane) are opened between the arterial branches to the optic chiasm and pituitary stalk. The internal carotid artery may be gently elevated and pushed laterally with the suction tip. This maneuver may expose the posterior communicating artery so that the real size of the PcoA, the thalamoperforating diencephalic branches, and the medial extension of the aneurysm can be identified. The surgeon can now gently mobilize the proximal part of the neck of the aneurysm posteriorly to identify the covered segment of the PcoA from above and dissect a small tunnel through the arachnoid layer between the PcoA and aneurysm (Figs 36 and 37).

In some cases, the origin of the posterior communicating artery will be hidden by the anterior clinoid process, and it will be advantageous to

Operative Technique 79

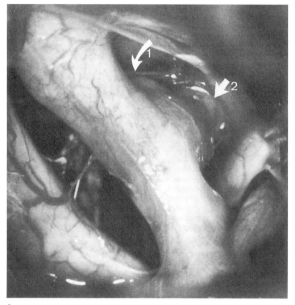
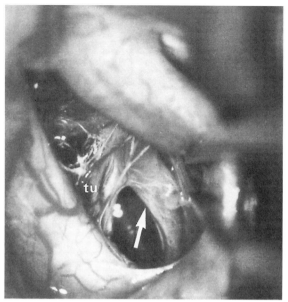
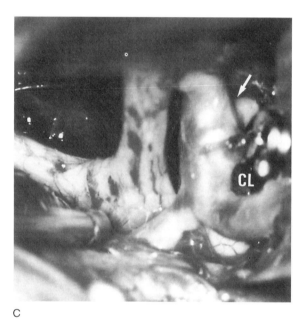

Fig 36A–C Only a trace of the posterior communicating artery (arrow 1) is visible on the top of the aneurysm (arrow 2) (**A**), but branches are clearly seen between the carotid artery and the right optic nerve with retraction of the carotid artery (arrow) (**B**), these branches are quite well defined. tu = tuberomammillary branches. Following clipping, the posterior communicating artery (arrow) is better seen in (**C**).

remove the process. This maneuver was described under ophthalmic aneurysms (page 45), and involves coagulation and incision of the dura, protection of the optic nerve and carotid artery with a strip of rubber glove, and removal of the anterior clinoid process with a high speed electric drill. It is not necessary to carry the removal of the bone as far medially, nor to unroof the optic canal. Removal of the anterior clinoid process was performed successfully in 16 cases to identify the PcoA and proximal part of the neck of the aneurysm (Fig **38A–E**).

The PcoA or the aneurysm itself may also be attached to the dura of the posterior clinoid process and require meticulous mobilization at this point.
Extension of the aneurysm proximally to the carotid canal and cavernous sinus has not been observed.

80 2 Internal Carotid Artery Aneurysms

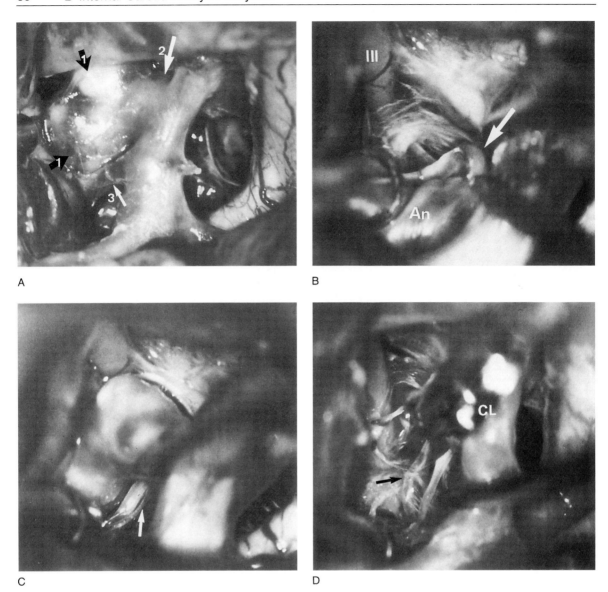

Fig 37A–D Left posterior communicating artery aneurysm (arrows 1) showing only a trace of posterior communicating artery (arrow 2), and the anterior choroidal artery (arrow 3). With retraction the pre-aneurysmal (B) and postaneurysmal (C) segments of the posterior communicating artery can be identified (arrows), and after clipping (D) its tubero-mammillary branches (arrow) can be seen.

Operative Technique

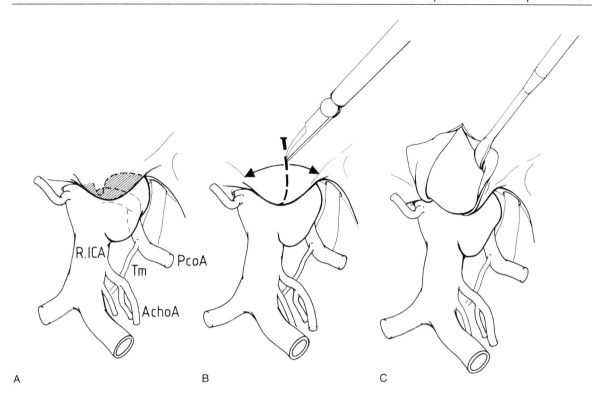

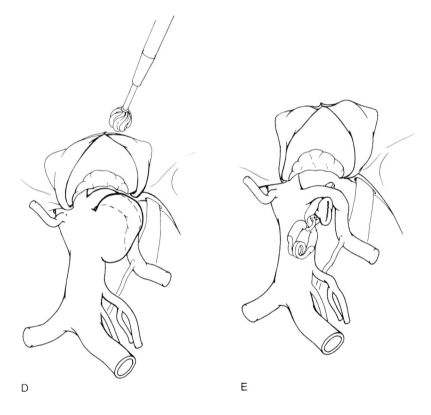

Fig **38A–E** The anterior clinoid process must be removed if the proximal wall of the aneurysm and the origin of the posterior communicating artery are covered. See description in text (p. 79).

Identification of the Anterior Choroidal Artery

With smaller aneurysms at this location, identification of the anterior choroidal artery or arteries may be no problem. One must remember that the AchoA will arise as two or more branches of the ICA in 30 per cent of cases. However, with larger aneurysms, the artery is commonly covered by and adherent to the fundus. Attention should be first directed to the area of the internal carotid artery bifurcation, where the uncal branches of the anterior choroidal artery may appear as medial striate arteries coursing beneath the bifurcation. Proximal striate arteries generally arise a few millimeters medial and lateral to the bifurcation on the anterior and middle cerebral arteries. Arteries coming directly beneath the bifurcation are usually branches of the anterior choroidal artery. These arteries are dissected and followed proximally to identify the anterior choroidal artery.

If the anterior choroidal artery cannot be visualized because the aneurysm is buried in the temporal lobe, subpial resection of a few millimeters of mesiobasal temporal lobe may prove useful. In addition freeing the aneurysm from the temporal lobe will release tension on the aneurysm associated with either retraction of the temporal lobe or dissection of the aneurysm neck. The pia around the fundus of the aneurysm is opened with bipolar coagulation and 5–6 mm of the cortex removed by gentle aspiration. Intratemporal hematoma is also removed, leaving a reasonable amount attached to the site of rupture. The AchoA can now be identified distally in the crural cistern between the uncus and the cerebral peduncle, and followed proximally, dissecting it from the wall of the aneurysm (Fig **39A–B**). The temporo-polar or anterior temporal artery may rarely originate from a very proximal part of the MCA and may be in the way of the lateral parts of the ICA. In such a case it should be dissected and mobilized from the temporal lobe over a few millimeters so that it will not be stretched by further necessary dissection in the crural cistern or by the application of the clip.

Identification of the Oculomotor Nerve

In 72 cases of the present series there were dense adhesions between the aneurysm and the oculomotor nerve and in another 46 cases, adhesions were found between the aneurysm and the edge of the tentorium. It is in this area that arachnoid adhesions are difficult to separate and

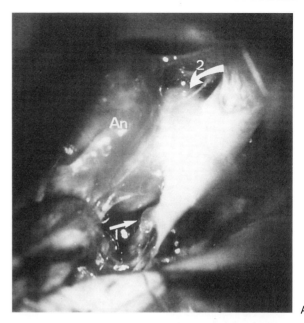

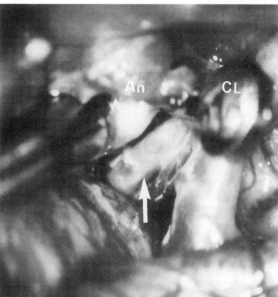

Fig **39A–B** In this proximal lateral wall aneurysm (An) the anterior choroidal artery (arrow 1) is immediately visible, while the posterior communicating artery (arrow 2) is not completely visualized (**A**) until after clipping (white arrow) (**B**).

one should not attempt to dissect these free. Rather one should go to the neck of the aneurysm and try to secure clip placement, then come back and coagulate, cut, and free the aneurysm from this area. It is better to cut through the aneurysm rather than try to remove it from the oculomotor nerve as this almost always leads to oculomotor palsy. If the fundus of the aneurysm is firmly attached to the III nerve and to the petroclinoid ligament, it should never be dissected. The neck of the aneurysm should be clipped first.

Dissection of Aneurysm Neck

With all important structures in the operative field now identified, the surgeon can proceed to the dissection of the neck itself. The key to separation of the aneurysm from the adjacent arteries is recognition of the arachnoid layers – the arachnoid of the carotid and interpeduncular cisterns, that separates the aneurysm from the posterior communicating artery, and the arachnoid of the carotid and crural cisterns that separates the aneurysm from the anterior choroidal artery. Only the lateral part that adheres to the III nerve should not be attacked.

A varying length of the posterior communicating artery will be incorporated into the neck of the aneurysm. The microtechnique is especially helpful in delineating the wall of the aneurysm and the parent arteries from arachnoid adhesions. A plane is gradually developed by gently spreading the bipolar coagulation forceps or with a small blunt dissector, and the arachnoid then sharply divided. The arachnoid should not be torn with a blunt instrument. The posterior communicating artery must be freed from possible adhesions to the posterior clinoid process.

It is important to make an effort to separate the posterior communicating artery from the aneurysm if possible rather than to place a clip across the neck of the aneurysm and the origin of the posterior communicating artery, for the following reasons:

1) A clip across the origin of the posterior communicating artery tends to kink the intima of the internal carotid artery compromising flow and perhaps serving as a nidus for thrombosis.
2) Perforating arteries arising from the posterior communicating artery may be compromised.
3) The posterior communicating artery may be the only, or an important source of blood supply to the ipsilateral posterior cerebral artery.
4) A clip applied closely to the base of the aneurysm on the internal carotid artery may leave a small corner of the aneurysm open to the lumen of the posterior communicating artery, so that the aneurysm is filled retrogradely (Fig **40**).

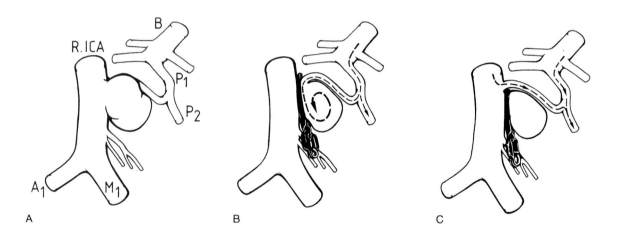

Fig **40A–C** Schematic illustration of the relationship between proximal lateral aneurysms and the posterior communicating artery as it affects the placement of a clip on the aneurysm. By failing to adequately dissect the posterior communicating artery from the aneurysm, a clip may be placed proximal to the artery allowing it still to distend the aneurysm.
A Aneurysm arising from the lateral wall of the internal carotid artery distal to the origin of the posterior communicating artery.
B Clip crossing both neck of aneurysm and posterior communicating artery allows the aneurysm to be filled from the basilar circulation.
C Proper clip placement. The aneurysm is excluded from the circulation and normal flow pattern is maintained.

Coagulation

In some cases some bulging parts of the neck can be coagulated and shrunk by bipolar coagulation. Coagulation of the whole neck is used in cases that have a well defined but broad neck but this is applied only after the dissection of the PcoA and its branches (Fig **41A–C**).

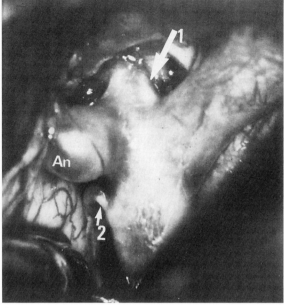

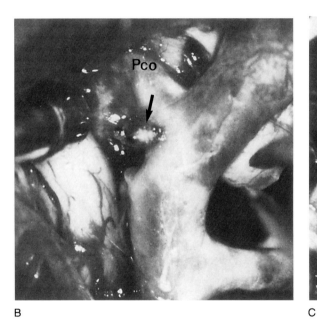

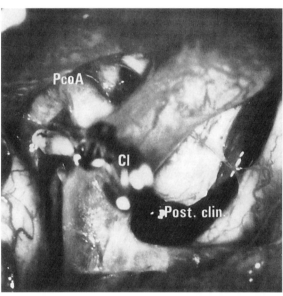

Fig **41A–C** Left posterior communicating artery aneurysm (An) arising at the origin of the posterior communicating artery (arrow 1) (arrow 2 shows the anterior choroidal artery) (**A**) after coagulation (arrow) (**B**) and clipping (**C**). Cl = clip, Post. clin. = posterior clinoid process.

Clip Application

When a 2 to 3 mm space has been created on the proximal and distal sides of the neck, a clip may be applied. The clip is usually introduced perpendicularly to the internal carotid artery with the blades pointing slightly laterally. The clip is closed slowly while the effect of closure on the internal carotid artery and the aneurysm is observed. Especially important is that the clip does not kink the internal carotid artery compromising its flow. The tips of the clip are noted beneath the aneurysm to see that they have not included the oculomotor nerve, the posterior communicating artery distal to the aneurysm, or the thalamoperforating arteries.

Fundus Resection and Closure

Following clip application, the fundus should be observed as to whether it gets bluish in color and whether it should be punctured with a small needle. If there is no blood flow the fundus is opened and thrombus removed. Successive coagulation of the cut edges of the aneurysm and clip reapplication is performed, until satisfactory clip placement is obtained. There are aneurysms with inferiorly bulging parts at the origin of the sac, that may escape obliteration by the primarily applied clip. The stepwise clipping, puncture, and resection of the saccule, with sealing of the cut edges of the aneurysm by repeated coagulation and replacement of the clip, eventually deliver the remaining portion of the aneurysm into the clip. In those cases with sclerotic, thick walls and partial or subtotal thrombosis, the fundus can be cut 2–3 mm distal to the clip and the technique of staging coagulation and clipping performed until a final clip can be applied. The cut fundus should be left in place if there are firm adhesions. If the fundus is attached to the oculomotor nerve, it should be transected to relieve tension, but attempts to remove the dome from the nerve should not be undertaken as oculomotor palsy usually follows this maneuver.

Papaverine is applied to the major arteries and the periadventitial sympathetic plexus over the superior wall of the ICA and the PcoA excised. After hemostasis, the wound is closed.

Intraoperative Rupture of the Aneurysm

Of the 173 cases, 21 (12.1%) ruptured at the time of operation. One case early in the series (1967), sustained rupture of the aneurysm during clip application (see page 91). Bleeding could not be controlled and the lesion was trapped between clips placed on the internal carotid artery and on the posterior communicating artery. The patient remained in poor condition (see Table **34**, No. 18). In 8 cases (4.6%), temporary clips were applied to the internal carotid artery to control a rupture and allow further dissection. Occlusion time varied from 20 seconds to 3 minutes and was well tolerated in all patients.

In 1 case, the internal carotid artery was repaired primarily over a 4 mm rent with microsutures while temporary clips were applied for 22 minutes and this patient did well. In the other 12 cases, bleeding could be controlled with suction, coagulation, or clip application to the aneurysm. Suzuki et al. (1979) reported the use of temporary clips on the parent artery in 74 per cent of their cases.

Ligated Aneurysms

In the first three years of this series, 8 patients were treated by ligating the neck of the aneurysm with a silk ligature. Since replaceable and non-slipping clips have been available, the ligature technique has not been used.

Bilateral Aneurysms

When the lamina terminalis and chiasmatic cisterns are fully opened the surgeon is able to examine the contralateral internal carotid and anterior cerebral arteries and may be able to clip incidental aneurysms present on these. Good success has resulted with internal carotid-ophthalmic and internal carotid artery bifurcation aneurysms that were clipped from the contralateral side. On rare occasions (2 cases), even a contralateral proximal middle cerebral artery aneurysm may be clipped. Aneurysms arising from the lateral wall of the internal carotid artery, however, do not lend themselves well to contralateral clipping. The internal carotid artery itself blocks the neck of the aneurysm and the origins of the posterior communicating and anterior choroidal arteries from the surgeon's view.

In 1 patient with bilateral large aneurysms of posterior communicating arteries it was possible from a right sided pterional approach to clip first the right PcoA and then to reach and clip a contralateral large aneurysm of the left PcoA. She also had a large anterior communicating artery aneurysm which was clipped through the same approach. This patient has done well. The reason for the one-session operation was to save the 67 year old lady from a second operation (see Fig

165A–G, page 324). In 9 other cases, 5 operated from the right side and 4 from the left side, 1 underwent a prophylactic second operation without incident, 2 sustained subarachnoid hemorrhage from the contralateral lesion and underwent successful second operation. One patient suffered a subarachnoid hemorrhage 3 months after the first operation from rupture of the contralateral posterior communicating aneurysm and was left hemiparetic and aphasic. The other 5 patients refused a second operation, but none has had further difficulty and they remain in good health (Fig **42A–B**).

"Kissing" aneurysms: In 2 patients (both female) the angiograms showed 2 aneurysms of the lateral wall of ICA. Operative exploration confirmed two adherent aneurysms with separate origins at the level of PcoA and anterior choroidal arteries. In both cases, the proximal aneurysms had ruptured. The dissection and clipping of these aneurysms succeeded finally, but the accomplishment was very difficult and hazardous in both cases (Figs **43** and **44A–E**).

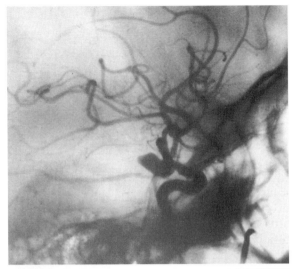
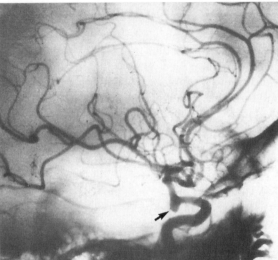

Fig **42A–B** Bilateral posterior communicating artery aneurysms – the right (**A**) had ruptured and was clipped, while the left (arrow) (**B**) remains asymptomatic after 8 years.

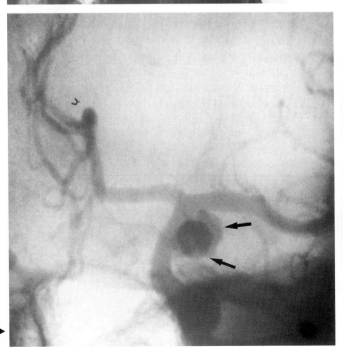

Fig **43** Left sided 'kissing' aneurysms of both the proximal and distal lateral wall as seen at angiography (arrows).

Operative Technique

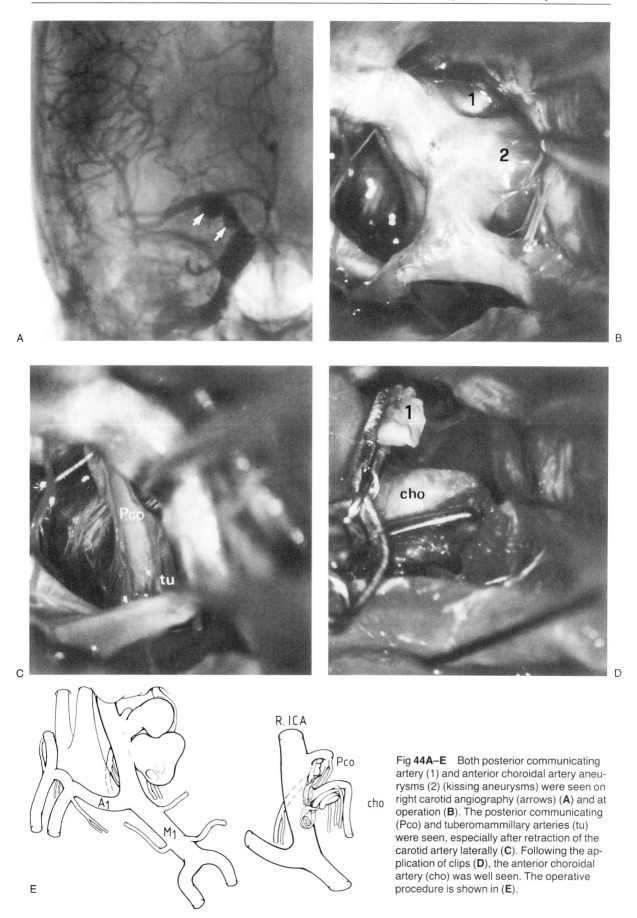

Fig **44A–E** Both posterior communicating artery (1) and anterior choroidal artery aneurysms (2) (kissing aneurysms) were seen on right carotid angiography (arrows) (**A**) and at operation (**B**). The posterior communicating (Pco) and tuberomammillary arteries (tu) were seen, especially after retraction of the carotid artery laterally (**C**). Following the application of clips (**D**), the anterior choroidal artery (cho) was well seen. The operative procedure is shown in (**E**).

Summary

In summary, the steps involved in clipping an aneurysm at this location include:
1) Frontotemporosphenoidal craniotomy,
2) Opening of the proximal Sylvian fissure across the internal carotid artery bifurcation,
3) Opening the medial carotid and interpeduncular cistern,
4) Opening the lamina terminalis cistern over the anterior cerebral arteries and optic nerves,
5) Dissection of the internal carotid artery proximal and distal to the aneurysm to gain control,
6) Identification of the posterior communicating artery and its branches, and dissection from the dura of the posterior clinoid process, if adhesions are present,
7) Identification of the anterior choroidal artery and its branches,
8) Removal of the anterior clinoid process if necessary,
9) Mediobasal temporal lobe incision if necessary,
10) Identification of the oculomotor nerve,
11) Dissection of the aneurysm neck,
12) Clip application,
13) Opening of fundus, coagulation, and clip replacement as indicated,
14) Fundus left attached to oculomotor nerve,
15) Routine hemostasis and closure.

Clinical Presentation and Operative Results

Background

While several publications have discussed the problem of internal carotid artery aneurysm (Black and German 1953; af Björkesten 1958; Höök and Norlén 1964a; Gurdjian et al. 1965; Kempe 1968; Kak et al. 1973; Hollin and Decker 1977) few reports have specifically addressed aneurysms arising from the origin of the posterior communicating artery. Harris and Udvarhelyi (1957) performed craniotomy on 12 patients and cervical carotid artery ligation on 66 patients with no mortality in the craniotomy group, but high morbidity in both groups. McKissock and associates (1960b) experienced a 67 per cent mortality rate in their 9 cases operated directly, but Paterson (1968) was able to bring this down to a 10 per cent mortality rate in 77 patients. Jeffreys and Holmes (1971) found a 4 per cent mortality and 8 per cent morbidity in 51 patients subjected only to cervical carotid ligation. Suzuki et al. (1979) reported 9.2% poor results and 7.0% mortality in 213 patients.

Presenting Features

In the present series, 173 patients underwent operation for aneurysm of the ICA-PcoA. In 8 cases the neck of the aneurysm was ligated and in 165 cases it was clipped. Of these, 46 (26.6%) were male and 127 (73.4%) female. Ages ranged from 12 to 73 with 62 per cent of patients between the ages of 40 and 60 (Table **23a**). The aneurysms were located on the right side in slightly less than 60 per cent of cases in both males and females (Table **23b**).

Of the 173 patients, 154 (89.0%) presented with subarachnoid hemorrhage. 2 patients presented with incidental aneurysms, one in association with a tumor and the other with a contralateral oculomotor palsy and bruit. One presented with a seizure. At operation 7 asymptomatic patients were found to have had a subarachnoid hemorrhage localized to the carotid cistern. Only 10 patients (5.8%) at surgery had not suffered a subarachnoid hemorrhage. The frequency of symptoms in the 173 patients is given in Table **24a** and **b**. Overall, 75 patients (43.3%) presented with an oculomotor palsy, 33 patients (19.1%) with hemiparesis, and 21 patients (12.1%) with speech difficulties. Considering only left sided aneurysms, 28.8 per cent of the patients were dysphasic. Seizures occurred in 9 per cent and in 1 patient a bruit was audible. 97 of the patients gave a history of severe headache in the past, unrelated to the current subarachnoid hemorrhage.

Table 23a Age and sex of 173 patients with aneurysms of the proximal lateral wall of the internal carotid artery

	Male	Female	Total	%
11–20 y	–	1	1	0.6
21–30	4	11	15	8.7
31–40	9	22	31	17.9
41–50	17	46	63	36.4
51–60	13	31	44	25.4
61–70	3	14	17	9.8
over 70	–	2	2	1.2
Total	46 (26.6%)	127 (73.4%)	173	100.0

Table 23b Sex and site of aneurysm

	Male	Female	Total	
Left	20	53	73	(42.2%)
Right	26	74	100	(57.8%)
	46	127	173	

Table 24a Symptomatology in 173 patients with aneurysms of the proximal lateral wall of the internal carotid artery

	Male	Female	Total	%
SAH only	26	45	71	41.0
SAH + III pr.	12	35	47	27.2
SAH + hpr.	3	18	21	12.1
SAH + III. pr. + hpr.	1	10	11	6.3
SAH + IV. pr.	1	1	2	1.2
III. pr. only (no bleed at operation)	1	9	10	5.8
(Expl. proved SAH)	1	6	7	4.0
Hpr. only (Expl. proved SAH)	–	1	1	0.6
Seizure disorder only (Expl. proved SAH)	1	–	1	0.6
Asymptomatic	–	2**/°	2	1.2
	46	127	173	100.0

** Meningioma 64 y
° bruit 70 y

Table 24b Incidence of symptoms

Symptom	Cases	%
Headache	165	95.4
Altered LOC	98	56.6
Vomiting	86	49.7
Diplopia	76	43.9
Hemiparesis	33	19.0
Dysphasia	21 (L. side)	28.8
Seizures	8	4.6

Outcome of Oculomotor Palsy

Oculomotor palsy presented with and without subarachnoid hemorrhage in 75 patients (43.3%). The incidence was slightly higher in women (Table **25a**). The degree, lateralization, and outcome of oculomotor palsy is noted in Table **25b**. Out of a total of 75 patients, 8 died. Of the remaining 67, there was full recovery in 55 (82.1%) and partial recovery in 7 (10.4%) occurring over weeks to months. In 5 patients (7.5%) there was no recovery after many months or years had elapsed and the damage was considered irreversible. There were no cases with permanent III palsy caused by operation, but in 12 cases transient palsies were seen.

Table **25a** IIIrd nerve palsy

Symptoms	Male	Female	Total	%
III + SAH	12	35	47	27.2
III + SAH + Hpr.	1	10	11	6.3
III + Local SAH	1	6	7	4.0
Only III	1	9	10	5.8
	15	60	75	

Table **25b**

Severity of palsy		
Total	45	60.0%
Subtotal	10	13.3%
Partial	12	16.0%
Mild	8	10.7%
Side of palsy		
Left	30	40.0%
Right	45	60.0%
Recovery		
Complete	55	82.1%
Partial	7	10.4%
None	5	7.5%
Died	8	

Table **25c**

Large hematomas	No palsy	Palsy
Cisternal	11	12
Subdural	10	7

Operative Results

Operative results are related to preoperative grade in Table **26a–b**. Of the 173 patients, 144 (83.2%) have made complete recoveries. 17 (9.8%) are in fair condition, 2 (1.2%) in poor condition, and 10 (5.8%) have died. Results will be discussed in relation to preoperative grade:

Grades 0a to IIb

131 patients presented in grades 0a to IIb. In this group, 124 (94.6%) made good recoveries. One of these patients developed an ischemic complication appropriate to the side of the aneurysm that resolved over 3 months. The other 123 cases had smooth postoperative courses and were for the most part discharged within 2 weeks of operation. 7 cases are categorized as fair. All were in grades IIa or IIb at the time of operation (see Table **34**). One of these patients (No. 4) required a ventricular shunt and did not improve to full working status. Another patient (No. 6) had a seizure disorder and left hemiparesis which were unchanged after operation. The other 5 patients suffered ischemic deficits. One (No. 7) had a left hemihypesthesia preoperatively that extended to a left hemiparesis in the postoperative period, and the other 4 were first found to have hemiparesis and/or speech difficulty in the postoperative period. In 2 cases operated upon since 1976, a CT scan has demonstrated a cerebral infarction appropriate to the neurological deficits.

Table 26a Surgical results related to preoperative grade

	Total No.	Good	Fair	Poor	Death
0a	2 (1.2%)	2 (100 %)	–	–	–
0b	10 (5.8%)	10 (100 %)	–	–	–
Ia	45 (26.0%)	45 (100 %)	–	–	–
IIa	56 (32.4%)	51 (91.1%)	5	–	–
IIb	18 (10.4%)	16 (88.8%)	2	–	–
IIIa	14 (8.1%)	12 (85.7%)	–	–	2 (14,3%)
IIIb	16 (9.2%)	6 (37.5%)	6	1	3 (18.7%)
IV	10 (5.8%)	2 (20.0%)	4	1	3 (30.0%)
V	2 (1.2%)	–	–	–	2
	173	144 (83.2%)	17 (9.8%)	2 (1.2%)	10 (5.8%)

Late follow up of these 131 cases revealed one man who was addicted to amphetamines and who ruptured a previously undetected middle cerebral artery aneurysm and died suddenly.

Grade IIIa

14 patients presented in Grade IIIa. Of these 12 (85.7%) went on to a complete recovery. 2 patients in the good category required ventricular shunts (see Table 32). One man (No. 2) developed a mild hemiparesis post-operatively that improved considerably after ventricular draining and a ventriculo-atrial shunt. The second patient (No. 3), a woman, developed over 7 months a progressive syndrome of drowsiness, headache, depression, and mental deterioration. Her symptoms were relieved within 4 weeks by ventricular shunting.

The other 2 patients died (see Table 35). In one 65 year old woman (No. 1), the middle cerebral artery was injured at operation, as the temporopolar branch was avulsed by the clip applicator, and an extracranial-intracranial anastomosis had to be performed. She, nevertheless, went on to cerebral infarction, was bed ridden and died three and a half years after operation. A 64 year old male patient (No. 2) (operated 1968) accumulated an epidural hematoma in the postoperative period and succumbed despite early reoperation and evacuation of the hematoma.

Grade IIIb

Of 16 cases in Grade IIIb, only 6 (37.5%) made a full recovery. Of these 6, two required ventricular shunts (see Table 33), 1 in the preoperative period (No. 4) and 1 postoperatively (No. 5). All have now returned to full activity.

6 patients (37.5%) were left in fair condition (see Table 34, Nos. 8–13). All had hemiparesis and/or aphasia prior to operation and none was made worse by operation. 2 required ventricular shunts

Table 26b

0a–0b–Ia–IIa–IIb =	131 cases = 75.7%	Results
	Good	124 cases (94.7%)
	Fair	7 cases (5.3%)
IIIa–b =	30 cases = 17.3%	
	Good	18 cases (60.0%)
	Fair	6 cases (20.0%)
	Poor	1 case (3.3%)
	Death	5 cases (16.7%)

in the postoperative period and 2 of the patients (Nos. 10 and 12), a 67 and a 68 year old woman died 9 and 6 months after operation from medical causes.

One patient is listed in poor condition (see Table 34, No. 18). This was the first aneurysm patient operated upon in Zurich with microsurgical techniques (January, 1967). Preoperatively she was in condition IIIb, somnolent with a right hemiparesis. The clips (Scoville) then available would not occlude the aneurysm and during further manipulation, the neck was torn. The internal carotid artery was clipped above and below the lesion and another clip applied to the posterior communicating artery. She was left with a hemiplegia and aphasia from which she only partially recovered. 3 patients died (18.7%) (see Table 35). One lady (No. 3) sustained 2 recurrent subarachnoid hemorrhages from an aneurysm that could not be completely obliterated with a clip, and a second lady was making good progress when she developed gastrointestinal hemorrhage and died at laparotomy (No. 5). The third patient (No. 4) had a lumbar drain inserted for hydrocephalus. This became infected with a gram negative organism, she developed meningitis, septicaemia, and died.

Grade IV

10 patients were in grade IV. Two patients (20.0%) made complete recoveries despite severe preoperative deficits (see Table **33**, Nos. 7 and 8). Both of these patients required ventricular shunts, however, in the postoperative period.

4 patients are in fair condition (see Table **34**, Nos. 14–17). Each has improved since operation, but remains with some pre-existing deficits. 2 have required ventricular shunting (Nos. 14, 16). There is 1 patient in poor condition (Table **34**, No. 19). This lady was admitted with marked somnolence, right hemiplegia and aphasia following subarachnoid hemorrhage. The operation was uncomplicated, but she showed no improvement and remains in a rest home.

3 patients have died (see Table **35**) (30.0%). 2 patients (Nos. 6 and 7) with large subdural hematomas were taken to theatre 1 day after rupture of their aneurysm. They remained comatose postoperatively, and died 2 days and 4 weeks later. A third lady (No. 8) remained in poor condition following operation, and had a ventricular shunt inserted, but she went on to die in a nursing home 17 months later.

Grade V

2 patients presented in grade V and both died. One 25 year old lady (see Table **35**, No. 10) presented in coma with a large subdural hematoma after her fourth subarachnoid hemorrhage. She remained in coma after operation and died in a nursing home 2 ½ years later. The other patient (No. 9) suddenly deteriorated on the ward, with extensor posturing and non-reactive pupils. She was taken immediately to the operating room and a large subdural hematoma was evacuated. She survived in a state of akinetic mutism postoperatively and died 10 weeks later.

Mortality and Morbidity Analysis

An analysis of the factors contributing to postoperative morbidity and mortality was made, with the following results (see Tables **34** and **35**).

Preoperative Grade

The preoperative condition is without question the most important factor determining postoperative mortality and morbidity. Of 131 cases presenting in grade 0a to IIb, there were no mortalities or poor results, and all but 5.3 per cent made a complete recovery.

Of 30 cases in grade IIIa–b, there was a 14.3 per cent mortality in grade IIIa, and 18.7 per cent in grade IIIb. Morbidity was 14.2 per cent in the IIIa group, but was found in 43.7 per cent of the IIIb group. In grade IV there was a 30 per cent mortality and a 50 per cent morbidity, and in grade V both patients died (Table **28**).

Hypertension

40 patients (23.1%) with internal carotid-posterior communicating artery aneurysms had a history of hypertension. Hypertension is related to sex, preoperative grade and postoperative result in Table **28**. It is noted that both the patient's condition at the time of operation and the postoperative result are adversely affected by the presence of hypertension. Overall 32.6 per cent of males and 27.6 per cent of females were hypertensive.

Hematoma

There were 23 patients (13.3%) who had hematomas of significant size. 17 of these had subdural hematomas (9.8%). In 8 patients there was only subdural hematoma, while in other 9 subdural hematomas were associated with intracerebral hematoma. 15 patients (8.7%) had an intracerebral hematoma that was associated

Table **27** Posterior communicating artery aneurysms. Length of hospital stay related to preoperative grade

	Grade 0–I	Grade II	Grade III	Grade IV
under 5 days	1	–	–	–
6–10 days	30	26	3	–
11–14 days	23	31	5	–
2– 4 weeks	3	16	15	6
1– 3 months	–	1	2	1
	57	74	25	7

Total 163 Patients
10 deaths excluded
173 patients

Table 28 Relationship of hypertension to sex, preoperative grade, and surgical result in 173 patients with aneurysms of the proximal (ICA-PcoA) lateral wall of the internal carotid artery

		Good	Fair	Poor	Death	Tot. Hyp.	Tot. Pat.	%
Grade I	Male	3	1	–	–	4	57	7.0
	Female	–	–	–	–			
Grade IIa–b	Male	5	2 (1)	–	–	16	74	21.6
	Female	6	2 (2)	1 (1)	–			
Grade IIIa–b	Male	1	1	–	–	11	30	36.7
	Female	3	3 (2)	–	3 (2)			
Grade IV	Male	–	–	–	2 (2)	8	10	80.0
	Female	1	3 (2)	1 (1)	1 (1)			
Grade V	Male	–	–	–	–	1	2	50.0
	Female	–	–	–	1			
Total with hypertension		19	12	2	7	40		23%
Total Patients		144 (13%)	17 (71%)	2 (100%)	10 (70%)		173	

( ) = b-group

Table 29 Relationship of hematoma to preoperative grade and surgical result in 173 patients with proximal lateral wall internal carotid artery aneurysms

	Good	Fair	Poor	Death	Tot. Hem.	Tot. Pat.	%
Grade I	–	–	–	–	0	57	0
Grade IIa	4 (SDH only-2) (icH only-1) (icH+ivH-1)	1 (icH only-1)	–	–	5	74	6.7
Grade III a 4 b 4	6 (SDH only-4) (SDH + icH-2)	1 (icH only-1)	–	2 (SDH + icH-2)	9	30	30
Grade IV	–	4 (SDH only-1) (icH only-1) (SDH + icH-2)	–	3 (SDH only-1) (icH only-1) (SDH + icH-1)	7	10	70
Grade V	–	–	–	2 (SDH + icH -2)	2	2	100
Total with hematoma	10 (7%)	6 (35%)	0 (0%)	7 (70%)	23 (13.3%)		
Total Patients	144	17	2	10		173	

with a subdural hematoma in 9 and an intraventricular hematoma in 1. Intracranial hematomas are related to preoperative grade and postoperative results in Table 29.

The presence of a hematoma appears to correlate better with the preoperative grade than with the postoperative results although mortality was certainly adversely affected by the presence of hematoma.

Number of Subarachnoid Hemorrhages

The number of subarachnoid hemorrhages is compared to the postoperative results in Table 30. This did not seem to be a significant factor – 71.5 per cent of patients with 1 bleed, 21.7 per cent of patients with 2 bleeds, and all 3 patients with 3 bleeds made good recoveries. All of the patients, however, who presented without bleeding including those found to have minimal local hemorrhage at operation made full recoveries.

2 Internal Carotid Artery Aneurysms

Table 30 Number of bleeds related to postoperative results

No. of bleeds	Good	Fair	Poor	Death
1	94 (65.3%)	13 (76.4%)	2 (100%)	6 (60%)
2	28	4	–	3
3	3	–	–	–
4	–	–	–	1
No bleeding	9	–	–	–
(bleeding proved by exploration)	(7)	–	–	–
Asymptomatic	3	–	–	–
	144	17	2	10

Hydrocephalus

12 patients (6.9%) required ventricular shunting, 1 preoperatively (Table **31a–b**), the other 11 in the postoperative period. Hydrocephalus is related to the preoperative grade and the postoperative result in table **31b**. There is a tendency for those patients in poorer grades eventually to require a ventricular shunt. Noteworthy is the 4.2 per cent incidence of shunts in the good recovery group and the 29.4 per cent incidence in the fair recovery group.

Table 31a Shunt statistics

		Age	Sex	Condition	No of SAH	Date of operation	Side	Time	Results
1.	C	61	F	IIIb	1	1967	R	2 m	Good, POS improved
2.	Sch	66	M	IIIb	2	1970	R	pre.	Good, Hpr. improved
3.	M	50	F	IVb	2	1970	R	6 w	Fair, POS improved
4.	K	25	F	V	3 + SDH + icH	1971	R	2 m	Poor, Died 3½ ys. later
5.	Z	60	M	IIIb	1	1972	R	2 w	Good, Hpr. improved
6.	R	61	F	IV	2	1973	L	4 w	Fair, Hpr. and POS improved
7.	W	49	F	IIa	1 + icH	1974	R	4 m	Good, POS improved
8.	H	39	F	IV	1 + icH	1974	L	2 w	Fair, died 17 months later from renal Ca
9.	F	38	F	IIIb	1	1976	R	3 w	Fair, POS improved
10.	L	53	F	IV	1	1977	L	4 w	Good, POS and Hpr. improved
11.	W	68	F	IIIb	1	1976	R	2 w	Fair, Hpr. and POS improved
12.	S	60		IIIb	1	1968	R	4 w	Good, Hpr. and POS improved

Table 31b Relationship of hydrocephalus to preoperative grade and postoperative result

Condition	Good	Fair	Poor	Death	Total Shunts	Total Patients	%
I	–	–	–	–	–	57	0.0
IIa	1	–	–	–	1	56	1.8
IIb	–	–	–	–	–	18	0.0
IIIa	1	–	–	–	2	14	14.3
IIIb	3	2	–	–	4	16	25.0
IV	1	3	–	–	4	10	40.0
V	–	–	–	1	1	2	50.0
Total with hydrocephalus	6 (4.2%)	5 (29.4%)	– (0%)	1 (10.0%)	12 (6.9%)		
Total Patients	144	17	2	10		173	

Seizure Disorder

8 patients presented with a seizure disorder (4.6%). In 6 patients this was first noted in the postoperative period. 2 of these patients died. The other 4 had only transient seizures and none requires anticonvulsant medication at present. 2 patients with preexisting epilepsy are unchanged.

Timing of Operation

Of the 161 patients who sustained subarachnoid hemorrhage (Table 32), only 4 underwent operation within the first 3 days. Each of these patients was moribund in grade IV or V and none survived. 23 patients underwent operation between 3 and 7 days. Of these 16 were in grades Ia to IIa; 14 (87.5%) had a good result and the other 2 a fair result. 1 patient in grade IIIa had a good result, and of the 4 patients in grade IV there were 2 fair results, 1 poor result, and 1 death. 50 patients were operated upon between 8 and 14 days. 28 were between grades Ia and IIa and all had good results. 15 other patients in poorer grades also had good results. 4 grade IIIa and b patients died and 2 had fair results. Thus a total of 77 patients underwent operation within the first 2 weeks after subarachnoid hemorrhage. 60 of these (77.9%) made complete recoveries, 9.1% showed fair results.

84 patients underwent operation more than 2 weeks after subarachnoid hemorrhage. Of these 72 (85.7%) made complete recoveries.

Patients in poorer grades made variable recoveries. No difference is seen in outcome between patients in good condition undergoing operation in the first two weeks and those going to surgery from 2 weeks to over 3 months after subarachnoid hemorrhage.

Operation

Finally an analysis was made of the effect of the operation itself on outcome. Of 173 patients undergoing operation, 144 (83.2%) are symptom free and have had their aneurysms treated. 24 of these patients had focal neurological deficits in the preoperative period from which they have recovered. Only 1 of these 144 patients had an episode of ischemia related to operation, and she has fully recovered.

19 patients remain with some neurological deficit and 10 have died. Of the 19 patients with postoperative morbidity, 13 showed deficits preoperatively and none of these was worsened by operation. In the other 6, deficits were either first noted or were more severe after operation. 5 of these patients were in grades IIa and IIb. In 1 case the aneurysm ruptured during dissection, but bleeding was easily controlled. Nevertheless, she awakened from anesthesia with a hemiparesis which did not completely recover. A second patient had a hemisensory deficit preoperatively that increased to a hemiparesis over the first 3 days postoperatively, then began to recede but did not completely disappear. The other 3 patients had the onset of ischemic deficits 3 days, 4 days, and 7 days after operation without a clear etiology. 3 of the 5 patients suffered a cerebral infarction verified by CT scan. The sixth patient was in grade IIIb at the time of operation, but required intracranial clipping of the internal carotid artery to control bleeding during operation and remained in poor condition afterwards.

Of the 10 deaths in this series, 5 were operated upon in extremis and never improved. 3 patients died from complications directly related to operation. In 1 patient the middle cerebral artery was injured, the patient sustained a massive cerebral infarction and died 3½ years later. In a second

Table 32 Timing of surgery and results in 161 patients with ruptured aneurysm of the posterior communicating artery

	Good						Fair				Poor		Death			
	Ia	IIa	IIb	IIIa	IIIb	IV	IIa	IIb	IIIb	IV	IIIb	IV	IIIa	IIIb	IV	V
1–3 d	–	–	–	–	–	–	–	–	–	–	–	–	–	–	2	2
4–7 d	2	12	2	1	–	–	2	–	–	2	–	1	–	–	1	–
1–2 w	10	18	7	6	1	1	–	1	2	–	–	–	2	2	–	–
2–4 w	21	10	6	4	3	1	2	–	2	1	1	–	–	1	–	–
1–3 m	8	8	1	1	2	–	1	1	2	1	–	–	–	–	–	–
> 3 m	4	3	–	–	–	–	–	–	–	–	–	–	–	–	–	–
	45	51	16	12	6	2	5	2	6	4	1	1	2	3	3	2
			132					17			2			10 = 161		

patient, the neck was broad and could not be suitably fashioned to perfectly accept the clip. Muscle was placed beneath the clip, but she nevertheless sustained 2 additional subarachnoid hemorrhages from this site and died. The third patient developed an epidural hematoma postoperatively which led to tentorial herniation. 2 patients developed complications in the postoperative period. One had a lumbar drain inserted for communicating hydrocephalus. This became infected, she developed meningitis, and died. The other was doing well when she developed gastrointestinal hemorrhage from peptic ulcer disease and died at laparotomy. Thus, of 173 patients there are 6 patients in whom an increase in morbidity was observed following operation (3.5%), and 5 patients (2.9%) in whom death might have been preventable. Compared to the expected incidence of mortality and morbidity in untreated cases, these numbers seem small. Nevertheless these 11 patients challenge the surgeon to continue to perfect operative techniques that can bring this incidence closer to zero (Tables **33–35**).

Table 33 Proximal lateral wall internal carotid artery aneurysm patients – delayed recovery

Patient	Age	Sex	Year	SAH	Site	Exam	Grade	Time	Operation	Postop	Time to full recovery
1. Ph	32	F	1972	1	Right	Normal	Ia	2 m	Clip	L. hemiparesis	3 m
2. Zb	60	M	1972	1	Right r. MCA	Somnol.	IIIa	10 d	Clip	L. hemiparesis shunt 2 w, recovery	2 m
3. Fe	38	F	1976	1	Right	Somnol.	IIIa	3 w	Clip	Headache POS shunt 7 m, recovery	1 y
4. Sch	66	M	1970	2	Right	Preop. shunt l. hemip.	IIIb	6 w	Clip	Same shunt revis.	4 m
5. St	60	F	1968	I	Right	Somnol. l. hemip. Cist. Hem.	IIIb	6 w	Clip Evac Hem.	Same shunt 4 w	6 m
6. Da	38	F	1975	1	Right l. cav.	After angio obtunded r. hemip. aphasia	IV	3 w	Clip	R. hemiparesis aphasia, recovery	3 m
7. M	50	F	1970	2	Right	Obtund. l. hemip. incontin.	IV	6 w	Clip	Same shunt 3 w	1 y
8. L	53	F	1977	1	Left l. MCA	Obtund. r. hemip.	IV	4 w	Clip Clip	Same shunt 7 w	6 m

Clinical Presentation and Operative Results 97

Table 34 Posterior communicating artery aneurysms – morbidity

Patient	Age	Sex	Year	SAH	Site	Mult.	Hematoma	Grade	Time	Operation	Remarks	Results
Fair Results												
Grade II patients:												
1. Hu	41	F	1972	1	Right	–	–	IIa	17 d	Clip	Postop. hpr. part. resolved	Fair
2. Me	45	F	1972	2	Right double	+	–	IIa	3 w	Clip	Postop. hpr. part. resolved	Fair
3. Go	46	F	1972	1	Right		Intratemp.	IIa	2 m	Clip Evac. hem.	Postop. l. hpr.	Fair
4. We	49	F	1974	1	Right l. P. com. A. + AcoA	+	Large icH	IIa	7 d	Clip	Required shunt postop. POS	Fair
5. BE	41	F	1975	1	Left		–	IIa	6 d	Clip	Postop. aphasia epilepsy	Fair
6. Za	41	M	1974	1	Right	–	–	IIb	6 w	Clip	Epilepsy, Alcoholism	Fair
7. Fr	62	F	1977	1	Right		–	IIb	10 d	Clip	Preop. l. sensory defic. Postop. l. hpr.	Fair
Grade III patients:												
8. Cs.	61	F	1967	1	Right l. AchoA	+	–	IIIb	10 d	Clip	Preop. l. hpr. POS Required shunt. Selfsufficient and working now.	Fair
9. Ma	50	M	1969	1	Left	–	Cisternal	IIIb	13 d	Ligature	Inc. hpr. post-op. and aphasia. part. resolved works on farm.	Fair
10. Am	67	F	1969	1	Left	–	–	IIIb	2 w	Clip	Preop. r. hpr. and aphasia	Fair * Died 9 ms.
11. Mi	37	M	1971	1	Left l. A$_1$ l. ICB	+	–	IIIb	6 w	Clip	Alcoholism preop. r. hpr. postop. epilepsy not working	Fair
12. We	68	F	1976	1	Right	–	Intratemp. SDH, cisternal, icH	IIIb	4 w	Clip	preop. l. hpr. required shunt	Fair Died 6 ms.
13. Ga	25	F	1977	2	Left		–	IIIb	2 w	Clip	Preop. r. hpr. aphasia Postop. improved but epilepsy 11 ms.	Fair
Grade IV patients:												
14. Mü	50	F	1970	2	Right	+	Cisternal	IV	6 w	Clip	preop. hpr. incontinence and POS. Postop. required shunt. Working 50%	Fair
15. Ke	37	F	1970	1	Left		–	IV	7 d	Clip	Preop. r. hpr. aphasia, Postop. improved	Fair

Continuation Table 34 p. 98

Table 34 (Continuation) Posterior communicating artery aneurysms – morbidity

Patient	Age	Sex	Year	SAH	Site	Mult.	Hematoma	Grade	Time	Operation	Remarks	Results
16. Re	61	F	1973	1	Left	–	–	IV	4 w	Clip	Preop. hpr. and aphasia required shunt	Fair
17. Ca	50	M	1976	1	Left		Intratemp.	IV	6 d	Clip Evac. hem.	Preop. r. hemiplegia, aphasia Postop. improved	Fair
Poor results												
18. Me	53	F	1967	1	Left	–	Cisternal	IIIb	4 w	Intracr. trapping	Incr. hpr. aphasia postop.	Poor
19. Mü	40	F.	1970	1	Left	–	Cisternal	IV	7 d	Clip	Preop. r. hpr. aphasia	Poor

Table 35 Proximal lateral wall internal carotid artery aneurysm patients – mortality

Patient	Age	Sex	Year	SAH	Site	Hematoma	Grade	Time	Operation	Remarks	Death
1. R	65	F	1968	1	Right	–	IIIa	3 w	Clip	Right MCA injured EIA, demented, left hemiparetic	3½ y
2. De	64	M	1968	1	Right	Cisternal	IIIa	2 w	Clip	Epidural hematoma	3 w
3. H	46	F	1969	1	Right	–	IIIb	2 w	Clip	Rerupture of aneurysm – 1 m.	6 w
4. St	48	F	1975	1	Right	Cisternal Intracer.	IIIb	3 w	Clip Evac. hem.	Diabetes, hypertension, lumbar drain infected with E. Coli-meningitis	2 w
5. Fr	43	F	1977	1	Left	Subdural Cisternal Intracer.	IIIb	10 d	Clip Evac. hem.	Preop. hemiparesis, hypertens. bleeding duodenal ulcer – 2 abdominal operations	3 w
6. Mi	47	F	1967	2	Left	Subdural Cisternal Intratemp.	IV	1 d	Clip Evac. hem.	Remained in coma preop. hypertension	2 d
7. St	56	M	1974	2	Left	Subdural Cisternal Intratemp.	IV	1 d	Clip Evac. hem.	Remained in poor condition	4 w
8. H	39	F	1974	1	Right	Subdural Intratemp.	IV	5 d	Clip Evac. hem.	Reexplored – Cerebral edema. Required shunt	17 m
9. M	53	F	1968	2	Right	Subdural Cisternal Intratemp.	V	1 d	Clip Evac. hem.	Remained in coma preop. hypertension	10 w
10. K	25	F	1971	4	Right	Subdural	V	1 d	Clip Evac. hem.	Required shunt, remained in coma 2½ years	2½ y

Anterior Choroidal Artery Aneurysms

Anatomical Relationships

Incidence

21 patients had ruptured aneurysms arising from the internal carotid artery at the origin of the anterior choroidal artery, comprising 6.6 per cent of the patients with internal carotid artery aneurysms and 2.1 per cent of the entire series. 10 aneurysms were on the right internal carotid artery and 11 on the left (see Table **40**).

Relationship to the Anterior Choroidal Artery

In about 70 per cent of cases, the anterior choroidal artery arises as a single trunk from the internal carotid artery and branches into a smaller group of arteries that go to the adjacent uncus and a single larger artery, that supplies the optic tract, diencephalon, and cerebral peduncle before entering the choroidal fissure to supply the choroid plexus. Branching may occur early or not until the artery is well within the crural cistern. In the other 30 per cent of cases there will be 2 or 3 or even 4 branches from the internal carotid artery. In these instances the larger branch usually originates proximally and follows the principal course of the anterior choroidal artery into the crural cistern, while the smaller branches go to the mediobasal portion of the temporal pole, especially the uncus. The anterior choroidal artery was never found to originate from the middle cerebral artery.

An aneurysm may arise in conjunction with any of the branches. The location of the aneurysm in relation to the internal carotid and anterior choroidal arteries in the present 21 cases is shown in Fig **45**. It should be noted that it was only very rarely possible to distinguish anterior choroidal aneurysms from posterior communicating aneurysms angiographically.

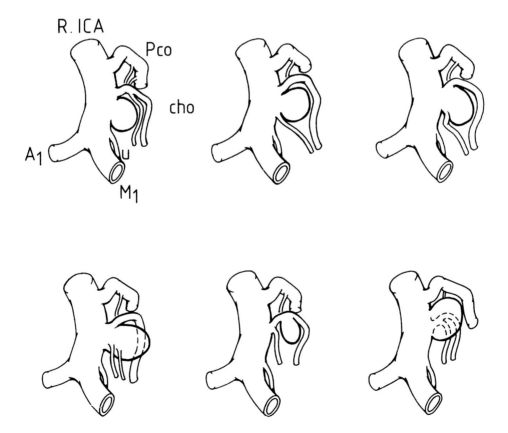

Fig **45** Schematic representation of distal lateral wall and true anterior choroidal aneurysms as related to the anterior choroidal artery and uncal artery.

Relationship to the Uncus and Tentorium

As these aneurysms project supero-, postero- and inferolaterally they are in intimate relationship with the mesial temporal lobe and are not infrequently partially buried in the uncus. Some small resection (1 × 1 cm) of mesobasal temporal lobe may be required to expose the aneurysm and the anterior choroidal artery branches. The aneurysms generally lie above the tentorium and are away from the oculomotor nerve, which lies deeper in the interpeduncular cistern at this point, but in 6 cases the fundus of the aneurysm was adherent to the oculomotor nerve.

Multiple and Bilateral Aneurysms

Of these 21 patients with aneurysms at the origin of the anterior choroidal artery, 11 (55%) had one or more additional aneurysms (Table **36a–b**). One patient had bilateral aneurysms of the internal carotid at the anterior choroidal artery. In this patient a left sided pterional approach was used to clip the left aneurysm first, then the right sided aneurysm was approached between the left and right optic nerves. It was possible in this case to reach the aneurysm and clip it because the fundus was hanging down (Fig **46A–C**). In 2 patients with ruptured aneurysms of PcoA there was an additional aneurysm proximal to the origin of anterior choroidal artery, a so-called "kissing aneurysm". The dissection and clipping of these aneurysms is very challenging (see Fig **44**).

Table **36a** Multiple and bilateral aneurysms (11 cases)

Side	No. of cases		Opposite AchoA	PcoA	ICB	M_1	MCB	AcoA	Total
Left	6	Micro	–	1	–	–	–	–	1
		Macro	–	2	2	–	–	–	4
Right	5	Micro	–	1	2	1	–	1	5
		Macro	1	–	1	–	1	1	4
	11		1	4	5	1	1	2	14

Table **36b**

		No. of Aneurysm
Single aneurysm	10 patients	10
1 additional aneurysm	9 patients	18
2 additional aneurysms	1 patient	3
3 additional aneurysms	1 patient	4
	21	35

Anatomical Relationships 101

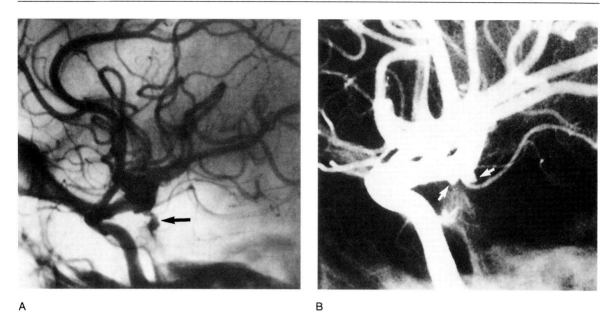

Fig **46A–C** Bilateral anterior choroidal artery aneurysms (arrows) demonstrated on left (**A**) and right (**B**) carotid angiography.

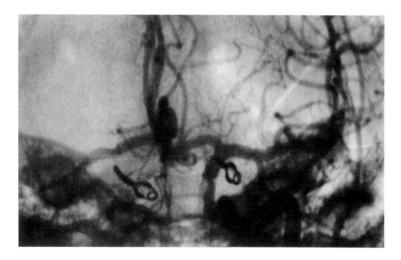

C Both aneurysms were approached from a single left pterional approach (the left sided aneurysm had ruptured) and were clipped as shown on post-operative angiography (Case 17, Table **40**).

9 patients had an additional aneurysm at the carotid bifurcation (2), posterior communicating (2), middle cerebral (2), or anterior communicating (1) arteries. One patient had 2 additional aneurysms (carotid bifurcation and anterior communicating) and one patient had 3 other aneurysms (bilateral carotid bifurcation and posterior communicating). Thus a total of 35 (21 anterior choroidal plus 14 additional) aneurysms were seen in this group. All of the anterior choroidal and 8 of the additional macroaneurysms were clipped while 5 microaneurysms were wrapped with muscle.

In addition to this group of ruptured anterior choroidal aneurysms, 35 cases of unruptured aneurysms of the anterior choroidal artery were found (and clipped in 14 cases) during procedures for symptomatic aneurysms at other locations. A further 21 microaneurysms at the origin of anterior choroidal artery were coagulated and wrapped (see Table **129**).

Operative Technique

Initial Exposure

A standard fronto-temporosphenoidal craniotomy is performed. The carotid and interpeduncular cisterns are opened to release spinal fluid and to gain control of the internal carotid artery proximal to the aneurysm. The proximal Sylvian cistern is opened toward the internal carotid artery bifurcation. If the aneurysm fundus is directed laterally into the temporal lobe, dissection may be continued across the bifurcation, releasing the arachnoid fibers across the origins of the anterior and middle cerebral arteries. If the fundus is directed superiorly into the area of the internal carotid artery bifurcation, dissection in this area should be deferred.

The lamina terminalis cistern is next opened over the anterior cerebral – anterior communicating complex to allow the orbital surface of the frontal lobe to fall away from the basal cisterns, and to evaluate collateral circulation through the anterior communicating artery. It is especially important with these aneurysms that retraction pressure on the frontal lobe not be transmitted to the aneurysm dome buried in the temporal lobe. Therefore, no retraction of the temporal lobe should be used initially, and retraction on the frontal lobe should be minimized until the arachnoid attachments between the frontal and temporal lobes have been severed.

Dissection of the Carotid Cistern

The posterior communicating artery is identified and its relationship to the aneurysm noted. If not enough internal carotid artery can be exposed between the posterior communicating artery and the aneurysm to allow placement of a temporary clip, the first few millimeters of posterior communicating artery should be dissected free so that in the event of premature rupture, bleeding could be controlled with temporary clips proximal on the internal carotid artery and on the posterior communicating artery. The oculomotor nerve is noted beneath the posterior communicating artery and its course beneath the aneurysm deduced.

The area of the internal carotid artery bifurcation is next examined. Depending on the size of the aneurysm, it may involve the origin of the middle cerebral, anterior temporal, or medial striate arteries. Branches of the anterior choroidal artery are sought in the area of the internal carotid artery bifurcation. They are seen emerging beneath the bifurcation of the ICA or beneath the origins of the anterior or middle cerebral arteries. These branches are dissected to define the course of the anterior choroidal artery.

Dissection of the Aneurysm Neck

With exposure of the internal carotid artery bifurcation above the aneurysm and the internal carotid and posterior communicating arteries proximal to the aneurysm, the anterior choroidal artery is next freed from the neck of the aneurysm. The neck of the aneurysm may overlie the anterior choroidal artery, and an incision into the mesiobasal temporal lobe will be required to adequately define the anterior choroidal artery and its relationship to the neck of the aneurysm. The pia around the aneurysm is opened with bipolar coagulation and 5–6 mm of cortex aspirated with gentle suction. The pia and any hematoma directly attached to the aneurysm fundus are left undisturbed. The anterior choroidal artery is identified in the crural cistern and followed back to its origin, freeing it from the aneurysm. It must be remembered that there may be more than one origin of the anterior choroidal artery. The arachnoid is separated until there are a few millimeters on either side of the aneurysm neck to allow placement of a clip.

Clip Application

A clip is slowly introduced over the neck of the aneurysm with the proximal blade passing between the anterior choroidal artery and the base of the aneurysm, and the distal blade sliding close to the aneurysm neck. While the clip is being allowed to close, the surgeon inspects the aneurysm and internal carotid artery to check for kinking or distortion. Broad or irregular necks usually require bipolar coagulation, or other methods to reduce the size of the neck as previously described. Following clip application the aneurysm is punctured and the collapsed sac mobilized. The AchoA and its branches are then inspected and their condition checked.

The fundus may be collapsed down or cut and then coagulated until the aneurysm is fully shrunken and there are no bulging parts left. In this stage the final clip can be applied. Any remaining hematoma is removed and hemostasis assured. Papaverine and periadventitial sympathectomy of the superior surface of major arteries is carried out, and the wound closed.

Summary

The steps in treating an aneurysm near the origin of the anterior choroidal artery include:
1) Frontotemporosphenoidal craniotomy,
2) Opening the carotid cistern to gain control of the internal carotid artery,
3) Opening the Sylvian cistern to come to the internal carotid artery bifurcation,
4) Opening the lamina terminalis cistern for better relaxation of the frontal lobe,
5) Identification of the PcoA and its branches and the possible variations (2 PcoA),
6) Idenfitication of the oculomotor nerve,
7) Inspection of the internal carotid artery bifurcation,
8) Identification of the anterior choroidal artery and its variations,
9) Cortical resection of the uncus if necessary,
10) Dissection of the aneurysm neck,
11) Clip application, coagulation, and clip reapplication after full shrinkage of the sac,
12) Application of papaverine and local sympathectomy,
13) Closure.

Clinical Presentation and Operative Results

Background

Previous publications concerning aneurysms of the internal carotid-anterior choroidal artery include Pertuiset et al. (1962), Otomo (1965), Drake et al. (1968a), Perria et al. (1971), and Viale and Pau (1979). Results have varied considerably with Drake et al. reporting a 43 per cent mortality and 14 per cent morbidity. Perria et al. a 10 per cent mortality and no morbidity, and Viale no mortality, but a 28 per cent morbidity. Suzuki et al. (1979) did not observe any cases of AchoA aneurysms in the series of 1,000 patients with intracranial aneurysms.

Presenting Features

In the present series of 21 patients, 10 were men and 11 women. Ages ranged from 25 to 64, with 9 of 21 patients (42.9%) under the age of 40. This is a somewhat younger group than that seen with internal carotid-posterior communicating artery aneurysms (Table 37a–b). All patients had sustained a subarachnoid hemorrhage, but it was determined in one man that the hemorrhage had been a hypertensive type and his aneurysm had not ruptured. 4 patients presented with hemiparesis and 2 of these with a right hemiparesis were also aphasic.

Table 37a Age and sex in 21 patients with aneurysms of the distal lateral wall of the internal carotid artery

Age	Male	Female	Total
21–30	2	1	3
31–40	3	3	6
41–50	3	4	7
51–60	2	2	4
61–70	–	1	1
	10 (47.6)	11 (52.3%)	21 (100%)

Table 37b Site and sex

Right	10	7 F / 3 M
Left	11	4 F / 7 M

Operative Results

Operative results are related to preoperative grade in Table **38**. 16 patients were discharged in good condition (76.2%), and they all have returned to regular work. One patient (No. 7) had a left hemiparesis preoperatively which improved only slightly after surgery and shunting. Another patient (No. 20) was in grade IIIb prior to operation with a right hemiparesis and aphasia. Computerized tomography showed a temporal hematoma. Postoperatively he improved over 2 years to a fair condition. He is now working part time with a mild right hemiparesis and aphasia. The one poor result was also grade IIIb prior to operation. This patient demonstrated left sided weakness but this was increased postoperatively and angiography showed that the anterior choroidal artery had been lost at operation (see Table **40**, No. 3). He remains with a severe left hemiparesis and memory deficit and is not self-sufficient (Fig **47A–D**).

2 patients in this group died (9.5%). One patient (No. 9) entered the hospital in grade IIIa but following angiography became semicomatose with a right hemiplegia and probable aphasia (grade IV). At operation the brain was markedly swollen. The aneurysm of the left anterior choroidal artery could be clipped but the bone flap was not replaced. She failed to recover from anesthesia and died 6 weeks later. Autopsy later confirmed a massive infarct of the left hemisphere.

A final patient (case 14), a 37 year old hypertensive, sustained an intracerebral hemorrhage and was found to have a right ICA – AchoA aneurysm (1975). CT scan had not then been implemented in Zurich. He underwent operation in grade 0a and the unruptured aneurysm was clipped without difficulty. In the postoperative period, he lapsed into coma with a left hemiparesis and at reexploration was found to have both old and new intracerebral hematomas in the area of the caudate nucleus with no apparent connection to the subarachnoid space. He went on to die and at autopsy no cause for the intracerebral hematoma was found.

Apart from this 1 patient who apparently died of causes unrelated to his aneurysm, patients in grades Ia to IIb have done well. 2 patients with preoperative deficits have not fully recovered, and 1 with a massive left cerebral infarct died. The 1 patient who was made worse by operation and remains in poor condition had occlusion of the anterior choroidal artery, demonstrating the importance of preserving this artery in treating aneurysms at this location.

Table 38 Preoperative condition and operative results

Grade	Total No.	Good	Fair	Poor	Death
0a	1	–	–	–	1
Ia	6	6	–	–	–
IIa	8	8	–	–	–
IIb	1	–	1	–	–
IIIa	2	2	–	–	–
IIIb	2	–	1	1	–
IV	1	–	–	–	1
	21	16	2	1	2
		76.2%	9.5%	4.8%	9.5%

Clinical Presentation and Operative Results 105

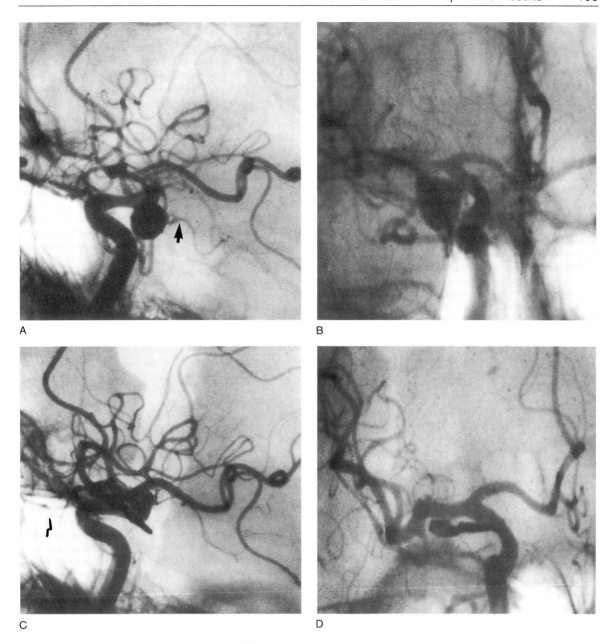

Fig **47A–D** Right carotid angiography (**A** and **B**) showing a lateral wall carotid aneurysm (arrow) that was thought to be proximal (posterior communicating). At operation the aneurysm was believed to be on the posterior communicating artery. Following inadequate dissection it was clipped, unfortunately including the anterior choroidal artery in the clip (**C** and **D**) and resulting in a markedly impaired patient (1971) (Case 3, Table **40**).

Operative Timing

Of the 20 ruptured aneurysms in this group, 9 were operated upon within the first 2 weeks (Table 39). 7 patients (78%) had good results. 1 patient (grade IIIb) suffered a poor result due to occlusion of the anterior choroidal artery, and 1 patient (grade IV) died of massive cerebral infarction. 11 patients were operated upon after the first 2 weeks with good results in 9 (82%). The other 2 patients had fair results with persisting preoperative deficits. As with other groups, no relationship between operative results and surgical timing are evident. Good grade patients and poor grade patients with hematomas should be operated upon early. Surgery is delayed only in poor grade patients without mass-producing hematomas.

Table 39 Timing of surgery and results in 20 patients with ruptured aneurysm of the anterior choroidal artery

	Good			Fair		Poor	Death	
	Ia	IIa	IIIa	IIb	IIIb	IIIb	IV	
1–3 d	–	1	1	–	–	–	–	
4–7 d	2	2	1	–	–	–	1	
1–2 w	–	–	–	–	–	1	–	
2–4 w	2	5	–	–	–	–	–	
1–3 m	2	–	–	–	–	–	–	
> 3 m	–	–	–	1	1	–	–	
	6	8	2	1	1	1	1	= 20

Summary

21 cases (Table 40) of internal carotid-anterior choroidal artery aneurysms were operated upon with good results in 16 (76.2%) and with 2 deaths (9.5%). The 1 poor result was related to occlusion of the anterior choroidal artery by the clip with resultant infarction. Two anatomical principles require recognition by the surgeon approaching these lesions. First the anterior choroidal artery is frequently doubled or tripled (30%). The relationship of the aneurysm to each vessel must be recognized to avoid occlusion and subsequent infarction. Second, in most cases only a presumptive localization of the aneurysm in respect to its anatomic relationship to the anterior choroidal and posterior communicating arteries can be gained on angiography. The precise definition of aneurysmal topography in this circumstance is often only revealed at operation (Figs **48A–C, 49A–B**).

Summary 107

Fig **48A–C** Aneurysm arising between the anterior choroidal and uncus arteries (arrows) (**A** and **B**). The operative procedure is shown in (**C**).

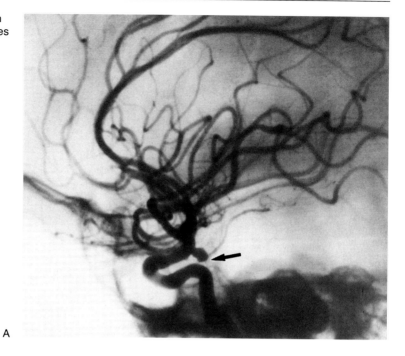

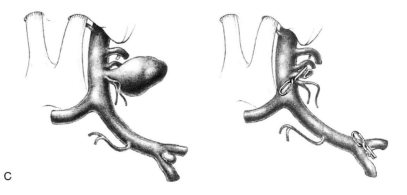

2 Internal Carotid Artery Aneurysms

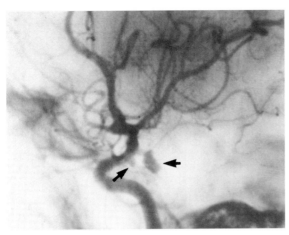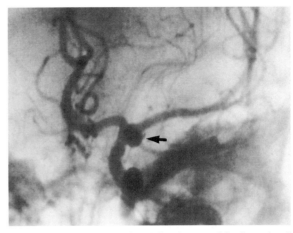

Fig 49A–B Left carotid angiography showing two aneurysms (arrows) of both proximal and distal parts of the lateral wall (**A** and **B**). The distal aneurysm had ruptured. Notice the azygous A_2 segment.

Table 40 Anterior choridal artery aneurysms

Name	Age Sex	Side	Condition	Interval before surgery	Other aneurysms	Date	Operation	Results
1. Gl	50 F	R	IIa	21 ds	–	30 March 1967	Clipped	Good
2. Fl	26 F	L	Ia	7 ds	–	15 Dec. 1967	Clipped	Good
3. Hä	51 M	R	IIIb, hpr. temp. + ventricular hematomas	9 ds	Micr: int. carot.-bifur.	19 Febr. 1971	Clipped/Biobond accidentally also AchoA clipped	Poor; hpr, POS Hydroceph.-shunt
4. Be	35 M	L	Ia	4 ws	–	9 Oct. 1972	Clipped	Good
5. Le	39 M	L	Ia	4 ms	–	23 Febr. 1973	Clipped	Good
6. Ap	46 F	R	IIa	7 ds	–	23 Nov. 1973	Clipped	Good
7. Br	51 F	R	IIb lt. hpr	5 ms	Micr: int. carot.-Bif P co A	13 Febr. 1975	Clipped/muscle/ clipped	Fair, hydroceph.-shunt
8. Be	64 M	L	IIa	27 ds	Micr: P co A	28 Febr. 1975	Clipped	Good
9. Ma	56 F	L	IV rt. hpr aphasia	8 ds	Carot. bif. rt. Micro: car. bif.lt./P co A rt.	23 Febr. 1976	Clipped/clipped, both from left side	Death, 6 weeks
10. Pa	44 F	R	Ia	3 ms	–	13 July 1976	Clipping of partially thrombosed large	Good
11. Gr	61 F	L	IIa	21 ds	P co A lt.	23 Sept. 1976	Clipped/clipped	Good
12. Pa	33 F	R	IIIa	5 ds	Middle cer.-bifurcation	16 June 1977	Clipped/clipped	Good, hydroceph.-shunt
13. Me	39 F	R	IIIa, temp. icH, ivH	3 ds	A co A	14 Sept. 1977	Clipped/clipped evacuation of hematomas	Good
14. Ka	37 M	R	Oa	5 ws	Micr: ant. temp. art.	12 June 1975	Clipped, post-operative i.c.H., reoperation	Death, 3 weeks
15. Yü	25 M	L	Ia	3 ws	Int. carot. bifurc. lt.	30 Sept. 1977	Clipped/clipped	Good (surgeon, fully working)
16. Mi	48 F	R	IIa	2 ws	–	16 Nov. 1977	Clipped	Good
17. Hö	33 F	L	IIa	7 ds	A cho A rt.	13 Febr. 1978	Clipped/clipped from left side	Good
18. No	45 M	L	IIa	1 m	P co A lt.	23 Febr. 1978	Clipped/clipped	Good
19. He	30 M	R	Ia	7 ds	–	2 May 1978	Clipped	Good
20. La	50 M	L	IIIb, Hpr. aphasia CT: lesion Infarct. and icH	2 ms	–	3 May 1978	Clipped, evacuation of hematoma	Moderate, fair as before
21. Fä	45 M	L	IIa	1 d	–	25 June 1979	Clipped	Good

Aneurysms of Internal Carotid Artery Bifurcation (ICBi-Aneurysms)

Anatomical Relationships

Incidence, Laterality

Bull (1962) in a study of 1769 aneurysms collected by McKissock over a period of eleven years, found 110 such cases (6.2%). Locksley (1966) found 118 (4.43%) of these aneurysms out of a total of 2659 intracranial aneurysms. Perria et al. (1968) found ICBi-An in 9%. Lassman (1979) reported 20 cases (7.1%) out of a series of 281 intracranial aneurysms. Suzuki (see Kodama et al. 1979) reported 29 cases (2.9%) out of a series of 1,000 intracranial aneurysms.

In the present series, 55 patients presented with symptomatic aneurysms of the internal carotid artery bifurcation, representing 17.2 per cent of internal carotid artery aneurysms and 5.4 per cent of all patients in the series (see Table 45). In 29 cases (52.7%) the aneurysm arose from the left internal carotid artery and in 26 cases (47.3%) from the right (see Table 41).

Size and Direction of Fundus

Aneurysms at this location varied in size from a small lesion of only 3 millimeters, (that had bled), to a truly giant aneurysm (Fig 50). There were 4 cases of giant aneurysm greater than 25 mm and none of these had ruptured. 2 of these were subtotally thrombosed.

These aneurysms can be quite broad-based. They usually sit more on the middle cerebral or anterior cerebral artery, although a specific relationship to the size of the arteries was not recorded. There are 3 general directions of fundus projection.
1) *Superiorly* into the lateral fronto-orbital gyrus or the base of the olfactory tracts,
2) *Posteriorly* into the anterior perforated substance, the lateral portion of the lamina terminalis cistern, or the Sylvian cistern,
3) *Inferiorly* into the carotid and interpeduncular, or even the ambient and crural cisterns (if a large aneurysm is more inferolaterally directed).

Relationship to Subarachnoid Cisterns

Around the internal carotid artery bifurcation is the point of convergence for several of the cisterns of the anterior and middle fossa. The aneurysms will initially be covered by the arachnoid of the carotid, olfactory, lamina terminalis, and Sylvian cisterns to a varying degree depending on the exact position of the aneurysm on the bifurcation. As the aneurysm encroaches on the Sylvian and lamina terminalis cisterns, the middle and anterior cerebral arteries will be compressed and their perforating branches will be displaced around the enlarging fundus.

Growth in a posterior direction will come to involve the crural and interpeduncular cisterns and particularly the diencephalic branches of the anterior choroidal and posterior communicating arteries. Strict attention to the cisternal boundaries will orient the surgeon to the proper planes of dissection.

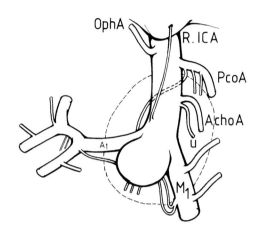

Fig 50 Schematic representation of carotid bifurcation aneurysms and their relationship to surrounding vessels as they grow.

Arterial Relationships

There are 10 arteries or groups of arteries (Fig 50) which must be identified prior to coagulation or clipping of an aneurysm at the internal carotid artery bifurcation:
1) Internal carotid artery,
2) Anterior cerebral artery,
3) Middle cerebral artery,
4) Perforating arteries from proximal anterior cerebral artery,
5) Recurrent artery of Heubner,
6) Medial striate arteries from proximal middle cerebral artery,
7) Lateral striate arteries (lenticulostriate arteries,

8) Temporal branches of middle cerebral artery,
9) Anterior choroidal artery and branches,
10) Diencephalic branches of the posterior communicating artery.

Generally, with growth of an aneurysm the middle cerebral artery will be displaced laterally and the anterior cerebral artery medially. However, the arteries may be displaced inferiorly or superiorly, depending on the direction of growth of the fundus. Because the arteries are bound by their cisternal walls, a large aneurysm may compress the origin of one or both of these arteries (Fig **51A–D**).

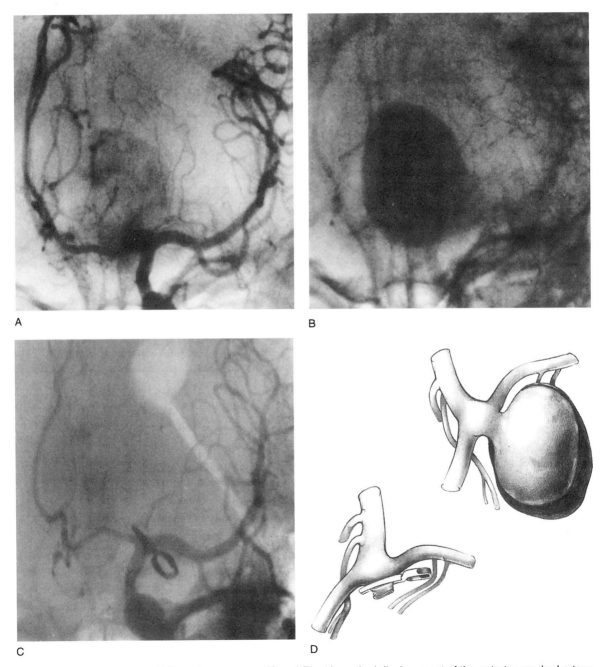

Fig **51A–D** Giant left carotid bifurcation aneurysm (**A** and **B**) with marked displacement of the anterior cerebral artery. This partially thrombosed lesion had a narrow neck and was clipped (**C**) with good results (Case 27, Table **45**). The operative procedure is shown in (**D**).

Perforating arteries including the striate groups, the recurrent artery of Heubner, and branches of the anterior choroidal and posterior communicating arteries are usually found on the posterior wall of the aneurysm. Striate arteries run a recurrent course and their origins may be further from the neck of the aneurysm than is at first apparent (Figs 52–54). An artery running directly beneath the internal carotid artery bifurcation is generally a branch of the anterior choroidal artery. Thalamoperforating arteries converge medially to penetrate the diencephalon and are, therefore, on the posteromedial aspect of the aneurysm when the lesion has extended into the interpeduncular cistern. Temporal arteries are involved with those large bifurcation aneurysms which grow into the Sylvian fissure. Arterial relationships are shown in Fig 50.

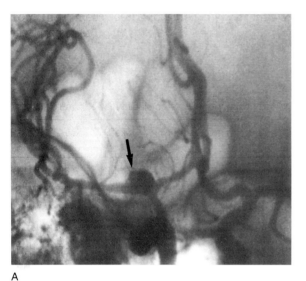

A

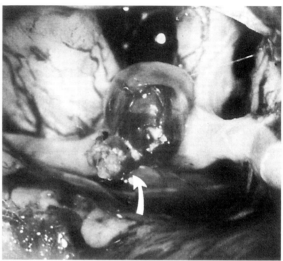

B

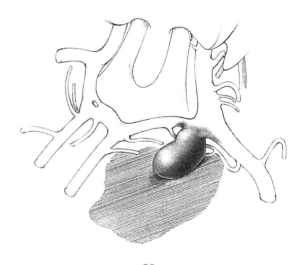

C

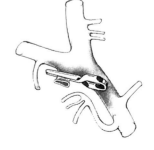

D

Fig 52A–D Right carotid bifurcation aneurysm (arrow) (**A**). As seen at surgery after bipolar coagulation of the posteriorly directed ruptured fundus (arrow) before (**B**) and after (**C**) final clipping. The aneurysm and local hematoma are pictured in (**D**) (Case 47, Table **45**).

2 Internal Carotid Artery Aneurysms

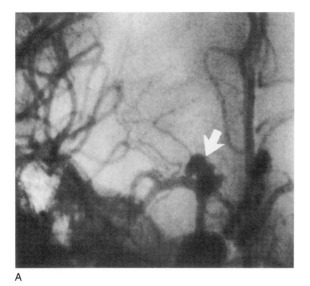
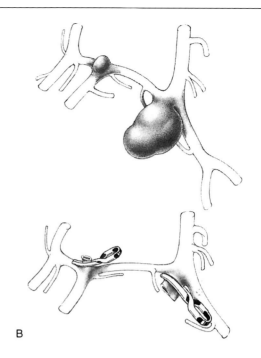

Fig **53A–B** The relationship between a right carotid bifurcation aneurysm and medial and lateral striate vessels on angiography (**A**) and at surgery (**B**) (Case 46, Table **45**).

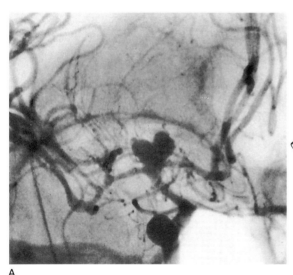
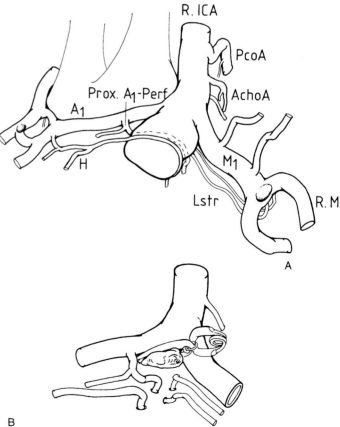

Fig **54A–B** Angiographic (**A**) and schematic (**B**) example of the close relationship between a carotid bifurcation aneurysm and perforating vessels including both Heubners' (H) and striate (Lstr) arteries from A_1 and M_1 (Case 48, Table **45**).

Venous Relationships

The area of the internal carotid artery bifurcation is also the point of convergence of much of the anterior and Sylvian venous system. Superficial middle and anterior cerebral veins may run over or under an aneurysm at the internal carotid artery bifurcation to reach the sphenoparietal or cavernous sinuses. The deep venous system, including the anterior and deep middle cerebral veins and the basal vein of Rosenthal, is on the inferior side of an aneurysm at this location.

Operative Technique

Initial Exposure

The aneurysm is approached through a pterional craniotomy. With the dura retracted and fixed anteriorly over the orbit, the laterobasal frontal lobe is retracted just enough to expose the carotid cistern which is opened. The small artery running from the internal carotid artery to the dura of the anterior clinoid process is coagulated and divided. The origins of the posterior communicating and anterior choroidal arteries are identified, and consideration given to where a temporary clip might be placed if premature rupture of the aneurysm occurs, or if a giant aneurysm must be decompressed before clipping. In such a case, ideally a clip should be placed distal to the anterior choroidal artery so that its perfusion is not compromised.

The course of the posterior communicating and of the anterior choroidal arteries is determined and the relationship of branches to the fundus of the aneurysm noted. With small aneurysms these branches will usually be free, but they may be involved with large or giant lesions. If the brain is tight, the interpeduncular cistern between the internal carotid artery and optic nerve or even the lamina terminalis may be opened to release cerebrospinal fluid.

Dissection of the Sylvian Fissure

The proximal Sylvian cistern is opened on the frontal side of the superficial middle cerebral veins, and dissection proceeds proximally toward the internal carotid artery bifurcation, with identification of the lenticulostriate and medial striate arteries. The fundus of the aneurysm is often adherent to, or buried in, the orbitobasal frontal lobe, and retraction of the frontal lobe must be minimal during this dissection. Temporopolar and anterior temporal arteries should be mobilized over a few millimeters, so that they will not be torn on retraction. The size and direction of the aneurysm fundus will determine how far proximally dissection on the middle cerebral artery may proceed.

Dissection of the Lamina Terminalis Cistern

The anterior cerebral arteries are exposed by opening the lamina terminalis cistern medially and crossing the mid-line to the opposite side. Then one can proceed proximally along the anterior cerebral artery toward the bifurcation. It is important for 3 reasons that the lamina terminalis cistern be adequately opened:

1) Retraction of the laterobasal frontal lobe will stretch bands of arachnoid across the anterior cerebral artery compromising its flow, and may transmit tension to the aneurysm fundus.
2) Perforating arteries and the recurrent artery of Heubner need to be identified prior to clipping the aneurysm.
3) The aneurysm may arise more towards the anterior cerebral or more towards the midddle cerebral artery side of the bifurcation and a decision may have to be made whether to sacrifice the origin of the anterior cerebral artery to adequately clip the aneurysm if an avulsion occurs (in 1 case in the present series). The relative sizes of the two A_1 segments and circulation through the anterior communicating artery will dictate the feasibility of this maneuver, and this should be assessed at the operating table.

The recurrent artery of Heubner is identified near the anterior communicating artery, and this artery is followed distally. It will generally lie within the lamina terminalis cistern posterior to the anterior cerebral artery. It may loop beneath the anterior cerebral artery, however, and be hidden behind the aneurysm. With dissection laterally, the medial striate perforating arteries, especially one good sized vessel, are identified and dissected from the neck of the aneurysm. Arachnoid adhesions between the aneurysm neck and the anterior cerebral artery itself are opened. The operating microscope is very helpful in delineating the extent of involvement of the aneurysm with the parent artery. The optic tract may abut the aneurysm fundus, and this should be separated from the wall of the aneurysm and from the anterior cerebral artery by inserting a small cottonoid sponge to displace the tract medially. If hematoma is present in the orbitobasal frontal lobe the pia should be incised and hematoma gently sucked away from the aneurysm to create additional operating space.

Dissection beneath the Bifurcation

With the middle cerebral artery and the anterior cerebral artery and their branches freed from the aneurysm, it still remains to inspect the posteroinferior wall of the aneurysm prior to applying a clip. The surgeon should identify the recurrent artery of Heubner, lenticulostriate arteries, the diencephalic arteries arising from the posterior communicating artery and the branches of the anterior choroidal artery as well as the deep venous system, particularly the vein of Rosenthal. As the overlying aneurysm hides this area the neck of the aneurysm must be retracted first to one side then to the other with a fine suction tip to allow a view of these structures. Following application of a temporary clip, puncture and collapse of the sac, this area can again be inspected.

Occasionally, the sac of the aneurysm may be partially or fully buried in the frontoorbital lobe. The pia will then be opened around the aneurysm dome and a few millimeters of subpial tissue resected. Freeing the aneurysm from the frontoorbital area will release tension on the aneurysm precipitated either by retraction of the frontal lobe or dissection or clipping of the aneurysm neck. In these cases retraction of the frontal lobe should be avoided or kept to a minimum.

Ligature and Clip Application

Between 1967 and 1970 the technique of applying a silk ligature around the neck of the aneurysm was utilized in 5 cases. Later the application of a clip to the neck of the aneurysm in 49 of 50 cases was possible. In most of these cases however, it was necessary to shrink the neck with bipolar coagulation before and after clipping as the neck tends to be broadbased with aneurysms at this location (see Fig **55A–C**). The clip is generally best introduced downward across the neck of the aneurysm, slowly wiggling the blades between the neck of the aneurysm and the anterior and middle cerebral arteries and their branches. As the clip is slowly closed, these arteries are inspected for kinking, twisting, and compromised flow. If temporary clips are applied to allow removal of atheroma and thrombus, an attempt should be made to place them proximal to the perforating arteries of the anterior and middle cerebral arteries, and distal to the anterior choroidal artery on the internal carotid artery. This will preserve flow in these smaller arteries.

In 1 case, the anterior cerebral artery was avulsed from its origin during dissection. A clip could be placed across the neck of the aneurysm to include

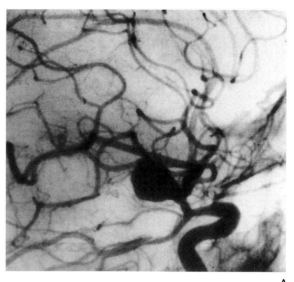

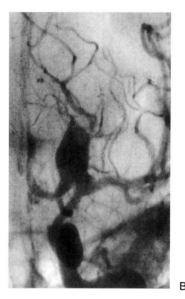

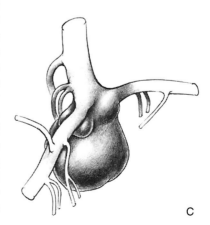

Fig **55A–C** Left carotid bifurcation aneurysm (**A** and **B**) intimately related to branches of the anterior choroidal artery (**C**) (Case 32, Table **45**).

the origin of the anterior cerebral artery and maintain satisfactory flow to the middle cerebral artery. A second clip was placed on the A_1 segment proximal to the medial striate perforating arteries. Good cross-filling through the anterior communicating artery was present.

In 5 cases the aneurysm was treated with a silk ligature. The ligature was passed beneath the internal carotid artery and the ends brought out beneath the anterior and middle cerebral arteries and between the perforating arteries and the neck of the aneurysm. As a result the knot could be tied on top of the aneurysm.

In 1 further case, a giant partially thrombosed aneurysm at the internal carotid artery bifurcation was associated with a contralateral hemiparesis. Following angiography there was spontaneous total thrombosis of the aneurysm and the ipsilateral internal carotid artery. Only a superficial temporal artery-middle cerebral artery anastomosis was performed in this case. (This case is discussed in Chapter 5, Vol. 1, Fig **252**.)

Fundus Resection and Closure

Following application of the clip, the fundus is punctured and the collapsed sac mobilized, coagulated, transsected, and removed. It is important to inspect the tips of the clip to be sure that they have not caught branches of the anterior choroidal or posterior communicating artery, and that the blades of the clip have completely crossed the neck of the aneurysm. Part of the fundus will often bulge inferiorly and escape the blades of the clip. This will require sealing the cut edges of the aneurysm by coagulation and delivering the remaining portion of aneurysm into the clip. This maneuver is repeated until the entire aneurysm is eliminated. In one case (No. 36) from the present series, a patient developed a new aneurysm at the site of a previously clipped internal carotid artery bifurcation aneurysm. As a result the staging technique of coagulation and reapplication of clips was developed.

Hematoma is removed from the cisterns and any additional hematoma in the frontal lobe is also removed. Papaverine is applied to the major arteries and a periadventitial sympathectomy carried out. With good hemostasis the wound is closed.

Summary

In summary, steps in the operative treatment of an aneurysm at the internal carotid artery bifurcation include the following:
1) Frontotemporosphenoidal craniotomy,
2) Opening the carotid cistern to gain control of the internal carotid artery,
3) Opening the Sylvian cistern and dissection of the middle cerebral artery and its branches,
4) Identification of the posterior communicating artery and its branches,
5) Identification of the anterior choroidal artery and its branches,
6) Opening the lamina terminalis cistern and dissection of the anterior cerebral arteries,
7) Identification and dissection of the recurrent artery of Heubner,
8) Protection of the optic tract,
9) Identification of the diencephalic arteries, anterior choroidal artery, and deep venous system beneath the bifurcation,
10) Dissection of striate arteries of A_1 and M_1 segments from the aneurysm,
11) Removal of hematoma from the frontal lobe if present,
12) Opening of pia around the dome of aneurysm if it is buried in the fronto-basal lobe,
13) Clip application, fundus resection, coagulation and replacement of the clip,
14) Final inspection,
15) Closure.

Bilateral and Multiple Aneurysms

Of these 55 cases of carotid bifurcation aneurysms, 18 (33%) had additional aneurysms. In 2 cases the carotid bifurcation aneurysms were bilateral. In both cases the left sided aneurysm had ruptured, and both aneurysms were clipped through a left pterional approach (cases No. 50 and 51). In these cases after clipping the ruptured left sided aneurysm, a small tunnel over the chiasm along the opposite A_1 segment to the carotid bifurcation was developed, allowing access for the coagulation and clipping of these nonruptured aneurysms (Fig **56A–G**). 9 other cases had one additional aneurysm, 5 cases had 2 other aneurysms and 2 cases had 3 additional aneurysms. The distribution of these additional aneurysms is noted in Table **41a** and **b**. Overall a total of 82 aneurysms were seen in these 55 patients.

Of the 27 additional aneurysms 11 were satisfactorily clipped while the other 16 microaneurysms were coagulated and covered with muscle at the same operation.

A further 39 patients presented with incidental aneurysms at this location in conjunction with another ruptured aneurysm (see Table **129**). In 18 cases microaneurysms have been coagulated and wrapped, in 21 cases asymptomatic aneurysms of the carotid bifurcation were clipped.

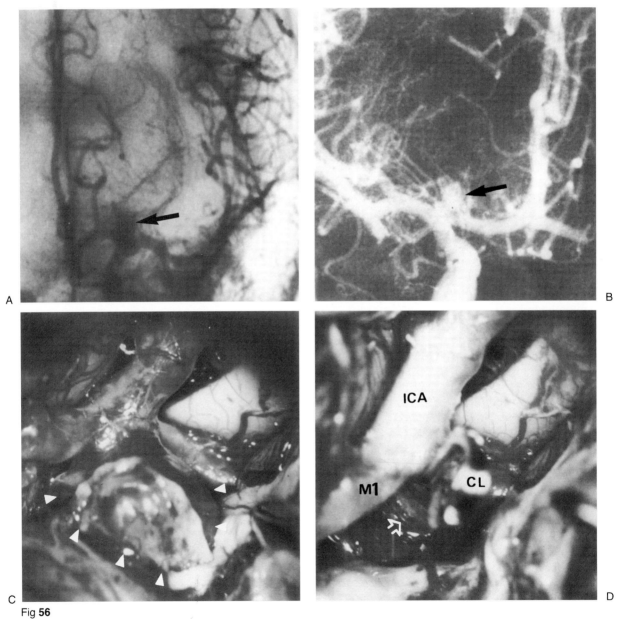

Fig 56

Bilateral and Multiple Aneurysms 117

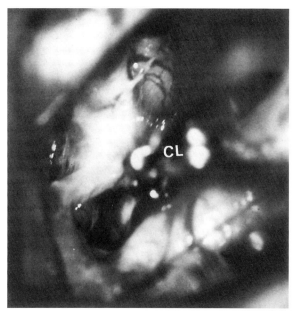

E

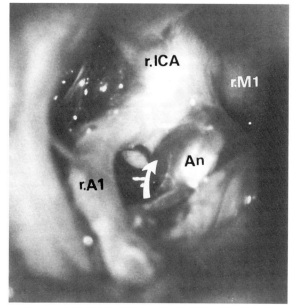

F

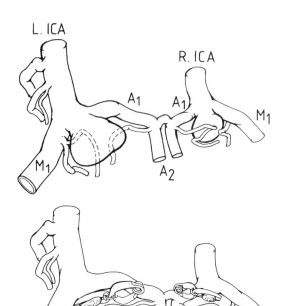

G

▲
◀ Fig 56A–G Bilateral carotid bifurcation aneurysms (arrows) (**A** and **B**) that were approached from the ruptured left side (arrow heads) (**C**). The left sided aneurysm was first clipped (the arrow shows the large striate artery underneath the aneurysm) (**D**), then dissection above the optic nerves and chiasm to the right sided aneurysm followed. This could also be clipped (**E** and **F**) (Case 50, Table **45**). The operative procedure is detailed in (**G**).

2 Internal Carotid Artery Aneurysms

Table 41a Internal carotid artery bifurcation aneurysms

				Lig.	Clip	Muscle	EIA
55 cases	Left 29						
	Right 26						
37 cases	Single aneurysms	= 37	L. 20 R. 17	5	31	–	1
11 cases	2 aneurysms	= 22			18	4	–
5 cases	3 aneurysms	= 15			9	6	–
2 cases	4 aneurysms	= 8			2	6	–
18 cases	Multiple aneurysms Total aneurysms	= 45 82		5	60	16	1

Table 41b Multiple aneurysms

Total No.		C–C	Opth	PcoA	AchoA	Oppos. ICB	M_1	MCB	AcoA	Ba	Total
Left 9 cases	Micro	–	–	1	1	–	1	1	–	–	4
	Macro	–	1	1	–	–	2	–	1	–	5
Right 9 cases	Micro	–	–	1	2	–	1	4	4	–	12
	Macro	–	–	2	–	2	–	1	1	–	6
											27

Clinical Presentation and Operative Results

Background

Discussions of aneurysms of the internal carotid artery bifurcation have been included in several publications concerning aneurysms at various locations, but few publications have specifically addressed themselves to aneurysms at this site. David and Sachs (1967) presented 10 cases with 1 death and 2 neurological deficits, and Perria et al. (1968) presented 10 cases of which 9 underwent direct operation and 2 died. Their only patient treated by carotid artery ligation also died.
Recently Sengupta et al. (1975b) have presented a series of 9 patients with no mortality and only 1 neurological deficit. Lassmann (1979) reported 11 successfully clipped cases adding to the series of Sengupta without a single mortality. Kodama et al. (1979) presented a series of 29 aneurysms that were all amenable to clipping, though their series did not include giant aneurysms. 1 patient died and in 3 cases the result was poor.

Presenting Features

Of 55 patients with aneurysms of the internal carotid artery bifurcation in the present series, 31 (56.4%) were male and 24 (43.6%) female. Especially striking in this group of patients was the young age, with 16 patients under the age of 20, and 29 patients under the age of 30 (Table **42**). In the entire series of 1012 patients, only 41 were under 20 years old and 16 of these 39% had aneurysms at the internal carotid artery bifurcation.
51 patients (92.7%) presented with subarachnoid hemorrhage. The other 4 patients presented with symptoms of mass lesions, including seizures and hemiparesis. In 1 patient subarachnoid hemorrhage was associated with a head injury.

Operative Results

With the exception of 1 totally thrombosed giant aneurysm, the aneurysms have been clipped in all 54 cases (including 3 cases of giant aneurysms). Operative results are related to preoperative grade in Table **43**. The table has been arranged to

Table 42 Sex and age in 55 patients with aneurysms at the internal carotid artery bifurcation

Age	Male	Female	Total
0–10	1*	1**	2 (3.6%)
11–20	9	5	14 (25.5%)
21–30	5	8	13 (23.6%)
31–40	9	4	13 (23.6%)
41–50	5	3	8 (14.5%)
51–60	1	3	4 (7.3%)
61–70	1	–	1 (1.8%)
over 70	–	–	–
	31 (56.4%)	24 (43.6%)	55

* 10 y
** 9 y
16/55 = 29% below 20 y

Table 43 Preoperative condition and operative results

	No. of cases	Good	Fair	Poor	Death
0b	4	2	2	–	–
Ia	24	24	–	–	–
IIa	13	13	–	–	–
IIb	3	3	–	–	–
IIIa	5	5	–	–	–
IIIb	3	–	2	–	1
IV	2	2	–	–	–
V	1	–	–	–	1
	55	49	4	–	2

show that all 43 patients without focal neurological deficit from grade Ia through IV had a good result. In addition 6 of 12 patients with focal neurological deficit also had a good outcome; thus totalling good results in 49 of 55 patients (89.1%). One patient (No. 22) suffered a recurrent subarachnoid hemorrhage 9 years after operation for a right sided bifurcation aneurysm. Angiography demonstrated a new left ICA-bifurcation aneurysm that was clipped in 1982. The patient has returned to full working capacity.

4 patients, (7.3%) remain in fair condition. 2 of these patients (No. 5 and 10) had large unruptured aneurysms with focal neurological deficit from mass effect (grade 0b) and the other 2 patients (No. 30 and 38) underwent operation after subarachnoid hemorrhage in grade IIIb, one with a right hemiparesis after epileptic seizures. All of these patients have shown some improvement postoperatively, and in fact, 2 of the 4 are working (see Fig 149).

2 patients died (3.6%). One of these patients (case No. 36) with cirrhosis, was in grade IIIb at the time of operation. The aneurysm was clipped, but in the postoperative period (2 weeks later) he sustained a recurrent hemorrhage, and reexploration revealed the formation of a new aneurysm at the base of the clip. This was again clipped. He developed hydrocephalus and required a ventricular shunt, and finally died of gastrointestinal hemorrhage. The other patient (case No. 46) entered the hospital in grade IIa, but suffered 2 recurrent hemorrhages while in the hospital and was taken to the operating room as an emergency in grade V. Hematoma was removed and the aneurysm clipped, but she did not wake from anesthesia and died 4 days later.

2 patients (38 and 39 year old males) were operated upon in grades IV respectively (cases No. 47 and 48). Both patients improved rapidly from preoperative hemisyndromes and made good recoveries. In these cases the rapid evacuation of intracranial hematomas was lifesaving.

Timing and Results

The timing of operation in 51 patients who sustained subarachnoid hemorrhage as related to preoperative grade and outcome is given in Table 44. 8 patients, 4 in grade IIa, 1 in grade IIb, 2 in grade IIIa and 1 in grade IV underwent operation in the first week with good results. 2 patients in grade IIIb undergoing operation in the first week had fair results, and 1 patient in grade IIIb operated in the second week died of gastrointestinal hemorrhage. A grade V patient treated the day of hemorrhage died. Outcome in these patients is related only to the clinical grade and not to the timing of operation (Table 45).

Table 44 Timing of surgery and results in 51 patients with ruptured aneurysm of the bifurcation of the internal carotid artery

	Good					Fair	Death		
	Ia	IIa	IIb	IIIa	IV	IIIb	IIIb	V	
1–3 d	–	2	–	2	–	1	–	1	
4–7 d	–	2	1	–	1	1	–	–	
1–2 w	5	5	1	2	1	–	1	–	
2–4 w	8	4	1	1	–	–	–	–	
1–3 m	4	–	–	–	–	–	–	–	
> 3 m	7	–	–	–	–	–	–	–	
	24	13	3	5	2	2	1	1	= 51

Table 45 Internal carotid bifurcation aneurysms

		Age Sex	Date	SAH	Time	Condition	Hypertension	Site	Size mm	Base	Others	Operation	Result
1.	Vi	26 M	1967	1	11 ds	Ia	(+)	R	20	Broad	–	Lig.	Good
2.	Fä	29 M	1967	1	3 ws	Ia	(+)	R	3	Broad	Intracavern. left	Lig.	Good
3.	Zü	43 F	1967	1	5 ds	IIa	+	L	8	Broad	A₁ left	Clip/clip	Good
4.	Zu	19 F	1968	– Epi + Hpr.	1 y	0b	–	R	50	Broad Thrombosed	spontaneous thromb. of ICA	EIA	Good
5.	Ri	47 M	1968	Epi	1 y	0b	–	R	40	Broad Part. thromb.	–	Lig.	Fair Hpr.
6.	Po	53 F	1969	1	3 ms	Ia	+	L	8	Broad	–	Lig.	Good
7.	Hü	13 M	1970	1	2 ws	Ia	–	L	10	Broad	–	Clip/lig.	Good
8.	Ac	37 M	1970	3/3 ws	12 ds	IIIa	+	R	8	Narrow ICH	–	Clip	Good
9.	Vi	44 m	1970	1	4 ws	IIa	–	L	20	Broad	–	Clip	Good
10.	De	19 F	1970	Epi	6 ms	0b, Epi + Hpr.	–	R	50	Broad	–	Clip	Fair Epi/mild Hpr.
11.	Sh	18 M	1970	1	24 ds	Ia	–	L	20	Broad	–	Clip	Good
12.	Ko	23 F	1971	1	3 ms	Ia	–	L	8	Broad	–	Clip	Good
13.	Me	33f	1971	1	10 ds	IIb diabetes insipid.	+	R	10	Broad Subdural hematoma	–	Clip	Good
14.	He	15 m	1972	2/1 y	3 ds	IIIa	–	L	8	Broad Large ICH	–	Clip	Good

Table 45 (Continuation)

	Age Sex	Date	SAH	Time	Condition	Hypertension	Site	Size mm	Base	Others	Operation	Result
15. Wy	35 M	1972	3/2 ms Epi.	10 ds	IIIa	+	L	7	Narrow	–	Clip	Good
16. Pa	28 M	1972	1	22 ds	Ia	–	L	5	Broad	–	Clip	Good
17. Si	19 M	1972	2	26 ds	Ia	–	R	8	Broad	–	Clip	Good
18. Me	21 F	1972	2	14 ds	Ia	–	L	8	Narrow	1 Micro.	Clip	Good
19. Ga	46 F	1972	1	23 ds	IIa	+	L	20	Broad	–	Clip	Good
20. Sa	9 F	1972	2	34 ds	Ia	–	L	8	Broad	– ICH small	Clip	Good
21. Sch	15 M	1972	2	8 ds	IIa	–	L	5	Broad	–	Clip	Good
22. Av	22 M	1973	1	2 ms	Ia	–	R	20	Broad Thrombosed	– ICH small	Clip	Good
23. Fo	36 F	1973	2	2 ds	IIIa	–	R	4	Narrow	–	Clip	Good
24. Me	36 M	1972	1	3 ds	IIa	–	L	6	Broad	–	Clip	Good
25. Cu	22 M	1973	2	5 ms	Ia	–	L	25	Broad	–	Clip	Good
26. Bü	55 F	1973	1	1 m	IIIa	+	L	5	Broad	3 micro. ICH	Clip	Good
27. Wi	63 M	1973	Epi + Hpr.	1 y	0b	–	L	50	Narrow Part. thromb.	–	Clip	Good
28. Fa	17 F	1973	1	3½ ms	Ia	–	R	10	Broad	–	Clip	Good
29. Te	10 M	1973	3	10 ds	Ia	–	R	6	Broad	– medium, ICH	Clip	Good
30. Pa	39 F	1973	1	3 ds	IIIb Hpr/HA	–	L	10	Broad	–	Clip	Fair
31. Bi	47 M	1973	1	15 ds	Ia	–	R	10	Broad	–	Clip	Good
32. Tr	45 M	1974	1	9 ds	IIa	–	L	10	Broad Sclerotic	temp.	Clip	Good
33. Be	44 M	1974	1	4 ms	Ia	–	L	10	Broad	1 micro	Clip	Good
34. Bl	31 M	1974	1	8 ds	IIa	–	R	10	Broad	ACA	Clip/clip	Good
35. Gr	20 M	1973	2/1 y	1 y	Ia	–	L	8	Broad	post. comm. left middle (sphen.)	Clip/clip/clip	Good
36. Me	53 M	1974	1	12 ds	IIIb Hpr. l.	–	R	6	Broad	rerupture, reoperation	Clip	RR Death
37. v. H	28 F	1974	1	2 ms	Ia	–	R	5	Broad	A₁ left	Clip	Good
38. Dü	22 F	1974	1	7 ds	IIIb Hpr. l.	+	R	8	Broad	3 micro m-bif./ant. chor. ACA	Clip	Fair
39. Zo	38 M	1975	1	4 ds	IIb Hpr. l. mild	–	R	20	Broad Part. thromb.	–	Clip	Good
40. Zd	37 M	1975	2	4 ms	Ia	+	R	20	Small Part. thromb.	–	Clip	Good
									2 micro.			
41. Pi	14 F	1976	1	14 ds	IIa	–	R	10	Broad	small ICH	Clip	Good
42. Fi	53 F	1976	1	23 ds	IIa	+	R	5	Broad	2 micro	Clip	Good

Table 45 (Continuation)

	Age Sex	Date	SAH	Time	Condition	Hypertension	Site	Size mm	Base	Others	Operation	Result
43. Ci	38 M	1976	1	26 ds	IIa	–	R	8	Narrow	–	Clip	Good
44. Sa	22 F	1976	2	6 ms	Ia	–	L	6	Broad	2 micro	Clip	Good
45. Fr	17 M	1976	1	2 ws	Ia severe local spasm	–	L	8	Broad	sphen. l.	Clip/clip	Good
46. Zg	24 F	1977	3/10 ds	1 d	V	–	R	10	Broad	ACA	Clip/clip	Death
47. De	39 M	1977	1	10 ds	IV ICH	–	R	8	Broad	ACA micro	Clip	Good
48. Zw	38 M	1977	1	6 ds	IV Hpr. l.	–	R	10	Broad	–	Clip	Good
49. Sch	36 F	1978	1	4 ds	IIa	–	L	6	Narrow	–	Clip	Good
50. Zi	28 F	1978	1	3 ws	Ia	–	L/R	10/8	Narrow	bil. right	Clip/clip bilateral	Good
51. Mu	13 M	1978	1	8 ds	IIa	–	L/R	6/4	Broad	bil. right	Clip/clip bilateral	Good
52. St.	14 m	1978	1	3 ws	Ia	–	L	10	Broad	–	Clip	Good
53. R	15 F	1978	1	3 ws	Ia	–	L	6	Broad	–	Clip	Good
54. Sa	42 F	1979	1	4 ws	IIb	–	L	8	Broad	opht. l. ICH rt.	Clip/clip	Good
55. Ca	31 F	1979	1	1 d	IIa	–	R	8	Broad	middle rt. post cer.	Clip/clip clip	Good

Summary of Internal Carotid Artery Aneurysms

Internal carotid artery aneurysms were among the first intracranial aneurysms to be clinically recognized. When located in the cavernous sinus or proximal on the intracranial internal carotid artery their characteristic symptomatology made diagnosis possible even before the advent of cerebral angiography. In addition, treatment was possible by cervical carotid artery ligation with acceptable results (Fig 57A–B).

Of 1012 patients in the present series 319 (31.5%) underwent operation for internal carotid artery aneurysms. Overall results for operation are given in Table 46. While aneurysms of the internal carotid artery generally form a family, each specific location of aneurysm has its individual profile of age and sex incidence, clinical presentation, association with other aneurysms, anatomical features, operative problems, and prognosis.

There are six regular sites for these aneurysms, all are found along a 2–3 cm segment of the ICA; groups 4 and 5 (Table 46) are very rare.

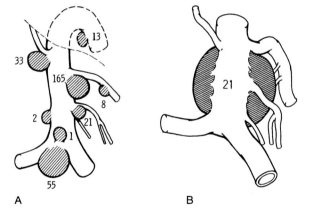

Fig 57A–B Schematic illustration of the site and frequency (numerals) of treated aneurysms of the internal carotid artery. **A** Saccular, **B** fusiform inferior wall aneurysms.

Table 46 Aneurysms of internal carotid artery and operative results

	Total No. of cases	Clip	Lig.	Tr.	M	EIA	Good	Fair	Poor	Death
1. Cavernous	13	–	13	–	–	(2)*	12	1	–	–
2. Ophthalmic	33	27	1	–	4	1 (only)	32	–	–	1
3. Inferior	21	14	3	2	2	(2)*	18	–	1	2
4. Medial	2	2	–	–	–	–	2	–	–	–
5. Superior	1	1	–	–	–	–	1	–	–	–
6. PcoA	173	172	–	1	–	–	144	17	2	10
7. AchoA	21	21	–	–	–	–	16	2	1	2
8. Bifurcation	55	54	–	–	–	1 (only)**	49	4	–	2
	319	291 91.2%	17	3	6	2 (4)* 0.6%	274 85.9%	24 7.5%	4 1.3%	17 5.3%

* also trapped, ligated or wrapped
** Case 4, Table **45**

Excluding 13 intracavernous aneurysms, a total of 306 cases of ICA aneurysms were operated upon with clipping in 95.1%, trapping in 1.0%, wrapping with muscle in 2.0% and ligating the cervical ICA in 1.9%. In 3 cases the intracranial portion of the ICA was inadvertendly trapped.

The direct operative approach with clipping of an ICA aneurysm within a triangular-shaped narrow field has some advantages and some disadvantages. In about 50% of the cases, the neck of the aneurysm presents itself to the surgeon at the beginning of dissection. For example it may extend from the ICA medially (ophthalmic aneurysms), laterally (aneurysms of the PcoA and AchoA) or posteriorly (aneurysms of the ICA bifurcation). In the other 50%, however, either the size of the aneurysm, its fusiform shape, or its bulging parts cover the parent arteries or their branches thereby making the dissection extremely difficult. Not only the narrowness of the operating field, but also the very limited mobility of the structures in the vicinity (like the clinoid processes, the petroclival ligament, the optic and oculomotor nerves, the pituitary stalk and infundibular parts of hypothalamus, the medio-basal part of hippocampal gyrus, and the ICA itself) complicate the proper dissection of the aneurysm neck and the proper application of the clip.

The surgeon has to adopt a meticulous technique to perform precise and decisive manipulations in such an inflexible, narrow space, in order to reach the neck of the aneurysm. If a premature rupture occurs, he must be ready to control the situation properly. The surgeon must be prepared to face all types of difficulties each with a possible hazardous outcome all occurring within this morphologically challenging space surrounded by physiopathologically delicate structures.

Knowing the microsurgical anatomy of the ICA and its variations and memorizing the positions of the aneurysmal neck and fundus, permit about 90% of these aneurysms to be clipped successfully. Fusiform and inferior wall aneurysms remain challenging problems.

3 Middle Cerebral Artery Aneurysms

Anatomical Relationships

Incidence, Laterality, Multiplicity

In the present series, 184 patients underwent operation for aneurysms of the middle cerebral artery, representing 18.2 per cent of the entire series. Aneurysms were equally divided between the right and left middle cerebral arteries, with 92 on each side.

In 59 cases (32.1%) there were additional aneurysms, totalling 280 aneurysms in the 184 patients; of these 225 could be clipped while 51 (microaneurysms) were merely coagulated and covered with muscle and acrylic glue. The distribution of multiple aneurysms is noted in Table **47**. 14 patients (7.6%) had bilateral aneurysms with 6 aneurysms on the opposite internal carotid artery and 8 symmetrical aneurysms on the opposite middle cerebral artery. It could be noted that contralateral aneurysms may present problems both in deciding which lesion has bled and in determining proper operative treatment for the incidental lesions.

68 patients presented with incidental aneurysms of the MCA in conjunction with another ruptured aneurysm (see Table **129a**, page 312). In 36 cases microaneurysms have been coagulated and wrapped, in 32 patients the aneurysms were clipped.

Table 47 Middle cerebral artery aneurysms. Multiplicity

Multiplicity		Inf.	Oph. A.	PcoA	AchoA	ICB	MCB	AcoA	PeA	Ba	Total
Left 27	Micro	–	–	4	4	4	14	1	1	–	28
	Macro	–	1	3	1	4	6	4	1	2	22
Right 32	Micro	–	1	4	2	–	13	3	–	–	23
	Macro	1	–	2	3	2	9	5	–	1	23
59											96

184 patients presented 280 aneurysms

			No. of aneurysms	Clipped	Not clipped
Single aneurysms	125 patients		125	124	1 (fusiform)
1 additional aneurysm	41 patients	82			
2 additional aneurysms	6 patients	18			
3 additional aneurysms	6 patients	24	155	90	51 (microaneurysm)
4 additional aneurysms	5 patients	25		11 contralateral	3 (contralateral)
5 additional aneurysms	1 patient	6			
			280	225	55

Size and Morphology

Of the 184 symptomatic aneurysms, 46 were bilobular, 25 trilobular, and 7 truly multilobular. In 5 cases, 2 aneurysms took independent origin from the same place on the middle cerebral artery (Fig 58A). In 41 cases the aneurysms were larger than 15 mm and in 3 cases they were larger than 25 mm (Fig 58B). Large and giant aneurysms were more common on the right side (29.3%) than on the left (14.1%). No sclerosis was present in 12 of these large aneurysms, moderate sclerosis in 27, and 2 lesions were almost entirely calcified with prominent vasa vasorum growing into the wall of the aneurysm.

Relationship to the Subarachnoid Cisterns

Aneurysms arising from the middle cerebral artery are contained within the Sylvian cistern. As described in the section on cisternal anatomy, this cistern is quite variable in its width, length, and depth, and also in its density of trabeculae. When the Sylvian fissure is shallow, the aneurysm may be very superficial and may even attach to the dura over the lateral sphenoid wing.

Aneurysms within the Sylvian cistern are more confined by the brain than aneurysms at other locations. The operculae of the frontal, parietal,

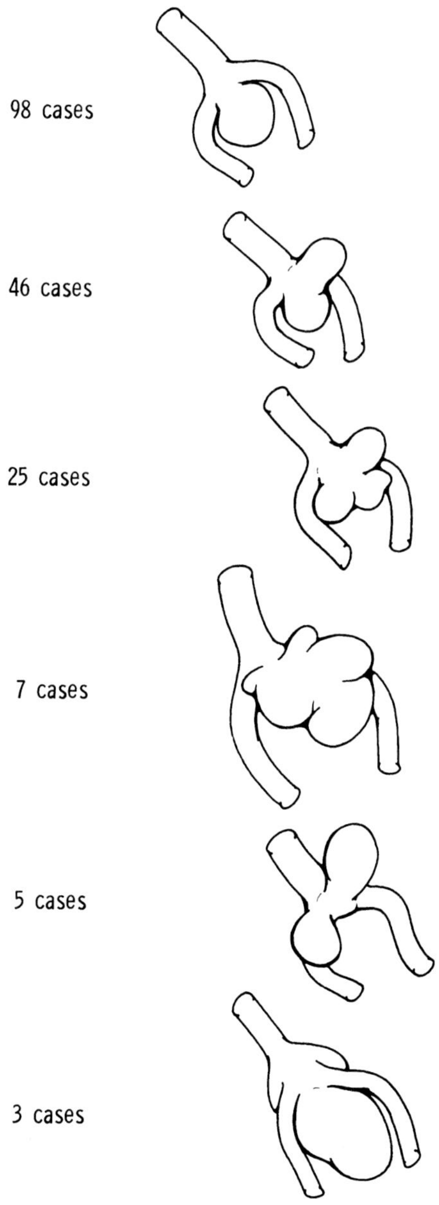

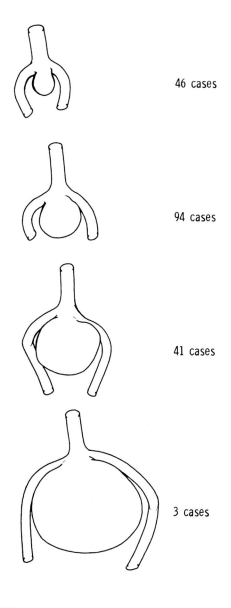

Fig 58A Schematic presentation of the various shapes of middle cerebral bifurcation aneurysms in own 184 cases.

Fig 58B Schematic representation of the effects of various sized middle cerebral bifurcation aneurysms on the superior and inferior trunks.

3 Middle Cerebral Artery Aneurysms

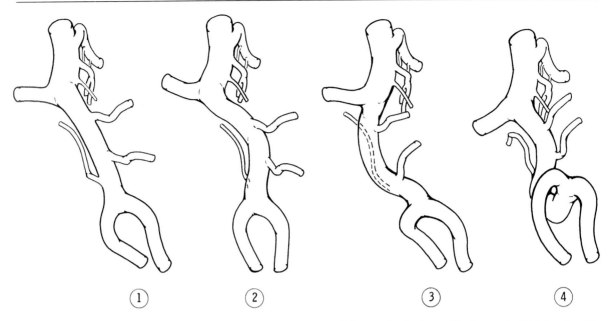

Fig 59 Schematic representation of the different courses of middle cerebral artery; (1) diagonal, (2) laterally, (3) medially, (4) anteriorly curved.

and temporal lobes usually cover both the insula and the aneurysm and thus play a part in containing a rupture of these aneurysms. The cistern may be quite distended by hematoma without rupturing into the brain or into the subdural space. Nevertheless, intracerebral hematoma is a common occurrence with aneurysms at this location (34.1%).

Relationship to the Middle Cerebral Artery

The course of the middle cerebral artery is quite variable. The artery may course diagonally (1) along the sphenoid ridge or may run laterally (2), superiorly or posteriorly, medially (3) or anteriorly (4) (Fig 59).

The anatomy of the middle cerebral artery was discussed in detail in Chapter 1, Vol. I, pages 72–91. The primary bifurcation of the middle cerebral artery is at a relatively constant length from the internal carotid artery bifurcation and is located at the anterior edge of the island of Reil (limen insula). Early branching of the large anterior temporal or operculofrontal artery may create the appearance of an early bifurcation, or if the main middle cerebral trunks distal to the primary bifurcation divide early a pseudobifurcation or even a more complex branching arrangement may be formed.

There are 5 principal locations on the middle cerebral artery system where aneurysms commonly arise (Fig 60, Table 48):

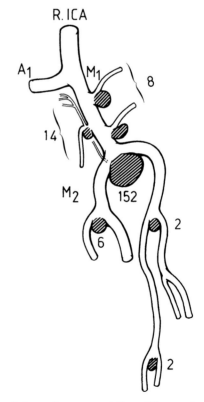

Fig 60 Schematic representation of the varying locations of middle cerebral artery aneurysms and their frequency (see Table 48).

Table 48 Localization of middle cerebral artery aneurysms

	Left	Right	
Ant. temp.	5 (1 multiple)	3 (1 multiple)	8
Lenticulostr.	8 (4 multiples) (4 singles)	6 (2 multiples) (4 singles)	14
Bifurcation	72	80	152
2nd Bif.	5	1	6
Distal	2	2	4
	92	92	184

Lateral Wall of Proximal Middle Cerebral Artery

In 8 cases, aneurysms were found on the temporal side of the M_1 segment, 5 on the left side and 3 on the right. These aneurysms arise at the origin of the temporopolar or anterior temporal branches of the middle cerebral artery and project into the adjacent temporal lobe. In some cases, the anterior temporal artery is especially large, giving the impression that the bifurcation of the middle cerebral artery is very near the internal carotid artery bifurcation. Other temporal branches may be adherent to the fundus of the aneurysm, and the lenticulostriate branches are often seen just opposite the aneurysm on the medial aspect of the middle cerebral artery (Fig **61A–B**).

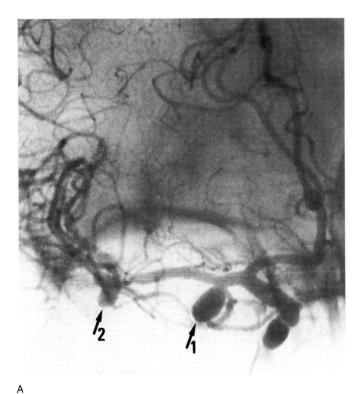

A

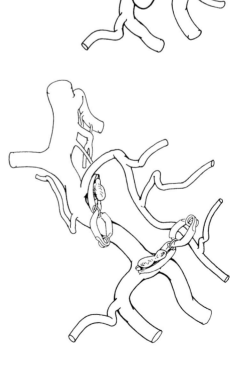

B

Fig **61A–B** Unruptured aneurysm of the right middle cerebral artery at the bifurcation (arrow 2) and a ruptured aneurysm (arrow 1) at the origin of the anterior temporal artery on angiography (**A**) and at operation (**B**).

Medial Wall of Proximal Middle Cerebral Artery

In 14 cases, 8 on the left and 6 on the right, aneurysms arose at the origins of the lenticulostriate branches of the middle cerebral artery and projected into the laterobasal frontal lobe. In 4 cases, the aneurysm arose from a common origin of the striate group and a lateral fronto-orbital artery that began proximal to the middle cerebral artery bifurcation. In 2 of these cases, the lateral frontoorbital artery was especially large, again giving the impression of an early middle cerebral artery bifurcation. The striate arteries are usually behind the aneurysm in these cases (Figs **62, 63A–B**).

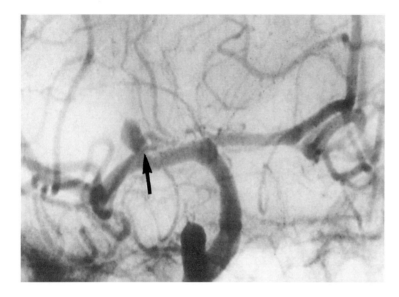

Fig **62** Right M_1 segment aneurysm (arrow) arising at the origin of the fronto-orbital and lateral striate arteries.

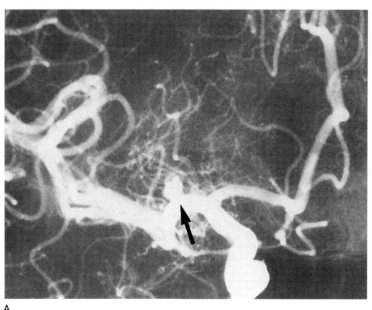

Fig **63A–B** Right M_1 segment aneurysm at the origin of the lateral fronto-orbital and lateral striate arteries as it appears on angiography (arrow) (**A**) and at surgery (**B**).

Middle Cerebral Artery Bifurcation

This is by far the most common location of an aneurysm on the middle cerebral artery accounting for 152 of 184 cases (82.6%). 72 aneurysms were on the left middle cerebral artery and 80 on the right. An aneurysm is usually based more on one major trunk than the other, usually the larger one. There are 3 principal directions of fundus projection with middle cerebral artery bifurcation aneurysms;
1) Anterosuperior (medially or laterally) toward the surface of the Sylvian fissure (sometimes adherent to or even overlying the dura of the sphenoid wing),
2) Posterior between the two major trunks of the bifurcation; and
3) Inferior toward the insula (Fig **64**).

With aneurysms at this location, lateral distal striate arteries are often found to arise from the area of the bifurcation or from the proximal few millimeters of the superior or inferior trunk (Figs **65, 66A–B, 67A–D**). These arteries are also usually on the larger trunk and therefore are on the inferomedial aspect of the aneurysm neck. It is important that these arteries be identified prior to coagulation or clipping of an aneurysm, especially in cases where the fundus is extending inferiorly.

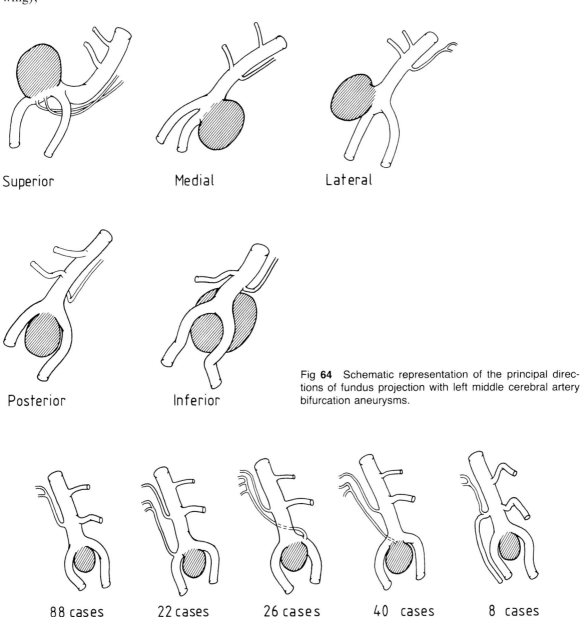

Fig **64** Schematic representation of the principal directions of fundus projection with left middle cerebral artery bifurcation aneurysms.

Fig **65** Schematic representation of the relationship between middle cerebral bifurcation aneurysms and the distal lateral striate arteries (right side).

130   3 Middle Cerebral Artery Aneurysms

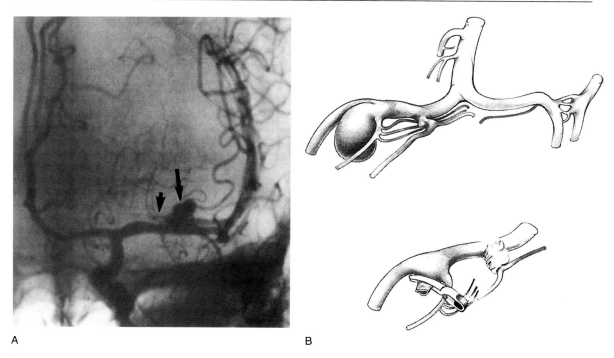

Fig 66A–B Left middle cerebral bifurcation aneurysm (large arrow) with its relation to the distal lateral striate arteries (short arrow) arising from the superior trunk as seen on angiography (**A**) and at surgery (**B**).

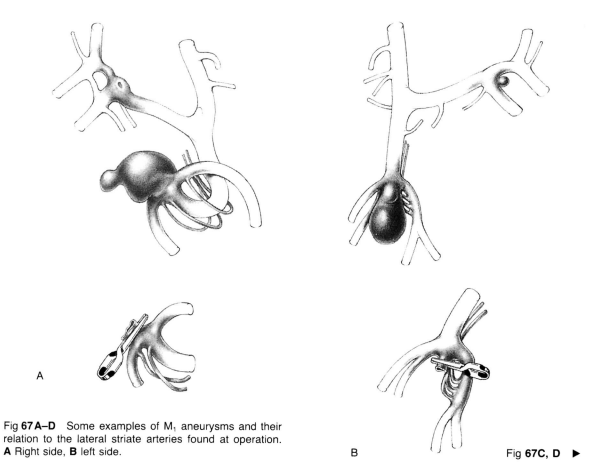

Fig 67A–D Some examples of M_1 aneurysms and their relation to the lateral striate arteries found at operation. **A** Right side, **B** left side.

Fig **67C, D** ▶

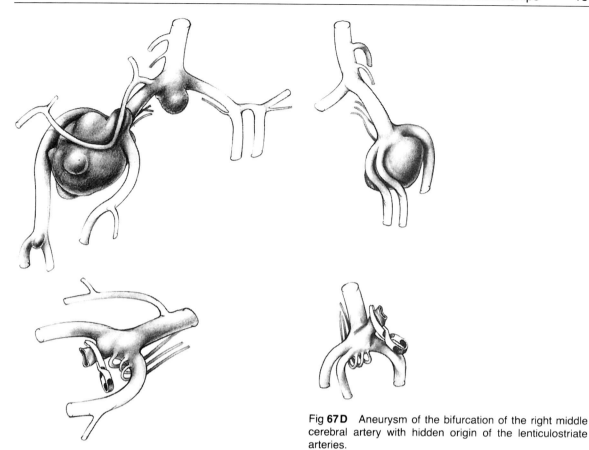

Fig 67C Left middle cerebral bifurcation aneurysm with the origin of lenticulostriates at the bifurcation of middle cerebral artery.

Fig 67D Aneurysm of the bifurcation of the right middle cerebral artery with hidden origin of the lenticulostriate arteries.

Secondary Middle Cerebral Artery Bifurcation

In 6 cases, 5 on the left and 1 on the right, aneurysms arose from a second bifurcation of the middle cerebral artery still within the Sylvian cistern (Fig 68).

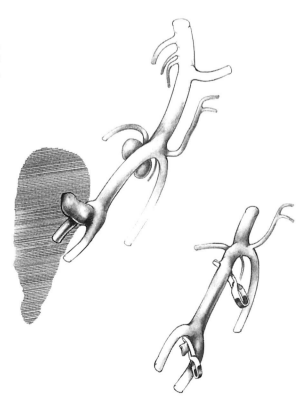

Fig 68 Schematic representation of a ruptured aneurysm of a second middle cerebral artery bifurcation with a temporal hematoma, and an unruptured aneurysm at the first bifurcation.

3 Middle Cerebral Artery Aneurysms

Distal Middle Cerebral Artery Branches

There were 4 cases of aneurysm arising from the peripheral branches of the middle cerebral artery, 2 on the right and 2 on the left. None of these aneurysms could be verified histologically to be mycotic, but this was suspected in at least 1 case where the patient developed a second peripheral aneurysm after the first had been clipped. This subsequently ruptured and left her hemiparetic. In 2 cases the aneurysm was thrombosed (see Vol. I, Fig **255**) and in 2 cases rupture of the aneurysm caused large intracerebral hematomas (Fig **69**).

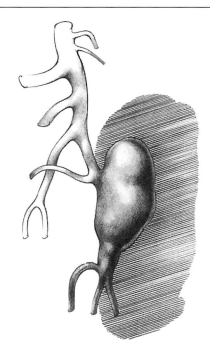

Fig **69** Schematic representation of a ruptured fusiform aneurysm of the distal right middle cerebral artery (M$_3$) with a temporal hematoma.

Operative Technique

Initial Exposure

A standard pterional craniotomy will expose aneurysms located at or proximal to the middle cerebral artery bifurcation. Some aneurysms more peripherally placed may be approached by extending this craniotomy posteriorly onto the temporal and parietal bones, while those aneurysms out of the Sylvian cistern will require an appropriately placed parietotemporal craniotomy. Special care must be taken when opening the dura with middle cerebral artery aneurysms, as the aneurysm may point superficially and be attached to the dura along the sphenoid wing (Fig **70A–C**).

The decision as to where to enter the Sylvian cistern and begin dissection of the middle cerebral artery and its branches depends on the radiographic anatomy of the aneurysm and associated hematoma, on the fullness of the brain at the time of exposure, on the course of the middle cerebral artery, and to some extent on the experience and confidence of the operating surgeon. The area of dissection may be schematically divided into three parts:

Area I: at the base of the Sylvian fissure where the Sylvian cistern communicates with the basal cisterns,

Area II: over the proximal middle cerebral artery up to its bifurcation (usually the location of the aneurysm "packet"); and

Area III: over the peripheral branches of the middle cerebral artery beyond the bifurcation (Figs **68** and **69**).

With the aneurysm presenting at the middle cerebral artery bifurcation, the brain moderately full, and no large hematoma present, the approach should start in area I. With the dura opened, the laterobasal frontal lobe is gently retracted medially to expose the optic nerve and internal carotid artery. The carotid cistern is opened to release cerebrospinal fluid and dissection is continued distally to the internal carotid artery bifurcation. Here, the thickened bands of arachnoid across the origin of the middle cerebral artery that separate the carotid and Sylvian cisterns are divided with scissors. These bands will constrict the origin of the middle cerebral artery when the retractor is applied to the frontal lobe. The lamina terminalis cistern is opened over the anterior cerebral arteries to allow the frontal lobe to be retracted. This helps to open the Sylvian fissure and to minimize retraction pressure on the frontal lobe. If the brain is specially tight, the interpeduncular cistern may be opened to release cerebrospinal fluid.

Operative Technique

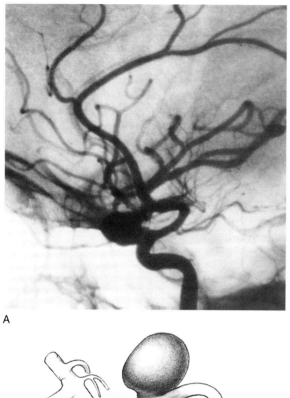

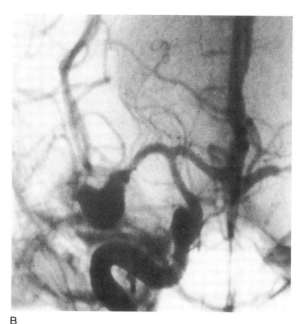

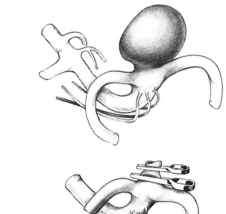

Fig 70A–C Right middle cerebral bifurcation aneurysm with antero-superior extension and adhesions to the dura along the sphenoid wing (A–C). The operative findings are shown in (C).

The Sylvian cistern is opened over the proximal middle cerebral artery distal to the internal carotid artery bifurcation. Dissection should stay on the frontal side of the superficial Sylvian veins. In the most medial part of the cistern, there are usually several small frontal veins that cross the cistern from the area of the anterior perforated substance to the mesial temporal lobe in order to join the middle cerebral veins. At times, these veins can be freed from their pial attachments to allow retraction, but often they must unavoidably be sacrificed. No apparent harm has been noted from taking these veins.

The goal of dissection in area II is to expose and protect the anterior temporal and lenticulostriate arteries while gaining proximal control on the middle cerebral artery trunk. Numerous arachnoid trabeculations are present in the proximal portion of the Sylvian cistern, and the cistern is quite variable in size. Separation of the frontal and temporal lobes may be difficult if there are pial adhesions. If the plane of the Sylvian fissure is lost, it is wise to identify a cortical artery on the frontal or temporal lobe and follow it into the fissure.

If the aneurysm originates from the M_1 segment dissection of the neck is now ready to proceed. For aneurysms located at the bifurcation, dissection is carried distally until the bifurcation is approached. The middle cerebral artery trunk is exposed so that a temporary clip can be placed if required, preferably beyond the largest striate arteries. Further dissection in area II is deferred, leaving the aneurysm untouched until the major branches have been identified distally.

To approach area III, an incision is made in the arachnoid of the Sylvian cistern 1 or 2 centimeters beyond the limen insulae on the frontal lobe side of the superficial middle cerebral veins. The fissure is opened to expose the major trunks of the bifurcation and their branches. The variability of branching within the Sylvian cistern has been discussed in Vol. I, Chapter 1. It is especially important that the surgeon inspect beneath the temporal operculum to be certain that the branches have been properly identified. A second self-retaining retractor may be useful to elevate the temporal operculum and help to open the Sylvian fissure, although retraction must be limited to avoid disruption of the aneurysm and strangulation of small vessels within the cistern by crossing arachnoid bands. If the arteries within the Sylvian cistern appear spastic, it is advisable to apply papaverine to them prior to beginning dissection of the aneurysm neck. Arachnoid, pia and clot adherent to the fundus of the aneurysm are left undisturbed until all important arteries have been identified.

When the aneurysm is small and the brain is adequately decompressed at the beginning of the operation, dissection may begin in area III to expose the branches of the middle cerebral artery within the Sylvian fissure and follow these proximally toward the bifurcation and aneurysm with its associated structures. When these are identified, the cistern is opened over area II, coming down on the trunk of the middle cerebral artery bifurcation. This approach avoids dissection in the more proximal basal cisterns, but gives less control of the middle cerebral artery initially and must therefore be evaluated in the light of the surgeon's experience and the radiographic appearance of the aneurysm.

If hematoma is present in either the temporal or frontal lobe, it is best to remove the major portion of the clot through an incision of the superior temporal or inferior frontal gyrus, leaving some hematoma and pia around the aneurysm. This will help relax the brain and create more working space, and the surgeon may be able to avoid extensive dissection in the basal cisterns. Hematoma can be followed to the temporal horn where it will usually end, and this will allow the temporal lobe to collapse away from the Sylvian fissure. If removal of hematoma does not adequately decompress the brain, attention is turned to area I and a standard dissection performed.

Dissection of the Aneurysm

With aneurysms arising from the proximal middle cerebral artery, dissection is generally not complicated, especially with those aneurysms arising from the lateral wall of the artery. One must keep in mind the recurrent course of the lenticulostriate arteries and ascertain that they are free of the aneurysm neck before a clip is applied.

With bifurcation aneurysms, the first problem of dissection is correct identification of the superior and inferior trunks of the bifurcation. It is easy to mistake a secondary branching in the area of the bifurcation as a principal bifurcation and especially to miss the inferior trunk which may be hidden under the temporal operculum.

A plane of dissection is developed between the superior trunk and the aneurysm wall and this followed proximally until the neck is defined and a 2 to 3 mm space developed for placement of the clip. A similar method of dissection is employed on the inferior trunk separating it from the aneurysm wall until the neck is defined and a suitable space exists to allow passage of a clip blade. Dissection should proceed parallel to the arteries to avoid tearing or avulsing a corner of the aneurysm.

The second problem is to identify the striate arteries arising in the area of the bifurcation. As the arteries generally arise from the base of the larger trunk, or from the middle of the bifurcation when the two trunks are of equal caliber, they will be beneath the neck of the aneurysm. Their usual course is recurrent on the middle cerebral trunk, proximal to the origin of the aneurysm. They may be identified, therefore, just below the middle cerebral artery bifurcation and followed toward the carotid bifurcation; gently depressing the neck of the aneurysm with the suction tip may help to identify their origin. In 1 case the branches were superior to aneurysm fundus and covered the aneurysm.

The final problem prior to clip application is to free the lateral orbitofrontal, or anterior temporal arteries that may be adherent to the aneurysm fundus, so that these will not be torn or stretched when the aneurysm is clipped (Fig **71A–B**). Dissection of these arteries can be extremely difficult as they can be quite adherent and the aneurysm very thin-walled. It is sometimes necessary to create enough space on the aneurysm neck to apply a clip, then come back to free these arteries and readjust the clip.

Operative Technique 135

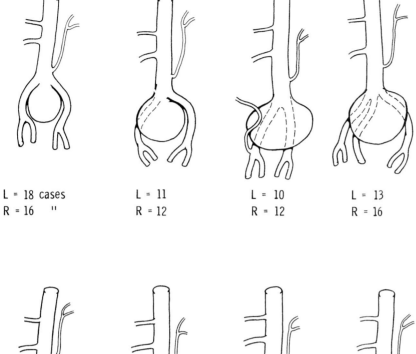

L = 18 cases
R = 16   "

L = 11
R = 12

L = 10
R = 12

L = 13
R = 16

Fig 71 A Schematic representation of the relationship between middle cerebral artery bifurcation aneurysms and the position of the superior and inferior trunks.

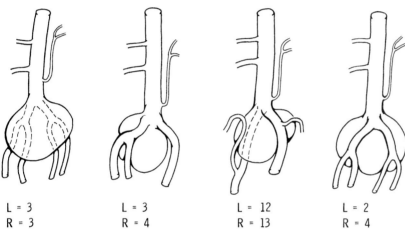

L = 3
R = 3

L = 3
R = 4

L = 12
R = 13

L = 2
R = 4

Fig 71 B Schematic representation of the relationship between middle cerebral artery bifurcation aneurysms and the position of temporal and fronto-orbital arteries.

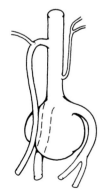
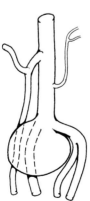
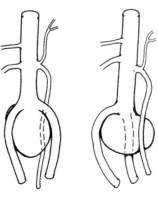

L = 12
R = 13

L = 12
R = 11

L = 4
R = 5

L = 3
R = 4

Temporal artery   Fronto - orbital artery

Clip Application

If the neck is well defined and narrow enough to accept the clip following dissection, the clip is introduced over the top of the aneurysm neck, taking care not to include the lenticulostriate arteries within the blades. The clip is closed slowly while the surgeon observes the middle cerebral artery and its branches to verify that they are not being compromised or distorted. More commonly, however, the neck is broad, or the aneurysm lobulated and bulbous, and one of the several techniques discussed in Vol. I, Chapter 3, will have to be employed. Successive bipolar coagulation and clipping has proved the most useful technique at this location. As the aneurysm shrinks, a neck is created allowing clip placement (Fig **72A–D**).

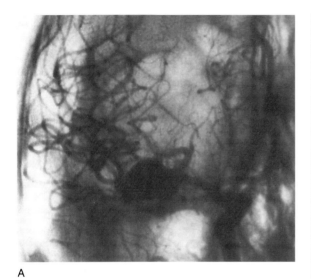

A

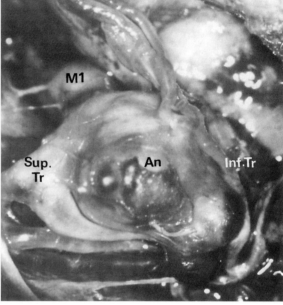

B

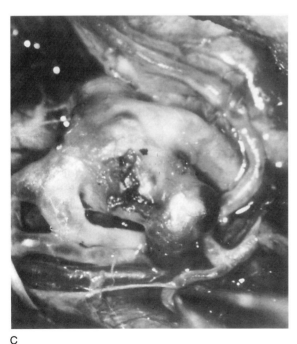

C

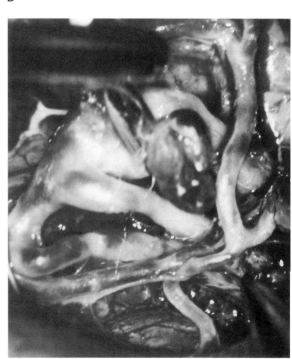

D

Fig **72A–D** Large right middle cerebral bifurcation aneurysm (An) (**A**) as seen at operation (**B**) with progressive coagulation (**C**) and final clip placement (**D**). Sup. Tr = superior trunk, Inf. Tr = inferior trunk.

For those aneurysms where atheroma or thrombus prevents application of a clip and makes bipolar coagulation ineffective, a temporary clip to the middle cerebral artery may be required. The temporary clip should be distal to the larger lenticulostriate arteries if possible. When these arise too far distally, such as from an M_2 segment, clip time must be kept to an absolute minimum. If there is significant backbleeding when the aneurysm is opened, temporary clips should be placed on the major trunks beyond the bifurcation to prevent a sump effect on distal collateral circulation. With the aneurysm opened, thrombus and atheroma are removed, a neck is created with bipolar coagulation and a clip applied.

Following clip application, the fundus is resected and the placement of the clip checked. The clip should be optimally seated, although the shape of the aneurysm and the bifurcation often makes it difficult to include all of the aneurysm in the clip without compromising the parent arteries. This is especially true when the aneurysm is directed inferiorly. Successive bipolar coagulation, resection, and clip replacement may allow the clip to be moved down to the base of the aneurysm. Muscle and sponge should be placed around any unclipped portion of the neck (Fig **73A–G**).

Of the 184 patients undergoing operation, only one had a true fusiform aneurysm which could not be clipped. This extended along the whole length of the M_1 segment and also affected the A_2 segment of the anterior cerebral artery (see page 287, Fig **227**, Vol. I). Following completion of this series, a 13 year old girl came to operation with a fusiform aneurysm confined to the left M_1 segment. This was successfully treated with an extra-intracranial anastomosis and excision (see Vol. I, p. 291, Fig **230**).

2 cases were treated early in the series by silk suture ligation. 4 cases required direct repair with microsutures. 2 of these were large, sclerotic lesions and the clip would not hold. Temporary clips were applied, the lesion opened, the sclerotic plaques removed, and the aneurysm successfully repaired with 8-0 sutures. In the third case, the inferior trunk was injured when the aneurysm was avulsed at its base. The repair with microsutures required that the middle cerebral artery be clipped for 32 minutes. The patient did poorly postoperatively. In the fourth case there was a large, partially thrombosed aneurysm which had simply too much wall to enclose in a clip. Temporary clipping was used for 30 minutes while the aneurysm was resected and the rent repaired with 8-0 sutures. The patient showed no postoperative symptomatology. In all other cases, a clip could be applied to the neck of the aneurysm. Incidental "baby" aneurysms were generally treated by electrocoagulation and covered with muscle.

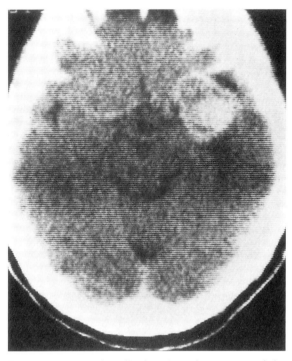

Fig **73A** Large subtotally thrombosed aneurysm of the right middle cerebral artery on CT scan.

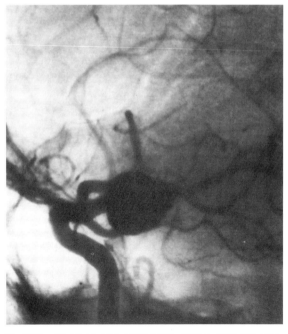

Fig **73B** Right carotid angiogram shows only the non-thrombosed portion of the aneurysm sac.

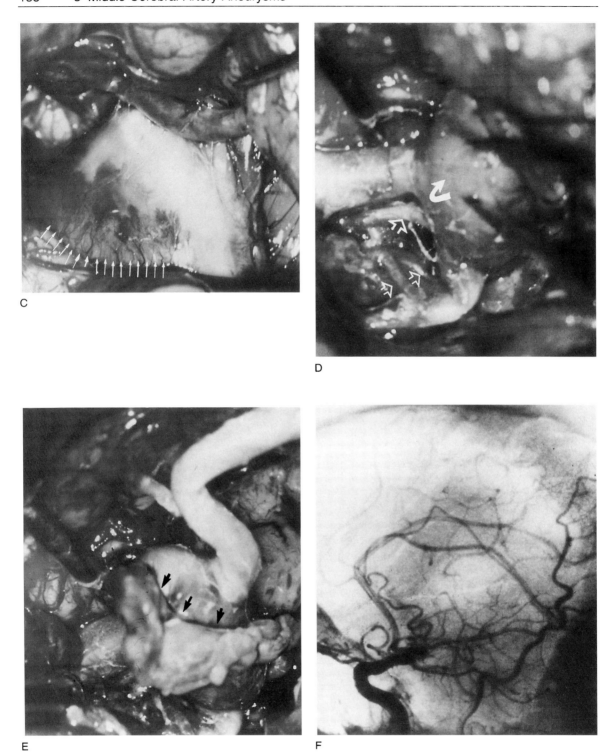

Fig **73C–F** At operation the aneurysm was seen to have a sclerotic wall with visible vasa vasorum (arrows) (**C**). With retraction (**D**) the distal lateral striate arteries (arrow) were also visible. An aneurysmorrhaphy (arrows) (**E**) was performed and a small residual bulge wrapped, with a good postoperative result (**F**).

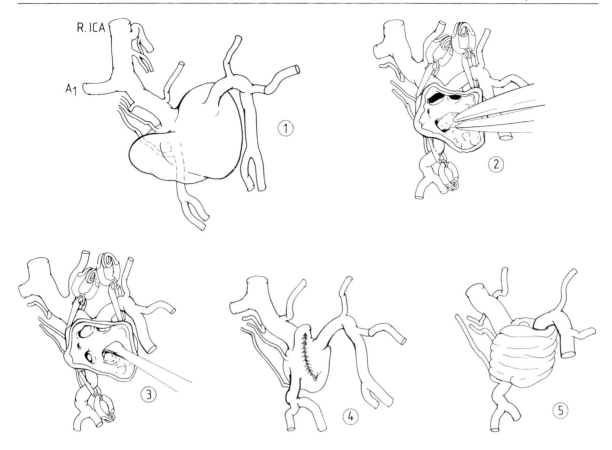

Fig 73G Schematic illustration of the operative procedure.

Closure

All hematoma is removed from the Sylvian cistern and from the adjacent temporal and frontal lobes, and papaverine is applied to the major arteries. The sympathetic plexus has routinely been removed from the arterial adventitia. With hemostasis secured, the wound is closed in the usual manner.

Summary of Operative Technique

1) Frontotemporosphenoidal craniotomy.
2) Opening of the carotid cistern to the internal carotid artery bifurcation.
3) Opening of the lamina terminalis cistern to allow retraction of the frontal lobe.
4) Removal of intracerebral hematoma if present.
5) Opening of the Sylvian cistern over the M_1 segment of the middle cerebral artery to gain proximal control.
6) Opening of the Sylvian cistern beyond the middle cerebral artery bifurcation to expose the major branches of the middle cerebral artery.
7) Separation of the middle cerebral artery branches from the neck of the aneurysm.
8) Identification and separation of the lenticulostriate arteries from the neck of the aneurysm.
9) Bipolar coagulation and clipping of the aneurysm with sequential clipping at the base, excision of the fundus, coagulation of the cut edges, and clip replacement until every part of the aneurysm is included in the clip.
10) Resection of the aneurysm fundus and inspection of clip placement.
11) Removal of remaining hematoma from the Sylvian cistern.
12) Application of papaverine and removal of adventitial sympathetic plexus from major arteries.
13) Hemostasis and closure.

Bilateral and Multiple Aneurysms

By opening the Sylvian fissure and carrying dissection into the basal cisterns across the carotid, lamina terminalis, and chiasmatic cisterns into the interpeduncular cistern, most of the common sites of aneurysm formation are exposed. In 23 patients, one or more additional aneurysms were present (ipsilateral to the middle cerebral artery aneurysm or in the midline) that could be clipped at one operation. 14 of these patients had one additional aneurysm, 6 had two additional aneurysms, and 3 had three additional lesions. Several of these patients in addition had smaller aneurysms which were coagulated and covered with muscle. Another 22 patients had only smaller or broader-based additional aneurysms which were again treated by the coagulation and muscle technique (Fig 74A–E).

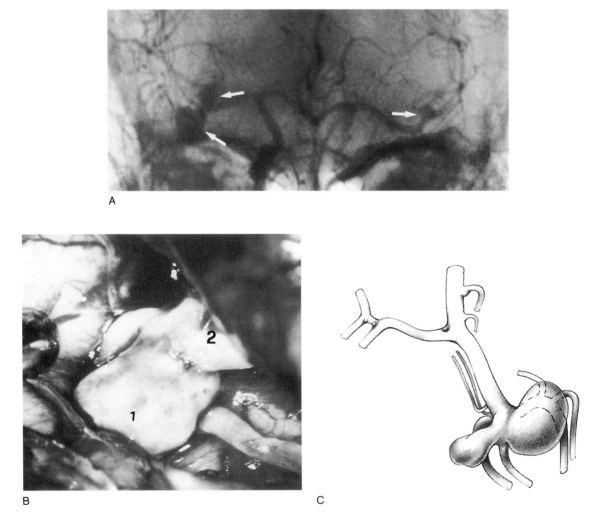

Fig 74 A–C   Right sided carotid angiography with cross compression showed bilateral aneurysms of middle cerebral artery bifurcation (arrows). On the right side the ruptured symptomatic aneurysm appears bilobular (**A**). At operation two aneurysms were seen arising from the same point (**B** 1 and 2). This situation is shown diagrammatically in (**C**).

Operative Technique

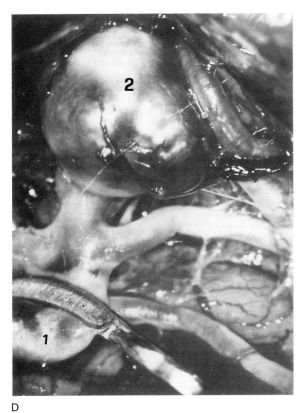
D

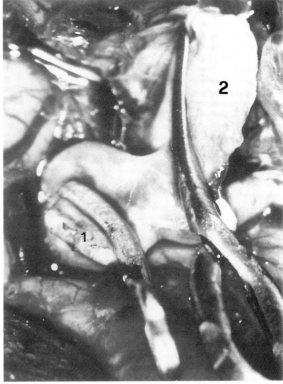
E

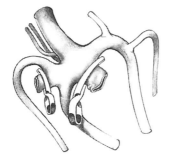
F

Fig 74 D–F First the medially directed unruptured aneurysm (1) was clipped (**D**) then the second, larger, ruptured aneurysm (2) with a temporally projecting fundus was dissected and clipped (**E**). The operative procedure is shown in (**F**).

More problematic are those cases in which additional aneurysms are located on the contralateral side. In 6 cases there were one or more aneurysms on the contralateral internal carotid artery. It is often possible to dissect and clip an aneurysm of the contralateral internal carotid artery bifurcation or of the medial wall of the internal carotid artery, but aneurysms of the lateral wall of the contralateral internal carotid artery are usually hidden from view by the optic nerve and by the artery itself. In 5 of these, a second operation was required to obliterate the aneurysm (Figs **75A–B, 76, 77A–G**). In 1 case it was possible following successful clipping of a right middle cerebral artery bifurcation aneurysm to clip aneurysms of the right and left internal carotid artery bifurcations and also an aneurysm arising from the proximal left middle cerebral artery at the origin of a striate artery. This latter procedure was attempted because the patient had several severe medical problems including a transplanted kidney and a second operation was risky. After clipping the right sided aneurysm, a subfrontal-suprachiasmal plane of dissection allowed access to the left M_1 segment and the aneurysm was clipped (Fig **78A–D**) (see also Chapter 7, Table **129**).

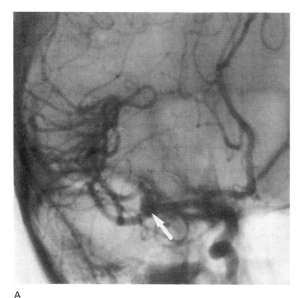
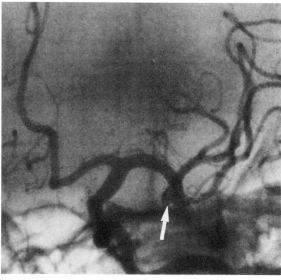

A   B

Fig **75A–B** Bilateral middle cerebral bifurcation aneurysms (arrows) (**A** right and **B** left) in a patient with left sided headaches and left sided changes on EEG. The right aneurysm was explored first because of its lobulation but was found to be unruptured. A second operation permitted clipping of the ruptured smaller left sided aneurysm.

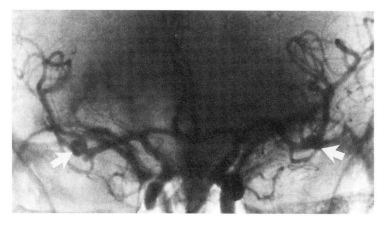

Fig **76** Symmetrical bilateral aneurysms (arrows) that were clipped in 2 separate procedures 3 months apart.

Operative Technique 143

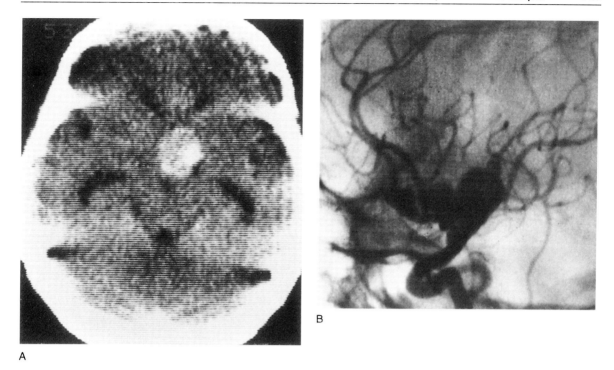

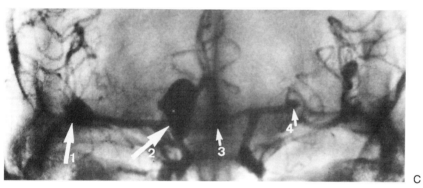

Fig 77A–G CT scan (**A**) of a 54 year old patient with a subarachnoid hemorrhage showing a large aneurysm. Angiography (**B** and **C**) showed aneurysms of the right middle cerebral bifurcation (1) and inferior wall of the internal carotid artery (2) the anterior communicating artery (3), and the left middle cerebral artery (4).

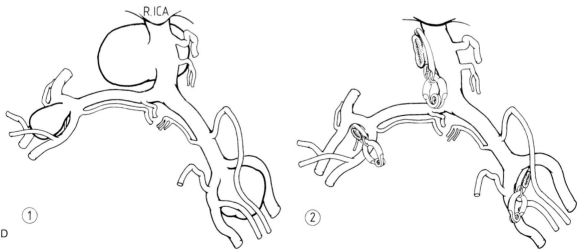

Fig 77D At operation (**D**) aneurysms of the right middle cerebral bifurcation and internal carotid-inferior wall and anterior communicating were clipped.

3 Middle Cerebral Artery Aneurysms

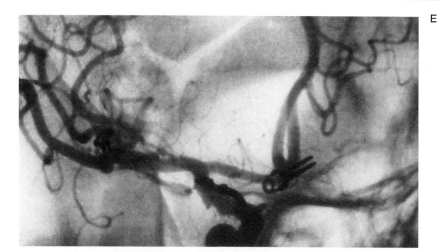

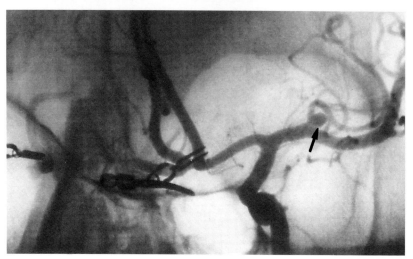

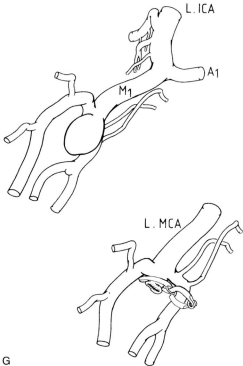

Fig **77 E–G** Postoperative angiography shows complete obliteration of the clipped right sided aneurysms (**E** and **F**) whereas the left sided aneurysm (arrow) of middle cerebral artery bifurcation is still unchanged. This was successfully occluded one year later at the insistence of the patient (**G**).

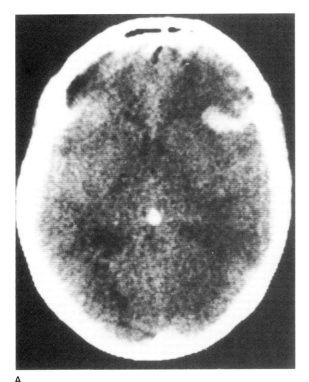

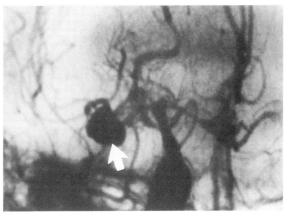

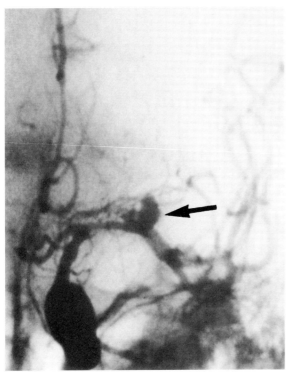

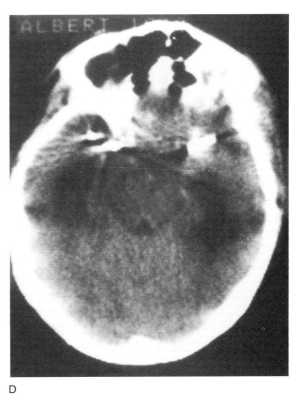

Fig **78A–D** Bilateral middle cerebral aneurysms seen on CT scan (**A**) and angiography (arrows) (**B** and **C**) in a 31 year old kidney transplant patient. The ruptured right aneurysm of the MCA-bifurcation was explored and clipped, as was the left sided M_1 aneurysm at the same right pterional approach. Postoperative CT scan (**D**) shows both clips in place.

Finally there are cases of bilateral symmetrical aneurysms of the middle cerebral artery bifurcation, of which there were 8 such cases in the present series. This situation presents two problems. First a diagnostic problem exists as to which lesion has bled. In 1 case, a patient showed bilateral middle cerebral artery bifurcation aneurysms larger on the right with no indication by symptomatology, angiography, or CT scan as to which aneurysm had bled. Only EEG suggested some left hemisphere disturbances. Because the right sided lesion was the larger it was done first and found to be unruptured. A second operation was required to treat the ruptured left sided aneurysm (Fig **75A–B**).

The second problem concerns the appropriate treatment of the unruptured aneurysm. Of these 8 cases 4 underwent a second operation within a few months to 2 years for treatment of the unruptured aneurysm. Three remain untreated and asymptomatic. The final patient had bilateral giant aneurysms (see below).

Giant Aneurysms

Giant aneurysms (greater than 25 mm diameter) occasionally arise from the middle cerebral artery and may give rise to ischemic symptoms or seizures. Most of these lesions will contain considerable thrombus and this thrombus may partially occlude the lumina of the parent arteries. If possible, the aneurysm should be shrunk with bipolar coagulation, forceps compression, or ligature, and then clipped in stages while resecting portions of the fundus. If the lesion is very large and subtotally thrombosed, it is sometimes possible to open the fundus and begin resecting thrombus as if it were tumor. This is continued until bleeding is encountered. Temporary clips are then applied. This maneuver shortens the time of temporary clipping and by removing much of the bulk makes the aneurysm much more manageable. When there is a question of either preexisting ischemia or anticipated use of temporary clips, an extracranial-intracranial arterial anastomosis may be indicated as was done in 1 case in the present series (see Fig **79A–H**, see also Vol. I, Fig **230**).

H. Le., a 44 year old man, (see Table **54**, case No. 6) complained of left frontal headaches, syncope, and gradual deterioration of memory and concentration over a 1 to 2 year period. Plain skull roentgenography revealed a larger ring-shaped calcification in the area of the left Sylvian fissure, and computerized tomography showed this to be a large, subtotally thrombosed aneurysm. A smaller aneurysm was present in the corresponding area on the right side. Angiography confirmed the presence of these aneurysms as well as a small aneurysm on the left internal carotid artery bifurcation. At operation on 15 November, 1976, the aneurysm was resected with a short segment of the left middle cerebral artery, and an end-to-end anastomosis of the superficial temporal artery to the inferior trunk of the middle cerebral artery performed. The left internal carotid bifurcation aneurysm and a tiny aneurysm on the anterior communicating artery were also clipped. The postoperative course was uneventful. Computerized tomography performed one year later demonstrated the right middle cerebral artery aneurysm to have grown almost to the size of the former left middle cerebral artery aneurysm. The patient was working and preferred to postpone a second operation. In October, 1978, he ruptured the right middle cerebral artery aneurysm and underwent emergency surgery at another hospital. He was left with a left hemiparesis (Fig **79A–H**).

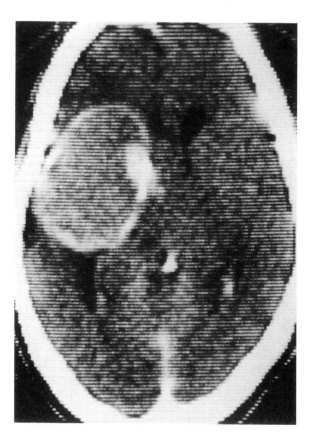

Fig **79A** Giant middle cerebral artery aneurysm on CT scan.

Operative Technique 147

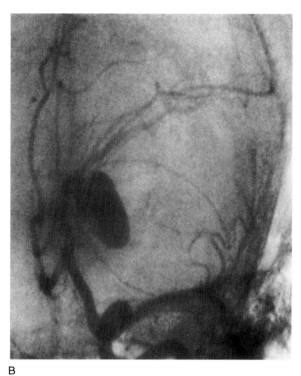

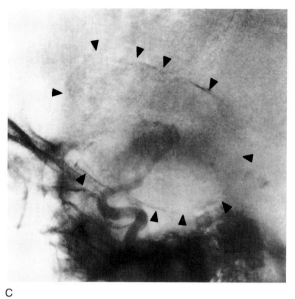

Fig 79 B–D Left sided giant, right sided large aneurysms of the middle cerebral artery (**B, C, F, G**). The calcified wall of the left sided aneurysm is outlined (arrow heads) (**C**). This subtotally thrombosed symptomatic aneurysm with mass effect was first explored and could be attacked only after trapping and EC-IC anastomosis. Additional aneurysms on the left carotid bifurcation and anterior communicating artery have been clipped (**D** 1–2).

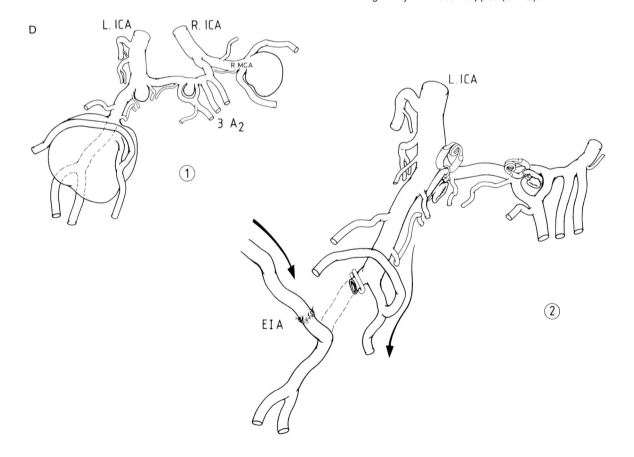

148   3 Middle Cerebral Artery Aneurysms

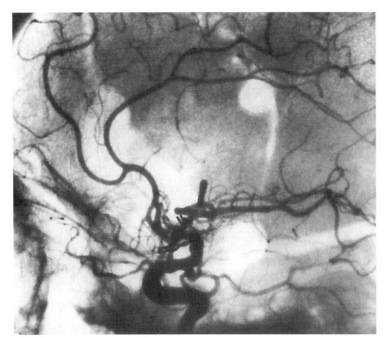

Fig 79 E The postoperative course was uneventful. Postoperative left sided angiography showed that the giant aneurysm had been eliminated and there was a patent anastomosis.

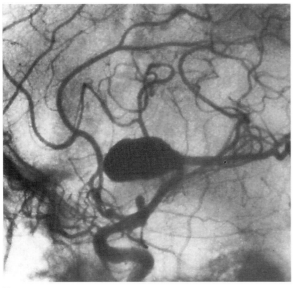

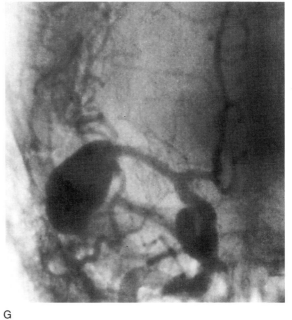

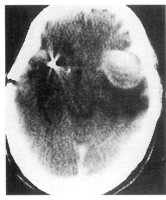

Fig 79 F–H Two years after operation the patient had an intracerebral hemorrhage from the right middle cerebral artery aneurysm. Right sided carotid angiograms (F and G) and CT scan (H). The patient underwent emergency surgery at another hospital.

Clinical Presentation and Operative Results

Background

When the morphology of cerebral aneurysms was less well understood and excision of the lesion seemed necessary, the ensuing mortality and morbidity of operation were forbidding (Dandy 1944). Nevertheless, Swain (1948) was able to report 4 intracranially operated patients in which there were no deaths and only one patient had a residual hemiparesis. Campbell and Burklund (1953) reported 6 cases in which an aneurysm of the middle cerebral artery had been excised. One of these died and three were left with a neurological deficit. It was clear that while collateral circulation might be sufficient in some cases, the routine sacrifice of the middle cerebral artery did not represent satisfactory treatment of these lesions.

Petit-Dutaillis and Pittman (1955) reported on 9 cases 4 of whom had died, and felt that under favorable circumstances it should be possible to exclude the aneurysm and leave the middle cerebral artery circulation intact. This opinion was echoed by Cabiesas and Landa (1956) and by Gass and associates (1958). The first large series of middle cerebral artery aneurysms was that of Höök and Norlén (1958) in which 64 patients underwent operation with a 9 per cent mortality and 25 per cent morbidity. McKissock and associates (1962) published a series of 61 patients who were compared to a similar size group of non-operated patients. Poor and good risk patients were included and an attempt was made to randomize the treatment protocol. 17 cases (27.9%) in the operated group died and 15 (24.6%) showed some morbidity. While this represented some improvement over non-operated cases, neurosurgeons were left with the feeling that treatment of these lesions remained inadequate. Thus other methods of treatment were sought. Selverstone (1962) described 13 patients whose aneurysms were treated by plastic coating with no mortality and one residual hemiparesis.

In the last 15 years, several larger series of patients have been published. Sachs (1966) reported 52 cases operated intracranially with a 42 per cent mortality rate and Laine and co-workers (1970) reported 100 cases done over a 10 year period with 24 per cent deaths. Robinson (1971) reported a series of 84 patients done between 1947 and 1969 with an overall mortality of 18 per cent. He also showed that the mortality rate had been reduced from 37 per cent before 1955 to 8 per cent after 1955 with improved case selection and technique. Lipovsek (1973) reported a series of 30 cases with aneurysms of the proximal middle cerebral artery treated by cervical carotid artery ligation only with mortality and morbidity rates of 20 per cent each, and Peerless (1974) reported on 28 middle cerebral artery aneurysm patients undergoing operation with a 7 per cent mortality and 14 per cent morbidity rate. These series of middle cerebral artery aneurysm patients are summarized in Table 49.

Table 49 Published series of middle cerebral artery aneurysm patients

Authors and year of publication	Time span of series	Method of operation	Cases	Mortality	Morbidity
Swain (1948)	not given	Intracran	4	0	25%
Campbell and Burklund (1953)	1947–1951	Intracran	6	17%	50%
Petit-Dutaillis and Pittman (1955)	1946–1954	Intracran	9	44%	22%
Cabiesas and Landa (1956)	1953–1955	Intracran	5	40%	0
Gass et al. (1958)	not given	Intracran	14	21%	7%
Höök and Norlén (1958)	1934–1955	Comb	64	9%	25%
McKissock et al. (1962)	1958–1961	Intracran	61	28%	25%
Selverstone (1962)	1958–1962	Intracran	13	0	8%
Sachs (1966)	1954–1965	Intracran	52	42%	17%
Laine et al. (1970)	1959–1969	Intracran	100	24%	20%
Robinson (1971)	1947–1969	Comb	84	18%	26%
Lipovsek (1973)	1957–1971	Car Lig	30	20%	20%
Peerless (1974)	1969–1972	Intracran	28	7%	14%

Intracran	all patients had an intracranial procedure
Car Lig	all patients had cervical carotid artery ligation
Comb	patients had either one or both of the above procedures

Presenting Features

Of the 184 patients undergoing operation for aneurysms of the middle cerebral artery, 113 (61.4%) were women and 71 (38.6%) men. Ages ranged from 14 to 71 with 80 per cent of patients between the ages of 30 and 60 (Table 50). The incidence of middle cerebral aneurysm is only slightly higher in women in patients under age 50, but is almost 4 times that of men in patients over 50. Thus much of the increased frequency of middle cerebral artery aneurysms in women is accounted for in the later age groups.

Rupture of a middle cerebral artery aneurysm occurred in 170 of the 184 patients (92.4%). Of the 14 patients with unruptured aneurysms, 3 were incidental findings (see Table 52) while all the others had neurological symptoms such as seizures, hemiparesis, aphasia or mental deterioration on the basis of mass effect. Of those patients presenting with subarachnoid hemorrhage, about half exhibited hemiparesis of variable severity, and about one third showed some speech disturbance.

Operative Results

Overall operative results for the 184 patients are related to preoperative grade in Table 51, 154 patients (83.7%) had a good result which means that they returned to their former activities with no deficit. 15 patients (8.1%) were left in fair condition, and 6 patients (3.3%) remained in poor condition. 9 patients (4.9%) died. Operative results are more meaningful, however, when discussed in relation to preoperative condition. In the following presentation, preoperative grades with similar outcomes have been grouped together to avoid repetition.

Table 50 Age and sex of 184 patients with middle cerebral artery aneurysms

Age	Total		%	Male		Female	
11–20	4		2.2	1		3	
21–30	20	133	10.9	9	60	11	73
31–40	47	(72.3%)	25.5	20	(84.5%)	27	(64.6%)
41–50	62		33.7	30		32	
51–60	38		20.6	10		28	
61–70	11	51	5.9	1	11	10	40
over 70	2	(27.7%)	1.1	–	(15.5%)	2	(35.4%)
	184			71 (38.6%)		113 (61.4%)	

Grades 0a, Ia, and IIa

This group includes 74 cases, 71 with subarachnoid hemorrhage and 3 with incidentally discovered aneurysms (Table 52). There were no deaths in this group of patients. All but 1 made complete recoveries. 3 patients experienced postoperative deficits (hemiparesis and aphasia in 2 and aphasia only in 1) but recovered over 2 weeks to 6 months. Temporary clips were not used in any of these 3 patients. 2 of the patients awoke with hemiparesis implying some injury to the brain occurring at operation. The third patient developed hemiparesis on the fifth postoperative day. CT scan was not yet available at the time these patients underwent operation. It is pre-

Table 51 Operative results related to preoperative grade in 184 patients with aneurysms of the middle cerebral artery

Grade	Total No.	(%) of 184	Good	Fair	Poor	Death
0a	3	1.6	3	–	–	–
0b	11	6.0	8	2	1	–
Ia	42	22.8	41	1	–	–
Ib	2	1.1	2	–	–	–
IIa	29	15.8	29	–	–	–
IIb	40	21.7	36	4	–	–
IIIa	7	3.8	6	1	–	–
IIIb	32	17.4	25	6	–	1
IV	9	4.9	4	1	3 (2*)	1
V	9	4.9	–	–	2 (1*)	7
	184		154 (83.7%)	15 (8.1%)	6 (3.3%)	9 (4.9%)

* died later

Table 52 Non ruptured asymptomatic aneurysms (Oa). 3 cases			Age	Sex	
	1. Cu	1975	55	F	The son of the patient (MD) performed an angiogram, because her sister died of a ruptured aneurysm. The angiograms showed an aneurysm of the right middle cerebral artery bifurcation. The operation was uneventful with a good outcome
	2. Ja	1977	49	M	Right sided Horner's syndrome indicated vertebral angiography. Accidental visualization of the right posterior communicating artery and internal carotid artery showed a well developed bilobular aneurysm of the right middle cerebral bifurcation. The patient (MD) insisted on operation. The clipping was successful without any side-effect.
	3. Sch.	1978	37	M	After successful operation on a hemorrhagic AVM of the right occipital lobe, a thin-walled large aneurysm of the right middle cerebral bifurcation was clipped at a second operation with a good result.*

* 9 other none ruptured aneurysm cases associated with hemorrhagic AVM's are presented in Table 25, page 310, Vol. I

sumed that each patient suffered some degree of cerebral infarction although each went on to make a full recovery.

One patient required temporary clipping of the middle cerebral artery to handle a large, sclerotic aneurysm and he has recovered to only a fair condition.

Or., a 41 year old man, had undergone a right frontal craniotomy for repair of a spontaneous cerebrospinal fluid fistula in 1962. On 5 Febuary, 1975, he sustained a subarachnoid hemorrhage and presented in a stable neurological condition. Angiography revealed an aneurysm on the right middle cerebral artery bifurcation with associated spasm of the internal carotid and middle cerebral arteries on the right. At operation on 18 February, 1975, the aneurysm was found to be large and broad based, and was especially sclerotic with calcification in the wall. It was necessary to apply temporary clips to the right middle cerebral artery twice for periods of 5 minutes each time. The aneurysm was finally successfully clipped and after coagulation muscle was applied to an associated small aneurysm at the origin of the right posterior communicating artery. The patient awoke with a left hemiplegia which has improved to a moderate hemiparesis. He is working at about 50 per cent capacity (Fig **80A–D**).

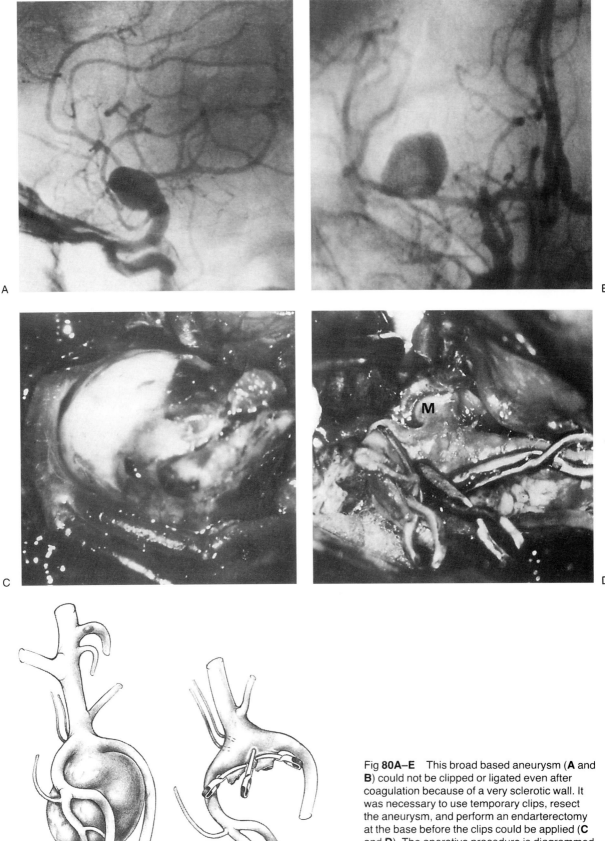

Fig 80A–E This broad based aneurysm (**A** and **B**) could not be clipped or ligated even after coagulation because of a very sclerotic wall. It was necessary to use temporary clips, resect the aneurysm, and perform an endarterectomy at the base before the clips could be applied (**C** and **D**). The operative procedure is diagrammed in (**E**). Unfortunately the patient awoke with a permanent hemiparesis.

The neurological deficit in this patient is attributable to the temporary clipping of the middle cerebral artery that was necessary to control the large, difficult aneurysm. In 6 other patients, 1 in grade Ia and 5 in grade IIa, temporary clipping of the middle cerebral artery was used for shorter periods of time – 30 seconds to 3 minutes – with no adverse effects.

One patient making a good recovery required re-operation when he remained drowsy after operation. Upon re-exploration only a subdural hematoma was found. 1 other patient experienced transient pulmonary emboli with no sequelae. The remainder of patients (68 out of 74) making good recoveries had a completely uncomplicated postoperative course with no hydrocephalus, seizures, or infection. The lengths of stay in the hospital and time prior to their return to work are given in Table 53.

Grades 0b, Ib, and IIb

There were 53 patients in these 3 grades, including 11 patients with unruptured aneurysms associated with neurological deficits (grade 0b). Again there were no deaths among these patients. 46 patients (86.7%) made a good recovery with preoperative neurological deficits resolving (Table 54).

Grade 0b: There were 11 patients who presented with unruptured large aneurysms associated with neurological deficits. None of these patients died and 8 made complete recoveries. One (No. 2)

Table 53 Length of hospital stay and time to return to work in 74 of 75 grade 0a–Ia–IIa patients with good results following operation for middle cerebral artery aneurysm*

Length of hospital stay	Cases	(%)
1–2 weeks	54	72.0
2–3 weeks	15	20.0
3–4 weeks	5	6.6

Time to return to work	Cases	(%)
1–2 months	55	73.3
2–3 months	10	13.3
3–6 months	9	12.0

* 1 patient remains in fair condition working at about 50 per cent capacity

Table 54 Non ruptured, but symptomatic aneurysms (0b)

Patient	Age	Sex	Year	Initial symptoms	Angiography	Aneurysm	Operation	Result	
1. Ru	58	M	1973	Insult + Hpr. r + aphasia	Stenosis ICA l.	Medium, MCA l.	Clip	Good	Full recovery
2. Ca	42	F	1975	Insult + Hpr. r. + aphasia	Stenosis ICA l.	Medium, MCA l.	Clip	Fair	Mild hpr. + dysphasia
3. St	36	M	1974	Insult + Hpr. l. + aphasia	Subtotal occl. of MCA r.	Fusiform MCA r.	Muscle	Poor	Unchanged Hpr. + aphasia
4. Ma	53	M	1977	Insult + Hpr. r. + aphasia	–	Small l.lent.str.	Clip	Good	Full recovery
5. Tu	57	M	1978	Seizures + Mild Hpr. l.	Subtotal Occl. of MCA l.	Large, MCA r.	Microsut.	Good	Full recovery
6. Le	44	M	1976	Seizures + Mild hpr. r. POS	4 aneurysms	Giant l.	Clip EIA Resection		2 ys later right MCA aneurysm ruptured since then hpr. l.
7. Mi	30	M	1973	Seizures + Mild arm paresis r.	–	Distal MCA aneurysm l. thrombosed	Clip Resection	Good	Full recovery
8. Ma	56	M	1978	Seizures + Mild hemisyndrome r.	–	Medium, MCA l.	Clip	Good	Full recovery
9. Ge	44	F	1974	Seizures + Dysphasia	–	Small, MCA l.	Clip	Good	Full recovery
10. D.	41	M	1979	Seizures + Hpr. r. + aphasia	–	Large, MCA l.	Clip	Good	Full recovery
11. C.	45	M	1979	Seizures + Mild hemisyndrome l.	–	Large, MCA r.	Clip	Good	Full recovery

showed improvement after surgery but remained with some neurological dysfunction and is listed in the fair category. One other patient (No. 6) had a contralateral middle cerebral artery bifurcation aneurysm for which he declined treatment. 2 years after operation he sustained a subarachnoid hemorrhage from this aneurysm and underwent operation at another hospital (see page 146).

One patient with a large fusiform aneurysm remains in poor condition:

L. St., a left-handed male seen in 1974 at age 36, had awakened on 31 March, 1963, with a left hemiparesis and aphasia. Subsequent angiography demonstrated an aneurysm of the right middle cerebral artery and a fusiform dilatation of the A_2 segment of the anterior communicating artery. At operation on 8 May, 1963, the middle cerebral artery was found to show a fusiform dilatation of the bifurcation and was wrapped with muscle. The anterior communicating artery was not explored. Although hindered by a mild left hemiparesis, the patient returned to full time work, married, and was active until 6 May, 1974, 11 years after the first operation, when he suddenly developed a complete left hemiplegia and a non-fluent aphasia. There was no associated headache and lumbar puncture was negative. Angiography showed continued presence of the previously noted aneurysms with occlusion of the right anterior cerebral artery and occlusion of the main branches of the right middle cerebral artery. He underwent surgery on 10 July, 1974, with the thought that perhaps some occluded vessels could be opened or an arterial bypass anastomosis performed. At operation the right frontal and temporal lobes were atrophic. The rest of the dilated A_2 was clipped, but nothing could be done with the thrombosed middle cerebral artery branches and the fusiform aneurysm was again wrapped in muscle.

He remained hemiparetic and dysphasic, with a fairly well-controlled seizure disorder. He is unable to work (see Vol. I, Fig **227**).

None of these 11 cases was made worse by operation. These large unruptured lesions present the problems of both a mass lesion and of an aneurysm.

Grades Ib and IIb: There were 42 patients in these 2 grades. Of these 38 (90.5%) made a good recovery. There were no deaths or poor results in these patients. Preexisting neurological deficits generally resolved within 4 to 12 weeks. 2 patients developed osteomyelitis of the bone flap and required subsequent cranioplasty. 2 patients have a seizure disorder, one of whom had seizures preoperatively and the other experiencing seizures first in the postoperative period. Both patients are well-controlled on anticonvulsant medication. Length of hospital stays and time to return to work are given in Table **55**.

4 patients, all in preoperative grade IIb, are categorized as fair results. 2 of these improved

Table **55** Length of hospital stay and time to return to work in 46 of 53 grades 0b–Ib–IIb patients with good results following operation for middle cerebral artery aneurysm*

Length of hospital stay	Cases	(%)
1–2 weeks	38	82.6
2–4 weeks	8	17.4
	46	

Time to return to work	Cases	(%)
1–3 months	14	30.4
3–6 months	32	69.6
	46	

* 6 cases are in fair condition and 1 in poor condition

with respect to their preexisting deficits, and 2 remained unchanged. Each of these patients had suffered cerebral infarction prior to operation, and while having the threat of recurrent hemorrhage removed, were not expected to be improved by operation, per se. None of these patients with acute or chronic infarction but with a fairly good level of consciousness was made worse by operation. 3 patients had seizures both pre- and postoperatively. 1 patient required ventricular shunting (Table **56**).

Grade IIIa

There were 7 cases in grade IIIa. All were women. 6 of these cases recovered to good condition, 6 patients were home within 2 weeks and 1 by 2 months. All have returned to full activity. 1 patient had pre- and postoperative seizures which have been controlled by medication. It is interesting that 3 of these 6 patients had fairly large intracerebral hematomas despite the lack of focal neurological deficits.

The seventh case had a complicated postoperative course, and died of an independent cerebrovascular lesion 3 months after operation:

M. H., a 34 year old woman with a ventricular septal defect, had complained of severe headaches associated with menses for years. On 13 July, 1974, she suffered a subarachnoid hemorrhage and was admitted in drowsy condition with minimal left hemiparesis. Angiography disclosed multiple aneurysms including lesions on both middle cerebral artery bifurcations and a larger aneurysm on the right M_1 segment. At operation on 27 July, 1974, a ruptured aneurysm of the right M_1 segment at the origin of a lenticulostriate artery was clipped as were 2 additional aneurysms on the right middle cerebral artery and an aneurysm of the anterior communicating artery. A small additional aneurysm of the right

Table 56 Patients in grade IIb with fair postoperative results

Patient	Age	Sex	Year	SAH	Side	Mul-tipl.	Hema-toma	Preoperative deficit	Grade	Time post SAH	Opera-tion	Course
Gi	35	M	1967	5	R	–	–	L. hpr.POS r. MCA sten.	IIb	6m	Clip	Preoperat. cerebral atrophy. VA shunt. Mild improvement, partially working
Su	31	M	1968	1	L	–	–	R. hpr. l. MCA sten.	IIb	6m	Clip	L. MCA stenosis. Moderate improvement, partially working
Be	31	F	1971	1	R	–	–	L. hpr.	IIb	2m	Clip	Moderate improvement, partially working
Si	43	M	1978	1	R	–	–	L. hpr.	IIb	8m	Clip	Moderate improvement, partially working

anterior temporal artery was covered with muscle. There was marked sclerosis of the middle cerebral artery and the major trunks. Her postoperative course was uneventful.
3 months later she succumbed to an intracranial hemorrhage. Autopsy surprisingly showed an unruptured left middle cerebral artery aneurysm, but rupture of a pontine cavernous malformation, which had taken the patient's life.

In this case the patient was recovering after surgery and would have achieved at least fair status had she not succumbed to a second hemorrhage from an independent source.

Grade IIIb

32 patients (25 females, 7 males) presented in a stuporous, confused state with hemiparesis and/or aphasia. Of these, 17 (56%) had an intracerebral hematoma and 1 had both an intracerebral and a subdural hematoma. Of these 25 patients (78.1%) made a good recovery, but this generally required more time than with the better grade patients. All 25 were back to full activity by the end of 6 months. None of these cases required reexploration, but 2 required ventricular shunts. Interestingly, only 1 of the 25 developed seizures.
6 patients recovered to fair status. These cases are summarized in Table 57. Again, failure to recover

Table 57 Patients in grade IIIb with fair operative results

Patient	Age	Sex	Year	SAH	Side	Mul-tipl.	Hema-toma	Preoperative deficit	Grade	Time post SAH	Opera-tion	Course	Result
1. Fü	51	F	1967	1	R	–	ICH	L. hemip. Hypertens. Diabetes	IIIb	13 d	Clip	Mod. improvement	Fair
2. Sc	51	F	1974	1	R	–	–	L. hemip. L. hemian.	IIIb	4 w	Clip	Req. VA shunt Hemip. improved Hemian. same	Fair
3. Ho	63	M	1975	L	R	–	–	L. hemip. L. hemian. Hypertens.	IIIb	10 d	Clip	Hemip. improved Hemian. same	Fair
4. Bo	48	F	1977	1	R	–	–	L. hemip. L. hemian.	IIIb	8d	Clip	Hemip. improved Hemian. same	Fair
5. Mo	62	F	1978	1	L	–	–	R. hemip. Aphasia	IIIb	5w	Clip	Mod. improvement	Fair
6. Re	37	M	1972	1	R	–	–	R. hemip. 3ds. after angiogr.	IIIb	2 m	Clip	Mod. improvement of r. hemip. Left normal CT does not show infarct	Fair

from preexisting deficits accounted for the morbidity in these cases.

One patient died of cerebral infarction:
Tr., a 48 year old female, suffered a subarachnoid hemorrhage on 18 November, 1969, with a resultant left hemiparesis and sensory deficit including a visual field deficit. Angiography showed a small aneurysm of the right middle cerebral artery and a 2 mm aneurysm of the posterior communicating artery origin. At the time of transfer on 21 November, 1969, the patient was somnolent, and at operation on 24 November, the brain was voluminous. The aneurysm on the right middle cerebral artery was clipped and the small aneurysm on the origin of the posterior communicating artery was coagulated and covered with muscle. The patient awakened slowly from anesthesia and continued to demonstrate a left hemiparesis. By the following day, she was obtunded and hemiplegic and was returned to the operating room. The brain was more swollen and hemorrhagic. A wide bony decompression was carried out, but the patient remained in poor condition and died 4 days later. An autopsy revealed a large hemorrhagic infarction in the center of the right frontal lobe.

At present, if CT scan were to show a large acute cerebral infarct in such a patient, operation would be delayed.

Grade IV

9 patients underwent operation in grade IV. All these patients had large hematomas including 2 with subdural hematomas. 4 made good recoveries (2 female, 2 male, aged 30–37 years) (44.4%). Except for a somewhat prolonged recovery time, the postoperative courses of these 4 patients were uncomplicated. None has epilepsy and none has required a ventricular shunt. 1 patient showed improvement of a preoperative hemiparesis, 4 other patients showed no improvement (also after shunt procedures) and died 4, 9, and 2 years later. 1 patient is in a poor condition after 8 years.

Although the rate of good recovery is of course significantly less in grade IV patients than in those in better preoperative condition, it is noteworthy that almost half of these semicomatose patients with large hematomas were able to return to a normal life and to their previous occupations. Without removal of hematoma and decompression of the brain most if not all, of these patients would die. This might justify intervention in grade IV patients secondary to ruptured middle cerebral artery aneurysms who have intracerebral hematomas.

Grade V

8 younger patients underwent operation in grade V with fixed, dilated pupils and absent respirations. Operation was undertaken in the hope that such young patients might be able to recover after removal of large intracranial hematomas. None of the patients had an EEG performed prior to operation, nor any other type of formal death determination, because of their critical condition and the need for urgent intervention. The 8 patients were operated upon as emergencies within a day or two of hemorrhage, and each of them died (Table **58**). Another patient (60 year old man) reruptured his aneurysm during induction of anesthesia (1970) and promptly dilated both pupils. He could be salvaged, but only with a poor long term result:

It is not generally advisable to subject grade V patients to operation unless they are young and the time of brain herniation has been very short. The presently increasing literature on evaluation of brain death may contribute some guidelines to making this judgement (Table **58**) (Figs **81 A–B, 82A–B, 83**).

Table 58 Patients presenting in grade V with middle cerebral artery aneurysms

Patient	Age	Sex	Year	SAH	Side	Hematoma	Time post SAH	Grade	Spont. Respiration	Operation	Poor	Death
1. Ma	37	F	1969	2	L	Front. ICH	Same day	V	+	Clip	–	6 w
2. De	30	M	1970	1	L	Temp. ICH Ins. ICH	Same day	V	0	Clip	–	2 d
3. Pi	31	M	1971	3	L	Temp. ICH ivH	Same day	V	0	Clip	–	1 d
4. Mi	37	M	1973	2	R	SDH Front. ICH Temp. ICH ivH	Same day	V	0	Clip	–	1 d
5. Sp	32	F	1974	3	R	Temp. ICH	Next day	V	0	Clip	4 years*	–
6. Gu	37	F	1974	1	R	SDH Temp. ICH ivH	Same day	V	0	Clip	–	1 d
7. Ma	35	M	1974	2	R	Temp. ICH ivH a. angularis thrombosed	Same day	V	0	Clip	–	6 w
8. Bu	23	F	1975	1	L	SDH Temp. ICH ivH	Same day	V	0	Clip	–	1 d
9. Tr	60	M	1970	2	L	Temp. ICH ins.	Same day	V	+	Clip	9 years**	–

* died 4 years later
** alive

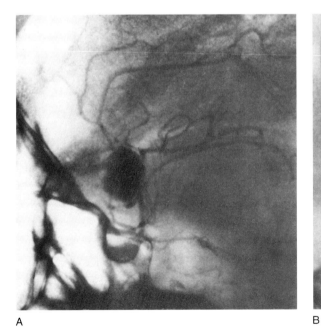 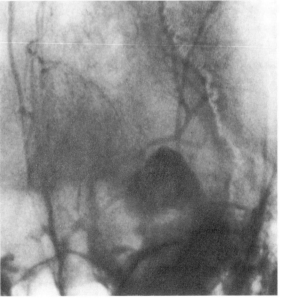

A B

Fig 81A–B 31 year old comatose patient, Case 3, Table 58, with marked spasm, mass effect, and a large middle cerebral aneurysm.

158   3 Middle Cerebral Artery Aneurysms

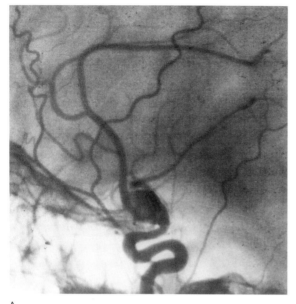

A

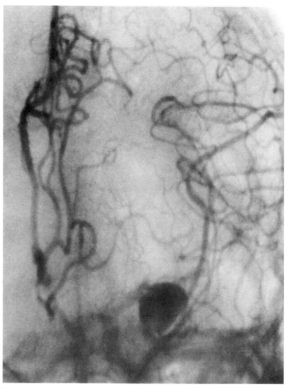

B

Fig 82A–B   30 year old comatose patient, Case 2, Table 58, with a middle cerebral aneurysm and marked mass effect.

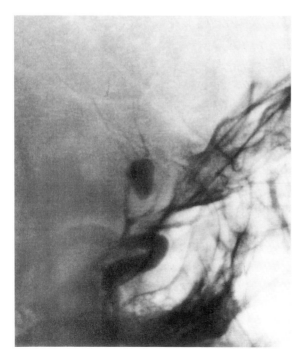

Fig 83   37 year old comatose patient, Case 4, Table 58, with severe spasm, non-filling of the middle cerebral artery branches, and an aneurysm at the left middle cerebral bifurcation.

Complications

Hydrocephalus

Of 184 cases undergoing operation, 10 (5.4%) required ventricular shunts, 1 in the preoperative period and 9 postoperatively. These patients are summarized in Table **59**. It is noted that 3 of the patients requiring shunts made good recoveries (in condition IIa–IIIb) while 3 others (in condition IV–V) died. The incidence of hydrocephalus with aneurysms of the middle cerebral artery is less than with other aneurysms as might be anticipated from their more lateral position away from the basal cisterns.

Epilepsy

11 patients (5.9%) developed epilepsy, either in the preoperative period (7) or in the immediate (3) or late (1) postoperative period. 9 cases have had preoperative hemiparesis (Table **60**). Only 1 patient (case No. 8) in an (a) category (without focal neurological deficit) developed a seizure disorder, and this was first seen in the preoperative period. The severity of hemorrhage does not appear to be an important factor in the production of epilepsy (as patients in Table **60** can be seen to range from grades 0b to IV) but infarction does seem to be a significant contributory factor.

Table 59 Patients with middle cerebral artery aneurysms requiring ventricular shunts for hydrocephalus

Patient	Age	Sex	Year	SAH	Side	Hemat.	Grade	Time of Operation	Result
1. G	35	M	1967	5	R	–	IIb	6 m	Fair
2. W.	50	F	1968	2	L	–	IIa	2 m	Good
2. W	50	F	1968	2	L	–	IIa	2 m	Good
3. St	46	F	1969	2	R	SDH	IV	1 d	Died 4 months
4. B	48	M	1970	1	R	ICH	IV	1d	Poor
5. F	62	F	1973	1	R	SDH + ICH	IV	3 w	Died 9 months
6. Sp	32	F	1974	3	R	ICH	V	2 d	Died 4 years
7. Sch	56	F	1974	1	R	–	IIIb	4 w	Fair
8. M	66	F	1975	1	R	–	IIIb	6 w	Good (shunt preop.)
9. M	61	F	1976	1	R	ICH	IV	5 d	Fair
10. U	62	F	1976	1	R	Cist.	IIIb	5 w	Good

5 cases with multiple SAH
6 cases with one SAH
4 cases with ICH
2 cases with SDH

Table 60 Patients developing epilepsy with middle cerebral artery aneurysms

Patient	Grade	Preop.	Transient postop.	Longterm postop.	Condition
1. Gi	IIb	+	–	+	Fair
2. V	IIb	–	+	–	Good
3. W	IV	–	+	–	Death
4. Su	IIb	+	–	+	Fair
5. Fa	0b	+	–	+	Good
7. Be	IIb	–	–	+	Fair
8. Go	IIIa	+	–	+	Good
9. Ho	IV	+	–	+	Good
10. Ep.	IIIb	+	–	+	Good
11. St	0b	+	–	+	Poor

Analysis of Results

Several factors were examined to evaluate their contribution to morbidity and mortality in the 184 patients with middle cerebral artery aneurysms:

Preoperative condition

The single most important factor in determining outcome was the preoperative condition. As was noted in Table **51** 98.6 per cent of patients in grades 0a, Ia, and IIa had a good result, while in grades 0b, Ib, and IIb only 86.8 per cent and in grades IIIa and b, only 79.5 per cent had a similar good outcome. Good results were seen in less than 45 per cent of grade IV patients and in no grade V patient. Similarly, mortality was 0 in patients from grades 0a to IIIa, but 3.1 per cent in grade IIIb, 11.1 per cent in grade IV, and 88.8 per cent in grade V. To accurately assess the importance of other factors it is necessary first to separate the patients into preoperative grades. With some factors this is possible, while with others the numbers are simply too small to be meaningful.

Age and Sex

Of the 184 patients in the present series 133 were under 50 years old and 51 were older than 50. Altogether 154 patients had a good outcome, including 112 of 133 patients under 50 (84.2%) and 42 of 51 (82.4%) over 50. There were 7 deaths (5.3%) in patients under 20 and 2 deaths (3.9%) in patients older than 50. While this might suggest no increase risk in older patients, it must be realized that much of the morbidity and mortality in younger patients is related to patients in very poor condition undergoing operation as a life-saving measure. An older patient in the same condition might be turned down for operation or not even transferred from the local hospital. Nevertheless, these figures do show that a substantial group of older patients can undergo operation for middle cerebral artery aneurysms with a favorable outcome (Table **61a–c**).

There were 113 women and 71 men in this series of patients. 98 women (86.7%) and 56 men (78.9%) had good results. Mortality rates between men and women were comparable, but morbidity figures are higher for men, and one is left with the impression that men withstand aneurysm rupture less well than women.

Table **61a** Age and sex

Age	Female		Male				
11–20	3		1				
21–30	11	73	9	60	F	73	
31–40	27	(64.6%)	20	(84.5%)	M	60	133 (72.3%)
41–50	32		30				
51–60	28		10				
61–70	10	40	1	11	F	40	51 (27.7%)
over 70	2	(35.4%)	–	(15.5%)	M	11	
	113		71			184	

Table **61b** Age, sex, and results

No. cases	Age	Sex	Good	Results Fair	Poor	Death	
133	under 50 y	F	64 (87.8%)	4	2 (2*)	3	73
		M	48 (79.7%)	6	2	4	60
51	over 50 y	F	34 (84.6%)	3 (7.7%)	1 (1*)	2 (7.7%)	40
		M	8 (75 %)	2 (16.6%)	1 (8%)	–	11
			154	15	6	9	184

Table 61c Sex, site, and results

	Good F	Good M	Fair F	Fair M	Poor F	Poor M	Death F	Death M	
Left	53	29	2	3	–	1	2	2	= 92 left
Right	44	28	6	4	3	2	1	4	= 92 right
	97	57	8	7	3	3	3	6	184
	154		15		6		9		

Timing of Operation

Timing of operation in the 170 patients who sustained subarachnoid hemorrhage is related to preoperative grade and operative results in Table 62. 14 patients (8.2%) underwent operation within 3 days of hemorrhage. 5 of these were in grade IV. 3 of these made full recoveries (60%), 1 remained in poor condition, and 2 died. 9 patients were in grade V. 7 of these died soon after operation, 1 still lives in poor condition after 12 years, and 1 remained in poor condition until her death 4 years later. Operation was performed as an emergency in all cases because of large intracranial hematomas. There were no good grade patients who underwent elective operation in the first 3 days.

31 patients had operation performed between 3 and 7 days after hemorrhage. Of these, 28 (90.3%) made good recoveries. 1 patient in grade IV recovered to a good condition and 1 grade IIIb patient died (see p. 156). 51 patients underwent operation between 8 and 14 days after subarachnoid hemorrhage. 1 patient in grade Ia was made worse by operation and 4 other cases in grades IIIa–b remained only in fair condition because of preexisting deficits, with 1 dying later from a pontine cavernous hemangioma.

Within the first 2 weeks, then, 56 patients in grades Ia to IIb underwent operation with 55 patients (98.2%) recovering completely and 1 patient achieving a fair result. From 2 weeks to over 4 months after hemorrhage, 57 patients in grades Ia to IIb were operated on, 53 patients (92.9%) recovered completely and 4 (all in grade IIb) were left in fair condition. This was primarily due to continuing neurological deficits from cerebral infarction. Grade Ia to IIa patients all did well, except 1 patient who underwent operation in the second week and suffered an ischemic deficit. Grade IIIb patients generally continued with their preexisting deficits or improved, except for 1 patient who underwent operation in the first week and died of cerebral infarction.

Thus mortality and morbidity do not appear directly related to timing of operation in this group of middle cerebral artery aneurysm patients. Some patients undergoing operation even months after the original ictus remained in only fair condition because of cerebral infarction which failed to improve over the time of delay. On the other hand, the proportion of good grade patients making a complete recovery does not seem to be adversely influenced by operation within the first week, and by operating early these patients are spared the risk of recurrent hemorrhage during the waiting period.

Table 62 Timing of surgery and results in 170 patients with ruptured aneurysm of the middle cerebral artery

	Good Ia	Ib	IIa	IIb	IIIa	IIIb	IV	Fair Ia	IIb	IIIa	IIIb	IV	Poor IV	V	Death IIIb	IV	V	
1–3 d	–	–	–	–	–	–	3	–	–	–	–	–	1	2	–	1	7	
4–7 d	3	–	9	6	3	6	1	–	–	–	–	1	1	–	1	–	–	
1–2 w	10	–	14	13	2	6	–	1	–	1	3	–	1	–	–	–	–	
2–4 w	11	1	5	13	1	8	–	–	–	–	–	–	–	–	–	–	–	
1–3 m	10	1	1	3	–	5	–	–	1	–	3	–	–	–	–	–	–	
>3 m	7	–	–	1	–	–	–	–	3	–	–	–	–	–	–	–	–	
	41	2	29	36	6	25	4 = 143	1	4	1	6	1 = 13	3	2 = 5	1	1	7 = 9	= 170

Number of Subarachnoid Hemorrhages

Operative outcome is related to number of subarachnoid hemorrhages in Table **63**. Of the 139 patients with only one documented subarachnoid hemorrhage 89.0 per cent made a good recovery and 2.9 per cent died, while of the 31 cases with two or more documented hemorrhages, only 58.0 per cent made a good recovery and 25.8 per cent died. It is, of course, difficult to know precisely how many times a patient has bled, and frequently in the history there will be suspicious episodes which cannot be proven. It would seem probable, however, that once a small bleed has filled a cistern and caused the arachnoid to adhere to the aneurysm fundus, the chance for the next hemorrhage to dissect into the brain is greater and hence would carry a higher mortality and morbidity rate.

Hematoma

Of the 170 cases with ruptured aneurysm, 58 (34.1%) had significant hematomas. The distribution of these hematomas is shown in Table **64**. The frequency of hematomas correlates well with preoperative grade and with operative outcome as noted in Table **65**. 50 per cent of all grade III patients and 100 per cent of grades IV and V patients had hematomas. This leads to the conclusion that depression of consciousness in these patients is secondary to herniation and mass effect rather than direct brain stem injury from the hemorrhage. This invites an earlier operative procedure to remove the mass.

Whether hematomas in better grade patients are directly contributing to focal neurological symptomatology is more difficult to answer. Clearly there is a higher incidence of hematoma in grade IIb than in grade IIa patients. Nevertheless, only 40 per cent of the patients in grade IIb with hemiparesis or aphasia actually had hematomas.

Table 63 Number of documented subarachnoid hemorrhages of aneurysms of the middle cerebral artery compared to operative outcome in 170 patients and unruptured aneurysms in 14 cases

Number of hemorrhages	Good	Fair	Poor	Death	Total
0	11	2	1	–	14
1	124	11	–	4 (2.9%)	139
2	16	2	2	6 (23.1%)	26
3	1	–	–	2 (66.7%)	3
4	1	1	–	– (0,0%)	2

Mortality rate for 0 hemorrhages = 0
Mortality rate for 1 hemorrhage = 2.9%
Mortality rate for mult. hemorr. = 25.8%

Table 64 Distribution of intracranial hematomas in 170 patients with ruptured aneurysms of the middle cerebral artery

Intracerebral hematomas	58	(34.1%)
Temporal	28	(3 with SDH)
Frontal	14	(3 with SDH)
Insular	7	
Temp. + Front.	0	
Temp. + Ins.	4	
Front. + Ins.	1	
Temp. + Front. + Ins.	4	(2 with SDH)
Subdural hematomas only	3 (1.8%)	

Table 65 Relationship of intracerebral hematoma in 58 cases to preoperative grade and outcome in 170 patients with ruptured middle cerebral artery aneurysms

Grade	Good	Fair	Poor	Death
Ia	2/ 41 (4.9%)	–/ 1	–	–
Ib	–/ 2	–	–	–
IIa	3/ 29 (10.3%)	–	–	–
IIb	14/ 36 (38.9%)	–/ 4	–	–
IIIa	3/ 6 (50.0%)	–/ 1	–	–
IIIb	14/ 25 (56.0%)	4/ 6 (67%)	–	–/1
IV	4/ 4 (100%)	1/ 1 (100%)	3/3 (100%)	1/1 (100%)
V	–	–	2/2 (100%)	7/7 (100%)
	40/143	5/13	5/5	8/9 = 58/170

No. of cases with intracerebral hematoma / Total No. of cases

Aneurysm Size

Of the 184 symptomatic aneurysms, 41 (22.3%) were considered large aneurysms, i.e. greater than 15 mm in diameter. In these patients, 82.9 per cent had a good result and 4.9 per cent died. Seen from the point of view of operative outcome, 34 of 154 patients (22.1%) with a good result, 5 of 15 patients (33.3%) with fair results, and 2 of 12 (16.7%) who died had large aneurysms. There seems to be, therefore, no added risk to patients with aneurysms of the middle cerebral artery greater than 15 mm over those with smaller lesions. Truly giant aneurysms (greater than 25 mm in diameter) form a separate class of lesion both with regard to pathophysiology and operative difficulty, but the number (3 cases) is too small to compare (Table 66).

Temporary Clipping of the Middle Cerebral Artery

Temporary clipping of the middle cerebral artery distal to the origin of the lenticulostriate arteries, was employed in 21 of the 184 patients undergoing operation (11.4%). The relationship of temporary clipping to preoperative grade and operative results is given in Table 67. In general, temporary clipping will be required when the aneurysm is difficult in configuration, or with large and sclerotic aneurysms of the 0b group (27.3%) or when there has been premature rupture or avulsion of an artery.

It is difficult with the figures presented to find a

Table 66 Large aneurysms (41 cases) of middle cerebral artery

	Good	Fair	Poor	Death
Right	22	3	–	1
Left	11	1	–	1
Bilat.	1	1	–	–
	34	5	–	2

generally deleterious effect of temporary clipping. For example, temporary clips were used in 8 of 29 grade IIa cases (27.6%), yet all had a good result, with the exception of the case described on page 152, Fig **80A–E**. In the group of patients without preoperative mental changes (0a–IIb) temporary clipping may be advocated, whereas the patients with mental changes (III–V) may react to the temporary clipping unfavourably. One must assume that the collateral circulation of the brain in patients of the latter group (III–IV) may gradually deteriorate and they should not be subjected to further adventurous manipulation.

Operation

Attempts were made to determine the effect of the operative procedure itself on outcome. 154 patients did well and are not discussed here. Of the 30 patients with fair or poor results or who died, 14 were in grades IV or V and underwent operation to try to preserve life. 12 of these died

Table 67 Use of temporary clips in 21 cases related to preoperative grade and outcome in 184 patients with middle cerebral artery aneurysms

Grade	Good	Fair	Poor	Death	Total	Percentage	
0a	–/ 3	–	–	–	–/ 3	0.0	
0b	2/ 8	1/ 2	–/1	–	3/ 11	27.3	
Ia	–/41	–/ 1	–	–	–/ 42	0.0	11.0%
Ib	–/ 2	–	–	–	–/ 2	0.0	
IIa	8/29	–	–	–	8/ 29	27.6	
IIb	2/36	1/ 4	–	–	3/ 40	7.5	
IIIa	–/ 6	–/ 1	–	–	–/ 7	0.0	
IIIb	2/ 25	1/ 6	–	1/ 1	4/ 32	12.5	12.3%
IV	–/ 4	–/ 1	–/1	2/ 3	2/ 9	22.2	
V	–	–	–/1	1/ 8	1/ 9	11.1	
	14/154 (9.1%)	3/15 (20.0%)	–/3	4/12 (33.3%)	21/184 (11.4%)		

No. of cases with temporary clip / Total No. of cases

and 2 were left in poor condition. At the same time, however, 4 other patients in equally poor condition made full recoveries and another is at least self-sufficient. 14 patients presented with focal neurological deficits in grades 0b, IIb or IIIb and these deficits have remained the same or have improved to some degree following operation.

This leaves 3 patients of 184 (1.6%) who were made worse by operation. 2 patients, one (page 151) in grade Ia and one in grade IIIb (page 156) developed cerebral infarction after difficult aneurysm dissections, in one case requiring prolonged temporary clipping of the middle cerebral artery.

The third patient in grade IV (see Table **59**, No. 3) had a cerebral infarct preoperatively and went on to die of uncal herniation postoperatively. With the CT scan this case would now have been delayed until cerebral edema had receded. The other 27 less than good results address the basic pathophysiological changes attending cerebral aneurysms.

Conclusion

In summary, experience in a group of 184 patients with middle cerebral artery aneurysms has shown that 80 to 85 per cent of aneurysms will arise from the primary bifurcation at the limen insulae, and that the other 15 to 20 per cent will occur at regular locations along the artery and its branches. A truly fusiform aneurysm of the middle cerebral artery which gives rise to branches from its fundus is quite rare, being encountered in only 1 of the 184 cases. Lenticulostriate arteries are frequently in close apposition to an aneurysm of the middle cerebral artery, even beyond the primary bifurcation from superior branches, and damage to these arteries probably accounts for much of the ischemic symptomatology appearing in the postoperative period. The variability of branching of the middle cerebral artery demands a thorough search to identify all arteries with special attention given to the temporal operculum.

The early mortality of middle cerebral artery aneurysm rupture is at least 20 per cent. Patients who are comatose (IV) or semicomatose (III) following rupture of a middle cerebral artery aneurysm will virtually always have a large hematoma and may thus benefit from early treatment. No grade V patient in this series has made a worthwhile recovery (Table **68**).

Hydrocephalus and epilepsy each have an incidence of about 5 per cent in patients with middle cerebral artery aneurysms.

Table **68** Results in 6 groups

		No. of cases	Good	Fair	Poor	Death
1.	Preop. good condition neurolog. and mental (0a+Ia+IIa)	74 (40.2%)	73 (98.6%)	1* (1.4%)	– (0%)	– (0%)
2.	Preop. neurol. deficits (0b+Ib+IIb)	53 (28.8%)	46 (86.8%)	6 (11.3%)	1 (1.9%)	– (0%)
3.	Preop. mental change (IIIa)	7 (3.8%)	6 (85.7%)	1 (14.3%)	– (0%)	– (0%)
4.	Preop. mental and neurol. deficits (IIIb)	32 (17.4%)	25 (78.1%)	6 (18.8%)	– (0%)	1 (3.1%)
5.	Semicomatose (IV)	9 (4.9%)	4 (44.4%)	1 (11.1%)	3 (2*) (33.3%)	1 (11.1%)
6.	Comatose (V)	9 (4.9%)	– (0%)	– (0%)	2 (1*) (22.2%)	7 (77.8%)

* died later

4 Anterior Cerebral and Anterior Communicating Artery Aneurysms

Introduction

Aneurysms arising from the anterior cerebral and anterior communicating arteries have presented considerable difficulty in adequate treatment. Their proximity to important midline brain structures gives rise to significant morbidity following rupture and poses challenging anatomical problems in their dissection.

Aneurysms originating from the anterior cerebral arteries can be divided into three general groups:
1) Proximal anterior cerebral artery (A_1 or precommunicating segment) aneurysms,
2) Anterior communicating artery aneurysms,
3) Distal anterior cerebral artery (pericallosal, postcommunicating, or A_2 to A_{3-4} segment) aneurysms.

Because of the different operative problems at each location, they will be discussed separately.

Proximal Anterior Cerebral Artery Aneurysms

Anatomical Relationships

There were 14 cases of ruptured aneurysm arising from the A_1 segment in the present series representing 3.4% of aneurysms on the anterior cerebral-anterior communicating artery complex and 1.4 per cent of the entire aneurysm series. In addition there were 6 unruptured aneurysms encountered during operation for aneurysms at other locations; these incidental aneurysms are not included in the present series. On completion of this monograph, another patient with an unruptured, asymptomatic aneurysm came to our attention (see Fig **2**, p. 2, Vol. II).

Aneurysms arose from the left anterior cerebral artery in 10 cases and from the right in 4. The aneurysm was located on the proximal third of the A_1 segment in 2 cases, on the middle third in 6 cases and adjacent to the anterior communicating artery in 6 cases. In 12 cases the aneurysm was typically saccular but in 2 cases consisted of a fusiform dilatation of the anterior cerebral artery (Fig **84A–D**).

In 11 cases the aneurysm was single while in 3 cases it was associated with additional aneurysms. (Cases 3, 11, 13, Tbl. **69**). In case 3 the additional aneurysm was on the left internal carotid bifurcation which was also clipped. In cases 11 and 13 the ruptured aneurysms on the left A_1 segment were explored and clipped using a right sided pterional approach. The additional aneurysms on the right MCA and ICB were also clipped.

Important anatomical relationships include perforating branches arising from the anterior cerebral artery and the recurrent artery of Heubner. In 2 cases larger aneurysms severely compressed the optic chiasm from its lateral aspect although in neither case was there clinical evidence of visual deficit. Hematoma may extend into the Sylvian and the olfactory cisterns as well as into the lamina terminalis cistern and back into the interpeduncular cistern.

Ba., a 15 year old boy presented with a 2 year history of bifrontal headaches, especially after physical exertion and amauroses occurring for a few seconds after rising from bed quickly. His visual acuity was normal. Plain skull films revealed left frontal calcification and CT scan showed a fronto-temporal hyperdense area. At surgery a calcified, partially thrombosed giant aneurysm of the left A_1 and A_2 segments was clipped and resected. Perforating vessels in this area had been chronically compromised by the aneurysm, but despite this his postoperative recovery was uneventful, with normal visual fields and acuity, and normal metabolic and endocrine functions (see p. 281, Vol. I).

4 Anterior Cerebral and Anterior Communicating Artery Aneurysms

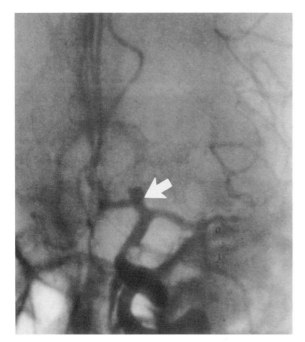

Fig **84A** Left proximal A$_1$ aneurysm (arrow).

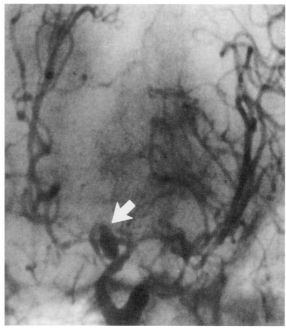

Fig **84B** Left bilobular proximal A$_1$ aneurysm (arrow).

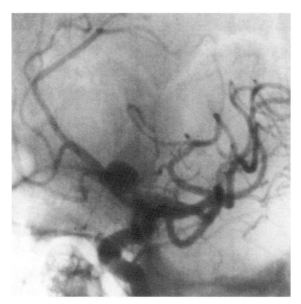

Fig **84C** Left distal A$_1$ aneurysm.

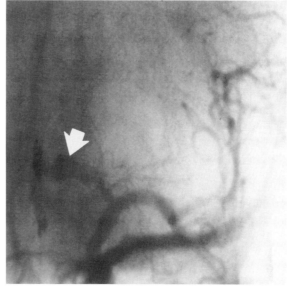

Fig **84D** Fusiform aneurysm left distal A$_1$ (arrow).

Operative Technique

Initial Approach

Aneurysms on the proximal anterior cerebral artery are approached through an ipsilateral frontotemporosphenoidal craniotomy. However in 3 of the 10 cases in this series, the operative approach to the left A_1 segment aneurysms was made from the right, either because the aneurysm appeared to be on the anterior communicating artery or as in 1 case, because the aneurysm was thrombosed and not recognized on angiography (see Table **69**, Case 11).

In these cases the dissection and clipping of the aneurysm was not especially difficult despite the contralateral approach.

Cisternal Dissection

The carotid cistern is opened back to the bifurcation of the internal carotid artery to expose the origin of the anterior cerebral artery. During this maneuver retraction on the frontal lobe must be minimal as the fundus of the aneurysm is often buried in the orbito-frontal cortex and excessive retraction may avulse it. The frontal lobe is mobilized by dissection of the chiasmatic cistern across to the contralateral A_1 segment. Then working back towards the aneurysm the surgeon has both proximal and distal control of the lesion. The anatomical relationship of the aneurysm to the optic chiasm and to the olfactory cistern will be appreciated at this time. In some instances it may be helpful to make a small cortical resection of the orbital gyrus over the aneurysm neck in order to facilitate the exposure.

Aneurysm Dissection

The most difficult and dangerous part of the dissection will be encountered when freeing adhesions between the perforating arteries and the aneurysm neck and fundus. Careful attention to arachnoidal planes of dissection and an appreciation of a variety of possible anatomical anomalies are important. When the aneurysm is directed inferiorly, perforating branches of the anterior cerebral artery may be adherent to the underside of the aneurysm.

Aneurysm Clipping

These aneurysms are often large and thrombosed or sclerotic. In 2 cases of the present series, the aneurysm was partially thrombosed and in 1 case it was totally thrombosed. Thus the application of temporary clips was necessary in order to open the aneurysm and evacuate its contents, before shrinking the lesion with bipolar coagulation and applying a permanent clip. In 1 case the anterior cerebral artery distal to the aneurysm was occluded by emboli from the aneurysm. With temporary clips applied, the embolus could be milked back into the opened aneurysm and removed before the aneurysm was clipped. In the 2 cases of fusiform aneurysms, a trapping procedure was used. Care was taken to avoid including perforating arteries between the clips. Fortunately, neither aneurysm was associated with hypoplasia of the contralateral A_1 segment and flow through the anterior communicating artery was good. Otherwise a trapping procedure would have been dangerous, and perhaps an anastomosis for collateral blood supply or simply a reinforcing procedure to the aneurysm would have been undertaken.

Clinical Presentation and Operative Results

Of the 14 cases with aneurysms of the proximal anterior cerebral artery, 12 were women and 2 were men. All patients presented with subarachnoid hemorrhage. 2 patients demonstrated right hemiparesis and aphasia, and one a left sided sensory disturbance. Ages ranged from 23 to 64 with over half of the patients between the ages 40 and 60 (Table **69**).

Surgical results in relation to preoperative grade are given in Table **70**. The prognosis of these aneurysms is good. There were no deaths in this group and 12 of 14 patients (85.7%) made good recoveries. This included all patients in grades Ia to IIIa. 2 patients presenting in grade IIIb showed some resolution of their preoperative deficits in the postoperative period and remain in fair condition.

2 patients underwent operation in the first week after subarachnoid hemorrhage and 3 in the 2nd week. 1 patient with a fair result underwent operation in the 3rd week and the other in the 2nd month after hemorrhage. Preexisting deficits rather than the timing of operation determined the outcome of these 2 cases (Table **71**). In 3 cases it was possible to clip additional aneurysms at the same operation.

Table **69** Proximal anterior cerebral artery aneurysm patients

Patient	Age	Sex	Year	SAH	Site	Grade	Hematoma SD	CIS	IC	Timing	Operation	Remarks	Result
1. Dö	64	F	1967	2	L. (m)	IIa	−	+	−	3 w	Trapping	Large, fusiform thrombosed, sclerotic	Good
21. Le	23	M	1968	1	R. (d)	Ia	−	−	−	2 w	Clip	−	Good
3. Zü	43	F	1967	1	L. (d) / L. ICB } 2	IIa	−	−	−	5 d	Clip/Clip	−	Good
4. Sch	39	F	1967	2	R. (d)	Ia	−	−	−	6 w	Clip	−	Good
5. Au	51	F	1969	1	L.	IIb	−	−	−	7 w	Clip	Thrombosed	Good
6. Fa	54	F	1970	1	L. (p)	IIa	−	+	−	2 w	Trapping	Fusiform	Good
7. Mü	40	F	1970	1	L. (d)	IIa	−	−	−	2 w	Clip	R. A$_1$ hypopl.	Good
8. Me	64	F	1972	2	R. (m)	IIIa	−	+	−	2 w	Clip	Spasm	Good
9. Bo	54	F	1973	1	L. (d)	Ia	−	−	−	6 w	Clip	−	Good
10. Me	60	M	1973	1	L. (d)	IIIb	−	+	−	5 w	Clip	Preop. R. hemipl. aphasia	Fair
11. Mo	39	F	1974	1	L. (m) / R. MCA } 2	Ia	−	−	+	4 w	Clip Clip	Thrombosed L. frontal hematoma	Good
12. Ci	28	F	1975	1	R. (m)	Ia	−	+	−	6 d	Clip	Embolus removed from A$_1$	Good
13. Ga	41	F	1978	1	L. (m) / R. MCA / R. ICB } 3	IIa	−	+	−	2 w	Clip Clip Clip	Sclerotic	Good
14. Gu	50	F	1978	1	L. (p)	IIIb	−	+	−	2 w	Clip	Double A$_1$, ischemia L. insula on CT	Fair

d = distal, M = middle, p = proximal A$_1$ segment

Table 70 Surgical results compared to preoperative grade in 14 patients with aneurysms of the proximal cerebral artery (A₁ segment)

Grade	Total No.	Good	Fair	Poor	Death
Ia	5	5	–	–	–
IIa	5	5	–	–	–
IIb	1	1	–	–	–
IIIa	1	1	–	–	–
IIIb	2	–	2	–	–
Total	14	12	2	–	–

Table 71 Timing of surgery and results in 14 patients with ruptured aneurysm of the A₁ segment

	Good				Fair	
	Ia	IIa	IIb	IIIa	IIIb	
1–3 d	–	–	–	–	–	
4–7 d	1	1	–	–	–	
1–2 w	1	2	–	–	–	
2–4 w	2	2	–	1	1	
1–3 m	1	–	1	–	1	
	5	5	1	1	2	= 14

Anterior Communicating Artery Aneurysms

Background

Although the successful operative management of an occasional anterior communicating artery aneurysm was reported (Tönnis 1936; Dandy 1942a), for many years these aneurysms were commonly regarded as the most dangerous on the anterior circulation. Norlén and Barnum (1953) first reported a substantial series dealing only with anterior communicating artery patients. Further reports followed and were summarized in a monograph edited by Krayenbühl (1959b). Many subsequent publications have described other series of patients with anterior communicating artery aneurysms.

Because of often unsatisfactory results following operations for anterior communicating artery aneurysms, several methods of treatment have been advised. Cervical carotid artery ligation has been recommended for those cases with a hypoplastic A₁ segment seen on angiography (Tindall and Odom 1969). Proximal anterior cerebral artery ligation on the dominant side was recommended by Logue (1956) and has continued to find favor with some neurosurgeons (Cook et al. 1965; Ahmed and Sedzimir 1967; Hugenholtz and Morley 1972; Scott 1973; Hockley 1975). Other techniques including wrapping and coating (Mount and Antunes 1975; Gillingham et al. 1976) operative and stereotactic thrombosis (Mullan et al. 1969; Alksne and Rand 1969; Mullan 1974; Alksne and Smith 1977) and catheterization with balloon occlusion (Serbinenko 1974; Debrun et al. 1978) have all been suggested as methods to avoid the difficult dissection required to adequately expose the neck of an anterior communicating artery aneurysm.

The introduction of the operating microscope to the treatment of these aneurysms has re-emphasized several basic surgical principles. First, a clear understanding of relevant anatomy is a prerequisite to effective operative treatment. The microsurgical anatomy of the anterior cerebral-anterior communicating artery complex was discussed in Vol. I, Chapter 1, and the pathological anatomy of aneurysms at this location will be discussed below. Second, an operative approach that gives adequate exposure of the lesion and surrounding structures without producing significant damage to the brain is required. A method of exposing and clipping these aneurysms that minimizes brain retraction and allows the relatively atraumatic handling of structures had to be developed. Finally, there are complications characteristic of aneurysms at this location that to some degree alter the indications and timing of operation as compared to aneurysms at other locations. This subject is discussed in the latter part of the chapter.

Anatomical Relationships

Incidence

The anterior communicating artery was the most frequent site of aneurysms in the present series with 375 patients (37.1%) presenting with aneurysms at this location. These aneurysms represent the vast majority of anterior cerebral artery complex aneurysms (91.2%). Another 56 patients had incidental aneurysms of the anterior communicating artery associated with ruptured aneurysms at other locations and are not included in this series, although these unruptured aneurysms have also been clipped in 32 patients, and coagulated and wrapped in 24 patients with microaneurysms.

Multiplicity

Additional aneurysms associated with ruptured lesions of the anterior communicating artery were found in 45 patients (12.0%). 35 patients had 1 additional aneurysm, 6 had 2 additional aneurysms, 2 cases had 3, and 2 cases had 4 additional aneurysms. In 15 of these patients, 2 independent aneurysms were present on the anterior communicating artery and in 4 cases 3 aneurysms were present on the anterior communicating artery each of which required separate clipping. The distribution of these multiple aneurysms is given in Table **72a** (Figs **85A–B, 86A–E**).

13 of these aneurysms were under 2–3 mm (microaneurysms). These aneurysms were always initially discovered at operation and were not visualized by angiography, so the incidence of such aneurysms at unexplored locations remains unknown. These microaneurysms were merely coagulated and covered with muscle. In addition 2 fusiform aneurysms of the anterior communicating artery and 2 aneurysms of the basilar artery bifurcation were covered with muscle. Thus of the 436 aneurysms in this group of patients 421 (96.6%) could be clipped (see Table **72b**).

In 8 patients additional aneurysms were located on the left middle cerebral artery or the lateral wall of the left internal carotid artery, and these required a left sided pterional craniotomy. This was performed primarily in 7 and as a second procedure in one. In another case left internal carotid-anterior choroidal artery and left internal carotid artery bifurcation aneurysms, in addition to the ruptured anterior communicating aneurysm, could be clipped from a right sided craniotomy (see also Table **129**).

Table **72a** Size and location of multiple aneurysms associated with AcoA aneurysms

			AcoA	OA L.	PcoA L.	PcoA R.	AchoA L.	AchoA R.	ICB L.	ICB R.	M$_1$ R.	MCB L.	MCB R.	PeA L.	PeA R.	Bas.	
Ruptured aneurysms	Left corner	< 2 mm Micro	2	–	1	–	–	–	–	–	–	1	–	–	1	= 5
		> 2 mm Macro	6	–	3	–	1	–	2	–	1	2	3	1	–	–	= 19
	Middle	Micro	1	–	–	–	–	–	–	–	–	–	–	–	–	–	= 1
		Macro	4	–	1	1	1	1	1	–	–	2	–	–	–	–	= 11
	Right corner	Micro	1	–	–	2	–	1	–	2	–	–	1	–	–	–	= 7
		Macro	5	1	1	3	1	–	–	2	–	–	1	–	2	2	= 18
			19	1	6	6	3	2	3	4	1	4	6	1	2	3	= 61

Table **72b** Obliterative technique employed in all aneurysms encountered in this group

	Cases	No. of aneurysms	Clipped	Muscle wrapping
Single aneurysm	330	330	328	2°
2 aneurysms	35 (15)	70	65	5
3 aneurysms	6 (3)	18	15	3
4 aneurysms	2	8	4	4 (1)
5 aneurysms	2 (1)	10	9	1 (1)
	375	436	421	15

( ) second or third aneurysm also on AcoA
° fusiform aneurysms

Anatomical Relationships

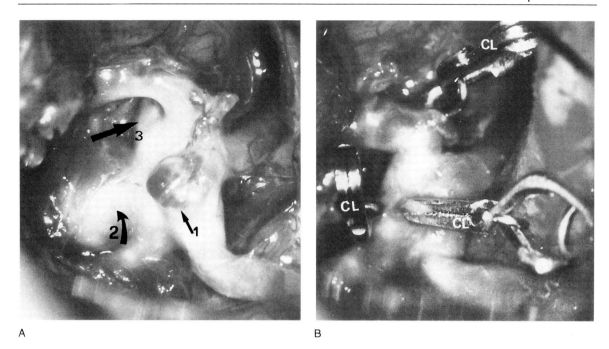

Fig **85A–B** Complex anterior communicating aneurysms with superior (arrow 1), posterior (arrow 2), and inferior (arrow 3) projections, before (**A**) and after (**B**) the application of three clips (CL).

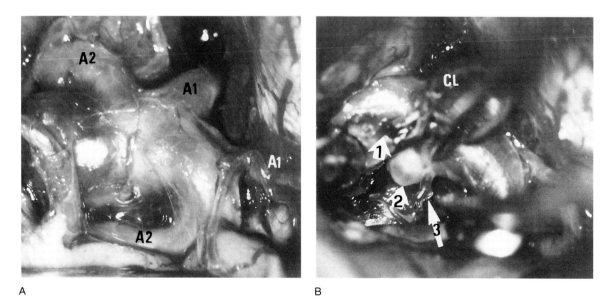

Fig **86A–E** Broad based aneurysm at the left corner of anterior communicating artery seen early in its dissection (**A**). During dissection looking for the hypothalamic arteries two further aneurysms were seen (**B**: arrow 1 = clipped aneurysm; 2 = further aneurysm; 3 = hypothalamic artery; Cl = clip).

Fig **86C–E** ▶

172   4 Anterior Cerebral and Anterior Communicating Artery Aneurysms

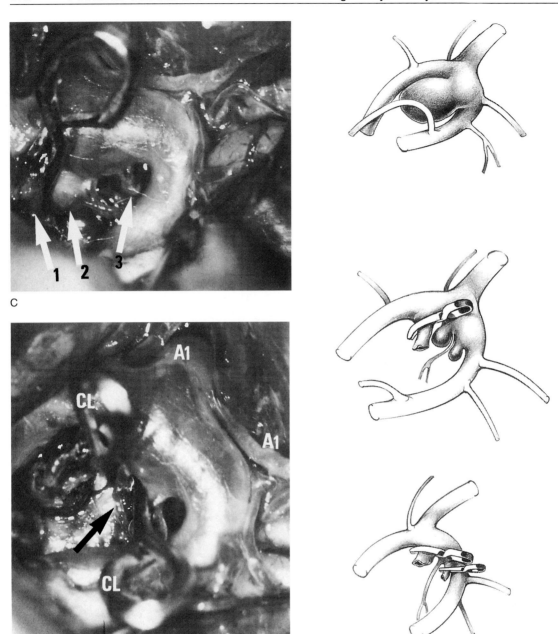

Fig **86 C**   The large aneurysm is clipped (arrow 1). Second aneurysm (arrow 2) third aneurysm (arrow 3).

Fig **86 D**   First and second aneurysms are incorporated in one clip and the third aneurysm needed a separate clip in between the hypothalamic arteries (arrow).

Fig **86 E**   Operative findings shown diagrammatically.

Location

Because the anterior communicating artery is a variable structure, an accurate description of its location and laterality requires some preliminary discussion. The proximal anterior cerebral arteries (A_1 segments) are equal in only about 20 per cent of patients with aneurysms of the anterior communicating artery. When one A_1 segment is severely hypoplastic, both distal anterior cerebral arteries will be supplied by only one internal carotid artery. In this situation the larger anterior cerebral artery may be thought of as a terminal branch of that internal carotid artery. Similarly the anterior communicating artery can be considered a continuation of the larger A_1 segment. This configuration has a fundamental relationship to the location of aneurysms on the anterior communicating artery (Figs **87, 88A–C**).

In the group of patients under discussion, all aneurysms except 1 were based primarily on the anterior communicating artery, the 1 exception arising from the A_2 segment just beyond the anterior communicating artery in a child. In 197 cases (52.5%) the aneurysm arose from the junction of the left A_1 segment and the anterior communicating artery, and in 108 cases (28.8%) from a similar position on the right corner. In 70 cases (18.7%), the aneurysm was based on the midportion of the anterior communicating artery. As a general rule, an aneurysm will arise from the side of the anterior communicating artery that receives the larger A_1 segment when the proximal anterior cerebral arteries are unequal, and will arise from the midportion of the anterior communicating artery when the proximal anterior cerebral arteries are equal. This was the case in 193 of 197 (98.0%) aneurysms of the left corner of the anterior communicating artery, 104 of 108 (96.3%) aneurysms of the right corner, and 67 of 70 (95.7%) midposition aneurysms (Table **73**).

Another anatomical point related to the location of aneurysms on the anterior communicating artery involves the presence of various anomalous formations of the anterior communicating artery itself. The anterior communicating artery is a multichanneled structure in the embryo which coalesces ultimately into a single channel joining the anterior cerebral arteries of the two sides. When this coalescence is incomplete, there may be more than one anterior communicating artery or there may be one or more fenestrations or bridges. Occasionally the primitive network persists (Figs **89A–C, 90A–C, 91A–B, 92**).

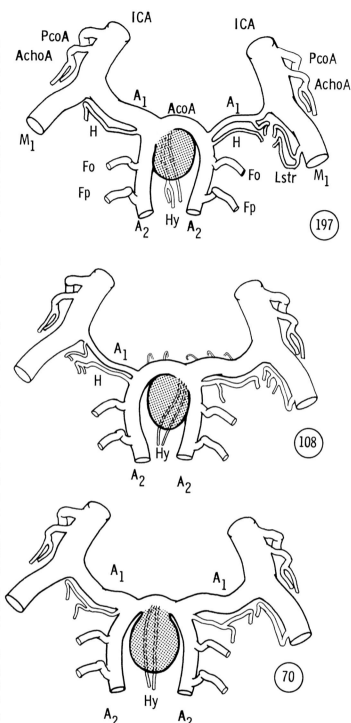

Fig **87** Schematic representation of the different positions of anterior communicating artery aneurysms as related to the size of the anterior cerebral arteries. The numbers of cases are shown encircled.

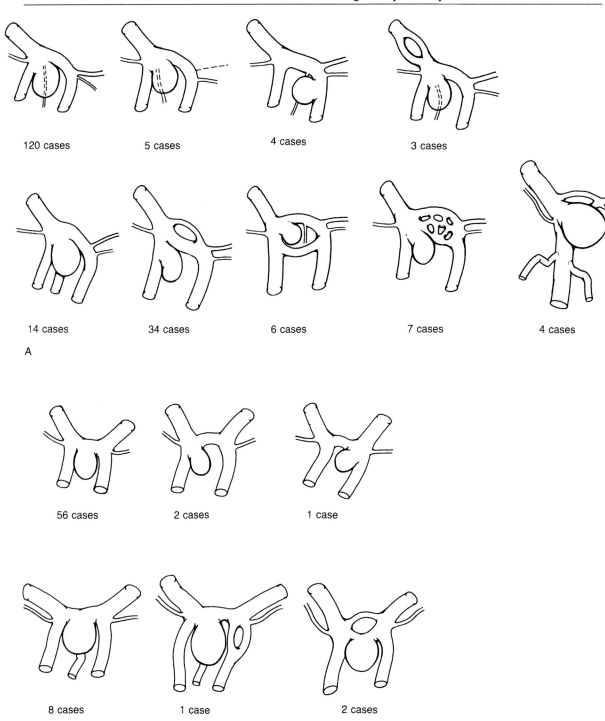

Fig **88A–C** Schematic representation of the relationship between anterior communicating artery aneurysms and anomalies of the A₁ segments.
A Hypoplasia right A₁.
B Equal A₁ segments.
C Hypoplasia left A₁.

Anatomical Relationships

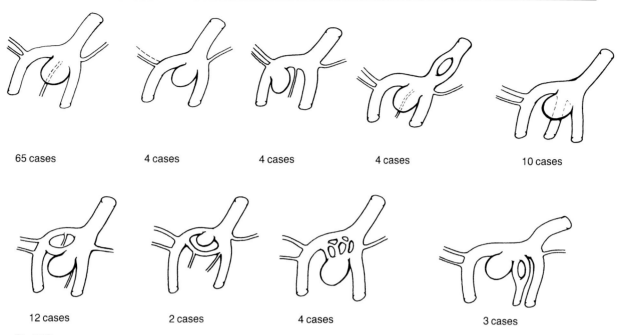

Fig 88C

Table 73 shows the relationship of aneurysms in the present series to the various anomalous formations of the anterior communicating artery. With full duplication the aneurysm is usually on the larger anterior communicating artery. In 56 cases of duplication, the aneurysm was on the proximal anterior communicating artery in 8 cases and the distal in 46. In 11 cases the aneurysm arose from a true network of small vessels. No cases were encountered where the anterior communicating artery was entirely absent although in 5 cases the 2 anterior cerebral arteries came together only over 1–2 millimeters.

Table 73 Relationship of cerebrovascular anomalies to 375 aneurysms of the AcoA

	No. of cases	Site of aneurysm	
Relation to A_1 segments			
Equal size	70 (18.7%)	Middle	67
		Left corner	2
		Right corner	1
Hypoplasia of one side	305 (81.3%)		
Left A > Right A	197 (52.6%)		
		Left corner	193
		Right corner	4
Left A < Right	108 (28.8%)	Right corner	104
		Left corner	4
Aplasia of A_1 segment	9 (2.4%)		
Right side 5 (1.3%)			
Left side 4 (1.1%)			
Fenestration of A_1 segment	7 (1.8%)		
Right side 4 (1.1%)			
Left side 3 (0.8%)			
Anomalies of the AcoA			
Aplasia	0		
Extreme hypoplasia	5 (1.3%)		
Fenestration	56 (14.9%)		
Duplicaion	32 (8.1%)		
Network	11 (3.0%)		
Anomalies of A_2 segment	43 (11.5%)		
1 A_2 segment	4 (1.1%)		
3 A_2 segments	17 (4.5%)		
Origin of frontopolar or callosomarginal at the corner A_1–A_2	19 (5.1%)		
Fenestration	4 (1.06%)		

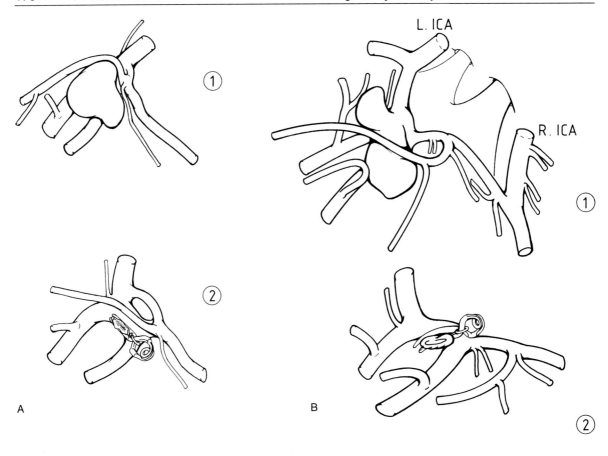
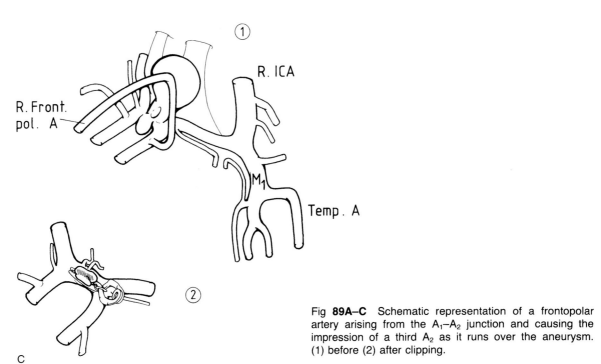

Fig **89A–C** Schematic representation of a frontopolar artery arising from the A_1–A_2 junction and causing the impression of a third A_2 as it runs over the aneurysm. (1) before (2) after clipping.

Anatomical Relationships 177

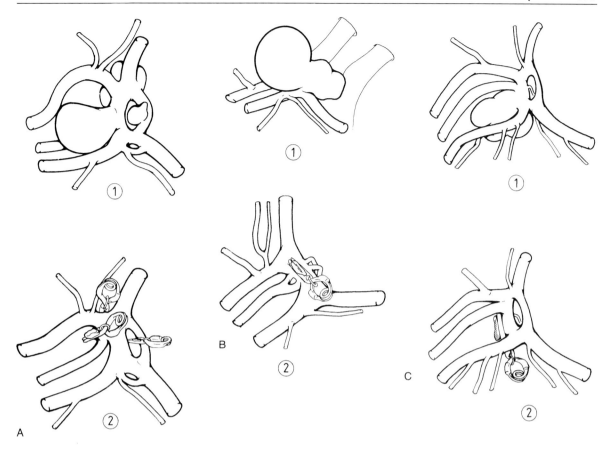

Fig **90A–C** **A** Three supero-postero-inferiorly directed aneurysms with fenestration of the anterior communicating artery and a third A_2.
B Bilobular (supero-anterior) aneurysm hiding a third A_2 with a fenestration.
C Postero-inferiorly directed aneurysm with complex topography due to a third A_2 and a duplicated anterior communicating artery.

Fig **91A** Unusual ring-shaped anterior communicating artery complex with a third A_2 and an aneurysm at the left corner.

Fig **91B** Aneursym originating on the second anterior communicating artery and hiding the third A_2.

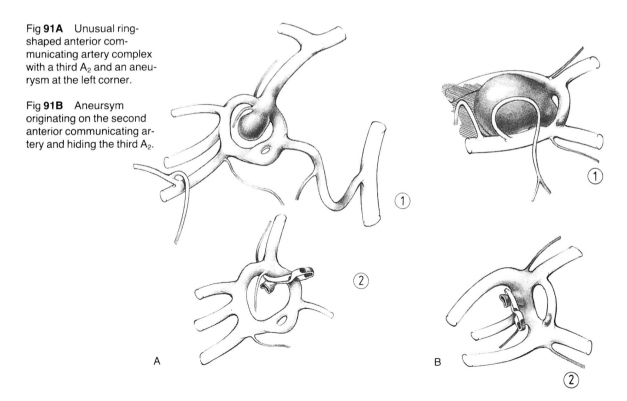

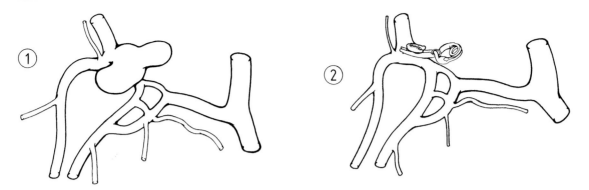

Fig 92 Fenestration of the right A₂ segment, before and after clipping.

Arterial Relationships

An aneurysm of the anterior communicating artery is related to 14 principal arteries or groups of arteries:

1) Right anterior cerebral artery (A₁ segment)
2) Left anterior cerebral artery (A₁ segment)
3) Anterior communicating artery (single, double or network)
4) Hypothalamic arteries
5) Right pericallosal artery (A₂ segment)
6) Left pericallosal artery (A₂ segment)
7) Right recurrent artery of Heubner (may be double)
8) Left recurrent artery of Heubner (may be double)
9) Right fronto-orbital artery
10) Left fronto-orbital artery
11) Right frontopolar artery
12) Left frontopolar artery
13) Proximal origin of callosomarginal arteries (occasionally)
14) Third A₂ segment.

The anterior cerebral arteries will be attached to anterior communicating artery aneurysms if the fundus of the aneurysm projects antero-laterally or infero-laterally. The contra-lateral A₁ segment may be hidden by an aneurysm that projects anteriorly or superiorly. With marked inequality of the A₁ segments, the smaller artery may be mistaken for a recurrent artery of Heubner or a fronto-orbital artery. The A₂ segments are regularly attached to the aneurysm fundus, especially with posterior projection.

The recurrent arteries of Heubner have a variable site of origin (Table **74**). The lateral course of these arteries results in their being attached to the aneurysmal fundus when it projects antero-later-

Table 74 Recurrent artery of Heubner

Bilateral	AcoA – corner	194	(51.7%)
Bilateral	A₁	9	(2.4%)
Bilateral	A₂	82	(21.9%)
Asymmetrical	A₁–A₂	90	(24.0%)
		375	
Aplasia			
Unilateral	Right	9	(2.4%)
	Left	5	(1.3%)
Bilateral		3	(0.8%)
Duplication	Right	7	(1.8%)
	Left	8	(2.1%)
	Bilateral	4	(1.1%)

ally or infero-laterally. They may also be attached to or hidden beneath the adjacent A₁ segments over several millimeters, thus making their identification difficult.

Medial fronto-orbital arteries generally arise a few millimeters proximal to the frontopolar arteries although a common origin is not usual. Either of these arteries may be attached to the aneurysm fundus within the lamina terminalis and corpus callosum cisterns.

Hypothalamic arteries have a close relationship to the anterior cerebral-anterior communicating artery complex, and thus to aneurysms at this location. These arteries arise from the side of the anterior communicating artery towards the larger A₁ segment when the A₁ segments are unequal and in the mid-portion of the anterior communicating artery when the A₁ segments are equal. Thus these arteries usually are just under the origin of the aneurysm and may be adherent to the fundus when it projects antero-inferiorly or postero-inferiorly (see Figs **96–103**).

Anatomical Relationships 179

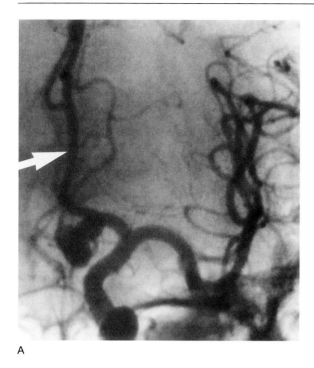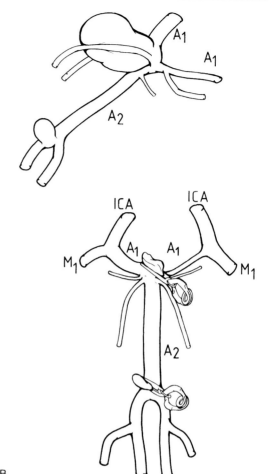

Fig **93A–B** A single A_2 segment (arrow) on angiogram (**A**) and schematic illustration (**B**).

In addition to the identification of the normally occurring 14 arteries just described, the surgeon must be aware of the several anomalies that can occur in this area (see Table **73**). While inequality of the A_1 segments is the rule with anterior communicating artery aneurysms, complete aplasia of an A_1 segment was seen in 9 cases (2.4%), 5 on the right and 4 on the left. Fenestration in the A_1 segment was present on the right side in 4 cases and on the left in 3. In one of these cases this was extensive enough to be considered as duplication. The A_2 segments are also variable. In 4 cases (1.1%) there was only one A_2 segment (Fig **93 A–B**) while in 36 cases (9.6%) there was a third A_2 segment. In 17 of these cases (4.5%), the artery appeared to be a true median callosal artery (three A_2), while in the other 19 (5.1%) it was an early origin of the frontopolar or callosomarginal artery.

This median A_2 segment may be as large as either pericallosal artery. In 1 case there was fenestration of the right A_2 segment, and in 3 cases fenestration of the third A_2 was found (see Fig **90B**).

Direction of Fundus

The aneurysm fundus may assume a number of configurations. While the most common shape is spherical, aneurysms of the anterior communicating artery have been seen that were either quite elongated or rather sessile in appearance. Additional lobulations or "daughter aneurysms" are frequently seen, and may be of sufficient size to give the aneurysm a bilobular or trilobular appearance (Figs **94A–D, 95A–L**).

The direction of the fundus is an important consideration in planning dissection. The fundus may be conveniently considered in any of 4 primary positions, although it is recognized that many aneurysms lie in an intermediate position and that some of the more complex aneurysms may occupy 2, 3, or all 4 of these primary positions.

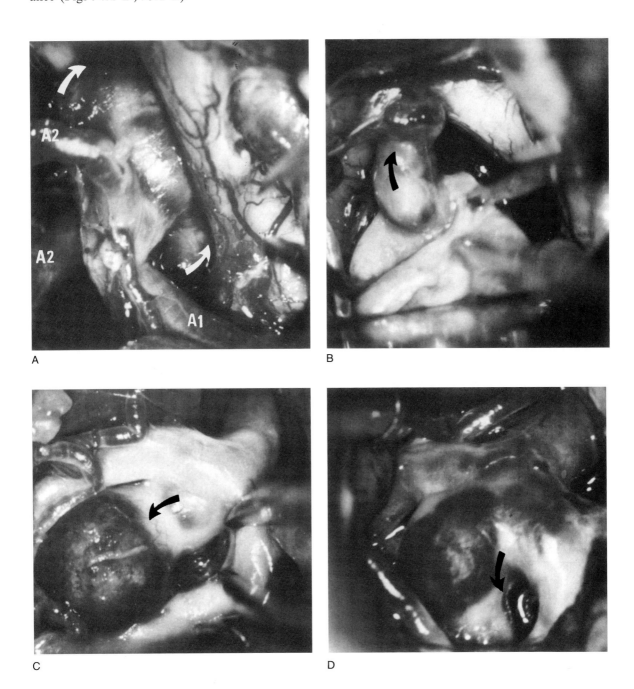

Fig **94A–D** Operative photographs of variably projecting anterior communicating aneurysms.
A Anterior (prechiasmatic). **B** Superior. **C** Posterior. **D** Posterior-inferior. Arrows indicate the direction of fundus.

Anatomical Relationships 181

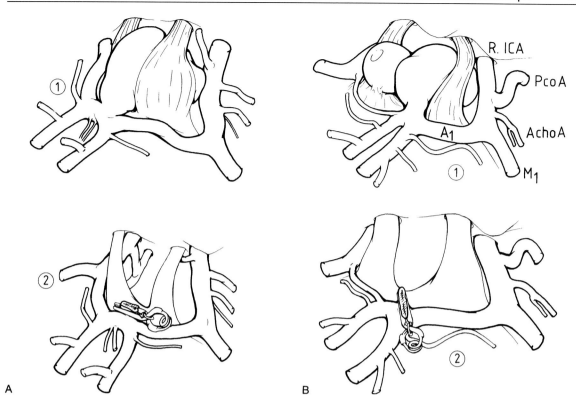

Fig 95A–L Schematic representations of anterior communicating aneurysm projections.
A Anterior (prechiasmatic). Equal A₁ segments. B Anterior with hypoplastic left A₁.

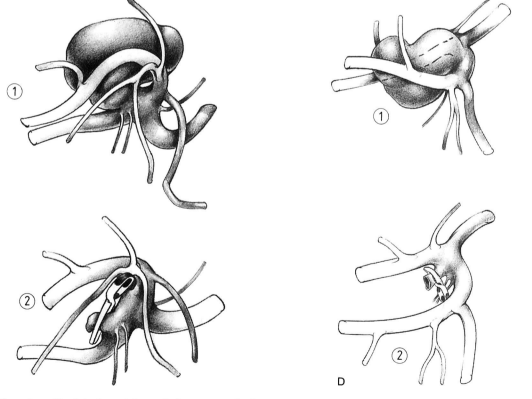

C Superior with distortion of the anterior communicating artery complex.
D Posterior – hiding the left A₂ segment.

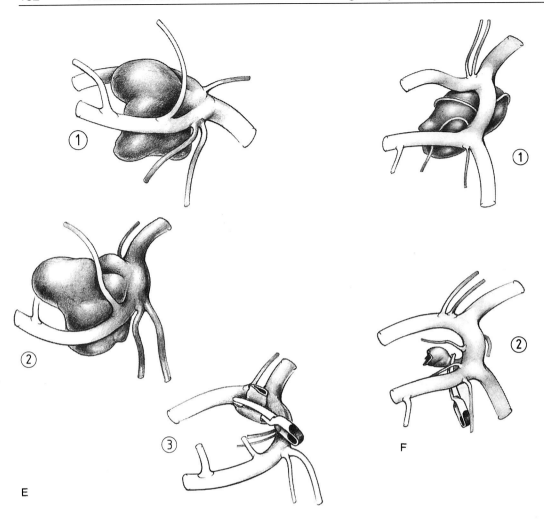

E Posterior-inferior – hiding the left A_2 segment.

F Inferior with the hypothalamic arteries draped over the aneurysm.

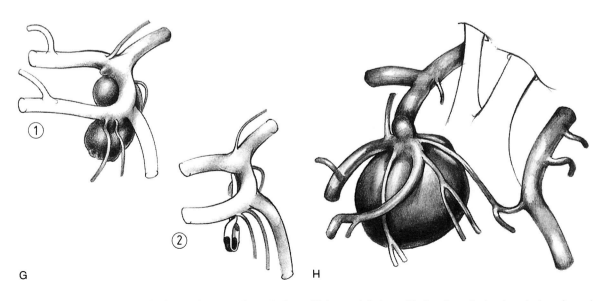

G Interior with the hypothalamic arteries over the anterior wall.

H Large inferior with the hypothalamic arteries draped over the wall.

Anatomical Relationships 183

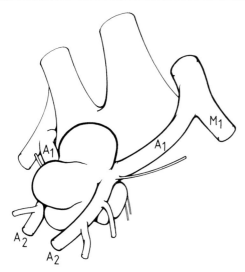

I Complex with superior-posterior-inferior and anterior extensions in all directions. Elimination of the lesion required 3 clips.

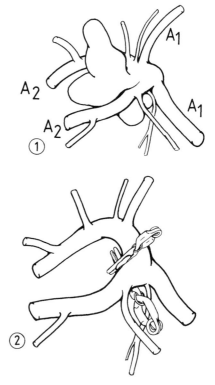

J Complex in three directions.

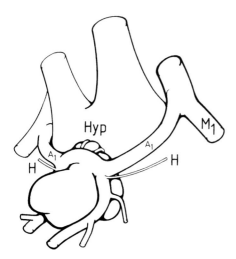

K Complex extending in all directions. 3 clips were needed to eliminate the aneurysm.

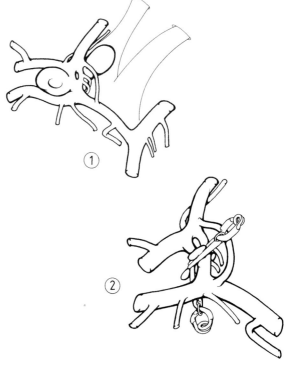

L Bilobed with posterior and anterior-inferior projections.

Anterior Projection: 48 Cases (12.8%)

Aneurysms projecting forward over the optic nerves will become invested with the arachnoid of the chiasmatic cistern and when large may be attached to the dura over the tuberculum sellae and limbus sphenoidale. In this position, the aneurysm may pull the entire anterior communicating artery complex forward out of the interhemispheric fissure. The aneurysm may compress the optic nerves from above or extend between them. In 1 case in the present series, an anterior communicating artery aneurysm grew between the optic nerves and presented laterally between the right optic nerve and right internal carotid artery. Large anteriorly projecting aneurysms will cover the opposite usually very hypoplastic A_1 segment from the surgeon's view and depress the pituitary stalk.

Superior Projection: 85 Cases (22.7%)

A second group of aneurysms project into the interhemispheric fissure anterior to the pericallosal arteries. The aneurysms may project more to the left or more to the right and be partially buried in the adjacent gyrus rectus. While these lesions are somewhat more favorably positioned from an operative point of view, the origin of the left pericallosal artery and left recurrent artery of Heubner may be hidden by the aneurysm, and the frontoorbital and frontopolar arteries are usually involved with the fundus.

Posterior Projection: 129 Cases (34.4%)

The largest group of anterior communicating artery aneurysms project posteriorly between the two A_2 segments. These aneurysms cover the opposite pericallosal artery and the origins of its branches: the frontoorbital and frontopolar arteries. These arteries are often adherent to the aneurysm wall. A fundus projecting posteriorly is hidden behind the ipsilateral gyrus rectus through a pterional craniotomy.

Inferior Projection: 53 Cases (14.1%)

This group of anterior communicating artery aneurysms proves most troublesome for the neurosurgeon. The fundus of the aneurysm projects into the lamina terminalis and is in close proximity to and usually covers the anteriorly or posteriorly displaced hypothalamic branches of the anterior communicating artery. It may also compress the anterior cerebral veins. The aneurysm lies behind the A_2 segment of the anterior cerebral arteries and beneath the A_1 segments and recurrent arteries of Heubner. With some lateral extension of the inferiorly projecting fundus, dissection of the A_1 segment and recurrent artery of Heubner can be extremely difficult.

Complex Projection: 60 Cases (16%)

This final group of anterior communicating artery aneurysms were distinctively bilobular or trilobular. The lobules projected superiorly, posteriorly, and inferiorly, and/or anteriorly. These aneurysms are usually large and their shape compounds the anatomical difficulties at operation.

The specific operative problems with the various fundus directions are discussed under Operative Technique.

Venous Relationships

The anterior cerebral veins possess the same general configuration but are deep to the anterior cerebral arteries, and thus covered from the surgeon's view by the aneurysm. These veins may be injured during dissection and create the impression that the aneurysm has ruptured. Smaller venous plexuses are found in front of the lamina terminalis, on the optic nerves, and near the cribriform plate. These may be a source of oozing blood during dissection. Finally, the confluence of veins forming the basal vein of Rosenthal is beneath the origin of the anterior cerebral artery and must be considered if a temporary clip is placed in this area.

Relationship to the Subarachnoid Cisterns

An aneurysm of the anterior communicating artery arises in the lamina terminalis cistern. Involvement of adjacent cisterns will depend on the direction of growth of the fundus. With anterior projection, the chiasmatic cistern will become applied to the fundus, with superior projection, the gyrus rectus and possibly the olfactory cistern, and with inferior projection the lamina terminalis itself. The arachnoidal walls are maintained with growth of the aneurysm, and provide the primary dissection planes for freeing the aneurysm from adjacent structures.

Operative Technique

Initial Approach

All anterior communicating artery aneurysms were approached through a pterional craniotomy, emphasizing removal of bone from the sphenoid wing and flattening the orbital roof. Under the operating microscope, this offers the shortest distance to the anterior communicating artery complex and requires the least brain retraction. A limited gyrus rectus resection is often required when this approach is used. For a right-handed surgeon, craniotomy is generally better performed on the right side. Exceptions to this include
1) Additional aneurysms of the left middle cerebral or left internal carotid arteries;
2) Significant hematoma in the left frontal lobe;
3) A giant thrombosed aneurysm arising from the left corner of the anterior communicating artery and projecting to the right side, thereby covering the approach to the left A_1 and A_2 segments (the surgeon will want to approach this from the side of the aneurysm neck).

With the dura retracted, the basal Sylvian cistern is opened on the frontal side of the Sylvian veins and the M_1 segment of the middle cerebral artery followed to the internal carotid artery bifurcation. The carotid cistern is opened and thickened arachnoid fibers over the origins of the anterior and middle cerebral arteries released. If the brain remains tight the interpeduncular cistern may be opened between the internal carotid artery and optic nerve or lateral to the internal carotid artery to release the cerebrospinal fluid. Hematoma in the interpeduncular cistern is common with ruptured anterior communicating aneurysms, and Liliequist's membrane must be opened with care. If an endostosis of the posterior clinoid process hinders the entrance to the interpeduncular cistern then the lamina terminalis should be opened to release CSF from the ventricle.

Ipsilateral Anterior Cerebral Artery
(A_1 Segment)

The lamina terminalis cistern is opened on the anterosuperior aspect of the proximal anterior cerebral artery. If the anterior cerebral artery pursues a straight course toward the interhemispheric fissure, it may be opened over its entire length. Often, however, the anterior cerebral artery curves beneath the orbito-frontal lobe and is covered by the orbital gyri and gyrus rectus. In this case it is not necessary to follow the artery posteriorly, but only to expose the first few millimeters of its origin so that a temporary clip could be placed in event of premature rupture. During dissection in the lamina terminalis cistern, the origins of perforating medial striate arteries are noted and the recurrent artery of Heubner identified.

Contralateral Anterior Cerebral Artery
(A_1 Segment)

Attention is next directed to the opposite anterior cerebral artery which is identified by opening the opposite side of the lamina terminalis cistern on the dorsal surface of the optic nerves and entering into the carotid cistern on the contralateral side. Numerous arachnoid trabeculations connect the lamina terminalis cistern to the chiasmatic cistern over the dorsal surface of the optic nerves. Division of these fibers allows the frontal lobes to fall a bit further away from the dorsal chiasm. The arachnoid over the opposite anterior cerebral artery is opened down to the carotid cistern and up to the optic foramen. The opposite internal carotid artery, the origin of the left M_1, the left A_1, and the course of the anterior choroidal and posterior communicating arteries can be identified. Perforating arteries of the A_1 segment are also identified and space created for the application of a temporary clip if required. In those cases where the fundus of the aneurysm projects anteriorly into the prechiasmatic area, it will be possible to prepare the opposite A_1 segment behind the fundus.

Exposure of the Anterior Communicating Artery Complex

If the fundus of an aneurysm is anteriorly or inferiorly directed, then the anterior communicating artery complex can be adequately exposed by opening the lamina terminalis cistern and by sharp dissection of the arachnoid membrane over the most proximal part of the interhemispheric fissure.

If the fundus of an aneurysm is superiorly or posteriorly directed, then it is advisable to perform a 7 to 10 mm resection of the ipsilateral gyrus rectus between the olfactory and medial fronto-orbital arteries. This exposes the A_2 segments as far as the origin of the frontopolar arteries.

In some cases both frontopolar arteries are very adherent to each other. Freeing them of their adhesions releases attachments to the opposite frontal lobe thus allowing a more gentle, effective retraction.

The pia over the gyrus rectus is opened with bipolar coagulation and microscissors. It may be necessary to dissect and mobilize the olfactory and medial fronto-orbital arteries away from the pia over a few millimeters to protect them from injury. Light suction will remove enough cortex to expose the interhemispheric fissure, the aneurysm, and associated arteries. The pia of the mesial surface of the gyrus and blood clot directly attached to the aneurysm should not be removed. With this resection, the anterior cerebral arteries distal to the aneurysm can be identified and retraction which might avulse the fundus of the aneurysm avoided. Although this procedure injures some cerebral cortex, this area of the gyrus rectus is frequently already damaged by the original rupture of the aneurysm. In a few instances, especially when the anterior communicating artery is located far posterior to the optic chiasm and additional retraction is necessary, the ipsilateral olfactory tract can be dissected free of its arachnoid attachments and also gently retracted anteriorly to avoid injury (see Fig **199K**, p. 233, Vol. I).

Dissection of the Aneurysm

With exposure of the anterior communicating artery complex, one needs to begin the identification of the 14 arteries mentioned above and their dissection from the neck of the aneurysm. The course of dissection will vary with the direction of the aneurysm fundus, and it is therefore appropriate to discuss dissection of the aneurysm under the four groups of fundus projection described under anatomical relationships.

Anterior Projection

Depending on the size of the aneurysm, the fundus may remain within the area of the lamina terminalis cistern, may extend into or between the optic nerves and chiasm, or may be attached to the dura on the anterior wall of the sella turcica over the tuberculum sellae. Anteriorly projecting aneurysms tend to be the larger lesions. Following preparation of the right anterior cerebral artery, the two distal anterior cerebral arteries and their branches are usually dissected without difficulty as the aneurysm is facing away from them. It is especially important to avoid retraction as the aneurysm may be fixed anteriorly. If the left anterior cerebral artery is hidden by the aneurysm fundus, it is best identified by following the left A_2 to the anterior communicating artery and then trying to identify the left A_1 at this point. The left recurrent artery of Heubner should also be identified at this time, and not misinterpreted as a hypoplastic A_1 segment. It may be the same size or larger than the opposite hypoplastic anterior cerebral artery and, on occasion, duplication may be present. This dissection must proceed until the surgeon is satisfied that all arteries have been properly identified and freed from the aneurysm in the area. Gentle depression of the aneurysm fundus with a sponge beneath the suction tip may help in some cases to expose this area during dissection.

On the inferior aspect of the aneurysm, space is developed between the neck of the aneurysm and the optic nerves and chiasm, using the arachnoid layer of the chiasmatic and lamina terminalis cisterns as a plane of dissection. If the fundus of the aneurysm compresses the optic nerves or seems to be buried within the substance of the optic nerves, no attempt should be made to dissect a plane between them and the wall of the aneurysm. This avoids any damage to the optic structures. The stalk will run inferiorly and the hypothalamic arteries postero-inferiorly away from the aneurysm in this situation (Fig **96A–B**).

The attachment of the aneurysm to the dura in the area of the tuberculum sellae does not need to be separated prior to the placement of a clip across the neck of the aneurysm. However, if this attachment is firm, application of a clip may pull the entire anterior communicating artery complex forward, putting tension on the anterior communicating artery and its branches, especially the hypothalamic arteries. Gentle squeezing of the neck of the aneurysm with forceps will warn that this is the case, and lead to further dissection.

Superior Projection

Aneurysms projecting superiorly in front of the pericallosal arteries (A_2 segments) are generally more easily handled than aneurysms projecting in other positions. They do present certain problems, however. When the aneurysm projects more to the right or to the left, it may be partially buried in one or both gyri recti. Retraction applied to the orbitobasal frontal lobe may be transmitted to the aneurysm fundus and lead to rupture. Therefore, gyrus rectus resection is helpful to further mobilize the aneurysm fundus as well as the frontal lobe and make visualization of the contralateral arteries easier.

The aneurysm may hide the proximal few millimeters of the contralateral A_2 segment and the origin of the left recurrent artery of Heubner. The left A_2 segment should be identified distally and followed to the anterior communicating artery, gently pushing the aneurysm forward until the corner of the anterior communicating artery is seen. Dissection can then proceed into the left A_1 segment to clarify the relationship to the aneu-

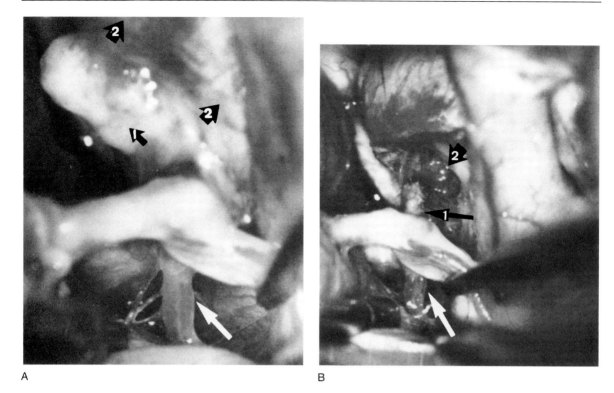

Fig **96A–B** A large anteriorly projecting aneurysm fixed in the prechiasmatic space:
A A small part of the subtotally thrombosed aneurysm is projecting postero-superiorly (arrow 1). Prechiasmatic large aneurysm (arrow 2). Hypothalamic arteries (white arrow).
B Neck of the aneurysm is clipped, coagulated, the clip removed, the neck fully coagulated (arrow 1) and finally clipped. The cut large thrombosed fundus is seen in the prechiasmatic space (arrow 2). Hypothalamic arteries (white arrow).

rysm of the recurrent artery of Heubner and the left anterior cerebral artery.

Especially troublesome with these aneurysms are firm attachments of the fronto-orbital and the frontopolar arteries to the wall of the aneurysm. In a few cases (7) it was not possible to save the fronto-orbital artery on the ipsilateral side and it was sacrificed with no apparent neurological deficit. One should try to preserve all cortical arteries, but this must be weighed against the likelihood of avulsing the aneurysm and damaging the major parent arteries when these attachments prohibit adequate dissection (Figs **97A–C, 98A–B**).

4 Anterior Cerebral and Anterior Communicating Artery Aneurysms

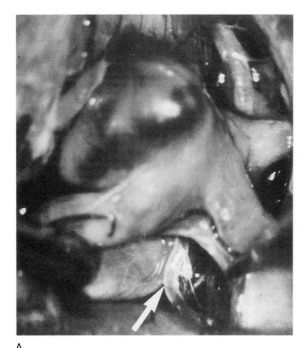

A

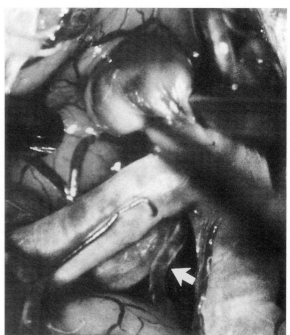

B

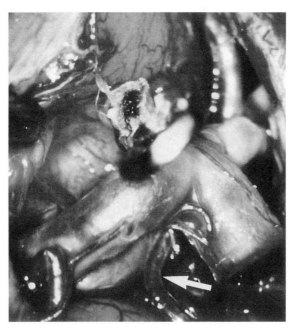

C

Fig 97A–C Operative photographs of a superiorly directed anterior communicating artery aneurysm (**A**), during coagulation (**B**), and after clipping (**C**). Hypothalamic artery (white arrows).

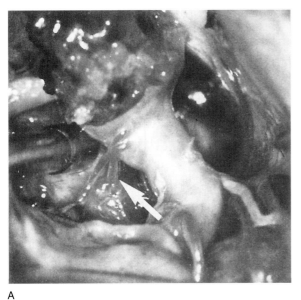 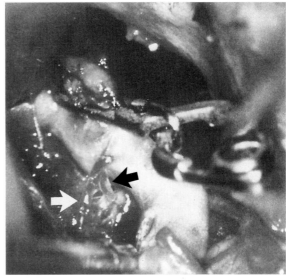

Fig 98A–B Operative photographs of a posterior-superior anterior communicating aneurysm before (**A**) and after (**B**) clipping. Notice the hypothalamic arteries (arrows).

Posterior Projection

An aneurysm in this location will almost always require an early incision into the ipsilateral gyrus rectus to adequately visualize the anatomical structures. The left A_2 segment is usually hidden behind the fundus of the aneurysm. Its identification and dissection generally require that the fundus be gently depressed with the suction tip, while the surgeon develops a plane between the aneurysm wall and the artery. Forceps should be spread in the direction of the artery to avoid tearing the base of the aneurysm or damaging the underlying hypothalamic arteries. The possibility of a single or third A_2 segment and early origin of callosomarginal arteries, must be kept in mind.

Adhesions between the aneurysm and the fronto-orbital and frontopolar arteries again present a problem with this group of aneurysms. If these are attached distal to the neck, their dissection may be postponed, but if adherent to the neck of the aneurysm, they will have to be engaged early in dissection. As previously mentioned, it may be more prudent in some cases to sacrifice an olfactory or fronto-orbital artery when it is adherent to the fundus, rather than risk tearing the aneurysm before the neck is adequately dissected. Even for those arteries attached distally, it is recommended that they be mobilized to some degree (2–5 mm) prior to clip placement. The squeezing of the aneurysm neck by the clip or coagulation of the neck may stretch these branches even to the point of avulsion from their parent arteries.

The hypothalamic arteries are identified on the inferior side of the aneurysm neck. These are hidden by the fundus of the aneurysm, but may be located from two directions:

1) The plane between the A_2 segment and the aneurysm neck may be further developed on the side of the larger A_1 segment. This may allow the surgeon to see the arteries if the aneurysm is gently retracted or depressed.
2) Dissection between the recurrent artery of Heubner and the fronto-orbital artery on the right side may permit the surgeon to elevate the right A_2 segment and look beneath it to see the arteries coursing back toward the hypothalamus (Figs **99A–B, 100A–B**).

190   4 Anterior Cerebral and Anterior Communicating Artery Aneurysms

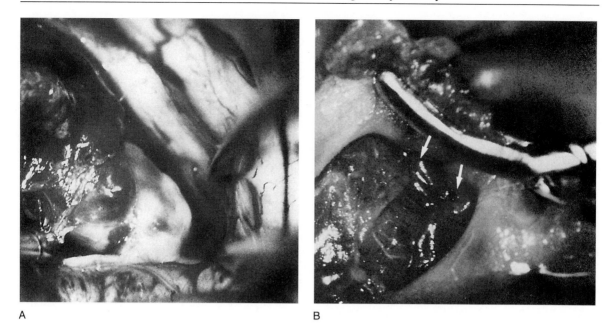

Fig 99A–B Superior-posteriorly directed aneurysm before (**A**) and after (**B**) clipping. Notice the two hypothalamic arteries (arrows).

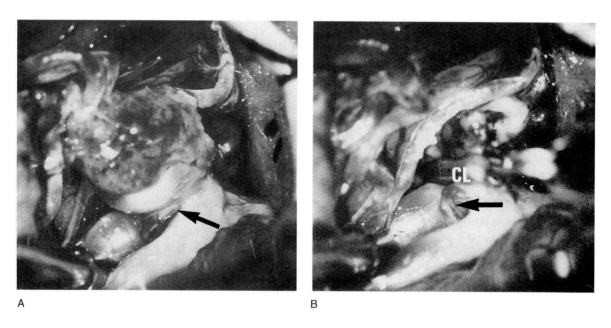

Fig 100A–B Superiorly directed aneurysm before (**A**) and after (**B**) clipping. Notice the hypothalamic arteries (arrows).

Inferior Projection

Aneurysms arising from the inferior wall of the anterior communicating artery and projecting downward toward the hypothalamus are among the most difficult to handle. Identification of the A_1 and A_2 segments is usually apparent, but the identification and dissection of hypothalamic branches and the clipping of the entire aneurysm without strangulating these branches can be an extremely difficult problem. The approach to this dissection of the hypothalamic branches can be directed from between both A_1 segments posteriorly, from between both A_2 segments anteriorly, or medially between the ipsilateral A_1 and A_2 segments along either the A_1 or the A_2 segment. The hypothalamic arteries are usually attached to the anterior wall of these aneurysms, although 4 cases were seen where these arteries were draped over the posterior wall. From either direction the aneurysm neck can be gently elevated with a fine suction tip so that these small arteries can be identified and dissected. If there is a third A_2 segment, then the hypothalamic arteries should not be dissected, because they take their origin from the inferior wall of the third A_2. If there is an infero-laterally projecting fundus (3 cases), the recurrent artery of Heubner and also the A_1 segment, are similarly attached to the fundus of the aneurysm making their identification quite difficult. Avoiding injury to them and to the hypothalamic branches requires meticulous dissection and considerable patience (Figs 101A–B, 102A–B).

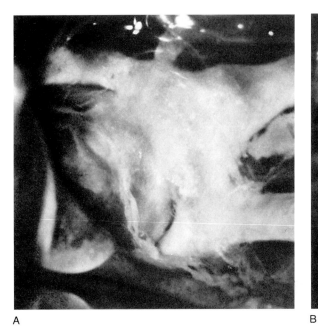
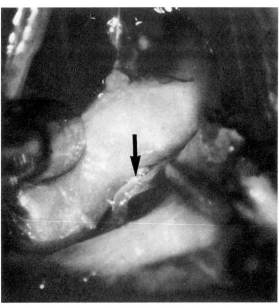

A   B

Fig **101A–B** Postero-inferior aneurysm before (**A**) and after (**B**) clipping with the hypothalamic artery (arrow) visible along its base.

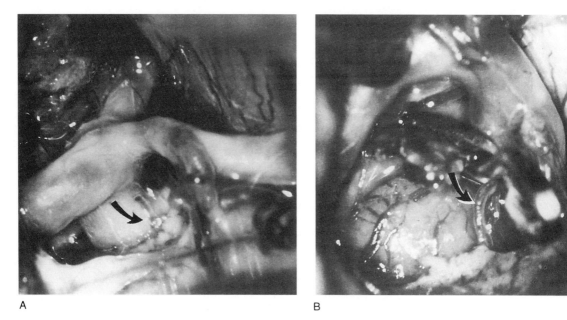

Fig 102A–B Inferiorly projecting aneurysm (arrow). Notice hypothalamic arteries (**A**). After clipping the A$_2$ segments are slightly elevated by the sucker. Notice the good visualization of the hypothalamic arteries (arrow).

Complex Projection

Complex anterior communicating artery aneurysms, of course, share the operative problems of each location, but the presence of additional loculations hinders the usual approaches to solving these problems. It has been especially useful in dissection of such aneurysms to employ successive bipolar coagulation, clipping, dissection, clip replacement, further coagulation, etc., until the entire aneurysm has been coagulated and the final clip applied. It is often possible with this technique to bring a menacing aneurysm to a straight forward clipping (Fig **103A–B**).

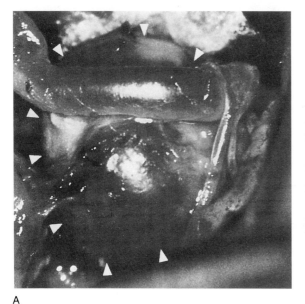
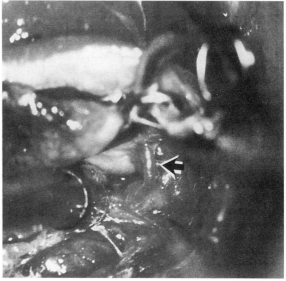

Fig **103A–B** A large complex aneurysm with bulging parts in all directions (**A**). The posteriorly projecting part is already coagulated (arrow heads). The clip is applied on the narrowed neck. The hypothalamic arteries are well visualized (arrow) (**B**).

Clip Application

When the 14 basic arteries, a true or false third A_2 (early origin of a large frontopolar or callosomarginal arteries), additional anomalies, the optic nerves and chiasm, the pituitary stalk, and the anterior cerebral veins have been identified and dissected from the aneurysm neck, the surgeon is ready to clip the aneurysm. The width, shape and direction of the neck are evaluated in deciding from which direction the clip should be applied. For aneurysms projecting anteriorly and superiorly, the clip is best introduced parallel to the anterior communicating artery, with the anterior blade sliding between the aneurysm and optic nerves and the posterior blade staying anterior to the opposite A_2 segment and recurrent artery of Heubner. Aneurysms projecting posteriorly are best approached between the two A_2 segments, with the clip applied more or less perpendicular to the anterior communicating artery. The base of the clip will usually be more to the right side and the tips of the blades a little more to the left. The blades of the clip will tend to point downward because of the angle of introduction through the craniotomy and care must be taken not to include the hypothalamic arteries, anterior cerebral veins or pituitary stalk (in cases of prechiasmatic localized large aneurysm) in the blades. Aneurysms which project inferiorly are especially difficult to clip. The clip may pass over the right A_2 segment but beneath the left, or it may be necessary to introduce the clip beneath the right A_2 segment between the anterior cerebral artery and the recurrent artery of Heubner. These general suggestions must, of course, be tailored to suit the specific situation encountered.

Few anterior communicating artery aneurysms have a neck that is immediately suitable for clipping. The surgeon may gain some idea of the effect of a clip to be applied by gently squeezing the neck of the aneurysm with forceps. This will demonstrate the pliability of the neck and the surgeon may assess the response of surrounding vessels to clip placement. If torsion or stretching is applied to adjacent arteries, further dissection may help. More often it will be necessary to reduce the size of the neck and shape it to accept the clip. Bipolar coagulation of the aneurysm has been most helpful in this situation, although compression of the aneurysm, use of a second clip, and occasionally a ligature have proved more useful in a few situations.

Temporary clipping of the anterior cerebral arteries is sometimes necessary. Often a clip to only the larger A_1 segment will be enough to control the bleeding or decompress the aneurysm. If the aneurysm is especially large and filled with thrombus, much of the thrombus can be removed before a temporary clip is applied, using the clip only when bleeding is encountered. The aneurysm should be as well dissected as possible before applying a temporary clip to minimize occlusion time.

If there is a large aneurysm with partial or total thrombosis of the fundus and severe sclerosis of the wall of the aneurysm, the application of a clip may lead to the strangulation of the anterior communicating artery, A_1 and the A_2 segments. In this case a clip can be applied to the neck and the aneurysm wall resected 2–3 mm distal to the clip. The cut edges can then be coagulated and secured with a second clip. The first clip is then removed or replaced until an ideal position is reached without strangulation of any artery. The fundus may be later extirpated or left untouched if it is firmly adherent to the surrounding structures.

It was possible in all but 3 cases to apply a clip to the neck of the aneurysm. In 1 case with a reruptured aneurysm the anterior communicating artery was repaired with microsutures (No. 7, Table **75**) to save the hypothalamic branches (Fig **104A–B**).

In 2 cases, the aneurysm had become truly fusiform and could only be covered with muscle (Figs **105–109**).

It is a common occurrence that even after coagulation and several readjustments of a clip, there is still a small portion of the aneurysm neck that bulges beneath the clip. That is to say that the weakness in the wall of the anterior communicating artery extends beyond what can be clipped without compromising flow through the parent arteries. This has been a particular problem with inferiorly projecting and complex aneurysms. In 7 cases in the present series there was formation of a new aneurysm either below or alongside the clip that led to recurrent subarachnoid hemorrhage, 4 of these fatal. These cases are summarized in Table **75**.

Up until 1976 a total of 7 patients (2.9%) of the 240 with anterior communicating artery aneurysms that were clipped, developed a new aneurysm around the clip. All these patients had muscle placed around the clip and the aneurysm neck, but this failed to provide enough support to prevent the development of a second aneurysm. None of the 135 patients operated upon from 1976–1979 nor the 79 patients from 1980–1982 have experienced recurrent aneurysm formation. It is felt that the staging technique of aneurysm coagulation, clipping, fundus resection, repeat coagulation and clip replacement is better able to bring all bulging corners into the clip, thereby preventing aneurysm recurrence.

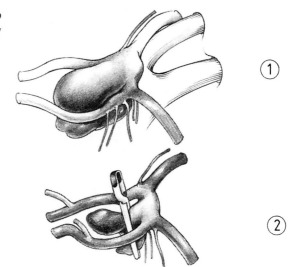

Fig **104A** Angiogram of a broad based anterior communicating aneurysm in a 46 year old patient that was clipped. **B** 3 weeks later the patient rebled and angiography was negative. Seven weeks later she suffered another subarachnoid hemorrhage and repeated angiograms were again negative. Nevertheless the patient was re-explored and a new aneurysm was found to have developed beneath the clip (3) necessitating an aneurysmorrhaphy (4) preserving the hypothalamic branches.

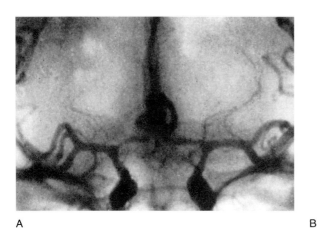

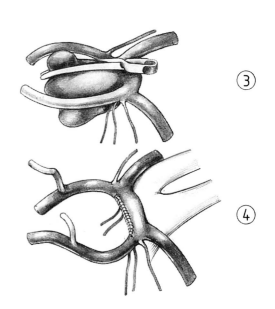

A   B

Table **75** Patients with rerupture of an aneurysm of the anterior communicating artery following clipping (7 cases)

Name	Age	Sex	Year	SAH	Grade	Post operative result	Recurrent SAH	Time	Reoperation	Final post op. outcome
1. Mu	36	M	1969	+	IIIa	Good	+	8 w	No	Death
2. Sch	43	M	1973	+	IIIa	Good	+	6 w	No	Death
3. Pe	44	F	1974	+	IIIa	Good	+	8 w	No	Death
4. H	47	F	1975	+	IIIa	Good	+	3 w	No	Death
5. Ja	40	M	1974	+	IIb	Good	+	8 d	Yes	Fair (L. hemiparesis)
6. Fi	42	M	1976	+	IIa	Good	+ (×2)	8 w, 11 w	Yes (× 2)	Fair (mild POS)
7. Cl	46	F	1973	+	IIa	Good	+ (×2)	4 w, 12 w	Yes (Repair of AcoA)	Good

Operative Technique 195

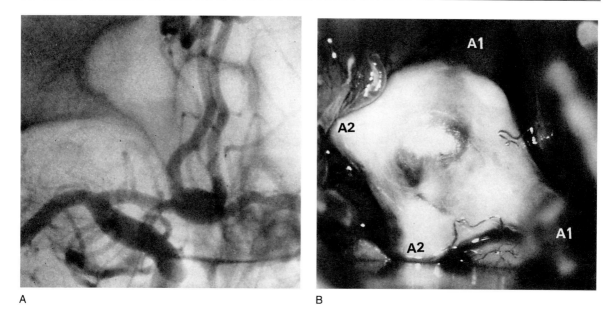

Fig 105A–B Fusiform anterior communicating aneurysm on angiography (**A**) and at surgery (**B**). The aneurysm could only be coagulated superficially and wrapped with muscle.

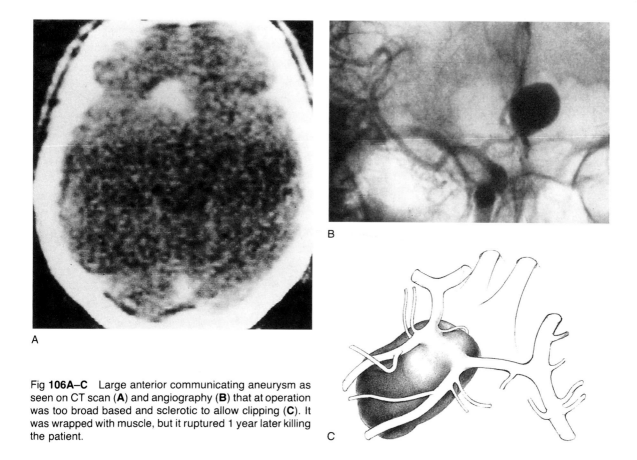

Fig 106A–C Large anterior communicating aneurysm as seen on CT scan (**A**) and angiography (**B**) that at operation was too broad based and sclerotic to allow clipping (**C**). It was wrapped with muscle, but it ruptured 1 year later killing the patient.

196   4 Anterior Cerebral and Anterior Communicating Artery Aneurysms

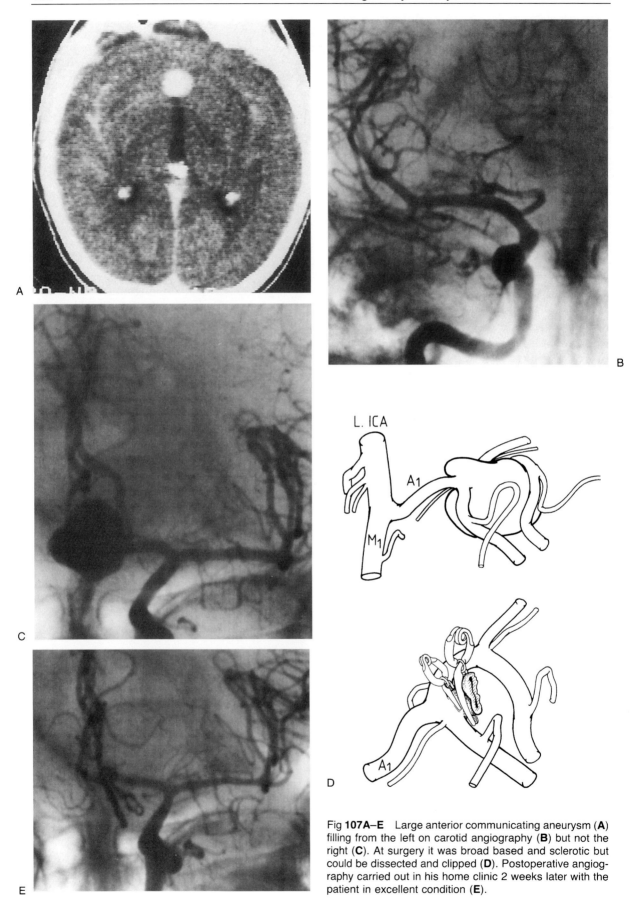

Fig 107A–E Large anterior communicating aneurysm (A) filling from the left on carotid angiography (B) but not the right (C). At surgery it was broad based and sclerotic but could be dissected and clipped (D). Postoperative angiography carried out in his home clinic 2 weeks later with the patient in excellent condition (E).

Operative Technique 197

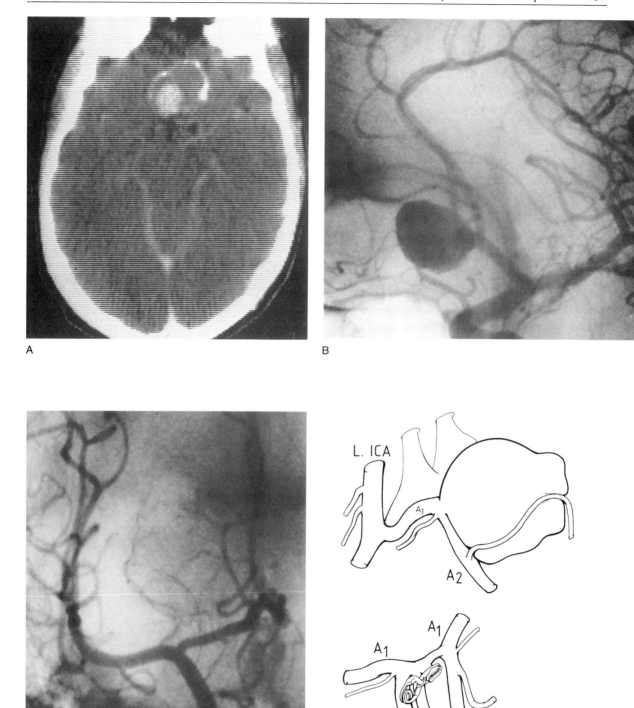

Fig 108A–E Giant anterior communicating aneurysm that was partially thrombosed on CT scan (**A**) filling from left on carotid angiogram (**B**) but not the right (**C**). At surgery the aneurysm had a rather short neck and could be clipped (**D**). Notice the third A_2. Normal postoperative CT scan (**E**).

Fig **108E** ▶

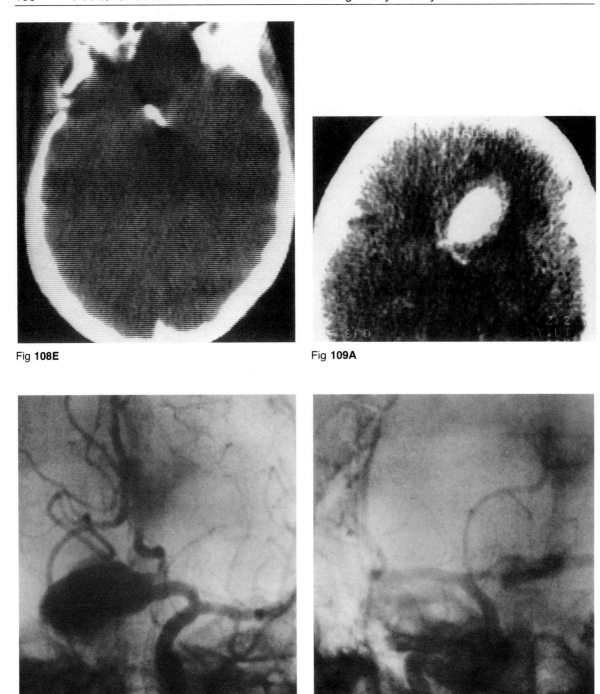

Fig 109A–E Giant partially thrombosed (**A**) anterior communicating aneurysm in a patient with psycho-organic syndrome. Angiography showed the aneurysm filling better from the left (**B**) than the right (**C**). At operation (**D**) a duplicated anterior communicating artery was found but the aneurysm was successfully clipped without residual deficit. Postoperative CT scan (**E**).

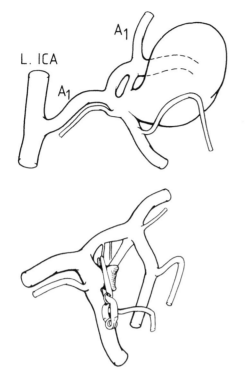
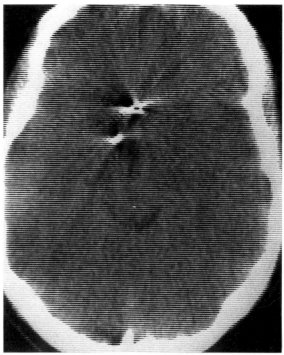

Fundus Resection

To ascertain that the clip is well-seated and that no normal structures are compromised, the fundus should be opened, thrombus removed, and the fundus resected. Following resection of the fundus, it is possible to seal the edges of the resected neck with bipolar coagulation and move the clip to a more favorable location if required. With the fundus removed, a better evaluation of the surrounding arteries and nerves can be performed. The clip should be so placed that with removal of the retractors there will be no torsion or traction on adjacent arteries, the optic nerve, or pituitary stalk.

Hemostasis and Closure

Papaverine is applied to the major arteries and the sympathetic fibers elevated from the superior wall of the arteries and resected. All hematoma is removed from the subarachnoid cisterns and any small bleeding points controlled. Careful inspection is required in the area of the cribriform plate, the dorsal surface of the optic nerves and chiasm, the lamina terminalis, and the orbitofrontal lobe beneath the retractor blade. With hemostasis secured, the wound is closed.

Summary of Operative Technique

(Sequence varies depending on fundus projection)

1) Frontotemporosphenoidal craniotomy (right side).
2) Opening the Sylvian, carotid, and interpeduncular cisterns.
3) Opening the lamina terminalis cistern and control of the right A_1 segment.
4) Dissection of the lamina terminalis cistern over the contralateral A_1 segment to the left ICA.
5) Ipsilateral partial gyrus rectus resection.
6) Identification of the A_2 segments and branches (there may be true or false 3 A_2).
7) Identification of the recurrent arteries of Heubner.
8) Dissection of the fronto-orbital and frontopolar arteries from the aneurysm.
9) Identification of the hypothalamic arteries.
10) Bipolar coagulation of the bulging parts of the aneurysm, or of the neck of the aneurysm.
11) Clip application to the properly prepared neck of the aneurysm.
12) Fundus resection.
13) Coagulation of the cut edges of the aneurysm distal to the clip, removal of the clip, coagulation of the entire base of the aneurysm, especially the inferiorly bulging parts of it.
14) Final clip application, after checking the position of hypothalamic arteries.
15) Check for adequacy of clip placement.
16) Papaverine and sympathectomy.
17) Hemostasis and closure.

Clinical Presentation and Operative Results

Presenting Features

The anterior communicating artery is the one common location for cerebral aneurysm that is more frequent in men than in women. Of the 375 patients with anterior communicating artery aneurysms, 231 (61.6%) were male and 144 (38.4%) female. Ages were between 15 and 73 with 64.5 per cent of patients under age 50 (see page 208). The average age of males was 45.1 years and of females 47.8 years. The age distribution did not differ from the age distribution of aneurysms in general.

Subarachnoid hemorrhage occurred in all but 4 patients. 2 of these 4 patients had incidental aneurysms in association with an astrocytoma and an arteriovenous malformation respectively, and 2 presented with a chiasmal syndrome and mental changes. In contrast to internal carotid artery aneurysms which not infrequently present with oculomotor palsies or visual disturbances, and middle cerebral artery aneurysms which can present with focal neurological deficits or epilepsy, anterior communicating artery aneurysms presented with rupture in all but 1.1 per cent of cases. Nevertheless, a wide variety of focal deficits accompanied hemorrhage in these patients.

The deficits can be grouped in relation to the position of the aneurysm. The blood flow distribution of the anterior cerebral arteries outlines a butterfly pattern on the inferior mesial and dorsal surface of the brain (see page 212, Fig 110). A list of possible neurologic findings includes:

1) Visual symptoms from optic nerve and chiasm compression.
2) Hypothalamic/endocrinological symptoms from hemorrhage and ischemia in the distribution of the hypothalamic arteries.
3) Psychoorganic syndrome due either to direct pressure on the orbitofrontal cortex by a giant aneurysm, to ischemia in the orbitofrontal septal and subcallosal cortex, along the anterior commissure, or to ischemia along the cingulate gyri in the distribution of the medial perforating, hypothalamic, frontoorbital and pericallosal arteries.
4) Paraparesis or hemiparesis from mesial hemisphere damage in the distribution of the pericallosal and callosomarginal arteries.
5) Extrapyramidal symptoms from basal ganglia damage in the distribution of the medial perforating arteries and the recurrent artery of Heubner.

The separation of focal deficits from alterations in consciousness is far more difficult in this group of patients than with those having aneurysms at other locations as the area of focal structural damage frequently includes neurons and tracts that are thought to form the neuroanatomical basis of consciousness, recent memory, and personality. In line with the other sections of this book, the separation of (a) and (b) in the grading system has been made on the basis of motor and sensory deficits. It must be realized that these 2 groups are somewhat more artificial than is the case with the more peripherally disposed aneurysms such as those on the middle cerebral artery. It will nonetheless be seen that morbidity does correlate with the presence of preoperative focal neurological deficits (b patients) although mortality is far better correlated with level of consciousness (Roman numeral grade) at the time of operation.

A further note of explanation is required concerning the grading of these anterior communicating artery aneurysm patients. Because they represent a group of aneurysm patients of special importance, several publications have come from this clinic relating the senior author's experience in the treatment of these lesions (Yaşargil et al. 1975, 1978). Many patients had been graded in their records in the earlier years by the system of Botterell and associates (1956) or Hunt and Hess (1968) and as such were downgraded for hemiplegia, medical complications, and so forth. An attempt has been made in this book to strictly grade all patients by the criteria set forth in Chapter 1 and each of the (1,012) records has been reviewed. Thus while the figures stated in this chapter may be at variance to some degree with earlier publications, they represent the most complete analysis that could be done on these patients and should take precedence over earlier publications. In almost all cases those patients whose grades were changed have been placed in a better grade. Hopefully the present grading system will portray as accurate a description as possible of the condition of these patients at the time they underwent operation.

Operative Results

In this large group of patients, it was possible to further refine the categories of operative results to provide a clearer picture of the postoperative course. Many patients (42) who went on to make full recoveries and who have now returned to normal lives, required additional time and perhaps a ventricular shunt or other therapy for

Table 76 The results of operation for anterior communicating artery aneurysms as related to the preoperative grade

	Grade	Total No.	Good	Good delayed recovery	Fair	Poor	Operat. death	Death other cause
No. SAH	0a	2	2	–	–	–	–	–
	0b	2	–	–	1	–	–	1
SAH	Ia	82 (1)*	80 (2)* (97,6%)	2 (2.4%)	–	–	–	–
	IIa	150	129 (86.0%)	17 (11.3%)	1 (0.7%)	–	1 (0.7%)	2 (1.3%)
	IIb	66	52 (78.8%)	8 (12.1%)	3 (4.5%)	1 (1.5%)	1 (1.5%)	1 (1.5%)
	IIIa	28	14 (50.0%)	6 (21.4%)	1 (3.6%)	1 (3.6%)	1 (3.6%)	5 (17.8%)
	IIIb	27	9 (33.3%)	9 (33.3%)	5 (18.5%)	2 (7.4%)	2 (7.4%)	–
	IV	17	–	–	–	9 (52.9%)	–	8 (47.1%)
	V	1	–	–	–	–	–	1 (100%)
		375	286 (76.3%)	42 (11.2%) (87.5%)	11 (oper. 0.5%) (2 cases) (preop. 2.3%)	13 (oper. 0.3%) (1 case) (preop. 3.2%)	5	18

( )* fusiform, muscle wrapping

Operative impairment

To fair	0.5%	
To poor	0.3%	
To death	1.3%	
Rerupture	1.1%	3.5%
Pulmonary emboli	1.1%	

complete recovery. For these patients a category of delayed recovery has been added. Patients who died have been divided into 2 groups – those in whom death could be related to operation, and those who died of later medical complications or died from the original hemorrhage in circumstances when the operation seemed to play no part in the postoperative course. These latter two groups of dead patients will be fully detailed in the following presentation.

Overall operative results are compared to the preoperative condition in Table **76**. Of the 375 patients undergoing operation, 328 (87.5%) had a good result, although in 42 patients (11.2%) there was some delay in recovery or a ventricular shunt was later required. 286 patients were home within 4 weeks, while the other 42 stayed from 4 to 12 weeks in the hospital. All 328 patients listed in good condition went on to a full recovery and are either fully employed or have returned to their former activities.

11 patients (2.9%) had a fair result, and 13 patients (3.4%) a poor result. 5 (1.3%) are listed as operative deaths and 18 (4.8%) as deaths from other causes. Less than good results were related to operative difficulties, preexisting morbidity, and medical complications especially prevalent in this group of aneurysm patients. Operative results are discussed in relation to the preoperative condition before attempting to separate out factors that contributed adversely to outcome.

Grade 0a

2 patients presented in grade 0a. Both of these anterior communicating artery aneurysms were associated with other lesions, an arteriovenous

malformation in a 35 year old man and an astrocytoma in a 64 year old man. Both patients did well from an operative point of view.

Grade 0b

2 patients with unruptured aneurysm but marked visual loss and mental changes underwent operation:

Ka., a 42 year old man noted onset of visual loss and headaches in 1972. Ophthalmological examination revealed optic atrophy and bitemporal hemianopsia. He was seen in this clinic in January 1975 where he was noted to be slowed and emotionally labile with poor recent memory. There was marked visual loss bilaterally. Angiography showed a large aneurysm of the anterior communicating artery extending over the optic chiasm and unusual fusiform dilatations of several branches of the right MCA. At operation this subtotally thrombosed aneurysm was totally extirpated. The postoperative course was uneventful and he returned home in 2 weeks. He improved somewhat both mentally and with regards to the vision in his left eye, but he remains unable to work (see Vol. I, Fig **228**).

This patient suffered both psychological and visual changes secondary to a large, subtotally thrombosed aneurysm filling the lamina terminalis cistern and pressing upon adjacent structures. His fair condition is a consequence of his preoperative deficits.

Pe., a 61 year old man, with a history of alcoholism and heavy smoking, complained of visual loss over 11 months and at the time of admission could only count fingers at 30 centimeters. There was bilateral optic atrophy. Angiography showed an aneurysm of the anterior communicating artery and hydrocephalus. At operation on 23 April, 1975, an unruptured small aneurysm was found on the right corner of the anterior communicating artery directed superiorly with no evidence of pressure on the optic nerves or chiasm. Marked cerebral atrophy was present with enormous subarachnoid cisterns. On 2 May, 1975, a ventriculoatrial shunt was inserted because of persistent cerebrospinal fluid accumulation beneath the skin flap. He was in the same neurological condition as when he had entered the hospital. However 2 days later he fell from bed and suddenly died before investigation could be undertaken. Autopsy showed hematomas in both cerebellar hemispheres.

This patient probably had toxic amblyopia but the presence of an aneurysm on angiography that was thought to be subtotally thrombosed led to an operation. His death was traumatic secondary to a fall from bed.

Grade Ia

There were 82 patients who underwent operation in grade Ia, and all had a good result. In 80 patients (97.5%) the postoperative course was smooth and they were discharged between 5 days and 4 weeks to home. In 2 patients (2.4%) there was a delayed recovery. One patient developed a postoperative epidural hematoma and required reoperation. The other patient required a ventriculoatrial shunt several weeks after operation. Both of these patients have returned to full employment. 6 of these patients underwent operation within the first 2 weeks, 29 between 2 and 4 weeks, and 47 after 1 month. This group contained 2 fusiform aneurysms of the anterior communicating artery which could not be clipped. There were no instances of subdural or intracerebral hematoma in these patients.

There were 10 patients, 6 men and 4 women, with ages ranging from 34 to 64 who presented with visual deficits. 5 of these patients had already undergone operation at another hospital and presented with either progressive visual loss or recurrent hemorrhage. Angiography generally revealed enlargement of the aneurysm over that present on the referring hospital's films.

The precise etiology of visual loss cannot be given. These 10 patients had large, sclerotic aneurysms usually partially or subtotally thrombosed. All 10 patients tolerated operation well and all recovered enough vision to allow them to return to full time work. This would imply that pressure on the optic apparatus was at least in part responsible for the visual loss. 11 other patients had similar sized aneurysms over the chiasm, but without visual symptomatology. These aneurysms tended to be less sclerotic with less thrombosis.

Grade Ib

No patients with anterior communicating artery aneurysms presented in grade Ib.

Grade IIa

150 patients (40.0%) were in grade IIa, the most common condition of patients coming to operation. Of these patients, 129 (86.0%) had an uncomplicated good result and were home within 2 to 4 weeks. 17 patients (11.3%) had a delayed good recovery. 10 of the 17 patients required shunts; 1 had porencephaly from a long-standing (10 years) frontal lobe infarct, and 3 had large intracerebral hematomas which took time to resolve. Overall 97.3 per cent of these patients made a complete recovery.

No. of cases	Good	Later good	Fair	Poor	Death
150	129	17 (10 shunt) (3 icH)	1 (RR)	–	3 PE (1.3%) surgical (0.6%)

RR = rerupture of aneurysm
PE = pulmonary embolism

One patient made only a fair recovery. This patient was 1 of 6 who sustained rerupture of a previously clipped aneurysm. There were no poor results in this group of patients.

3 grade IIa patients died (2.1%). 2 patients (41 and 50 year old men) were doing well after uncomplicated operations when they suddenly died 7 days and 2 weeks later of pulmonary embolism.

The third patient deteriorated after operation:

Sch., a 52 year old overweight man had a history of hypertension, diabetes, hypercholesterolemia, hepatitis, and recurrent thrombophlebitis. He was a heavy smoker. He sustained two subarachnoid hemorrhages, 10 days and 7 days before operation. Angiography showed an aneurysm of the anterior communicating artery. He was in grade IIa. At operation on 31 January, 1975, a bilobular aneurysm sat on the left corner of the anterior communicating artery. This could be shrunk with coagulation and clipped. Marked atherosclerosis of the internal carotid and middle cerebral arteries was noted. The systemic blood pressure was lowered to 80 torr systolic during the clipping. Immediately after operation the patient was found to have a left hemiparesis and was somnolent. He experienced gastrointestinal bleeding 10 hours later and the blood sugar was 600 mg%. The next day he showed no spontaneous movements. 4 days later he was re-explored where brain edema and spasm of the vessels was noted. He died the following day. Autopsy disclosed ischemic necrosis bilaterally in the watershed area between the areas supplied by the anterior and the middle cerebral arteries. Pulmonary emboli were present bilaterally.

This patient suffered ischemic infarction in the terminal areas of both distal anterior cerebral arteries during operation, possibly secondary to lowered blood pressure or to manipulation of the arteries. Subsequent cerebral edema led to his death. Thus the surgical death rate in this group of aneurysms is 1/150 (0.7%).

Grade IIb

66 patients presented in grade IIb. 60 of these made good recoveries (90.9%), although in 8 cases, the final recovery was delayed. 5 of these latter patients required ventricular shunts, 4 had large intracerebral hematomas which required time to resorb, and 2 presented with ischemic symptomatology. These latter two patients are interesting in that each had a neurological syndrome which has been ascribed classically to an infarct within the middle cerebral artery distribution. The first of these was a 63 year old man who presented with a left hemiparesis mostly involving the arm with a central left facial weakness and a complete left homonymous hemianopsia. The second patient was a 64 year old woman who demonstrated a discrete partial Gerstmann syndrome with acalculia and right-left disorientation without associated paresis, sensory disturbance or visual field deficit.

No. of cases	Good	Later good	Fair	Poor	Death
66	52 (1 icH)	8 (5 shunt) (4 icH) (2 infarct)	3 (1 RR) (1 epid. hem.) (1 infarct)	1	2

3 patients had fair results. 1 of these had a clipped aneurysm that ruptured (Table **77**, case No. 5). The second patient was a 56 year old man who underwent operation 2 years after two subarachnoid hemorrhages which left him mentally slowed and hemiparetic on the right. Operation was uneventful, but the preexisting deficits remained essentially unchanged. He works at about 50 per cent capacity.

The third patient's postoperative course was complicated by an epidural hematoma, which lay outside the original craniotomy site and was not easily visualized by angiography. The findings seemed explicable by cerebral ischemia and edema and thus removal of the hematoma was delayed three weeks. This type of eventuality is less likely in the age of computerized tomography, although the CT scan may not always show epi- and subdural hematomas clearly.

1 patient presenting in grade IIb condition remains in poor condition. This patient (a 57 year old female) demonstrated a progressive ischemic deficit beginning 2 days after a seemingly uncomplicated operation. She had evidence of impending infarction with bilateral weakness of the lower extremities in the preoperative period and should have had her operation delayed.

2 patients presenting in grade IIb died (3.0%). One, a 63 year old man with hypertension, had a severely sclerotic aneurysm that ruptured during clip placement and both A_1 segments had to be clipped to gain control. Nevertheless, he was making an excellent recovery and in fact returned to his home hospital just 6 days after operation. 3 weeks later he died of pulmonary embolism.

The second patient developed ischemic symptomatology and cerebral infarction one day after the anterior communicating artery was trapped and isolated from the circulation. This case was done early in the series, and it is not clear exactly what type of injury he sustained.

Grade IIIa

28 patients underwent operation in grade IIIa. Of these, 20 (71.4%) have had a good result. 6 of these had delayed recoveries, with 4 requiring shunts and with 4 requiring time for resolution of their intracerebral hematomas.

No. of cases	Good	Later good	Fair	Poor	Death
28	14	6	1	1	6

One patient had a fair result with an unusual postoperative complication following treatment of an anterior communicating artery aneurysm by trapping:

Ec., a 43 year old male engineer suffered a subarachnoid hemorrhage on 1 April, 1970, and angiography demonstrated an aneurysm of the anterior communicating artery. He underwent operation 12 days after hemorrhage in grade IIIa – he was somnolent, emotionally labile, disoriented, at times combative and showed marked meningism. The aneurysm sat on the right corner of the anterior communicating artery, inferiorly directed and was treated by trapping the anterior communicating artery. Postoperatively the patient recovered to a normal level of consciousness but showed a deficit for recent memory to the point that he could easily add rather complex numbers when presented on paper but he was unable to carry out the simplest calculations with figures presented orally. He simply could not remember the figures long enough. In addition he lost the desire to drink, and with no hint of diabetes insipidus carries a constant serum sodium of 160 meq/l. He needs persistent reminding by his wife to drink water. He is able to do some work, but has not returned to his former position as an engineer.

This patient suffered a hypothalamic injury that was partially present in the preoperative period, but was primarily noted after an operation that had sacrificed the hypothalamic arteries. Although some patients have had no apparent effect from trapping and isolation of the anterior communicating artery, it is important to avoid this if at all possible as demonstrated by the above case.

One patient has been placed in the poor category: This was a case in which the aneurysm ruptured just as the dura was being opened. A temporary clip on the left A_1 helped to control the bleeding and to dissect and to clip the aneurysm. He survived the operation, but required a shunt, which became infected and had to be revised. This patient has a severe psychiatric disorder with no other signs of neurological dysfunction.

6 patients presenting in grade IIIa died (21.4%). 4 of these were doing well after surgery but experienced rerupture of the clipped aneurysm with a fatal outcome (see Table **79**, p. 208). The 5th patient was a 57 year old lady who developed aspiration pneumonitis following rupture of an anterior communicating artery aneurysm and did not undergo operation until 10 weeks later. Operation was uncomplicated but she developed hydrocephalus requiring a shunt and died 5 weeks later of pulmonary embolism. The 6th patient, a 54 year old man, died of a postoperative complication. After the uneventful clipping of an aneurysm, this patient awoke from surgery but over the next 3 days he gradually deteriorated. At reexploration a large right subdural hematoma was found. Following removal of the subdural hematoma, the patient remained in a state of akinetic mutism with a left hemiparesis. He was later transferred to a local hospital where he died 5 months after operation. No autopsy was performed.

Grade IIIb

27 patients were grade IIIb at the time of operation. As might be anticipated, the morbidity rate was higher than with grade IIIa patients although mortality, setting aside the 4 reruptured patients in grade IIIa form a special group, was about the same. 18 patients (66.7%) had a good outcome although in half the cases, recovery was delayed. 6 of these delayed recovery patients required shunts in the postoperative period, 2 had large intracerebral hematomas, and 1 had an associated cerebral infarct with gradual resolution of symptoms.

Good	Later good	Fair	Poor	Death
9	9	5	2	2
18 (66.7%)		(18.5%)	(7.4%)	(7.4%)

5 patients are listed in "Fair" condition and these are summarized in Table **77**. 3 presented with fixed neurological deficits which showed only partial resolution. In 3 patients epidural hematomas caused delayed improvement.

2 grade IIIb patients are in poor condition. A 49 year old man confused and somnolent with a right hemiparesis and aphasia underwent operation 10 weeks after a subarachnoid hemorrhage. 2 months later he was involved in a motor vehicle accident and suffered a concussion. He subsequently developed hydrocephalus and required a shunt and has shown little improvement. He remains unable to work. The other patient, a 53 year old man, with hypertension and diabetes developed epilepsy and hydrocephalus in the postoperative

Table 77 The patients with a final „fair" result

Name	Age	Sex	Year	SAH	Time	Grade	Site	Hemat.	RE	Cause	Shunt	Follow-up	Work capacity
1. K.	47	M	1975	–	2 y	0b	Chiasm. Sy. POS	L. giant	–	–	–	4y unchanged	?
2. F.	42	M	1976	2/5y	9 d	IIa	POS	R. inf.	–	–	+ Rerupture reoperat.	3y neurol. no deficit, mild POS	50%
3. B.	33	M	1972	2/1w	2 m	IIb	POS, L. hpr.	L. sup.	–	Epid. hem.	+ 6w	7y L. hpr. mild, HA	50%
4. K.	56	M	1976	2/4m	2 y	IIb	R. hpr.	L. post.	–	–	–	3y unchanged	50%
5. J.	40	M	1974	1	8 d	IIb	R. hpr. mild	L. inf.	–	–	– Rerupt. 8d later, reop.	5y L. hpr., HA	50%
6. E.	43	M	1970	1	10 d	IIIa	POS	R. sup.	–	–	+	9y POS	50%
7. A.	36	M	1974	1	6 d	IIIb	L. hpr.	L. sup.	–	Epid. hem.	–	5y L. hpr. mild	50%
8. P.	38	M	1974	2/2w	2 m	IIIb	R. hpr., POS	M. post.	+	Epid. hem.	–	5y partially improved	50%
9. H.	29	M	1977	2/2w	3 w	IIIb	Paraplegia leg, aphas.	L. post.	Callos.	–	–	2y improvement no aphasia but parapleg.	50%
10. M.	41	F	1977	1	13 d	IIIb	L. hpr., POS	L. post.	Callos. front. R.	–	–	2y neurol. no deficit, mild POS	50%
11. K.	53	M	1978	1	7 m	IIIb	R. hpr., POS, aphasia	L. sup. L. ICB	+	–	–	1y improvement	50%

period. A shunt was inserted with little improvement. A recent CT scan has shown bilateral frontal lobe atrophy. Neither of these patients was able to recover from the initial brain injury and subsequent hydrocephalus.

2 of the grade IIIb patients with intracerebral hematomas had a fatal outcome (7.4%). Both patients died from bacterial meningitis. Both these cases were done early in the series (1967/1968) and were treated by trapping the anterior communicating artery. Both remained in poor condition postoperatively. Nevertheless, it was the superimposition of central nervous system infection that led to each patient's demise.

Grades IV and V

17 patients were in grade IV at the time of operation. None of these made a worthwhile recovery. 13 of these patients had intracerebral hematomas. 9 (52.9%) remain in poor condition (6 with hematomas) and 8 (47.1%) have died (7 with hematomas).

The one patient undergoing operation in grade V also died. These patients are summarized in Table **78**. Of those that died, only the grade V patient died in the immediate postoperative period. The others lived from 4 weeks to a year. These patients presented with apallic syndrome, more severe neurological deficits like hemiplegia, paraparesis, paraplegia, and tetraparesis.

With aneurysms at other locations, one sees a few patients presenting in grade IV who go on to make good recoveries. However, with this group of aneurysm patients, the removal of hematomas, ventricular shunting, prolonged nursing care, and time did not seem to be of much benefit. It is therefore recommended that operation only be performed in younger patients in grade IV who clearly have a hematoma with mass effect. Otherwise these patients should be treated with nursing care, corticosteroids, and observation until they show some evidence of recovery before operation is contemplated.

Analysis of Results

Those factors that might have contributed to a favorable or unfavorable outcome were analyzed in detail:

Preoperative Grade

As with aneurysms at other locations, preoperative grade is the single most important prognostic indicator of operative result. In the 371 patients with subarachnoid hemorrhage the preoperative grade has been related to results, with patients grouped to show percentages in the various categories (Table **79**). It is seen that there is a progressive decline in good results with each higher grade and conversely with the exception of grade IIIb a progressive increase in mortality related to the preoperative grade. In some patients, the deficit is fixed at the time of aneurysm rupture. Thus even perfect surgery, though preventing further deterioration from aneurysm rupture and though removing intracranial hematomas to reduce intracranial pressure and brain shifts, will never restore areas of irreversibly damaged brain.

Age and Sex

Age and sex are related to operative results in Table **80a** and **b**. There is a tendency for patients over 50 years old to have a less favorable course than those younger, but this is not dramatic. Good results were obtained in 88.4 per cent of patients under 50 and 85.7 per cent of patients over 50. Mortality in patients over 50 was twice that of younger patients, but this was based on only 23 cases who died. It is possible that patients who remain in fair and poor condition at younger age, might have succumbed at older ages, but this is not proven by the statistics presented.

A good outcome was obtained in 93.0 per cent of females and 84.0 per cent of males. Mortality rates were similar at 5.6 per cent and 6.5 per cent respectively. One is left with the impression that surviving women are perhaps more able to make a complete recovery than surviving men. A single factor such as age or sex in these patients has little predictive value, however, and these statistics are presented only to give a general feeling for the relationship between sex, age, and outcome.

Number of Subarachnoid Hemorrhages

Of the 371 patients with subarachnoid hemorrhage, 266 (71.7%) sustained 1 hemorrhage, 91 (24.5%) 2 hemorrhages, and 14 (3.8%) 3 or more hemorrhages. The number of hemorrhages is related to the preoperative grade and outcome in Table **81**. 91.7 per cent of patients with 1 subarachnoid hemorrhage had a good result as did 82.4 per cent of patients with 2 hemorrhages. Similar results were seen in only 50.0 per cent of patients with 3 or more hemorrhages. Mortality rates correspondingly increased with the increased number of hemorrhages.

Looking at the preoperative grade, 8 of 266 patients with 1 hemorrhage (3.0%), 5 of 91 with 2 hemorrhages (5.5%), and 5 of 14 with 3 hemor-

Table 78 Patients presenting in Grades IV and V with ruptured aneurysms of the anterior communicating artery

Name	Age	Sex	Year	SAH	Grade	Hematoma Cist	IC	IV	SD	Timing	Operation	Shunt	Survival Time	Result
Ci	40	M	1967	3	IV R. hpr., Epi	+	0	0	0	5 days	Trapping	0	12 years	Poor – r. hemiparesis aphasia, POS
We	60	F	1968	1	IV parapar.	+	+	0	0	4 weeks	Trapping	+	7 months	Death, hemiparesis
Lo	70	M	1968	2	IV L. hpr.	+	+	0	+	2 weeks	Trapping	0	6 weeks	Death
Fo*	60	M	1969	1	IV L. hpr., Epi.	+	+	0	0	2 weeks	Clip	0	4 weeks	Death – myocard. inf.
Ra*	58	M	1970	2	IV R. hpr.	+	+	0	0	1 day	Clip	+	1 year	Death
Ba	45	M	1970	3	IV parapl.	+	+	0	0	4 days	Clip	+	9 years	Poor – paraplegia, Nursing home
Pe	27	M	1970	2	IV tetrapar.	0	+	0	0	1 day	Clip	+	9 years	Poor – paraplegia, POS
Fi*	42	M	1971	1	IV L. hpr., Epi	0	0	0	0	3 weeks	Clip	0	8 years	Poor – POS, right hemiparesis, aphasia
Du	48	M	1972	3	IV l. hpr.	+	+	0	+	4 weeks	Clip	+	7 years	Poor – l. hemiparesis
Vi	42	F	1972	1	IV parapl.	0	+	0	0	3 weeks	Clip	+	6 months	Death
Vi	35	M	1973	1	IV L. hpr.	0	0	0	0	4 weeks	Clip	+	6 years	Poor – tetraspastic Parkinsonian, POS
Se	53	M	1973	3	IV R. hpr., Epi	0	0	0	0	3 months	Clip	+	6 years	Poor – POS, akinesia Parkinsonism
Sch	31	M	1974	1	IV R. hpr.	+	+	0	0	2 days	Clip	0	5 months	Death
St	64	F	1975	2	IV R. hpl., Epi	+	+	0	0	1 day	Clip	+	3 months	Death
He	47	M	1975	3	IV L. hpl., Epi	+	+	+	0	6 days	Clip	+	3 months	Death
Oe	45	M	1975	2	IV parapl.	+	+	+	+	5 days	Clip	+	4 years	Poor – paraplegia, POS
Lo	56	M	1977	1	IV L. hpl.	0	0	0	0	3 months	Clip	+	2 years	Poor – l. hemiparesis POS
Ge	51	F	1977	2	V tetrapar.	+	+	0	0	10 days	Clip	0	1 day	Death

rhages (35.8%) presented in grades IV or V. An increased number of hemorrhages does to some degree affect the preoperative status and outcome, perhaps because second and third hemorrhages tend to be more severe. However, this correlation is rather loose. As an example, 3 patients in grade IIa with 3 hemorrhages did well, while 3 patients in the same grade with only one hemorrhage died.

The time interval between hemorrhages varied considerably. 34 of the 105 patients (32.4%) known to have had more than one hemorrhage, sustained a second hemorrhage within the first 2 weeks. The other 71 patients had recurrent

Table 79 Operative results of ruptured anterior communicating aneurysms as related to preoperative grade

Grade	SAH Total No.	Good	Good Delayed recovery	Fair	Poor	Death			Total
Ia–IIa	232	209 (90.0%)	19 (8.2%)	1 (0.4%)	–	3	2 PE 1 surg.	(0.9%) (0.4%)	1.3%
IIb	66	52 (78.8%)	8 (12.1%)	3 (4.5%)	1 (1.5%)	2	1 PE 1 surg.	(1.5%) (1.5%)	3.0%
IIIa	28	14 (50.0%)	6 (21.4%)	1 (3.6%)	1 (3.6%)	6	1 PE 4 RR 1 surg.	(3.6%) (14.3%) (3.6%)	21.4%
IIIb	27	9 (33.3%)	9 (33.3%)	5 (18.5%)	2 (7.4%)	2	surg.		7.4%
IV	17	–	–	–	9 (52.9%)	8	natural		47.1%
V	1	–	–	–	–	1	natural		100.0%
Total SAH	371	284 (76.5%)	42 (11.3%)	10 (2.7%)	13 (3.5%)	22	5 surg. 4 PE 4 RR 9 natural	(1.3%) (1.1%) (1.1%) (2.4%)	5.9%

	SAH Total No.	Good	Fair	Poor	Death
Ia–IIa	232	98.3%	0.4%	0.0%	1.3%
IIb	66	90.9%	4.5%	1.5%	3.0%
IIIa	28	71.4%	3.6%	3.6%	21.4%
IIIb	27	66.7%	18.5%	7.4%	7.4%
IV	17	–	–	52.9%	47.1%
V	1	–	–	–	100.0%

Table 80a Relationship between sex, age, and final outcome in all anterior communicating artery aneurysm patients

Age	Sex	Good	Good Delayed recovery	Fair	Poor	Death	Total No.
15–20 y	M	7	–	–	–	–	7
	F	3	–	–	–	–	3
21–30 y	M	21	2	1	1 (1)	–	25
	F	11	–	–	–	–	11
31–40 y	M	36	8	4	3 (2)	2 (1)	53
	F	20	3	–	–	–	23
41–50 y	M	56	6	3	5 (4)	5 (1)	75
	F	35	6	1	–	3 (1)	45
51–60 y	M	38	7	2	3 (2)	5 (3)	55
	F	33	3	–	1	4 (1)	41
61–73 y	M	9	4	–	–	3 (1)	16
	F	17	3	–	–	1 (1)	21
		286	42	11	13 (9)	23 (9)	375

( ) In condition IV-V

Table 80b Relationship between sex, age over or below 50 and outcome

Sex	Age	Total	Good	Fair	Poor	Death
M	< 50	160	136 (85.0%)	8 (5.0%)	9 (5.6%)	7 (4.4%)
	> 50	71	58 (81.7%)	2 (2.8%)	3 (4.2%)	8 (11.3%)
		231	194 (84.0%)	10 (4.3%)	12 (5.2%)	15 (6.5%)
F	< 50	82	78 (95.1%)	1 (1.2%)	–	3 (3.7%)
	> 50	62	56 (90.3%)	–	1 (1.6%)	5 (8.1%)
		144	134 (93.0%)	1 (0.7%)	1 (0.7%)	8 (5.6%)
Combined	< 50	242	214 (88.4%)	9 (3.7%)	9 (3.7%)	10 (4.1%)
	> 50	133	114 (85.7%)	2 (1.5%)	4 (3.0%)	13 (9.8%)
		375	328 (87.5%)	11 (2.9%)	13 (3.5%)	23 (6.1%)

Table 81 The outcome as related to the preoperative condition and the number of subarachnoid hemorrhages

	Good 1×	2×	3×	Fair 1×	2×	3×	Poor 1×	2×	3×	Death 1×	2×	3×	No. of ruptures
Ia+b	67	15	–	–	–	–	–	–	–	–	–	–	82
IIa	114	29	3	–	–	–	–	–	–	3	1	–	150
IIb	46	14	–	1	2	–	–	1	–	1	1	–	66
IIIa	9	9	2	1	1	–	–	1	–	2	1	2	28
IIIb	8	8	2	3	2	–	2	–	–	1	1	–	27
IV	–	–	–	–	–	–	3	2	4	5	2	1	17
V	–	–	–	–	–	–	–	–	–	–	1	–	1
	244	75	7	5	5	–	5	4	4	12	7	3	371

1 bleed 266 cases, 2 bleeds 91 cases, 3 bleeds 14 cases.
Not only the number of SAH but also the severity of SAH is important

hemorrhages from 2 weeks to 17 years after the original hemorrhage. No particular pattern relating the outcome to the time of occurrence of the second or third hemorrhage emerged.

Hydrocephalus

The incidence of hydrocephalus was higher for anterior communicating artery aneurysm patients than for patients with aneurysms at any other location. Of 371 patients with ruptured aneurysms, 46 (12.4%) required ventricular shunts. In 6 patients, shunts were inserted in the preoperative period, and in the other 40, at varying times postoperatively. An additional 76 patients (20.3%) had evidence of mild to moderate hydrocephalus that resolved on its own.

Hydrocephalus requiring a ventricular shunt is compared to preoperative grade and operative result in Table 82. It is noted that there is a progressive increase in the percentage of patients requiring shunts, comparing 20.0 per cent of fair result patients and 76.9 per cent of patients with poor results who needed shunts. A shunt was inserted in 7 of 22 patients who died (31.8%), 2 of these preoperatively. As 27 of 46 patients went on to a good recovery after shunting, the other 19 patients presumably had no malresorptive hydrocephalus but additional brain impairments preventing their recovery.

Ventricular shunts were required in 30 of 231 men (13.0%) and 16 of 144 women (11.1%) suggesting no particular sex predilection. There was a slightly higher incidence in older age groups with 11.2 per cent of 197 patients between 31 and 50 requiring a shunt compared to 18.3 per cent of 131 patients between 51 and 70. Shunts were required in 12.5 per cent of patients with 1 hemorrhage, 8.2 per cent of patients with 2 hemorrhages, and 33.3 per

Table 82 Ventricular shunts in 46 patients out of 371 SAH cases

Grade	Total No.	Shunts	Good	Fair	Poor	Death
Ia	82	1 (1.2%)	1	–	–	–
IIa	150	10 (6.7%)	9	1	–	–
IIb	66	9 (13.6%)	7	1	–	1
IIIa	28	6 (21.4%)	4	–	1	1
IIIb	27	9 (33.3%)	6	–	3 (1)*	–
IV	17	11 (64.7%)	–	–	6 (4)*	5 (2)*
V	1	–	–	–	–	–
Total No. of SAH cases	371	46	27 (8.3%) 326	2 (20.0%) 10	10 (76.9%) 13	7 (31.8%) 22

( )* preoperative shunt

cent of patients with 3 hemorrhages. It is the severity of hemorrhage as determined by preoperative grade rather than the number of hemorrhages that seems to be an important factor in hydrocephalus.

Intracranial Hematoma

Of 371 patients with ruptured cerebral aneurysms, 39 (10.4%) presented with intracranial hematomas of varying sizes and locations (Table 83). 6 patients had only subdural hematomas (1.6%) and 5 patients had only intraventricular hematomas (1.3%), without associated intracerebral clots. A particular type of intracerebral hematoma extending along the corpus callosum was found in 4 patients (1.1%), these patients presenting with lower extremity dysfunction (paraplegia) and altered levels of consciousness and showing no improvement.

Of 371 patients with subarachnoid hemorrhage from ruptured anterior communicating artery aneurysms, 174 (46.9%) were operated upon within the first 2 weeks. In this group of patients, 39 (22.4%) were found to have large hematomas around the aneurysm, 51 (29.3%) had hematomas filling the basal cisterns (including the interpeduncular cistern), 52 (29.9%) had only small, localized hematomas, and 32 (18.3%) had no evidence of blood clot. Thus a significant proportion of these early operated patients can be expected to reveal significant hematomas at surgery.

The presence of hematoma is presented in relation to preoperative grade and surgical result in Table 84a and b. A progression of worsening preoperative grade is noted in the presence of hematoma (Table 84a). The incidence of hematoma in those making early good recoveries is 1.1 per cent, but increases to 28.5 per cent of those with delayed

Table 83 Location of hematomas in 39 patients with ruptured anterior communicating artery aneurysms

Hematoma	Cases
Subdural hematoma (6)	
Only subdural	3
+ intracerebral	3
Interhemispheric (6)	
Only interhemispheric	5
+ intracerebral	1
Intracerebral hematoma (27)	
Frontal (18)	
Only intracerebral	14
+ intraventricular	4
Corpus callosum	4
Intraventricular only	5
	39 = 10.4%

recoveries, 40.0 per cent of those with fair recoveries, 46.2 per cent of those with poor final results, and 59.1 per cent of those who died (Table 84b). Thus, while the presence of hematoma is tolerated well in some patients, it generally has an unfavorable effect on both preoperative condition and outcome.

The suspicion remains that hematoma plays less of a direct pathophysiological role with anterior communicating artery aneurysms than with middle cerebral artery aneurysms. All grade IV and V patients with ruptured middle cerebral artery aneurysms had hematomas and these were associated with severe brain shifts. Patients with ruptured anterior communicating artery aneurysms suffer more direct orbitofrontal and upper diencephalic damage, and the removal of the hematoma is less likely to salvage a patient in extremis.

Table 84a The presence of hematoma in relation to preoperative grade and surgical results

Preoperative condition		Postoperative result		Hematoma		
Ia	(82 cases)	Good	80	–		
		Delayed good	2	–		
		Fair	–	–		
		Poor	–	–		
		Death	–	–		
IIa	(150 cases)	Good	129	–		
		Delayed good	17	2		
		Fair	1	–	3	2 %
		Poor	–	–		
		Death	3	1		
IIb	(66 cases)	Good	52	1		
		Delayed good	8	4		
		Fair	3	–	6	9.1%
		Poor	1	–		
		Death	2	1		
IIIa	(28 cases)	Good	14	1		
		Delayed good	6	4		
		Fair	1	–	6	21.4%
		Poor	1	–		
		Death	6	1		
IIIb	(27 cases)	Good	9	2		
		Delayed good	9	2		
		Fair	5	4	10	37 %
		Poor	2	–		
		Death	2	2		
IV	(17 cases)	Good	–	–		
		Delayed good	–	–		
		Fair	–	–	13	76.4%
		Poor	9	6		
		Death	8	7		
V	(1 case)	Death	1	1	1	100 %
					39	

Table 84b Outcome of hematoma cases related to overall outcome results

	No. of cases	Hematomas	Per cent
Good recovery	284	4	1.1
Delayed recovery	42	12	28.5
Fair	10	4	40.0
Poor	13	6	46.2
Death	22	13	59.1
	371	39	

Cerebral Ischemia and Infarction

The area of distribution of the anterior cerebral-anterior communicating artery complex generally assumes the shape of a butterfly (Fig 110). The anterior cerebral arteries perfuse the anterior basal ganglia and hypothalamus. This distribution is supplemented by the recurrent arteries of Heubner, which while originating closer to the anterior communicating artery, actually supply an area of the internal capsule and basal ganglia more lateral and posterior than the anterior cerebral

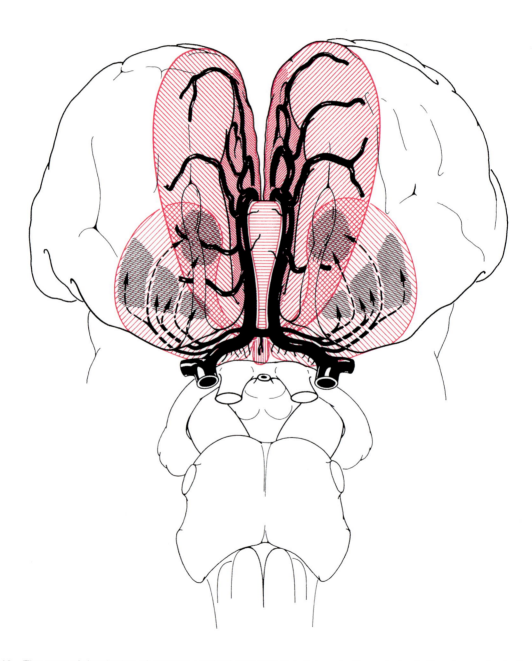

Fig 110 The area of distribution of anterior cerebral and anterior communicating arteries in the shape of a butterfly.

artery. The anterior communicating artery supplies the anterior hypothalamus and subcallosal area and the distal anterior cerebral arteries the corpus callosum and medial aspects of both hemispheres. As a result, ischemia in the distribution of one or more of these arterial segments and their well recognized variations may give rise to a variety of neurological symptoms.

For most patients in the present series, an area of cerebral infarction was assumed on clinical grounds, but in the last 7 years, many have been examined by computerized tomography. In 10 patients, frontal lobe ischemia that was silent clinically has been noted on CT scan, suggesting that ischemia is perhaps more common than recognized. A characteristic finding on CT scan with ruptured anterior communicating artery aneurysms is bilateral parasagittal areas of ischemia corresponding to the watershed areas of the distal anterior cerebral artery distribution. This may be associated with paraplegia and lower extremity sensory disturbances suggestive of a spinal lesion. Finally, some patients presented with symptoms usually referable to the distribution of the middle cerebral artery. Patients with hemiparesis often had the face and arm more severely affected than the leg. Aphasia has been seen, and 2 patients presented with homonymous hemianopsia. 1 patient developed a partial Gerstmann syndrome following rupture of an anterior communicating artery aneurysm with acalculia and right-left disorientation.

Ischemic events undoubtedly play a part in the mental changes seen with ruptured anterior communicating artery aneurysm. Infarction has been seen in the subcallosal area and in the cingulate gyri at operation or on CT scan in some of these patients. In many patients though, there is no apparent macroscopic infarction despite profound disturbances of memory, attention, and personality.

Patients in grades IIb and IIIb often had symptoms or CT scans suggestive of cerebral ischemia. 4 of 93 patients in these two groups died (4.3%). 1 of these was doing well and died of pulmonary embolism, leaving 3 (3.2%) dying from neurological and operative problems. In groups IIa and IIIa there were 178 patients. 9 (5.1%) of these died but 4 of the deaths related to recurrent subarachnoid hemorrhage and 3 to pulmonary embolism. Only 2 (1.1%) were related to neurological injury. Similarly, morbidity in grades IIb and IIIb was present in 11 of 93 patients (11.8%) while in grades IIa and IIIa, only 3 of 178 (1.7%) had neurological impairment. It appears that cerebral ischemia plays some role in both morbidity and mortality, although perhaps less than is sometimes implied by other series.

Electrolyte Disturbances

Assuming a normal range of serum sodium concentration from 135 to 145 meq/l, 182 patients showed hypo- or hypernatremia in the postoperative period (Table **85a–d**). In 5 patients serum sodium was greater than 150 meq/l, and in 22 it was less than 130 meq/l for periods from 1 to 10 days. Serum sodium concentrations are related to preoperative grade in Table **85a**. Only 5.9 per cent of patients in grade IV had a normal sodium concentration while 29.4 per cent had a sodium less than 130 meq/l. There is a tendency for an increasing incidence of hyponatremia to relate to a worsening preoperative condition. Although a few patients showed hypernatremia, only 4 patients developed diabetes insipidus, all of whom had their anterior communicating artery trapped at surgery. Of the other 11 patients undergoing isolation of their anterior communicating artery by trapping, 9 had some sort of electrolyte abnormality, while only 2 were normonatremic.

Table **85a** Preoperative natremia

Natremia	No. of cases	
Norm	301	(80.3%)
Hypo	68	(18.1%)
Hyper	6	(1.6%)

Table **85b** Postoperative natremia

Natremia	No. of cases	
Norm	193	(51.5%)
Hypo	152	(40.5%)
Hyper	25	(6.7%)
Hypo-Hyper	5	(1.3%)

40 patients (10.7%) have had pre- and postoperative electrolyte changes

Table **85c** Electrolyte disturbance and its duration

1 day	65 cases	35.7%
2 days	39 cases	21.4%
3 days	20 cases	11.0%
4 days	16 cases	8.8%
5 days	13 cases	7.1%
6–10 days	22 cases	12.1%
2–4 weeks	6 cases	3.3%
Permanent	1 case	0.5%
	182	

4 patients showed diabetes insipidus

Table **85d** The incidence of sodium abnormalities related to the postoperative condition

Post-operative grade	Total No.	Hyponatremia < 129	Hyponatremia 130–134	Normo-natremia 135–145	Hypernatremia 145–150	Hypernatremia 150 >
0a	2	–	–	2	–	–
0b	2	–	1	1	–	–
Ia	82	1 (1.2%)	28 (34.1%)	49 (59.8%)	3 (3.7%)	1 (1.2%)
IIa	150	7 (4.7%)	43 (28.6%)	91 (60.7%)	6 (4.0%)	3 (2.0%)
IIb	66	3 (4.5%)	23 (34.8%)	37 (56.1%)	3 (4.5%)	–
IIIa	28	3 (10.7%)	16 (57.1%)	6 (21.4%)	3 (10.7%)	–
IIIb	27	2 (7.4%)	16 (59.3%)	6 (22.2%)	3 (11.1%)	–
IV	17	5 (29.4%)	8 (47.1%)	1 (5.9%)	2 (11.8%)	1 (5.9%)
V	1	1	– (47.1%)	–	–	–
	375	22	135	193	20	5

Seizure Disorder

Postoperative transient seizures occurred in 8 patients. 6 of these had an associated intracerebral hematoma and 3 required shunts for persistent hydrocephalus. All patients with seizures underwent operation at a time when medication to reverse anesthesia was being given. Since this practice was discontinued 7 years ago there have been no further cases of postoperative seizures. A seizure disorder accompanying an anterior communicating artery aneurysm presently seems quite rare; occurring in 7 cases preoperatively in grades IIIb and IV (see Tables **78** and **92**) and only in 1 case postoperatively in a grade IIIb patient.

Psychoorganic Syndrome (POS)

It is well recognized that disorders of consciousness, memory, concentration, and personality can follow the rupture of an anterior communicating artery aneurysm. At times these symptoms appear first in the postoperative period and are presumed to have resulted from surgical damage to the orbitofrontal cortex or upper diencephalon. Lindqvist and Norlén (1966) examined 33 cases with operatively treated anterior communicating artery aneurysms. They found that 17 of the 33 patients (51.5%) had evidence for Korsakoff's syndrome (primary memory defect with confusion and confabulation in an otherwise alert patient). In 5 patients (15.2%) the condition was still present after months or years.

In the present series, 199 patients (53.1%) manifested some psychoorganic disturbance during the hospital course (Table **86a, b**). In 71 patients (18.9%) with normal mentation preoperatively, there was a transient POS postoperatively which resolved in days. In 5 patients (1.3%) changes first noted in the postoperative period were permanent. 123 patients (32.8%) demonstrated POS preoperatively; 85 (22.7%) improved after operation, 19 (5.1%) were left with permanent mental changes and 19 (5.1%) died. Of the 24 (6.4%) patients remaining with POS, 5 (1.3%) first developed the changes postoperatively and 19 (5.1%) had a continuation of preexisting deficits.

In relation to age, 15 of 242 patients under 50 (9.3%) and 4 of 133 patients over 50 (3.0%) had permanent psychoorganic syndrome. Taking the deaths into account revealed that 23 of 242 (9.5%) patients under 50, and 15 of 133 (11.3%) patients over 50 demonstrated persistent POS. Thus a definite relationship to age is not apparent.

Table **86a** Psychoorganic syndrome (POS) pre- and 6 months postoperatively in cases with aneurysms of anterior communicating artery (375 cases)

Preop. →	Normal	Normal	POS	Normal	POS	POS
Postp. →	Nomal	Transient POS	Improv.	Permanent POS	POS	Death
No of cases	176 (46.9%)	71 (18.9%)	85 (22.7%)	5 (1.3%)	19 (5.1%)	19 (5.1%)

(65.8)

(88.5%)   (1.3%) (surgical)   (10.2%)

Table **86b** Psychoorganic syndrome related to the outcome

Preop. → Postop. →	Normal Normal	Normal Trans. POS	POS Improv.	Normal Perm. POS	POS POS	POS Death
Good	173	61	52	–	–	–
Later good	–	9	33	–	–	–
Fair	–	–	–	4	7	–
Poor	–	–	–	1	12	–
Death	3*	1*	–	–	–	19
	176	71	85	5	19	19

* pulmonary emboli

Anatomical Factors

The location of the aneurysm on the anterior communicating artery and the projection of the fundus are compared to outcome in Table **87a** and **b**. Of 199 aneurysms on the left corner, 85.4 per cent of patients had a good result, of 67 in the midposition, 88.1 per cent a good result, and of 109 on the right corner 90.8 per cent a good result. Mortality also shows a little variation, with 7.0 per cent on the left, 7.5 per cent in the middle and 3.7 per cent on the right.

The projection of the fundus seems more important, however. Anterior, superior, and posterior had good results of 93.7 per cent, 91.8 per cent, and 88.4 per cent respectively, while patients with inferiorly projecting aneurysms had only 79.2 per cent good results and those with complex projection 81.7 per cent. Similarly, mortality was nil for the anterior projection, 2.4 per cent for the superior projection and 6.2 per cent for the posterior projection, but 11.3 per cent and 11.6 per cent for the inferior and complex projections respectively. These figures represent both the potential for damage during rupture with aneurysms directed toward the diencephalon and the increased operative difficulty.

Table 87a Site of aneurysms at the anterior communicating artery complex and results

Site	Total No.	Good	Fair	Poor	Death
Left	199 (53.1%)	170 (85.4%)	8	7	14 (7.0%)
Middle	67 (17.8%)	59 (88.1%)	1	2	5 (7.5%)
Right	109 (29.1%)	99 (90.8%)	2	4	4 (3.7%)
	375	328 (87.5%)	11 (2.9%)	13 (3.5%)	23 (6.1%)

Table 87b Position of aneurysms and results

	Total No.	Good	Fair	Poor	Death
Anterior	48 (18.8%)	45 (93.7%)	1	2	–
Superior	85 (22.7%)	78 (91.8%)	4	1	2 (2.4%)
Posterior	129 (34.4%)	114 (88.4%)	4	3	8 (6.2%)
Inferior	53 (14.1%)	42 (79.2%)	2	3	6 (11.3%)
Complex	60 (16.0%)	49 (81.7%)	–	4	7 (11.6%)
	375	328	11	13	23

Timing of Operation

The timing of operation in the 371 patients with subarachnoid hemorrhage is related to preoperative grade and postoperative result in Table **88**. 15 patients (4.0%) underwent operation within the first 3 days. 11 of these were in grades IIa to IIIb, and each of these had a good result. Of these 11 patients, 7 were physicians, medical students, or relatives of physicians who were transferred to the clinic very early. 1 patient was pregnant, 1 had an intracerebral hematoma, and 2 were done early because of approaching holidays. The other 4 patients underwent operation in grade IV for removal of hematoma. 3 of these died and 1 is in poor condition.

There were 52 cases (14.0%) done between the fourth and seventh day post hemorrhage. Of these, 49 were in grades Ia to IIIb and 46 made a good recovery (93.9%). 1 patient in grade IIIb was making a fair recovery when he developed an epidural hematoma which increased a preexisting left hemiparesis. Another patient in grade IIIa had a recurrent subarachnoid hemorrhage from a clipped aneurysm and died, and 1 patient with a poor result developed a delayed ischemic deficit in the first postoperative week. She had shown some evidence of cerebral ischemia preoperatively and her operation probably should have been delayed. 3 other patients were operated upon in grade IV with 2 poor results and 1 death.

107 patients (28.8%) underwent operation in the second week after hemorrhage, 104 were in grades Ia to IIIb and 94 (90.4%) made a good recovery. Of the 3 cases with fair results, 1 suffered rerupture of a previously clipped aneurysm, 1 had a hematoma and right frontal infarct that improved postoperatively, and 1 treated early in the series by trapping the anterior communicating artery, was unable to return to work. There were no poor results, but 7 patients died (6.7%). 3 patients in grade IIIa experienced rerupture of a previously clipped aneurysm and died, 1 grade IIIb patient died of bacterial meningitis, 1 grade IIIa patient died of postoperative subdural hematoma, 1 grade IIa patient succumbed to a hypothalamic injury noted after operation, and 1 grade IIb patient suffered a fatal cerebral infarction following a trapping procedure. 3 grade IV–V patients operated in the second week died.

Between 2 and 4 weeks, 110 patients (29.6%) underwent operation. Of these, 105 were in grades Ia to IIIb and 97 (92.4%) made a full recovery. 1 man in grade IIIb with a fair result was rendered immediately paraplegic by a corpus callosum hematoma and suffered an infarction in the parasagittal areas bilaterally. 2 patients remain in a poor condition, 1 in grade IIIa suffered rerupture of his aneurysm while the dura was being opened and later had an infected ventricular shunt, and another in IIIb with hypertension, diabetes, and hemiplegia showed ventricular enlargement and frontal lobe atrophy. 4 patients died, 3 of pulmonary embolism, 2 of whom were in preoperative grade IIa and were making good postoperative recoveries. 1 patient in grade IIb was left in fair condition after his aneurysm ruptured during anesthetic induction and 1 patient in grade IIIb developed bacterial meningitis. 5 cases underwent operation in grade IV with 3 poor results and 2 deaths.

87 patients underwent operation more than 4 weeks after hemorrhage, and 78 (89.6%) of these made a complete recovery. Of 4 fair results, 4 patients in grades IIb and IIIb had severe preoperative deficits that cleared to some degree after operation, and 1 patient in grade IIb accumulated an epidural hematoma postoperatively with a resultant hemiparesis. One grade IIIb patient with hydrocephalus had a poor result and 3 grade IV patients remain in poor condition. 1 patient in grade IIa died unexpectedly of pulmonary embolism following a shunt operation performed 2 months after her original aneurysm operation.

The chance of full recovery for patients in grades Ia to IIIb undergoing operation between 1 and 3 days was 100 per cent, between 4 and 7 days 93.9 per cent, between 8 and 14 days 90.4 per cent, between 15 and 28 days 92.4 per cent and after 28 days 92.9 per cent. Mortality rates for the same time periods were 0 for 1 to 3 days, 1.9 per cent for 4 to 7 days, 6.5 per cent for 8 to 14 days, 3.6 per cent for 15 to 28 days, and 1.2 per cent for after 28 days.

Table 88 Timing of surgery and results in 371 patients with ruptured aneurysm of the anterior communicating artery

	Good					Later good					Fair				Poor				Death					
	Ia	IIa	IIb	IIIa	IIIb	Ia	IIa	IIb	IIIa	IIIb	IIa	IIb	IIIa	IIIb	IIb	IIIa	IIIb	IV	IIa	IIb	IIIa	IIIb	IV	V
1–3 d	–	3	4	1	1	–	–	–	1	1	–	–	–	–	–	–	–	1	–	–	–	–	3	–
4–7 d	2	29	7	2	2	–	3	–	–	1	–	–	–	1	1	–	–	2	–	–	1	–	1	–
1–2 w	4	49	13	8	3	–	9	1	3	4	–	1	1	1	–	–	–	–	1	1	4	1	2	1
2–4 w	29	38	18	3	1	–	3	4	–	1	1	–	–	1	–	1	1	3	2	1	–	1	2	–
1–3 m	27	6	7	1	2	2	1	4	2	2	–	1	–	1	–	–	1	2	1	–	–	–	–	–
> 3 m	18	4	2	–	–	–	–	–	–	–	–	1	–	1	–	–	–	1	–	–	–	–	–	–
	80	129	51	15	9	2	16	9	6	9	1	3	1	5	1	1	2	9	4	2	5	2	8	1
			284					42				10				13					22			371

Table 89 Timing, grading and outcome (371 cases of ruptured anterior communicating artery aneurysms)

Total No.		1–3 d 15	4–7 d 52	1–2 w 107	2–4 w 110	> 4 w 87
Grade						
I–III	353 cases	11	49	104	105	84
Good		11 (100%)	46 (93.9%)	94 (90.4%)	97 (92.4%)	78 (92.9%)
Fair		–	1	3	2	4
Poor		–	1	–	2	1
Death		–	1	7	4	1
IV–V	18 cases	4	3	3	5	3
Good		–	–	–	–	–
Fair		–	–	–	–	–
Poor		1	2	–	3	3
Death		3	1	3	2	–

Mortality and morbidity rates for these time periods are comparable (Table 89). The only time period that stands out is the second week in which 7 patients in grades Ia to IIIb were lost. 3 of these patients had recurrent subarachnoid hemorrhages from a previously clipped aneurysm, 1 had a postoperative subdural hematoma, and 1 died of bacterial meningitis. This leaves just 2 patients in whom the cause of death could be related to the manipulation of arteries, technical problems, or possibly the timing of operation. Of the 174 patients undergoing operation within the first 2 weeks, 23 (13.2%) had less than a complete recovery. 10 of these were in grades IV and V and did no worse nor better than patients in the same grade done after 2 weeks. 6 patients suffered rerupture of a previously clipped aneurysm, with 2 left in fair condition and 4 dead. The relationship of timing of operation to these cases is not clear. 1 patient died of a postoperative subdural hematoma, and 1 patient was made worse by an epidural hematoma. Timing of operation was incidental in these patients. 1 patient died of an infection, again presumably unrelated to the timing of operation as related to the subarachnoid hemorrhage.

5 patients are left whose course may in some way relate to the timing of operation. 2 patients developed psychoorganic syndrome after trapping procedures performed early in the series. Operation conceivably could have been tolerated better at a later time, but there is no way to prove this. 2 patients developed delayed ischemic symptoms, 1 of whom had shown early evidence of ischemia preoperatively. The final patient had a frontal hematoma and infarct that improved after operation. The relationship of operative timing to the deficits in these last 3 patients can only be speculative.

Patients operated upon after 2 weeks showed similar deficits again on the basis of hematoma, infarction, infection, hydrocephalus, intracranial hematoma, or pulmonary embolism. Timing of operation, per se, does not seem to be an important factor in predicting operative result. Many other factors must be considered together to decide the proper time for operation.

Operative Procedure

The effect of the operative procedure itself was evaluated, both with regard to technical factors and with regard to complications.

Intraoperative rupture. 90 patients (24.0%) experienced rupture of the aneurysm sometime between the induction of anesthesia and the final clipping. The time of intraoperative rupture is related to operative results in Table 90. 5 of the

Table 90 Rupture of aneurysm

Rupture during	Total No.	Good	Fair	Poor	Death
Anesthesia	3	2	–	–	1 (IIa)
Craniotomy	2	1	–	1 (IIIa)	–
Dissection of aneurysm	46	42	1	2	1 (IV)
Coagulation of aneurysm	18	16	1	1	–
Clipping of aneurysm	21	18	1	1	1 (IIb)
	90 (24%)	79	3	5	3

aneurysms ruptured before the craniotomy was completed. Nevertheless, 4 of these went on to full recoveries; the other died later of pulmonary embolism after making a good recovery. This implies that the surgeon should not abandon the procedure when early rupture occurs.

In the remaining 85 patients, the aneurysm ruptured at some point during the exposure and clipping of the aneurysm. 46 occurred while the aneurysm was being dissected free. Of these 42 (91%) had a good result, while 3 (7%) had a fair or poor outcome, and 1 (2%) died. 18 aneurysms bled during coagulation and of these, 16 (89%) had a good result, while the other 2 suffered fair or poor results. The other 21 ruptured while the aneurysm was being clipped. In this group 18 (86%) had a good result, 2 (10%) had fair or poor results, and 1 (4%) died. In general bleeding could be controlled by the application of a pledget or muscle (67 cases), or with temporary clips (27 cases), because the anatomical relationships had already been clarified by dissection. The percentage of good results is the same as for all patients undergoing operation. It appears that the rupture of an aneurysm at this location is not a significantly adverse factor.

Temporary clipping was used in 45 patients (12.0%) in various combinations. These are related to outcome in Table **91**. Results show no increased morbidity or mortality associated for anterior communicating artery aneurysms. A trapping procedure in which clips are applied permanently to both sides of the anterior communicating artery was used in 15 cases (inferiorly bulging aneurysms) early in the series (1967–1970). In these patients 8 (53.3%) had good, 1 (6.7%) poor results while 6 (40%) suffered a fatal outcome. For this reason and because of associated electrolyte imbalances that occurred in many of these patients (see Table **85**), this procedure is to be avoided if at all possible.

Table 91 Temporary clipping of aneurysm

	Total No.	Good	Fair	Poor	Death
One – A_1	27 left 16 right 11	24	1	1 (IIIa)	1 (IV)
Two – A_1	14	12	–	1 (IV)	1 (IIb)
Both – A_1					
One – A_2	3	3	–	–	–
Both – A_1 – A_2	1	1	–	–	–
	45 (12%)	40	1	2	2

Trapping – 15 cases: 8 good – 1 poor – 6 death
(4%)

Operative Complications

286 patients (76.3%) had a completely smooth postoperative course. The remainder suffered some type of peri-operative complication such as diabetes insipidus, gastro-intestinal bleeding, pulmonary embolus, hepatitis, steroid psychosis, epilepsy, etc. (Table **92**). 14 patients (3.7%) required reoperation for such things as intracranial hematoma, brain edema, rhinorrhea, and infectious processes.

42 patients with anterior communicating artery aneurysms made delayed good recoveries. 39 of these were thought to have had hydrocephalus, preoperative intracerebral hematoma, or preexisting cerebral infarction. Only 3 were directly related to operative problems.

In the 11 patients making fair recoveries, 5 could be considered as being made worse by the operation. 2 patients with mild hemiparesis preoperatively developed postoperative epidural hematomas resulting in a more severe deficit. 1 patient developed a memory deficit and hypothalamic disturbances after the anterior communicating artery and its hypothalamic branches were isolated from the circulation. 2 patients experienced regrowth and rupture of previously clipped aneurysms.

Of the 13 cases with poor results, 1 patient who was in grade IIb with paraparesis deteriorated 2 days after operation with increasing somnolence and a left hemiparesis. CT scan confirmed an area of infarction in the right frontal area. She showed delayed improvement. A second patient (IIIa) sustained rerupture of his aneurysm during the opening of the dura. He remains in poor condition. The other 11 patients remain in poor condition on the basis of deficits existing preoperatively.

In the final group of 23 patients who died, 9 were admitted in grades IV or V and succumbed. 4 patients were making satisfactory recoveries and died of pulmonary embolism. 1 patient fell from bed in the postoperative period and sustained a fatal head injury. Death in the other 9 patients can be related to operative complications. In 4 patients, a new aneurysm arose from the area of clipping and reruptured with a fatal outcome. 2 patients developed bacterial meningitis and died 7 and 12 days postop. respectively. 1 patient treated with a trapping technique developed cerebral infarction and died 20 months after operation. Another patient developed a subdural hematoma postoperatively which was evacuated but he remained in poor condition and died 5 months later.

Table **92** Complications in 89 cases

Ia	2 cases	
IIa	19 cases	
IIb	13 cases	
IIIa	9 cases	
IIIb	18 cases	
IV	28 cases	
Hematomas:		
epidural	2	(1)
subdural	3	
intracerebral (intraventr.)	2	
Rerupture	7	(1)
Wound infection (soft tissue)	3	
Osteomyelitis	2	
Epidural empyema	1	
Bacterial meningitis	2	
Aseptic meningitis	1	
Rhinorrhea	2	
CSF collection (subgaleal)	13	
Hydrocephalus	46	
Hemiparesis:		
transient	11	
delayed	6	
permanent		
partial	4	
full	5	
Aphasia:		
transient	13	
delayed	1	
permanent	–	
POS:		
transient (1–3 d)	61	
delayed (4d–4w)	9	
permanent	5	
Steroid psychosis	2	
Hypothalamic disorder:		
transient	27	
permanent	4	
Epilepsy:	8	
transient	–	
permanent		
Gastro-intestinal bleeding	8	(3 gastric resection 4 conservative treatment 1 died)
Pulmonary emboli:		
mild	34	
severe	12	
total	5	
Hepatitis	2	

The final patient had damage to the hypothalamic arteries and died of gastrointestinal hemorrhage, hyperglycemia, and pulmonary embolism.

Thus of 375 patients undergoing operation, the operation itself was a factor in the outcome of 3 of 42 patients (7.1%) with delayed good result, 5 of 11 patients with fair result (45.5%), 2 of 13 patients who died (39.1%). Overall, operative factors contributed to the morbidity and mortality in 19 of the 375 patients (5.1%).

Medical Problems

Pulmonary embolism was the most common major medical complication occurring in 17 patients (4.5%). 4 of these were making good recoveries and suddenly died from pulmonary embolism between 1 and 4 weeks postoperatively. 13 patients with pulmonary emboli survived. No correlation between sex, age, grade, hypertension, fluid balance, or anesthesia could be found, but the 4 patients in good condition who died of pulmonary embolism had been on bed rest or reduced activity, 19 days, 3 weeks, 4 weeks, and 10 weeks respectively. Perhaps this prolonged period of bedrest contributed to their pulmonary embolism. Pulmonary embolism thus accounted for 4 of the 23 deaths (17.4%).

Gastrointestinal hemorrhage occurred in 8 patients. 3 were treated with a nasogastric tube and 4 with antacids and anticholinergic medications only. All 7 of these patients recovered. 1 patient had uncontrolled gastrointestinal bleeding, and was taken to theatre but died at laparatomy. Other medical problems included hepatitis in 2 patients, steroid psychosis in 2 patients, and thrombophlebitis.

Summary

In the present series, 375 patients underwent operation for aneurysm of the anterior communicating artery. There were multiple aneurysms present in 12 per cent of cases resulting in 421 aneurysms being clipped and an additional 15 covered with muscle. The successful operation of these aneurysms demands a thorough knowledge of the relationships of the aneurysm to the cisternal anatomy and to neighboring arteries and veins. These anatomical relationships are complex and many anomalies and variations have been described. Important factors include the exact location of the aneurysm, the projection and complexity of the fundus, the relationship of the 14 arteries or groups of arteries around the anterior cerebral-anterior communicating artery junction and the aneurysm, and the anomalies of the A_1 segment, anterior communicating artery and A_2 segments of the anterior cerebral arteries.

Operation is performed through a pterional craniotomy with removal of bone from the base of the skull and dissection through the subarachnoid cisterns. A general guide to the operation has been given with the qualification that each operation must to some degree be tailored to a particular set of circumstances.

Clinical findings and operative results are presented in detail. All but 4 patients sustained subarachnoid hemorrhage. Presenting symptoms reflect the central location of the anterior communicating artery and the complex area of distribution of the anterior cerebral arteries. Hematoma, cerebral ischemia, and hydrocephalus contribute to the presenting neurological deficits.

Overall, 328 patients had a good result (87.5%). In 286 (76.3%) the postoperative course was entirely smooth and the patients were home in less than 4 weeks. In another 42, more time for recovery, ventricular shunting, or other procedures were required before the patient could return to normal life. In 39 of these cases, delay was a result of inherent pathological processes, while in 3 operation played a part in slowing recovery.

11 patients (2.9%) had fair results, 6 on the basis of preexisting deficits, 1 from hypothalamic injury following a trapping procedure, 2 from postoperative intracranial hematomas and 2 from recurrent hemorrhage from the clipped aneurysm. 13 patients (3.5%) had a poor outcome. In 11 of these preoperative deficits decided the outcome. In 1 case the aneurysm ruptured during craniotomy. The patient was salvaged, but later developed a shunt infection and remains in poor condition. The other patient developed cerebral ischemia postoperatively. Thus of a total morbidity of 24 patients (6.4%), there were 7 (7.9%) in whom operation was in part responsible.

Of the 23 deaths, 9 patients were moribund at the time of operation. Another 4 died of pulmonary embolism in the postoperative period. 1 patient fell from bed and suffered a brain contusion. Of the remaining 9 patients, 4 experienced rerupture of a previously clipped aneurysm, 1 suffered hypothalamic damage at operation, 1 developed cerebral infarction postoperatively, 1 developed a

4 Anterior Cerebral and Anterior Communicating Artery Aneurysms

Table 93 Clinical details and causes of death in 23 fatal cases of anterior communicating artery aneurysm

Patient	Age	Sex	Year	SAH	Time	Grade			Hematomas			Site	Operation	Shunt	Follow-up	Cause of death	Survival time
								cist.	SDH	icH	ivH						
E.	63	M	1972	2/1w	4 w	IIb	POS, mild R. hpr.	–	–	–	–	L. mixed	Clip	–	Full recovery	Pulmonary emboli at home	4 w
M.	57	F	1973	1	10d	IIa	POS, hydroceph.	+	–	–	–	L. sup.	Clip	Postop.	Improvement	Pulmonary emboli	3 w
N.	41	M	1975	2/1y	19 d	IIa	–	+	–	+	–	L. post.	Clip	–	Good	Pulmonary emboli	2 w
G.	50	M	1975	1	3 w	IIa	Rupture in anesthesia before begin. of operation	++	–	–	–	L. post.	Clip	–	Fair	Pulmonary emboli	1 w
M.	36	M	1969	2/2w	2 w	IIIa	Somnolence, POS	+	–	–	–	L. inf.	Clip	–	Recovery, good	Rerupture 2m later Angiography negative	6 w
Sch.	43	M	1973	3/5w	10 d	IIIa	Somnolence, POS	+	–	–	–	L. mixed	Clip	–	Recovery, good	Rerupture twice 3w/6w later at home hospital	2 d
P.	44	F	1974	1	9 d	IIIa	Somnolence, POS	+	–	–	–	R. inf.	Clip	–	Recovery, good	Rerupture 8w later, Coma, Reoperation	1 d
H.	47	F	1975	3/3m	7 d	IIIa	Somnolence, POS	+	–	–	–	R. inf.	Clip	–	Recovery, good	Rerupture 3w later, Coma, Angiography negative	10 d
C.	59	F	1967	1	9 d	IIb	POS, mild hpr.	+	–	+	–	M. post.	Trapping	+	Apallic, poor	Ischemia	20 m
K.	53	F	1967	1	3 w	IIIb	R. hpr. since 5 y	+	+	+	–	M. inf.	Trapping	–	Fair	Meningitis	12 d
Sp.	44	M	1968	2/2w	2 w	IIIb	Somnolence, hpr., epilepsy, POS	+	–	+	–	M. post.	Trapping	–	Fair	Meningitis	7 d
Q.	54	M	1968	1	2 w	IIIa	Somnolence, POS	+	–	+	–	L. mixed	Trapping	–	Fair, rexpl. subdural	Apallic	5 m
Sch	52	M	1975	1	10 d	IIa	–	–	–	–	–	M. mixed 3 A$_2$	Clip	–	Poor	Gastrointestinal bleeding	5 d
P.	61	M	1975	unrup.	–	0b	Chiasm syndr. POS	–	–	–	–	R. ant.	Clip.	+ because of Liquid coll. under skin	Good	Accident	11

subdural hematoma, and 2 died of infection. This gives an operative mortality of 9/375 (2.4%) and a gross mortality of 23/375 (6.1%). Patients experiencing morbidity and mortality are summarized in Tables **93** and **94**.

A microsurgical approach to aneurysms of the anterior communicating artery has provided a method for safe and complete exclusion of the aneurysm from the circulation, with accurate dissection and minimal brain retraction. With a firm grasp of the detailed microanatomy in this area, vast experience should not be required to obtain a favorable result. However, laboratory experience in microsurgical techniques is required to effectively use these operative methods.

Table **94** Mortality

Patient	Age	Sex	Year	SAH	Time	Grade		cist.	Hematomas SDH	icH	ivH	Site	Operation	Shunt	Follow-up	Death cause	Survival time
W.	60	F	1968	1	4 w	IV	Apallic, tetrasp. tracheotomy	+	–	+	–	L. post.	Trapping	Preop.	Unchanged	Pneumonia	7 m
L.	70	M	1968	2/17y	2 d	IV	Apallic, tetrasp.	+	+	+	–	L. inf.	Trapping	–	Unchanged	Occlusion of femor. A.	6 w
F.	60	M	1969	1	2 w	IV	Apallic, R. hpl.	+	–	+	–	L. mixed	Trapping	–	Unchanged	Pulmonary emboli	64
R.	58	M	1970	1	1 d	IV	Apallic, tetrasp.	+	–	+	–	L. post.	Clip	Postop.	Apallic	Chron. unrin. inf.	1 y
V.	42	F	1972	1	3 w	IV	Apallic, tetrasp.	–	–	–	–	L. post.	Clip	Preop.	Apallic		6 m
St.	64	F	1975	2/11d	1 d	IV	Apallic, R. hpl.	+	–	–	–	R. post.	Clip	Postop.	Unchanged	Pneumonia	3 m
H.	47	M	1976	3/3m	6 d	IV	Apallic	+	–	+	+	R. inf.	Clip	Postop.	Unchanged	Bleeding ulcer	3 m
Sch.	31	M	1974	1	2 d	IV	Apallic, hpl. (Angiography in another hospital 2 hours after SAH thereafter Impairment.)	+	–	+	–	L. mixed	Clip	–	Unchanged	–	5 m
G.	51	M	1977	2/2w	10 d	V	Coma, tetrapl.	+	–	larg. call.	+	L. mixed	Clip	–	Unchanged	–	1 d

Distal Anterior Cerebral Artery Aneurysms (pericallosal artery aneurysms)

Anatomical Relationships

23 patients presented with ruptured aneurysms of the anterior cerebral artery distal to the anterior communicating artery and superior to the corpus callosum; therefore the term used is pericallosal aneurysm. 1 of these cases was a mycotic aneurysm. These represent 5.6 per cent of all aneurysms on the anterior cerebral – anterior communicating artery complex, and 2.3 per cent of all aneurysms in the series. In an additional 7 cases, there were incidental distal anterior cerebral artery aneurysms associated with ruptured aneurysms at other locations.

In 13 cases the ruptured aneurysm was on the left side and in 10 cases on the right. In 16 cases the aneurysm arose at the origin of the callosomarginal artery (CMA) and in 6 cases at the origin of the frontopolar artery (FPA). One of these arose from a point of quadrification of an enlarged single A_2 segment (see Vol. I, Fig **98**), and 1 case at the origin of the frontoorbital artery (Fig **111A–C**).

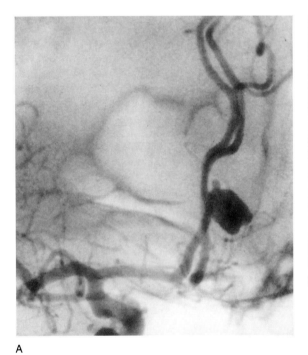

A

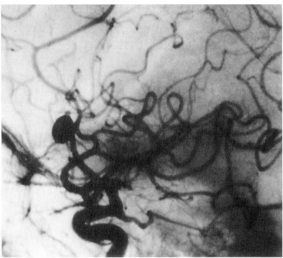

B

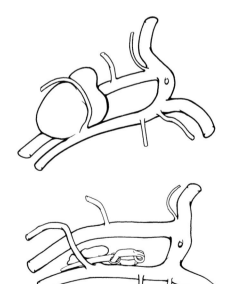

C

Fig **111A–C** Unusual case of a proximal A_2 aneurysm (**A** and **B**) that was clipped through a pterional approach (**C**).

Multiple aneurysms were present in 12 patients (52.2%). In 10 cases there was a small aneurysm in a mirror position on the contralateral distal anterior cerebral artery. 7 of these 10 aneurysms were not large enough to clip, but they were coagulated and covered with muscle. The other 3 larger aneurysms were clipped. Other additional aneurysms included an anterior communicating artery aneurysm, which was clipped and one middle cerebral and one basilar bifurcation aneurysm that were each also clipped during a combined frontal-paramedian and pterional craniotomy. Thus in the 23 patients with distal and anterior cerebral artery aneurysms there were a total of 36 aneurysms, 29 of which were clipped and 7 (micro) of which were merely coagulated and covered with muscle (Table **95**).

The pericallosal aneurysms present very special difficulties for the surgeon.

1) The interhemispheric fissure and the callosal cistern are very narrow. A lumbar drain is useful in gaining additional working space.
2) The depth of the falx may be short and, therefore, both cingulate gyri may be densely adherent.
3) Aneurysms at this location are commonly broad-based and frequently sclerotic. They involve the origins of the branching arteries to a varying degree.
4) Sclerosis of both the fundus of the aneurysm and of the opposite pericallosal artery may occur at a site of attachment between the two and this can lead to considerable difficulty in dissection.
5) At times it will be quite difficult to tell from which anterior cerebral artery the aneurysm is arising. Angiography may not be helpful in clarifying this.
6) The dome of the aneurysm may be densely fixed on the pia layer of the cingulate gyrus, or it may even be within the gyrus. Therefore, retraction of the frontal lobe should be careful and minimal.
7) The aneurysms may be located at the bifurcation of an azygos A_2.

Hematomas were present in 14 of the 23 patients (60.9%): in 1 case an interhemispheric subdural hematoma, in 6 cases a small intracerebral hematoma in the adjacent cingulate gyrus, and in 7 cases large hematomas in the corpus callosum and frontal lobe. 4 of the latter 7 cases had associated intraventricular hematomas. The tight confines of the corpus callosum cistern make hematomas more likely with aneurysms at this location. The side of the hematoma is not dependent on which pericallosal artery gives rise to the aneurysm as the fundus may be directed either medially or laterally.

Table 95 Multiplicity and bilaterality in 23 patients with ruptured distal anterior cerebral artery aneurysms

Side	Size	Ipsilat. Pericall.	Contralat. Pericall.	ACA	MCA	Bas.	Total
Left	Micro	–	5	–	–	–	5
	Macro	7	2	1	–	–	10
Right	Micro	–	2	–	–	–	2
	Macro	4	1	–	1	1	7
		11	10	1	1	1	24

		Total	
Single aneurysm	11 patients	11	
1 additional aneurysm	11	22	(6 micro)
2 additional aneurysms	1	3	(1 micro)
	23	36	(29 clipped, 7 coagulated)

Operative Technique

Initial Approach

The pterional approach was used in one patient with an aneurysm at the origin of the frontoorbital artery. In 19 cases a right paramedian frontal craniotomy was used to allow an interhemispheric approach to the aneurysm (Figs **112A–C, 113**, see also Vol. I, Fig **200A–D**). In cases where additional aneurysms were present, a combination of the usual smaller pterional craniotomy and the frontal paramedian craniotomy was used (3 cases) (Figs **114A–B, 115** and **163**). This approach provides good access to distal anterior cerebral aneurysms and associated internal carotid, middle cerebral or basilar bifurcation aneurysms. In the case of left sided additional aneurysms, the craniotomy is made on the left side.

A troublesome problem in the interhemispheric approach is that of ascending veins which often restrict the working area along the falx even though an exposure width of only 20 mm is sufficient. In cases where it is not possible to work between the veins, an attempt should be made to preserve the larger veins.

As the fundus of the aneurysm is usually buried in one or both cingulate gyri, it is very important to limit lateral retraction of the right hemisphere to a few millimeters, so as not to avulse the fundus away from the parent artery.

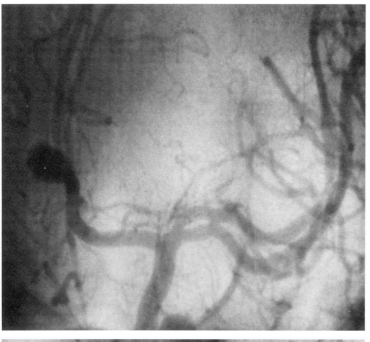
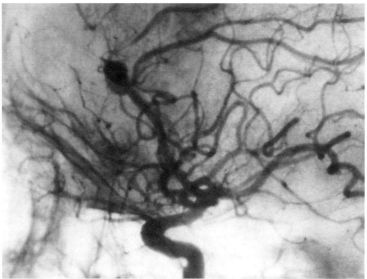
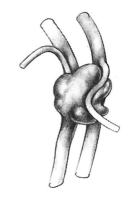
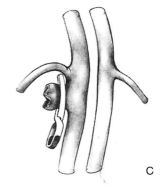

Fig **112A–C** Pericallosal aneurysm arising at the knee of the pericallosal artery. Notice the left accessory middle cerebral artery.

Operative Technique

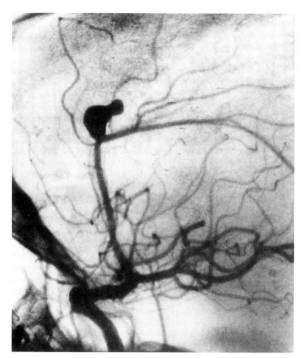

Fig 113 Supero-posteriorly directed aneurysm was found postero-inferior at operation.

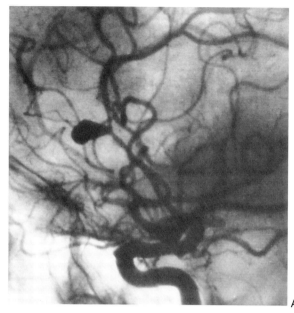

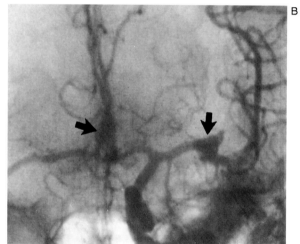

Fig 114A–B Anteriorly directed pericallosal aneurysm with perifocal spasm (**A**) and an incidental left middle cerebral bifurcation aneurysm (arrows) (**B**). At operation the superiorly directed pericallosal and middle cerebral aneurysms were clipped using a single left frontal paramedian and pterional approach.

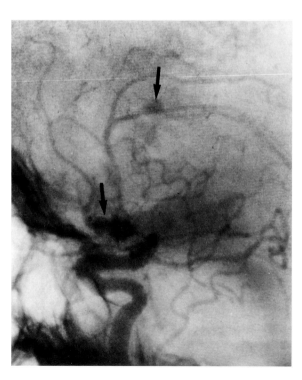

Fig 115 Ruptured pericallosal aneurysm and an unruptured anterior communicating aneurysm (arrows) which were both clipped using the same frontal paramedian approach.

Removal of Hematoma

Hematoma should be removed early in dissection to provide additional working room. If the hematoma has penetrated the ventricle, its removal will allow the ventricle to collapse and further decompress the brain. Hematoma immediately around the aneurysm, however, should be left until proximal and distal control of the parent arteries has been gained.

Identification of Parent Arteries

The depth of the falx will vary and cannot be used as a guide to identification of the corpus callosum cistern. When the falx is shallow, exposure may be more difficult as the adjacent gyri on each hemisphere tend to adhere by their pial surfaces.

Ideally, proximal control should be gained first, but in cases of distal anterior cerebral artery aneurysm this has usually not been possible. Exposing the aneurysm between the cerebral hemispheres generally brings the surgeon to the parent arteries distal to the aneurysm. Some confusion may be encountered distinguishing the pericallosal arteries from the frontopolar, callosomarginal or even more superficial arteries, as these arteries are paired and variable in size. The cingulate gyri may be very adherent and be mistaken for the corpus callosum. Identification of the pericallosal arteries depends upon the recognition of the corpus callosum cistern with its transversely running, parallel, white fibers.

By following a cortical artery proximally, one has good method for finding the pericallosal artery. With identification of the pericallosal arteries, dissection is continued within the corpus callosum cistern until the aneurysm is approached. Attention should then be directed to the proximal side of the aneurysm and both pericallosal arteries exposed to provide proximal control with temporary clips should premature rupture occur.

As the fundus of the aneurysm is usually extended to the right or left side and fixed to the cingulate gyrus, the exploration of the A_2 segments proximal to the aneurysm can be accomplished either by passing along the opposite cingulate gyrus or by dissecting the arachnoid and pia around the dome of the aneurysm and mobilizing it.

Aneurysm Dissection

With proximal and distal control of the arteries assured, the surgeon may begin dissection of the neck of the aneurysm. In situations where the aneurysm is covered by the cingulate gyrus, it may be helpful to perform a small subpial resection of the gyrus to expose the aneurysm fundus. Each pericallosal artery and each frontopolar or callosomarginal artery, as the case may be, must be separated from the neck of the aneurysm prior to the application of a clip. Sclerosis of the neck of the aneurysm and encroachment of the lumen of the aneurysm on the lumen of the arterial branches cause difficulty in adequately defining the neck of the lesion.

Aneurysm Clipping

As with aneurysms at other locations, the aneurysm is best clipped by a technique of successive bipolar coagulation followed by application of a clip, further coagulation as necessary, and reapplication of the clip, until satisfactory clip placement has been achieved. Because these lesions are often broad based and sclerotic, it may be advisable to use temporary clips, open the aneurysm to remove the atheromatous contents, coagulate, and then apply a permanent clip. Liberal use of papaverine to the anterior cerebral arteries is indicated throughout the procedure as these small arteries are especially vulnerable to spasm.

Fundus Resection

Following clipping, the fundus is resected, further bipolar coagulation performed as necessary, and adequate clip placement ascertained. All hematoma should be removed from the corpus callosum cistern and the arteries freed from any restraining attachments that might kink or distort them with release of retraction. With good hemostasis the wound is closed.

Summary

In summary, the steps in the treatment of a distal anterior cerebral artery aneurysm include:
1) Right paramedian frontal craniotomy. Left or right pterional and paramedian craniotomy, if additional aneurysms are to be clipped.
2) Dural flap retracted medially without compromise of superior sagittal sinus.
3) Preservation of ascending veins when possible. Release of 20–30 cc cerebrospinal fluid through a lumbar drain.
4) No more than a few millimeters (5–10 mm) retraction of the mesial right frontal lobe.
5) Identification of the pericallosal arteries in the corpus callosum cistern, distal to aneurysm.
6) Removal of intracerebral and intraventricular hematoma if present.
7) Exposure of the parent arteries proximal to the aneurysm.

8) Dissection of the aneurysm neck and identification of all arteries.
9) Separation of the adhesions between two pericallosal arteries.
10) Clipping of aneurysm neck, fundus resection, coagulation and replacement of the clip.
11) Liberal use of papaverine.
12) Hemostasis and closure.

Clinical Presentation and Operative Results

There have been a few reports in the medical literature discussing distal anterior cerebral artery aneurysms.
Of the 23 cases of ruptured distal anterior cerebral artery aneurysm in the present series, 15 patients were men (65.2%) and 8 women (34.8%). Ages ranged from 24 to 60 with a median age of 42 (Table 96). 2 cases described earlier (Cases 8 and 10, Yaşargil and Carter 1974) had incidental pericallosal artery aneurysms associated with ruptured aneurysms of the internal carotid-posterior communicating artery and middle cerebral artery respectively. These have not been included in this group, but rather in the appropriate symptomatic group of aneurysm patients. Another 7 patients also had unruptured distal anterior cerebral artery aneurysms associated with ruptured aneurysms at other locations (2 on PcoA, 2 on MCA and 3 on AcoA) and these aneurysms were clipped at the same operation.
All patients presented with subarachnoid hemorrhage and each patient had suffered only 1 hemorrhage. 6 patients had hemipareses and in 4 of these, the hemiparesis was ipsilateral to the anterior cerebral artery bearing the aneurysm. Presenting features are summarized in Table **99**.

Timing and Results

Operative results in relation to preoperative grade and timing of operation is given in Tables **97** and **98**. Of the 23 patients, 20 (87%) have made a good recovery. This includes all patients undergoing operation in grades Ia to IIIa. One patient in fair condition was a 44 year old man who ruptured a mycotic aneurysm and underwent operation in grade IV. 2 patients have had poor results, both presented in grade IIIb. One patient with a large intracerebral hematoma extending into the ventricle failed to improve after operation, required a shunt and is left with a seizure disorder. The other patient sustained occlusion of the pericallosal artery by atheromatous plaque fracture from the arterial wall by the clip. Reoperation restored patency to the artery, but he remained in poor condition.

Table **96** Sex and age in 23 patients with ruptured distal anterior cerebral artery aneurysms

Age	Total No.	%	Male	Female
0–20	0	–	–	–
21–30	3	13	2	1
31–40	3	13	–	3
41–50	10	43.5	8	2
51–60	7	30.4	5	2
	23	100	15 (65.2%)	8 (34.8%)

Table **97** Pericallosal aneurysm patients, grade and outcome

Grade	Total No.	Good	Fair	Poor	Death
Ia	5	5	–	–	–
IIa	6	6	–	–	–
IIb	2	2	–	–	–
IIIa	5	5	–	–	–
IIIb	4	2	–	2	–
IV	1	–	1	–	–
	23	20	1	2	0

Table 98 Timing of surgery and results in 23 patients with ruptured aneurysm of the pericallosal artery

	Ia	Good IIa	IIb	IIIa	IIIb	Fair IV	Poor IIIb
1–3 d	–	1	–	–	–	1	–
4–7 d	–	–	–	1	–	–	–
1–2 w	1	3	–	2	–	–	1
2–4 w	1	2	1	2	2	–	1
1–3 m	2	–	1	–	–	–	–
> 3 m	1	–	–	–	–	–	–
	5	6	2	5	2	1	2 = 23

2 patients in grades IIa and IIIa underwent operation in the first week after hemorrhage with a good result. The patient with a mycotic aneurysm underwent operation 3 days after hemorrhage in grade IV with a fair result. The other 2 patients with poor results underwent operation in the second and third week respectively. Of the 7 cases with large intracerebral hematomas, 6 presented with focal neurological deficits (b category), as did the patient with an interhemispheric subdural hematoma. The 3 patients with less than good results all had large hematomas. One of these patients (No. 5) developed hydrocephalus and required shunting. Despite this treatment, however, he remained in a poor condition (Table **99**).

Clinical Presentation and Operative Results 231

Table 99 Patients with distal anterior cerebral artery aneurysms (Pericallosal artery)

	Age	Sex	Year	SAH	Site	Mult.	Spasm	Hematoma	Condition	Day	Operation	Remarks	Result
1. De	36	F	1967	1	L. CMA	–	–	Frontal	IIIa	2 w	Clip	–	Good
2. Ca	53	M	1968	1	L. CMA	–	+	Small	Ia	6 w	Clip	–	Good
3. Sp	29	F	1969	1	R. FPA	–	–	–	IIa	2 w	Clip	–	Good
4. An	60	F	1969	1	L. FPA	–	+	–	IIIa	3 w	Clip	–	Good
5. Fe	24	M	1971	1	R. CMA	–	++	Large, corp. call. ivH	IIIb	11 d	Clip	Prop. R. hpr., R. VI palsy. Postop. L. hpr., POS, Epi. shunt	Poor
6. Mu	40	F	1972	1	R. CMA	–	+	Large, corp. call. ivH	IIIa	7 d	Clip Microsuture	–	Good
7. Ba	44	M	1972	1	R. CMA bilat.	+	–	Large, corp. call.	IV	3 d	Clip	Mycotic	Fair
8. Eg	53	M	1972	1	L. CMA bilat.	+	–	Small	Ia	2 w	Clip	–	Good
9. We	50	F	1972	1	L. CMA	+	–	Large frontal, ivH	IIb	6 w	Clip	Sclerotic aneurysm	Good
10. Co	47	M	1973	1	L. CMA bilat. AcoA	–	–	Small	IIIa	3 w	Clip Clip	–	Good
11. Cu	51	M	1973	1	R. CMA	+	+	Large frontal	IIIb	3 w	Clip	Thrombosis of R. pericall. A. Reexplored. Artery repaired with microsuture. Postop. L. hpr.	Poor
12. Ka	43	M	1973	1	L. CMA	–	–	–	IIa	3 w	Clip	–	Good
13. St	38	F	1975	1	R. FPA	–	++	Large frontal, callosal, ivH	IIa	11 d	Clip	–	Good
14. Ra	43	M	1975	1	R. CMA bilat.	+	–	–	IIa	3 w	Clip	Sclerotic aneurysm	Good
15. Pe	47	M	1976	1	L. FPA bilat.	+	–	–	Ia	9 m	Clip Clip	–	Good
16. Gr	54	F	1976	1	R. CMA Babi	+	–	Small	IIIa	9 d	Clip Clip	–	Good
17. Fi	41	M	1976	1	L. CMA bilat.	+	+	Small	Ia	6 w	Clip Clip	Postop. hpr. aphasia. Reexpl. 11d-epid. hemat. Recovered	Good
18. La	43	F	1976	1	L. FPA	–	–	–	IIa	3 d	Clip	Postop. hpr., Recovered	Good
19. So	43	M	1976	1	L. CMA bilat.	–	–	–	IIIb	3 w	Clip	Sclerotic aneurysm	Good
20. Wi	53	M	1976	1	L. CMA bilat.	+	–	Small	Ia	3 w	Clip	–	Good
21. Du	29	M	1977	1	L. FPA L. MCA	+	–	ivH	IIIb	3 w	Clip Clip	–	Good
22. Sch	42	M	1978	1	L. CMA bilat.	+	–	Interh., SDH	IIb	3 w	Clip	–	Good
23. F	59	M	1979	1	R. F. orb.	–	–	–	IIa	2 w	Clip	–	Good

5 Vertebrobasilar Aneurysms

Background

The successful operative treatment of vertebrobasilar aneurysms has come about more slowly than has the treatment of aneurysms of the anterior circulation. The first case of a successfully treated vertebrobasilar aneurysm was desribed by Schwartz (1948), although Höök and associates (1963) report that a posterior fossa aneurysm was successfully treated by Professor Olivecrona in 1932. Scattered reports of treatment of these lesions appeared over the next several years with the general conclusion that some lower vertebrobasilar aneurysms might be successfully treated, but that upper basilar and basilar bifurcation aneurysms were beyond operative treatment. Drake (1961b) and Jamieson (1964) reported their experiences with these aneurysms, and indeed mortality and morbidity rates were discouraging. Sahs and associates (1969) reviewed the reported operative cases through 1968 and found that the overall mortality rate was 38 per cent, with a mortality of 52 per cent for basilar bifurcation aneurysms. By 1968, however, Drake was able to report improved results and in the last 10 years he has been able to achieve a 7 per cent mortality rate in 408 vertebrobasilar aneurysms (Drake 1978). Other recent series have also shown improved results in these aneurysm patients.

In the present series, 97 patients (9.6%) had aneurysms of the vertebrobasilar circulation. The location and frequency of these aneurysms are listed in Table 100. It is noted that over half of these aneurysms arose from the basilar artery bifurcation and 49 aneurysms were on the basilar artery or its branches. These aneurysms are included in quite extensive anatomical boundaries and for various aneurysms, a variety of operative approaches were used through frontotemporosphenoidal, temporal, occipital, suboccipital, and transclival craniotomies. Aneurysms at each location will be presented separately so that the anatomical, operative, and clinical problems of each aneurysm location can be discussed together. A short summary of vertebrobasilar artery aneurysms is found at the end of the chapter.

Table 100 Frequency and location of aneurysms on the vertebrobasilar circulation in the present series

Location	Number	%
Basilar artery bifurcation	50	51.5
Upper basilar artery trunk (P_1-Sup. cereb. A.)	5	5.2
Posterior cerebral artery (P_1 segment)	5	5.2
Posterior cerebral artery (P_1/P_2 junction)	3	3.1
Posterior cerebral artery (P_2 segment)	3	3.1
Posterior cerebral artery (P_3-segment)	3	3.1
Distal superior cerebellar artery	2	2.1
Basilar artery trunk (saccular)	3	3.1
Basilar artery trunk (fusiform)	5	5.2
Vertebral artery – PICA origin (saccular)	10	10.3
Distal posterior inferior cerebellar artery	5	5.2
Vertebral artery trunk (saccular)	2	2.1
Vertebral artery trunk (fusiform)	1	1.0
Total	97	100

Basilar Artery Bifurcation Aneurysms

Anatomical Relationships

Incidence and Multiplicity

Aneurysms arose from the bifurcation of the basilar artery in 50 patients (51.5% of vertebrobasilar aneurysms, 5.0% of the entire series). Additional aneurysms were present in 18 cases (36.0%). There were 13 additional aneurysms on the internal carotid artery (7 macro clipped, 6 micro wrapped) 10 on the middle cerebral artery (4 macro clipped), 8 on the anterior cerebral-anterior communicating artery complex (6 macro clipped), giving a total of 81 aneurysms in these 50 patients (Table 101a and b). Another 10 patients also had unruptured aneurysms of the basilar bifurcation associated with ruptured aneurysms at other locations (1 ophthalmic, 1 PcoA, 1 pericallosal, 3 MCA, 3 AcoA, 1 PICA) which were clipped at the same operation.

Projection of Fundus

With aneurysms of the basilar artery bifurcation (Fig 116A–C), the direction of the fundus is an important factor both with regard to the technical difficulty encountered at operation and to the ultimate prognosis. Three primary directions of fundus projection are recognized:

Anterior and Antero-Superior Projection

The aneurysm projected forward toward the dorsum sellae in 5 of the 50 cases (10.0%). This is the most favorable situation from the operative point of view. The aneurysm may be attached to the dorsum sellae, but it is directed away from the perforating arteries and lies relatively free in the anterior portion of the interpeduncular cistern.

Superior and Supero-Posterior Projection

Aneurysms projected superiorly toward the posterior diencephalon in 14 cases (28.0%). These aneurysms can indent the posterior hypothalamus and third ventricle, but perforating arteries tend to course away from the neck.

Postero-Inferior and Inferior Projection

Most troublesome and unfortunately most common (31 cases – 62%) are aneurysms which project posteroinferiorly into the interpeduncular fossa. These aneurysms are partially covered by the cerebral peduncles and are intimately attached to the paramedian and circumflex arteries (superior cerebellar artery branches) as well as to the posterior thalamoperforating and posterior medial choroidal arteries arising from the P_1 segment of the posterior cerebral artery. These aneurysms are enclosed in a tight space within the interpeduncular cistern and may reach giant proportions without rupture (Fig 117A–E).

Table 101a Sites of multiple aneurysms in combination with basilar bifurcation aneurysms

	OA	PcoA	AchoA	ICB	MCB	M_1	AcoA	Total	
Basilar bifurcation									
Micro	1r	2r	1l	1l	3r	3r	1	14	
		1l					1		31
Macro	1r	2r	1r	2r	3r	1l	2	17	
	1l						4		

Table 101b

	No. of aneurysms
Single aneurysm in 32 Patients	32
1 additional aneurysm in 10 patients	20
2 additional aneurysms in 5 patients	15
3 additional aneurysms in 1 patient	4
4 additional aneurysms in 2 patients	10
Total 50 patients	81

5 Vertebrobasilar Aneurysms

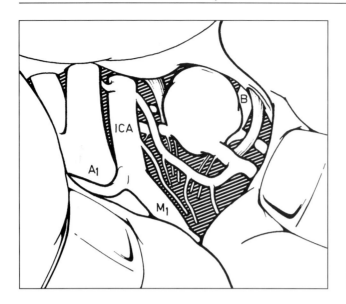

Fig 116A–C Schematic representation of basilar artery aneurysms and their relationship to the thalamoperforate arteries.

A Superoanteriorly projecting aneurysm at the basilar bifurcation. The thalamoperforators are free from the sac.

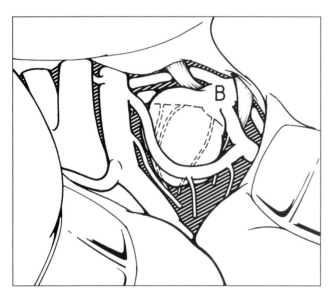

B Superoposteriorly directed aneurysm of the basilar bifurcation with the thalamoperforators hidden behind the sac. They may be closely adhering or relatively free from the sac.

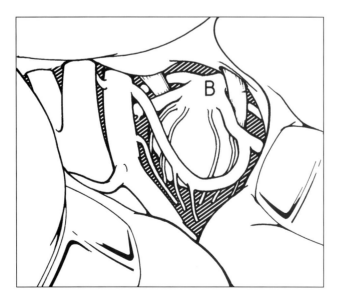

C Posteroinferiorly directed aneurysm of the basilar bifurcation with the thalamoperforators over the superolateral surface of the sac. These may be free from or very adherent to the sac.

Anatomical Relationships 235

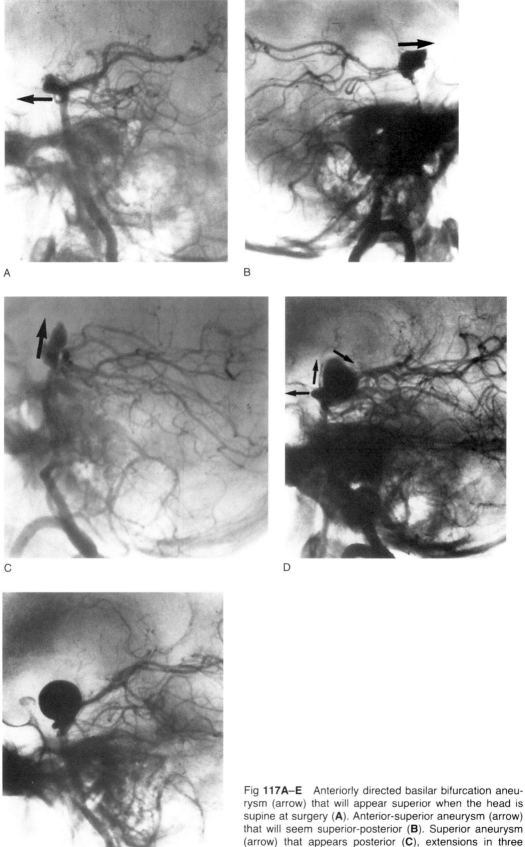

Fig 117A–E Anteriorly directed basilar bifurcation aneurysm (arrow) that will appear superior when the head is supine at surgery (**A**). Anterior-superior aneurysm (arrow) that will seem superior-posterior (**B**). Superior aneurysm (arrow) that appears posterior (**C**), extensions in three directions (arrows) (**D**) and a bulbous aneurysm that is similar in all planes (**E**).

While the above schematic outline serves as a guide to the basic anatomical relationships of a given aneurysm fundus, bilobularity, multiple loculations, "daughter aneurysms", and irregular shape are the rule rather than the exception with these aneurysms. Thus many aneurysms exhibit features of more than one of the above primary directions of fundus projection.

Size of Aneurysm

Aneurysms of the basilar artery bifurcation vary in size from small to truly giant lesions. In the present series, 9 aneurysms (18.0%) were small (less than 6 mm), 31 (62.0%) were medium sized (6–15 mm), 7 (14.0%) were large (15–25 mm) and 3 (6.0%) were giant aneurysms (larger than 25 mm). Larger lesions were most common with posteroinferiorly directed aneurysms (Table 102a). Thrombus and sclerosis were most evident in larger lesions, although some small to medium sized aneurysms showed marked sclerosis of the aneurysm wall as well as in the basilar and posterior cerebral arteries (Table 102b).

Relation to Posterior Communicating and Posterior Cerebral Arteries

The relative sizes of the posterior communicating arteries and the P_1 segments of the posterior cerebral arteries are important factors in making operative decisions and these should be carefully investigated by angiography and at operation. It is common with aneurysms of the basilar artery bifurcation that one or more of these arteries will be hypoplastic.

Relationship to the Dorsum Sellae

The relationship of the basilar artery apex to the sella turcica is also of importance in exposure of the neck of an aneurysm at this location. In 2 cases, there was an endostosis of the posterior clinoid process and it was not possible to see the upper basilar artery until the posterior clinoid process had been removed with a high speed drill (Fig 118).

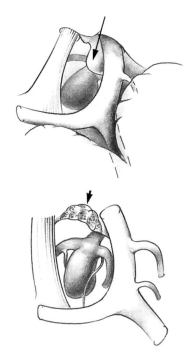

Fig 118 In cases of endostosis of the posterior clinoid process the approach to the basilar bifurcation will be hindered. The endostosis can, if necessary, be drilled off.

Table 102a Size of basilar artery bifurcation aneurysms related to direction of fundus projection

Fundus projection	Total	(%)	Small	Medium	Large	Giant
Antero-superior	5	10.0	3	2	–	–
Supero-posterior	14	28.0	4	9	1	–
Postero-inferior	31	62.0	2	20	6	3
Total	50	100.0	9	31	7	3
			18.0%	62.0%	14.0%	6.0%

Table 102b Success of aneurysm clipping related to aneurysm size

Aneurysm size	Number of cases	Number clipped	(%)
Small	9	9	100.0%
Medium	31	26	83.9%
Large	7	4	57.1%
Giant	3	1	33.3%
	50	40	80.0%

Operative Technique

Initial Approach

In the present series, the first 9 patients were treated by a subtemporal approach to the aneurysm as described by Drake (1961), Jamieson (1964) and others. Technical disadvantages to the subtemporal approach were recognized however in these 9 cases. In only 4 of the 9 cases could the aneurysm be clipped because the perforating arteries from the basilar trunk and from the P_1 segment opposite the craniotomy could not be adequately visualized or could not be separated from the wall. It has since been noted that on occasions, the thalamoperforating arteries may arise as a single trunk from one P_1 segment to supply both sides (see Figs **121, 122**). If this is from the side opposite the craniotomy, the entire posterior thalamic supply is jeopardized. In addition, retraction of the temporal lobe applies torque to the brain stem and the oculomotor nerve is often injured.

In many of the microsurgical procedures performed through a pterional craniotomy such as anterior circulation aneurysms and parasellar tumors, the proximity of the basilar artery bifurcation to the internal carotid artery and optic nerve had been noted. The area was often exposed when Liliequist's membrane was opened to allow release of cerebrospinal fluid from the interpeduncular cistern. Because the origins of both P_1 segments and their associated perforating and choroidal arteries were well visualized by this approach, it was reasoned that a pterional craniotomy might provide a more satisfactory anatomical exposure in cases of basilar artery bifurcation aneurysm. This method has been found satisfactory in most cases (Yaşargil et al. 1976). Nevertheless, the working area is confining and considerable experience with microsurgical techniques is necessary to fully utilize this approach to basilar artery aneurysms. The subtemporal approach to basilar apex aneurysm has been discussed in detail by Drake, and will not be repeated here (see Fig **119A–D**).

Pterional craniotomy requires modification to approach an aneurysm on the upper basilar artery or P_1 segments. It is important that the temporalis muscle be elevated from the zygomatic process of the frontal bone far enough inferiorly to allow adequate retraction of the muscle. The muscle should be released at least to the marginal tubercle just above the frontozygomatic suture. Additionally, more bone should be removed from the temporal squama than is the case for anterior circulation aneurysms. This will provide a little mobility for the temporal lobe should it be necessary to retract this laterally to come down along the tentorial edge in dissection.

The Sylvian cistern is opened on the frontal lobe side of the superficial cerebral veins and dissection carried across the confluence of cisterns above the internal carotid artery bifurcation to separate the frontal and temporal lobes and allow gentle retraction to be applied to the laterobasal frontal lobe. This will expose the carotid and chiasmatic cisterns.

Entering the Interpeduncular Cistern

After operating the Sylvian, lamina terminalis carotid and chiasmatic cisterns to allow release of cerebrospinal fluid, the surgeon must decide the direction of dissection he is to follow on the basis of the relationship of the optic nerve, internal carotid artery, oculomotor nerve and tentorial edge. Three possibilities for approach to the basilar bifurcation exist:

1) *At least 5 mm exists between the optic nerve and the internal carotid artery.* In especially favorable cases, the internal carotid artery will bow laterally to create a semicircular working area. In these cases Liliequist's membrane is opened into the interpeduncular cistern between the optic nerve and the internal carotid artery. The posterior communicating artery will be lateral to the dissection as it curves toward the posterior cerebral artery (Fig **119A**).

2) *The optic nerve and internal carotid artery are closely approximated.* In this case, the interpeduncular cistern is entered lateral to the internal carotid artery and medial to the oculomotor nerve. Dissection will be carried out circumferential to the posterior communicating artery as this artery is followed toward the posterior cerebral artery (Fig **119B**).

3) *The optic nerve and internal carotid artery are closely approximated and little space exists between the internal carotid artery and tentorial edge.* This is the most unfavorable circumstance in dissection. Dissection again must be performed lateral to the carotid artery, but additional space must be made. With the temporal pole retracted laterally and posteriorly, the tentorial edge is excised and the edges sutured to the dura over the greater wing of the sphenoid. Care must be taken not to injure cranial nerves III and IV (Fig **119C–D**).

Fig **119A–D** Schematic illustration of the basilar bifurcation by pterional approach.
A Standard pterional approach to the upper basilar artery through the carotid cistern medial to the carotid artery if the artery courses laterally.
B If the internal carotid artery courses medially, then the approach will be lateral to the carotid artery.

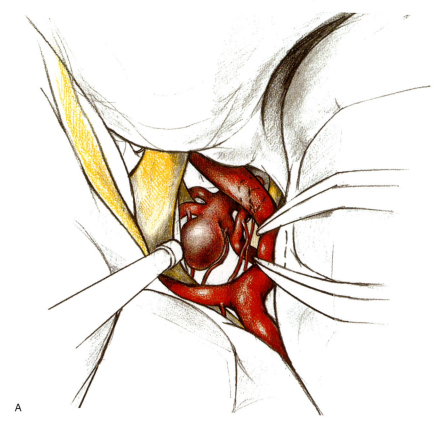

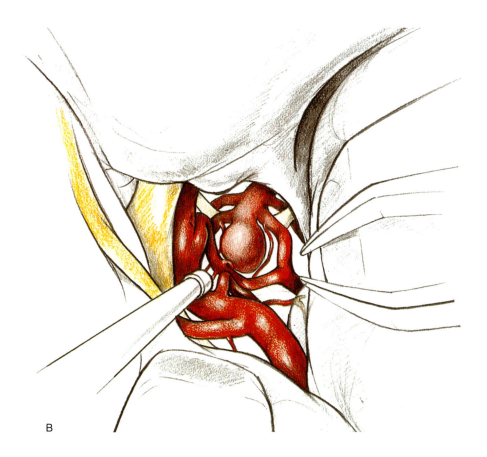

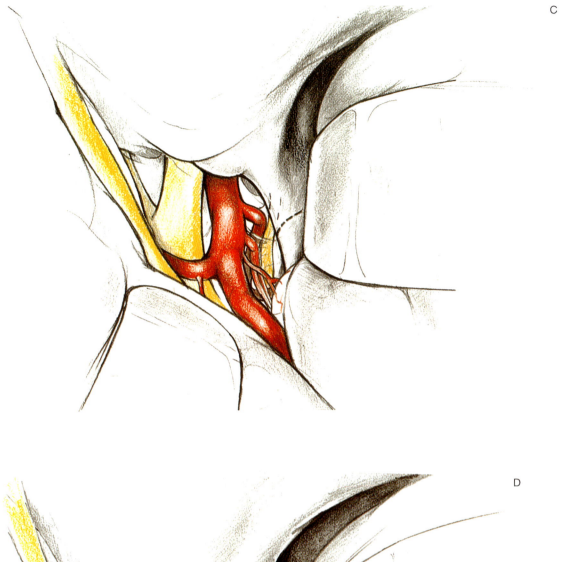

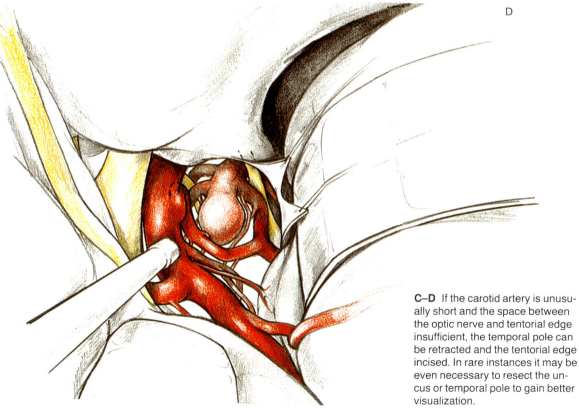

C–D If the carotid artery is unusually short and the space between the optic nerve and tentorial edge insufficient, the temporal pole can be retracted and the tentorial edge incised. In rare instances it may be even necessary to resect the uncus or temporal pole to gain better visualization.

Frequently, a combination of these maneuvers is required to adequately delineate the aneurysm and basilar artery bifurcation area. The small arteries running to the optic chiasm and pituitary stalk from the internal carotid artery can usually be mobilized and pushed out of the way, so these arteries should not be needlessly sacrificed. Veins running from the orbitofrontal and temporal lobes to the cavernous and sphenoparietal sinuses may also be in the way of dissection. At times they can be mobilized from the pia and nudged out of the way, but often small veins must be coagulated and divided. Finally, because there is unavoidable manipulation of the internal carotid artery, middle cerebral artery, A_1, posterior communicating artery and the anterior choroidal artery during dissection, possibly resulting in mechanically induced spasm, it is advisable to apply papaverine to the artery and remove some of the sympathetic plexus before entering the interpeduncular cistern.

Dissection of the Posterior Communicating Arteries

After the interpeduncular cistern is opened, the posterior communicating artery is followed posteriorly and the origins of the anterior thalamoperforating arteries noted. The opposite posterior communicating artery is also visualized from this angle, although with large aneurysms pointing superiorly, the more distal portion of the opposite posterior communicating artery may be hidden behind the fundus. This portion of the artery is often laterally displaced by the fundus of the aneurysm and it or its associated perforating arteries may be adherent to the aneurysm wall. The contralateral posterior communicating artery can be explored and checked through the prechiasmatic space (over or under the ipsilateral optic nerve and superior to the pituitary stalk).

Dissection of the Posterior Cerebral Arteries

The posterior cerebral arteries will be seen *en face* from a pterional approach. The arteries should be identified proximally at their junction with the posterior communicating arteries and the origins of the posterior medial choroidal and posterior thalamoperforating arteries noted during this dissection. The surgeon should be considering the various possible locations for temporary clip placement or even sacrifice of the P_1 segments. If possible, an area on the basilar artery proximal to the aneurysm should also be dissected for provisional temporary clip placement, although the bulk of the aneurysm fundus may make this impossible.

Dividing the Circle of Willis

On occasions, especially with large aneurysms, it will be advisable to divide the circle of Willis at some point to provide more working space. There are three possibilities for opening the circle of Willis while still preserving flow to all areas (Fig **120**):

1) *Posterior communicating artery.* If the posterior communicating artery is hypoplastic and the P_1 segment is well developed, the posterior communicating artery may be divided (11 cases). The point of division will depend on the relationship of the artery to the aneurysm and on the location of the anterior thalamoperforating (diencephalic) arteries. This may mean dividing the posterior communicating artery near the internal carotid artery or more commonly near the posterior cerebral artery. In some instances, the artery is best divided in its mid-portion, letting some of the perforating arteries go with each stump. Before one sacrifices the posterior communicating artery, it should be recognized that the ipsilateral P_1 segment may be injured during dissection of the aneurysm neck. It is, therefore, prudent to postpone deliberate sacrifice of the posterior communicating artery for as long as possible.

2) *Posterior cerebral artery.* In the converse situation, where the P_1 segment is hypoplastic and the posterior communicating artery stout, division of the P_1 may be considered. This situation will most commonly arise when the aneurysm is eccentrically seated on the larger contralateral P_1 segment and the surgeon feels he should include the hypoplastic P_1 in the clip rather than attempt separation of the artery from the neck of the aneurysm. In this case, of course, the clip must sit proximal to the posterior medial choroidal artery and the perforators arising from the P_1 segment. There may be substantial arteries even when the P_1 segment itself is quite hypoplastic (1 case). The other possible indication for sacrificing the P_1 segment is when damage occurs to it during dissection. Depending on the degree of back bleeding and the relative sizes of the P_1 and posterior communicating artery, the surgeon must decide if he is willing to sacrifice the artery or whether he should attempt microvascular repair.

3) *Anterior cerebral artery.* Finally, in 1 case in the present series, the anterior cerebral artery was

Operative Technique 241

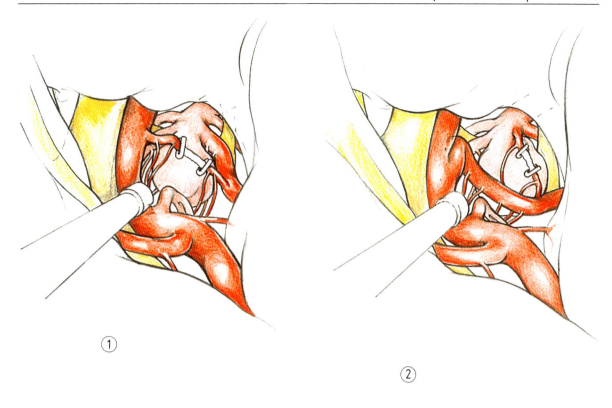

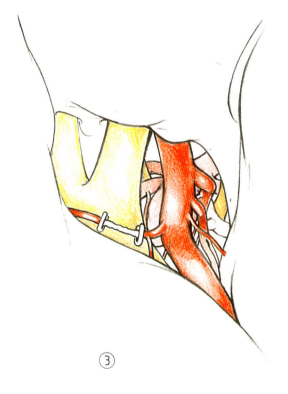

Fig 120 Dividing the circle of Willis in cases with large aneurysms in combination with hypoplastic segments such as
(1) Hypoplastic posterior communicating artery,
(2) Hypoplastic P_1 segment,
(3) Hypoplastic A_1 segment.

divided close to its origin from the internal carotid artery to allow better retraction of the internal carotid artery. In this case the A_1 segment was hypoplastic, the opposite A_1 and anterior communicating artery were well developed, and it was possible to leave the medial striate arteries with the anterior cerebral artery complex. No untoward reaction occurred following this maneuver.

Removal of the Posterior Clinoid Process

Occasionally, when the basilar bifurcation is low in relation to the dorsum sellae, the ipsilateral posterior clinoid process will partially hide the neck of the aneurysm and the opposite posterior cerebral artery (see Fig **118**). To complete the dissection, this process must be partially removed. The dura over the dorsum sellae is dissected with unipolar electrocoagulation applied to an insulated small blunt nerve hook. The posterior communicating artery is sometimes attached to the posterior clinoid process and this must be freed before coagulation is applied. The dura is incised and peeled back from the posterior clinoid process with a small periosteal elevator. The tip of the process is removed with a high speed electric drill with a diamond burr. The internal carotid artery should be protected with a small piece of sterile surgeon's rubber glove. Bleeding is controlled with electrocoagulation and bone wax.

Dissection of Aneurysm Neck

Depending on its origin and projection the neck of the aneurysm may be adherent to one or both posterior cerebral arteries, the posterior thalamoperforating or posterior medial choroidal branches of the P_1 segment, or the paramedian and circumflex branches of the superior, cerebellar and basilar arteries. Arteries do not originate from the fundus of the aneurysm and small branches must be followed to the area of the neck and the arachnoid separated to free them from the aneurysm. However, aneurysms in this location, especially those arising from the basilar artery bifurcation itself tend to balloon the adjacent sides of the P_1 segments and the upper basilar artery trunk to some degree. Furthermore, it is rare that a narrow, cylindrical neck is found. A second bulging is often present right at the interface of neck and parent artery. It is, therefore, often necessary to apply bipolar coagulation to portions of the neck to shrink and shape it so that a clip will seat properly. Often a lobule of the aneurysm must be coagulated before further separation of the P_1 segment or perforators from the aneurysm can be performed. If the opposite P_1 origin is hidden behind the aneurysm, it will be necessary to mobilize the fundus and gently depress or elevate it with the sucker tip over a small sponge until the origin of the artery and any perforating arteries can be visualized.

Clip Application

The clip will generally be introduced at an angle over the neck of the aneurysm between the two posterior cerebral arteries. As the clip is slowly closed, the surgeon observes the effect on the parent arteries. The clip blades must not include perforating arteries behind the aneurysm and must not twist or kink normal arteries. Most "tricks" described in Chapter 7, to occlude the aneurysm will at one time or another be employed in treatment of these upper basilar aneurysms. However, despite a variety of maneuvers, it is not infrequent that the aneurysm will still not accept a clip. 2 important causes are severe sclerosis and subtotal thrombosis of the aneurysm, and both of these entities prevent the clip from closing on the neck of the aneurysm. With large aneurysms of the anterior circulation, it is often possible to apply temporary clips, open the aneurysm, remove thrombus and plaque, and apply a clip. There has been an occasional case of basilar artery bifurcation aneurysm where clips could be applied to the basilar trunk below the aneurysm and to both P_1 segments to open the aneurysm. In general, however, this has not been technically feasible, and subtotal thrombosis and sclerosis remain a major obstacle to satisfactory operative treatment of these lesions (Figs **121A–C, 122A–D, 123A–C**).

Operative Technique 243

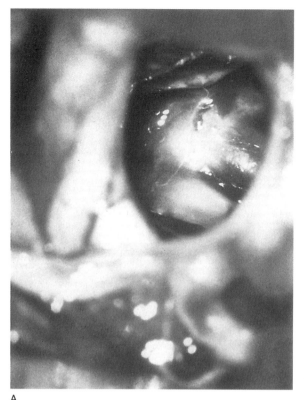

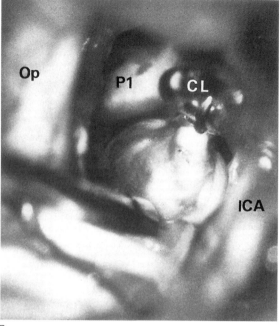

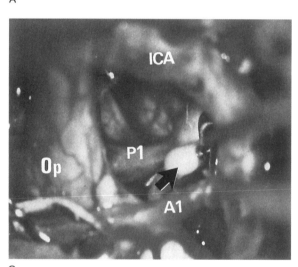

Fig **121A–C** Operative illustration of a basilar bifurcation aneurysm seen between (**A**) right internal carotid artery and right optic nerve before clipping, (**B**) after clip application, and (**C**) after coagulation (arrow).

244 5 Vertebrobasilar Aneurysms

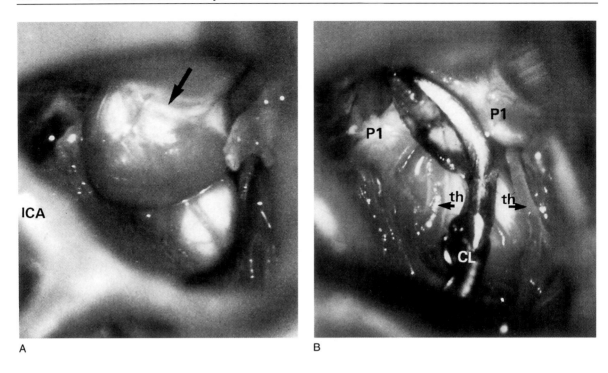

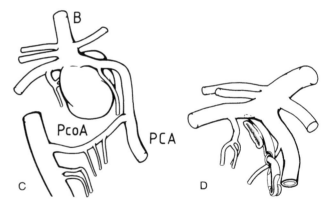

Fig **122A–D** Posteroinferiorly directed aneurysm seen lateral to the right internal carotid artery (**A**), after clipping and coagulation (**B**). Notice the thalamoperforators (th) (arrows). Schematic illustration (**C–D**).

Operative Technique 245

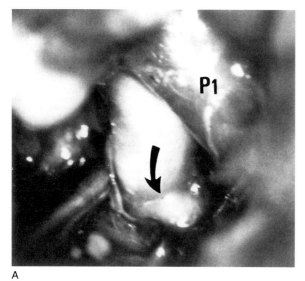

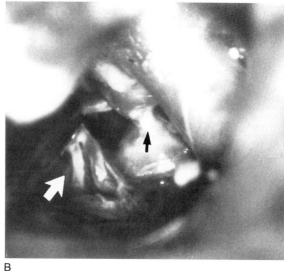

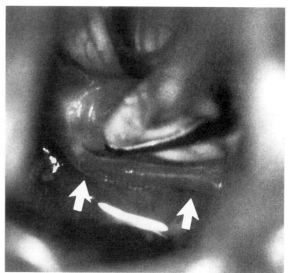

Fig 123A–C Posteroinferiorly directed aneurysm (large arrow) (**A**), after coagulation (black arrow), thalamoperforators (white arrow) (**B**), large thalamoperforating branch (white arrows), originating from the left P_1 (**C**). P_1 = right P_1 segment.

Of the 50 patients with basilar artery bifurcation aneurysms, it was possible in 39 to place a clip across the neck of the aneurysm and save all normal arteries. In another case, a giant aneurysm of the basilar artery bifurcation could be trapped between clips on the basilar artery and both P_1 segments (see Fig **125**). In 10 cases, it was either not possible or deemed too dangerous to apply clips and these aneurysms were covered with muscle and acrylic. The success of clipping is related to the size of the aneurysm (see Table **102b**, Fig **124**). It was found that 5 of the cases which were not clipped were medium sized aneurysms. These 5 cases were done early in the series, 4 through a subtemporal approach. It is probable that with increased operative experience in treating these lesions, they would be clipped if operated on today. The other 5 aneurysms, however, were large to giant aneurysms that were subtotally thrombosed and it was simply not possible to apply a clip. 2 of these cases each underwent 2 separate operations with no success in finding a way to clip their aneurysms. The patient with a giant aneurysm which was trapped had undergone a previous exploration when only muscle could be applied. Progressive neurological impairment led to a second procedure wherein the upper basilar artery was trapped (see Fig **125A–F**).

Even in those cases that had a clip applied to the neck of the aneurysm, there was often a small portion of the aneurysm that could not be included in the clip without compromising the parent arteries or adjacent perforating arteries. In 3 cases, there was a fair portion of the aneurysm

246 5 Vertebrobasilar Aneurysms

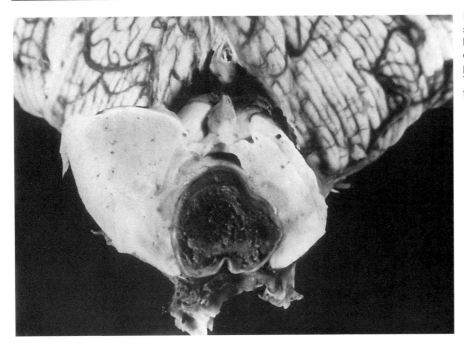

Fig **124** Pathological specimen of a giant basilar bifurcation aneurysm that eroded into the mesencephalon killing the patient. This is the inferior projection for the surgeon.

remaining and this was covered with muscle and acrylic. One of these patients reruptured the aneurysm 2 weeks later and died, while the other 2 are doing well up to the present time.

A similar case of rerupture after clipping is discussed under aneurysms arising from the upper basilar artery trunk.

Closure

All blood should be washed from the interpeduncular and other subarachnoid cisterns, and papaverine supplied to the major arteries of the carotid and basilar circulations. The craniotomy is closed in the usual manner.

Summary of Operative Technique

1) Frontotemporosphenoidal craniotomy.
2) Opening of the parasellar subarachnoid cisterns.
3) Decision as to where to open the interpeduncular cistern – medial or lateral to internal carotid artery.
4) Incision into the free edge of the tentorium if necessary.
5) Application of papaverine to the arteries.
6) Dissection of the posterior communicating and anterior choroidal arteries and branches.
7) Dissection of the posterior cerebral artery and branches.
8) Possible division of a hypoplastic segment of circle of Willis.
9) Preparation of areas on both P_1 segments and the basilar artery trunk for possible placement of the temporary clips.
10) Dissection of the aneurysm neck.
11) Possible removal of the posterior clinoid process.
12) Clip application.
13) Fundus resection.
14) Clip inspection, replacement.
15) Closure.

Clinical Presentation and Operative Results

Presenting Features

Of the 50 patients with aneurysms of the basilar artery bifurcation, 22 (44.0%) were men and 28 (56.0%) women. Ages ranged from 18 to 69, with 42 per cent of the patients between ages 41 and 50 (Table 103a and b). 48 patients (96.0%) experienced subarachnoid hemorrhage. About one third of these showed focal neurological deficits. Two patients with unruptured aneurysms presented with giant aneurysms and brain stem symptomatology.

Operative Results

Overall results for the 50 patients are related to preoperative grade in Table 104. Good results were obtained in 37 patients (74.0%), fair results in 4 (8.0%), poor results in 5 (10.0%) and 4 patients died (8.0%).

Grades Ia and IIa

28 patients were either alert at the time of operation or showed only mild alterations in level of consciousness. Some of these patients had an oculomotor palsy, but none showed hemiparesis or evidence of brain stem injury. The aneurysm could be clipped in 24 of these cases, and in 4, the lesion was wrapped with muscle. Good results were obtained in 27 patients (96.4%). None of the 4 patients treated with muscle wrapping had experienced recurrent subarachnoid hemorrhage over 3, 10, 11 and 13 years.

Table 103a Age and sex distribution in 50 patients with aneurysms of the basilar artery bifurcation

Age	Male	Female	Total	(%)
11–20	1	0	1	2.0%
21–30	3	3	6	12.0%
31–40	5	5	10	20.0%
41–50	9	12	21	42.0%
51–60	4	7	11	22.0%
61–70	0	1	1	2.0%
	22	28	50	
	44.0%	56.0%		100.0%

Table 103b Comparison of age and sex to operative result in 50 patients with aneurysms of the basilar artery bifurcation

Age	Good M	F	Fair M	F	Poor M	F	Death M	F	Total
11–20	–	–	–	–	–	–	1*	–	1
21–30	1	3	1 (1)	–	1 (1)	–	–	–	6
31–40	4 (2)	4	–	–	1 (1)	–	–	1	10
41–50	7	9 (1)	1	–	–	3	1 (1)	–	21
51–60	3 (1)	6 (1)	–	1 (1)	–	–	1	–	11
61–70	–	–	–	1**	–	–	–	–	1
Total	15 (3)	22 (2)	2 (1)	2 (1)	2 (2)	3	3 (1)	1	50

22 M
28 F } 68.2% 78.6% 9.1% 7.1% 9.1% 10.7% 13.6% 3.6%

( ) = aneurysms not clipped; covered with muscle and acrylic
* 18 year old male
** 69 year old female

Table 104 Operative results related to preoperative grade in 50 patients with aneurysm of the basilar artery bifurcation

Grade	Total	%	Good	Fair	Poor	Death
0b	2	4.0	1	–	–	1 (1)
Ia	12	24.0	12 (1)	–	–	–
Ib	2	4.0	1	–	–	1 (1)
IIa	16	32.0	15 (3)	1	–	–
IIb	7	14.0	5 (1)	1 (1)	1	–
IIIa	4	8.0	3	–	–	1
IIIb	7	14.0	–	2 (1)	4 (1)	1
	50	100.0	37 (5) 74%	4 (2) 8%	5 (1) 10%	4 (2) 8%

( ) aneurysm not clipped; covered with muscle and acrylic agent

One patient remains in fair condition. This 69 year old lady developed hydrocephalus in the postoperative period and required a ventricular shunt. She is able to care for herself.

Grade 0b

This special group includes 2 patients with large to giant unruptured aneurysms. One has made a good recovery and 1 has died:

C. P., a 24 year old male, complained of headaches from 1971, which were unsuccessfully treated with acupuncture. In July, 1975, he developed a progressive mental slowing, forgetfulness, emotional lability, dysarthria, dysphagia, perioral dysesthesia, tetraspasticity, visual difficulties, and hypertensive crises, and was found to have papilledema. Vertebral angiography showed a giant subtotally thrombosed aneurysm of the basilar artery bifurcation. A ventricular shunt was inserted on 2 August, 1975, with some improvement in level of consciousness. The patient subsequently developed tetraparesis and increasing clumsiness with intention tremor. He underwent exploration on 13 August, 1975, but it was not possible to apply a clip to this aneurysm and it was covered with muscle. He slowly deteriorated postoperatively, and was bedridden, requiring a tracheostomy. 3 months later, on 18 November, 1975, he underwent a second exploration and clips were placed across the basilar artery above the superior cerebellar arteries and across both P_1 segments to trap the aneurysm. The aneurysm was opened and emptied of the mass of thrombus. The postoperative course was surprisingly favorable. He made daily progress and 6 months after operation was able to return to work (Fig 125A–F).

E. E., a 42 year old man, presented with a 9 month history of progressive diplopia, ataxia, tremor, and difficulty with speech. He evidenced Parinaud's syndrome on examination and was unable to walk. At operation on 20 December, 1968, a giant aneurysm of the basilar artery bifurcation was approached subtemporally. It was not possible to place a clip or ligature without strangulation of the thalamoperforating arteries, and the lesion was covered with muscle and coated with acrylic. He remained unchanged postoperatively, and over the next 3 months was bedridden until his death. Autopsy showed that the large aneurysm had virtually replaced the mesencephalon.

Because of the progressive nature of these large aneurysms, a trapping procedure must be strongly considered in cases with well developed collateral circulation despite the risk of brain stem infarction.

Grades Ib and IIb

9 patients presented in grades Ib or IIb. Six of these (66.7%) made a good recovery. One of these was a 55 year old woman with a ruptured basilar artery bifurcation aneurysm and a large incidental left internal carotid-ophthalmic artery aneurysm. The carotid-ophthalmic aneurysm could be clipped but the basilar artery aneurysm could only be covered with muscle. She has improved to full working status and has experienced no recurrent subarachnoid hemorrhage. In the other 5 patients it was possible to clip the aneurysm. 1 patient (11.1%) remain in poor condition. One patient in this group died:

Eg., an 18 year old boy, suffered a subarachnoid hemorrhage on 6 October, 1971. Angiography revealed a large aneurysm of the basilar artery bifurcation and he underwent exploration on 8 November, 1971, through a subtemporal approach. The aneurysm was covered with muscle. In October, 1972, he again suffered a subarachnoid hemorrhage and presented in grade Ib. Angiography showed that the aneurysm had enlarged. A second operation was performed through a right pterional craniotomy on 14 December, 1972, but again it was not possible to apply a clip to the neck of the large aneurysm. The superior cerebellar and posterior cerebral arteries were now involved with the neck of the aneurysm. He remained well for 4 years, but CT scan performed during this time showed enlargement of the aneurysm. In 1976, he suffered a third subarachnoid hemorrhage and died.

Clinical Presentation and Operative Results 249

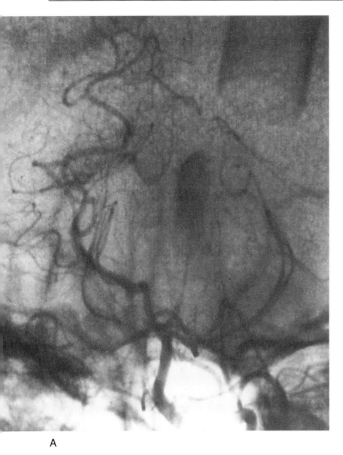

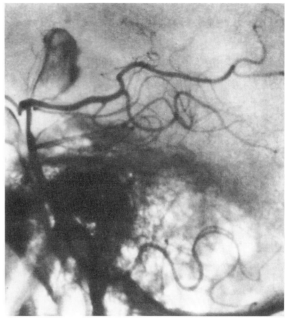

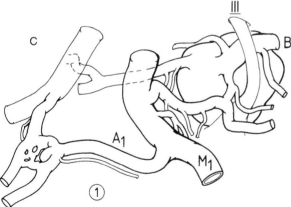

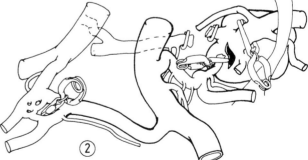

Fig 125A–F Giant partially thrombosed basilar bifurcation aneurysm (**A** and **B**) in a 24 year old tetraplegic, somnolent patient. Thought unclippable at operation, the patient was re-explored because he deteriorated, and the aneurysm was trapped and decompressed. Schematic illustration (**C**).

Fig 125D–F ▶

250 5 Vertebrobasilar Aneurysms

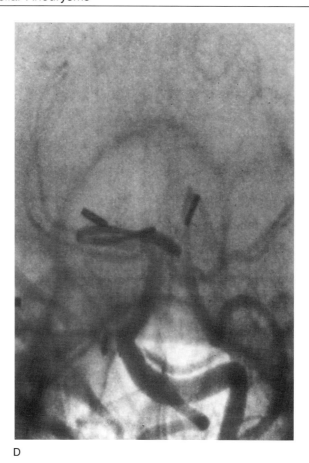

Fig 125 D–F The patient made a good recovery, and postoperative angiography showed occlusion of the basilar beyond the superior cerebellar arteries (D), with good posterior cerebral filling through the posterior communicating arteries on the right (E) and left (F) carotid angiograms (E and F).

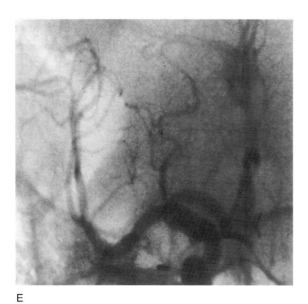

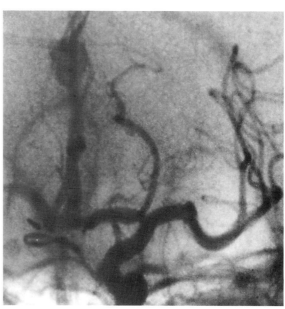

Grade IIIa

4 patients underwent operation in grade IIIa and in each case the aneurysm could be clipped. 3 patients (75.0%) made good recoveries and have returned to their former activities. In the fourth patient a large aneurysm could not be clipped properly and the patient died.

Gr., a 59 year old man with hypertension sustained 3 subarachnoid hemorrhages over a period of 3 years. A ventriculoatrial shunt was inserted in another hospital. He presented in grade IIIa, confused and ataxic. At operation on 6 August, 1973, a large aneurysm of the basilar artery bifurcation was approached through a left pterional craniotomy so that an aneurysm of the internal carotid-posterior communicating artery could be treated at the same time. The sclerotic aneurysm would not accept coagulation readily. With each attempt at coagulation the neck would shrink, but by the time the clip had been introduced into the operative field, the neck had again expanded to its original size, and would not accept the clip. Finally the clip was placed across the aneurysm neck, but some of the perforating arteries had been damaged by coagulation. The patient remained in coma after operation and died 3 days later of gastrointestinal hemorrhage. Unfortunately no larger clips were available at that time, they have only been developed after this painful experience.

Grade IIIb

7 patients underwent operation in grade IIIb. These patients were in poor condition with evidence of mesencephalic injury and yielded generally poor results. 2 patients had a fair outcome, 1 with a residual left hemiparesis present and shunted preoperatively and the other requiring a ventricular shunt 3 months after operation. 4 patients are in poor condition, each with persistent severe deficits present in the preoperative period. 2 had ventricular shunts inserted preoperatively. None was made worse by operation. In 3 patients the aneurysm could be clipped and in the other case it was covered with muscle. 2 of these patients are in nursing homes, but one is able to care for himself at home and occasionally does a small bit of work. 1 patient died. Her inferiorly bulging aneurysm could not be entirely clipped. She was making a good recovery but experienced rerupture of the unclipped portion of the aneurysm (No. 6, Table **105**). These 7 patients are summarized in Table **105**.

No patient underwent operation for basilar artery bifurcation aneurysm in grades IV or V.

Table **105** Clinical features of 7 patients presenting in grade IIIb with aneurysms of the basiliar artery bifurcation

Name	Age	Sex	Year	SAH	Size	Preop deficit	Grade	Timing	Operation	Postop course	Result
1. G	30	M	1968	2	Medium	Tetraparesis Confusion Somnolence	IIIb	10 days	Subtemp. Muscle	R. CN III palsy Epilepsy Hydrocephalus, *shunted*	Poor
2. Zi	24	M	1974	1	Giant	L. hemiparesis Parinaud Syn.	IIIb	7 days	Pterion Muscle	Improvement *shunt*	Fair
3. Ba	49	F	1974	1	Medium	R. hemiparesis Aphasia Hydrocephalus, *shunt* preop Somnolence 4 add. aneurysms	IIIb	3 weeks	Pterion Clip	Little improvement Bedridden	Poor
4. Bi	44	F	1975	2	Large	L. hemiparesis R. CN III palsy Somnolent R. MCA aneurysm	IIIb	10 days	Pterion Both clip	Epilepsy No improvement	Poor
5. Ki	44	F	1975	1	Medium	R. hemiparesis Akinetic Hydrocephalus, *shunt* preop	IIIb	3 weeks	Pterion Clip	No improvement	Poor
6. Ro	34	F	1977	1	Medium	Paraparesis Somnolent	IIIb	5 weeks	Pterion Part. Clip	Improvement, 2 w. later rerupture	Death
7. Sc	47	M	1977	2	Medium	L. hemiparesis Akinetic Hydrocephalus, *shunted*	IIIb	11 days	Pterion Clip	Epilepsy	Fair

Outcome of Oculomotor Paralysis

Minor paresis of one or both oculomotor nerves is a common postoperative finding that generally disappears within a few days. 12 patients (24.0%) had transient oculomotor palsies lasting days to weeks. 5 of these involved the right oculomotor nerve, 3 the left nerve, and in 4 patients both nerves were involved. In 4 patients (8.0%) oculomotor palsy was permanent. In one of these patients, the oculomotor nerve was thinned and virtually encased by the aneurysm. To gain access to the aneurysm neck the nerve was sacrificed. One of the patients later had a ophthalmological procedure to correct eye movement with a satisfactory result.

Analysis of Operative Results

The treatment of basilar artery bifurcation aneurysms is less satisfactory than that for aneurysms at other locations. The combined mortality and morbidity for these patients was 26.0 per cent, as compared with 16.8 per cent for internal carotid-posterior communicating artery aneurysm patients, 16.3 per cent for middle cerebral artery aneurysm patients, 10.9 per cent for internal carotid artery bifurcation patients and 12.5 per cent for anterior communicating artery aneurysm patients. Furthermore, in 10 patients it was not possible to clip the aneurysm and in another patient the aneurysm reformed and ruptured after it had been clipped. The factors contributing to operative difficulties and to the poorer outcome in these patients have been examined:

Age and Sex

Age and sex are related to outcome in Table **103a** and **b**. The mortality rate for patients under 40 years old is $2/17 = 11.8$ per cent, and for patients over 40 $2/33 = 6.1$ per cent. Morbidity rate for the same age groups is $3/17 = 17.6$ per cent, and $6/33 = 18.2$ per cent respectively. 3 out of 4 deaths occurred in males, but morbidity was about evenly divided between the sexes. As with aneurysms at other locations, women seem to have a slightly more favourable outcome.

Hydrocephalus

Of the 50 patients with basilar artery bifurcation aneurysms 10 (20.0%) required ventricular shunting for hydrocephalus, 3 in the preoperative period and 7 postoperatively. 6 of these 10 patients were in grade IIIb at the time of operation. Seen another way, 5 of the 7 patients presenting in grade IIIb required ventricular shunts. The presence of hydrocephalus is related to preoperative grade and surgical results in Table **106**.

Timing of Operation

A comparison of the timing of operation independent of grade with the operative results in the 48 patients who sustained subarachnoid hemorrhage with basilar bifurcation aneurysms is seen in Table **107**. 3 patients underwent operation in the first week after hemorrhage and all of these had a good outcome. 12 patients were operated in the second week with 8 good results, 2 fair results and 2 poor results. Between 2 and 4 weeks, 17 patients underwent operation, with 13 good results, 1 fair result and 3 poor results. Taking all patients operated on before 4 weeks and comparing these to those operated on after 4 weeks, there are 71.9 per cent good results and mortality rate of zero in the first group, and 81.3 per cent good results and a mor-

Table **106** Incidence of hydrocephalus related to preoperative grade and postoperative result in 50 patients with aneurysms of the basilar artery bifurcation

Grade	Good	Fair	Poor	Death	Total	(%)
0b	1/ 1	–	–	1/1	2/ 2	100.0
Ia	–/12	–	–	–	–/12	0
Ib	–/ 1	–	–	–/1	–/ 2	0
IIa	–/15	1/1	–	–	1/16	6.3
IIb	1/ 5	–/1	–/1	–	1/ 7	14.3
IIIa	–/ 3	–	–	1/1	1/ 4	25.0
IIIb	–	2/2	3/4	–/1	5/ 7	71.4
Total	2/37	3/4	3/5	2/4	10/50	
%	5.4	75.0	60.0	50.0	20.0	

Table 107 Timing of surgery and results in 48 patients with ruptured aneurysm of the basilar artery bifurcation

	\multicolumn{5}{c}{Good}	\multicolumn{3}{c}{Fair}	\multicolumn{2}{c}{Poor}	\multicolumn{3}{c}{Death}	
	Ia	Ib	IIa	IIb	IIIa	IIa	IIb	IIIb	IIb	IIIb	Ib	IIIa	IIIb
1–3 d	–	–	–	–	–	–	–	–	–	–	–	–	–
4–7 d	2	–	–	–	–	–	–	1	–	–	–	–	–
1–2 w	1	–	4	–	3	–	1	1	–	2	–	–	–
2–4 w	4	1	7	1	–	1	–	–	1	2	–	–	–
1–3 m	4	–	–	4	–	–	–	–	–	–	1	1	1
>3 m	1	–	4	–	–	–	–	–	–	–	–	–	–
	12	1	15	5	3	1	1	2	1	4	1	1	1
	\multicolumn{5}{c}{36}	\multicolumn{3}{c}{4}	\multicolumn{2}{c}{5}	\multicolumn{3}{c}{3}	= 48

tality rate of 18.7 per cent in the second group. Thirty out of 32 patients in the group (a) without preoperative neurological deficit showed good results (93.8%), 1 patient a fair result and 1 patient died (3.1%). In contrast to this group are the results in the group (b) with preoperative neurological deficits; only 6 out of 16 patients had a good result (37.5%), 3 cases fair (18.7%), 5 cases poor (31.2%), and 2 cases died (12.5%). There seems to be no detrimental effect of early operation on basilar artery bifurcation patients. However, the number of 48 patients is too few to calculate the percentage and to make a fair assessment.

Anatomical Problems

Direction and size of fundus. The direction and size of the aneurysm fundus are related to operative results in Table **108**. All but 1 of the patients with aneurysms directed anteriorly or superiorly had a good result, and all of these aneurysms could be clipped. Only 1 aneurysm in these 2 groups was larger than 15 mm in diameter (Table **102a**).

With aneurysms directed posteriorly, 2 were small and these could both be successfully clipped with a good outcome for the patients. In the other 29 aneurysms directed posteriorly 20 were medium size, 6 large and 3 truly giant aneurysms; only 15 patients (51.7%) had a good result and 4 of these could not be clipped. The 4 deaths and 5 poor results in patients with basilar artery bifurcation aneurysms were all in patients with posteriorly directed aneurysms. 5 of these patients presented in grade IIIb. Of the 29 aneurysms, only 19 could be clipped (65.5%), the rest being covered with muscle and cyanoacrylate. These larger, posteroinferiorly directed aneurysms represent an especially difficult operative challenge, and are associated with a high mortality and morbidity.

Table 108 Projection of aneurysm fundus related to operative results in 50 patients with aneurysms of the basilar artery bifurcation

	Total No.	Good	Fair	Poor	Death
Anterior					
Small	3	2	1	–	–
Medium	2	2	–	–	–
Superior					
Small	4	4	–	–	–
Medium	9	9	–	–	–
Large	1	1	–	–	–
Posterior (posteroinferior)					
Small	2	2	–	–	–
Medium	20 (5)	15 (3)	2 (1)	2 (1)	1
Large	6 (3)	1 (1)	1 (1)	2	2 (1)
Giant	3 (2)	1	–	1 (1)	1 (1)
	50	37	4	5	4

( ) not clipped

5 Vertebrobasilar Aneurysms

Thrombosis. In 7 patients the aneurysm was subtotally thrombosed. 4 of these aneurysms were large to giant. Only 1 of these could be clipped and 1 was trapped. The other 5 aneurysms were covered with muscle. 3 of these patients have had good results, one fair, one poor, and two died. Morbidity and mortality in the latter 4 patients was due in each case to an inability to adequately treat the aneurysm. In the 2 cases with morbidity, the aneurysm has enlarged, in 1 case the aneurysm enlarged and caused the patient's death, and in the fourth case the aneurysm reruptured after 4 years, taking the patient's life. These three factors of size, fundus direction, and amount of thrombosis are, of course, all interrelated. Except for 1 case in the present series, all aneurysms larger than 15 mm were directed posteroinferiorly and 7 of these 9 aneurysms were subtotally thrombosed. These large posteroinferiorly directed aneurysms accounted for 3 of the 4 deaths and 6 of the 10 patients not making a full recovery.

Operative Problems

Craniotomy and Approach

The craniotomy and approach to the aneurysm used in these 50 patients is related to operative results in Table **109**. The only distinctive finding here is the far higher morbidity in patients who had the aneurysm approached lateral to the internal carotid artery. This finding relates to the fact that posteriorly directed aneurysms must have a more lateral direction of approach since the neck is covered by the P_1 segments and basilar trunk *en face*.

Table **109** Operative approach

	Good	Fair	Poor	Death
Right subtemporal	4 (2)	–	1 (1)	2 (2)
Left subtemporal	1	–	–	–
Left pterional	–	–	–	1
Right pterional	32 (3)	4 (2)	4	1
	37 (5)	4 (2)	5 (1)	4 (2)

( ) Muscle wrapped

Removal of a portion of the posterior clinoid process between the optic nerve and ICA with an electric drill in 2 cases

Aneurysm Treatment

Patients whose aneurysms were treated only by muscle wrapping and the application of acrylic are compared with those whose aneurysms were clipped or trapped in Table **110**. While results are generally better in clipped or trapped lesions, it must be remembered that 7 of the muscle treated aneurysms were large or giant aneurysms. As muscle wrapping represents a failure to be able to apply a clip, it is not surprising that these aneurysms were the more difficult lesions to treat. Nevertheless, only 1 patient has died of rerupture of his aneurysm and another was killed by progressive enlargement of his aneurysm. On the other hand, 5 patients have had good results, these for periods of from 2 to 12 years. 2 of the 3 patients with morbidity have shown enlargement of their aneurysms. 1 patient with incomplete aneurysm clipping also reruptured and died. The prognosis, therefore, in an unclipped aneurysm of the basilar artery bifurcation is not good, but the patient's preoperative condition and age must be considered before undertaking a dangerous trapping procedure.

Table **110** Comparison of clipped and nonclipped aneurysms to preoperative grade and operative result in 50 patients with basilar artery bifurcation aneurysms

	Clipped Aneurysms					Nonclipped Aneurysms				
Grade	Good	Fair	Poor	Death	Total	Good	Fair	Poor	Death	Total
0a	1	–	–	–	1	–	–	–	–	0
0b	1	–	–	–	1	–	–	–	1	1
Ia	10	–	–	–	10	1	–	–	–	1
Ib	1	–	–	–	1	–	–	–	1	1
IIa	12	1	–	–	13	3	–	–	–	3
IIb	4	–	1	–	5	1	1	–	–	2
IIIa	3	–	–	1	4	–	–	–	–	0
IIIb	–	1	3	1	5	–	1	1	–	2
Total	32 80%	2 5%	4 10%	2 5%	40	5 50%	2 20%	1 10%	2 20%	10

Coagulation of Aneurysm Neck

The aneurysm neck was coagulated prior to placement of a clip in 20 of 40 cases (50.0%). 3 of these cases had poor results and 2 cases died. These figures are about the same as for aneurysms not coagulated prior to clipping. Aneurysms at other locations have been routinely coagulated with no apparent deleterious effect to the parent artery. It is only in the last few years that larger clips capable of occluding the neck of large basilar artery bifurcation aneurysms have been available. In many earlier cases, the clip would simply slip off the aneurysm neck, and pretreatment by coagulation was a necessity for clip placement, even when it appeared dangerous. Nevertheless, even with modern clips, bipolar coagulation of the aneurysm remains an effective method of achieving perfect clip placement.

Division of a Major Artery

In 11 cases the posterior communicating artery was divided to allow better access to the aneurysm neck. 8 of these patients had good results, 2 poor results and 1 died. Both patients with poor results were grade IIIb at the time of operation and the patient who died is one who reruptured a clipped aneurysm. There thus seemed to be no morbidity incurred by division of the posterior communicating artery. The A_1 segment of the anterior cerebral artery was divided near its origin in one case to allow more retraction of the internal carotid artery. This patient made an uncomplicated recovery.

Intraoperative Rupture

The aneurysm ruptured during dissection in 8 cases. 5 of the 6 patients in grades Ia to IIb have gone on to make full recoveries, but one grade IIb patient remains in poor condition and this is undoubtedly attributable to intraoperative rupture of the aneurysm and difficulties in getting the aneurysm clipped. 2 patitents in grade IIIb remain in poor condition, but did not seem to have been worsened by intraoperative rupture of the aneurysm.

Summary

50 patients had operative treatment of basilar artery bifurcation aneurysms. In 40 cases it was possible to clip the aneurysm, although in one of these clipping was incomplete. In the remaining 10 cases the lesions were covered with muscle and an acrylic bonding agent. A pterional approach to the upper basilar artery has been preferred to the subtemporal approach. This method allows better appreciation of the P_1 segments of the posterior cerebral arteries and their perforating branches bilaterally, and avoids retraction of the temporal lobe.

Anatomical problems include the large size of many of these aneurysms with sclerosis and partial to subtotal thrombosis, and the posteroinferior projection of the greatest number of these aneurysms. The relationship of the internal carotid artery to the optic nerve is important in this frontolateral approach to the aneurysm. The relative sizes of the posterior communicating and posterior cerebral arteries (P_1 segments) provide different options for interrupting the circle of Willis.

In this group of 50 patients, 37 made good recoveries (Table 111). These included patients from grades 0a to IIIa, but no grade IIIb patient made a full recovery, and no grade IV or V patients underwent operation. 32 of the 37 aneurysms could be clipped and the other 5 were covered with muscle. 2 patients required ventricular shunts before making a full recovery.

There were 4 fair results. 1 was an elderly lady who required a ventricular shunt in the postoperative period, but is self sufficient at home. 2 of the patients did not recover completely from neurological deficits existing preoperatively, and 1 of these has required a shunt and had epileptic seizures. None of these was made worse by operation.

5 patients had poor results. 4 of these were in grade IIIb and have not recovered from deficits present preoperatively. 1 patient presented in grade IIb, and following intraoperative rupture and temporary clipping of the basilar artery remains in a poor condition. In a final case, the aneurysm could not be clipped and has undergone progressive enlargement as noted by angiography and CT scan.

4 patients died. In 2 of these aneurysms could not be clipped. In 1 patient the aneurysm progressively enlarged and destroyed the mesencephalon, and in the other case the aneurysm enlarged and ruptured 4 years after 2 operative explorations and wrapping with muscle and cyanoacrylate. The third patient experienced rerupture of a partially clipped aneurysm, and the fourth patient remained in coma after a difficult clipping of a large, sclerotic aneurysm.

5 Vertebrobasilar Aneurysms

Table 111 Preoperative condition: Type of treatment and results

	Cases		Good	Fair	Poor	Death
Group 1 *Ia – IIa*						
12 (1) 16 (3)	= 28	24 Clip	23	1	–	–
		4 Muscle	(4)	–	–	–
Group 2 *0b – Ib – IIb*						
2 (1) 2 (1) 7 (2)	= 11	7 Clip	6	–	1	–
		4 Muscle	(1)	(1)	–	(2)
Group 3 *IIIa*	= 4	4 Clip	3	–	–	1
Group 4 *IIIb*	= 7	5 Clip	–	1	3	1
		2 Muscle	–	(1)	(1)	
			37 (5)	4 (2)	5 (1)	4 (2)

( ) = not clipped

Non clipped cases 10 treated with coagulation + muscle wrapping + acrylate

Size of aneurysm	Good	Fair	Poor	Death
Medium	3*	1**	1***	–
Large	1'	1''	–	1'''
Giant	1+	–	–	1++
	5	2	1	2

Observation time

Good   *   9y, 10y, 12y, ' 2y, + 6y
Fair   **   6m, '' 5y
Poor   *** 11y
Death   ''' 13y, ++ 3m

Upper Basilar Artery Trunk Aneurysms

Anatomical Relationships

In 5 cases the aneurysm was between the superior cerebellar artery and the posterior cerebral artery. Aneurysms arose from the right side of the basilar artery in 2 cases and the left side in 3. The oculomotor nerve was attached to the aneurysm in all 5 cases.

In one case the patient, who had an posterior communicating artery aneurysm clipped 10 years before, presented with a basilar artery trunk aneurysm in addition to a saccular aneurysm of the left middle cerebral artery bifurcation and a "baby" aneurysm of the right middle cerebral artery bifurcation.

Operative Technique

All aneurysms were approached through a pterional craniotomy. Consideration must be given to the side of craniotomy. To some degree it is more convenient to be working from the side opposite the aneurysm, because the angle is more favorable and the neck is not covered by the fundus of the aneurysm. Nevertheless, it is difficult for a right handed surgeon to work from the left side because the depth at which dissection must be performed demands an uncomfortable angle of approach. Generally then it is better to come from the right side unless there are special factors dictating otherwise.

In one case of an aneurysm between the superior cerebellar and posterior cerebral arteries it was possible to coagulate the neck of the aneurysm and place a clip across it. In the case of an aneurysm below the superior cerebellar artery it was also possible to clip the neck, although the oculomotor nerve which had been elevated and compressed to a transparent band by the aneurysm had to be sacrificed to completely expose the neck. In a third case, the aneurysm was trapped between a clip placed at an angle across the upper basilar artery including the origin of the posterior cerebral artery, but sparing the superior cerebellar artery. A small clip was then placed on the P_1 segment to trap the lesion. One perforating artery was included in the trapped segment. It was also possible in this case to clip an aneurysm of the left middle cerebral (M_1) through the same right sided approach. The patient had an uneventful postoperative course. In the fourth case the neck could

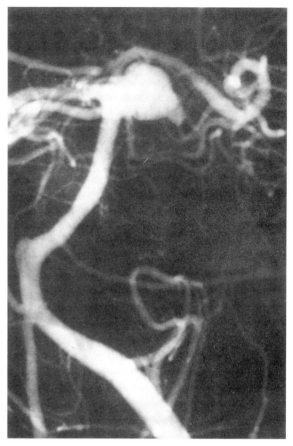

Fig 126 Broad based aneurysm between the origin of the left superior cerebellar artery and posterior cerebral artery. This could be clipped within 70 seconds of temporary clipping of the basilar artery proximal to the origin of the superior cerebellar artery. The 63 year old patient made a good recovery.

not be developed over a sufficient length. Clip application severely compromised the basilar artery and the clip would not close when placed more distally on the aneurysm. This lesion was treated with muscle wrapping and acrylic (Figs **126, 127A–C**).

258 5 Vertebrobasilar Aneurysms

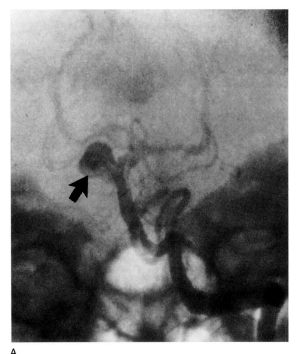

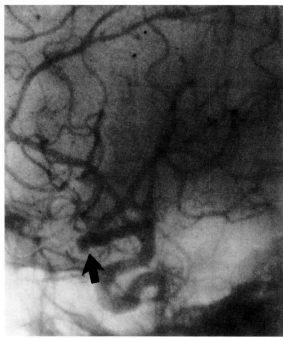

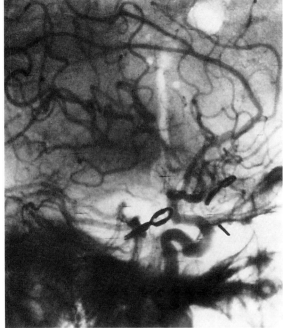

Fig 127A–C Right basilar artery aneurysm arising at the origin of the superior cerebellar artery (arrow) (**A**) with a second aneurysm at the right middle cerebral artery bifurcation (arrow) (**B**). Both were completely obliterated via a single right pterional approach as seen on postoperative angiography (**C**).

Clinical Presentation and Operative Results

These 5 patients were all men, ages 40 to 58. All 5 patients presented with subarachnoid hemorrhage (Table 112). 2 patients had oculomotor palsies. One of the patients had undergone craniotomy for clipping of an internal carotid-posterior communicating artery aneurysm 10 years earlier. Vertebral angiography had been performed at that time and there was no aneurysm present on the basilar artery. This lesion thus formed and ruptured within 10 years (case 5 Table 112, see also Fig 237A–E, Vol. I).

4 of these patients had good operative results.

One patient (No. 5) required a ventricular shunt in the preoperative period.

One patient (No. 2) has a permanent oculomotor palsy, but is otherwise capable of full activity. The fifth is the other patient (No. 3) in this series of vertebrobasilar aneurysms who reruptured an aneurysm after it had been clipped at operation 4 weeks before. Autopsy showed that the base of this aneurysm had bulged forming a new aneurysm and this had gone on to rupture.

This case re-emphasizes the need to strive for perfect clip placement. Nevertheless, there will be some cases where it is not possible to place a clip proximal to the weakness in the wall of the parent artery, and these patients remain at risk.

Table 112 Clinical features in 5 patients with aneurysms of the upper basilar artery trunk (SCA + PCA)

Name	Age	Sex	Year	Side	Addit. aneur.	SAH	Preoperative deficits	Grade	Timing	Operation	Postoperative course	Result
1. C.	55	M	1973	L	–	1	Recovered	Ia	3 m	Pterion Clip	Full recovery	Good
2 G.	58	M	1974	R	R. MCA	2	R. CN III palsy	Ib	18 d	Pterion Clip/clip	Full recovery Oculomotor palsy	Good
3. B.	40	M	1974	L	–	1	Drowsy Meningism	IIa	8 d	Pterion Clip	Doing well, then rerupture	Death
4. L.	56	M	1978	R	–	1	R. CN III paresis	Ib	2 m	Pterion Muscle	Full recovery	Good
5. G.	52	M	1978	L	R. PCA L. M$_1$	2	Confused, lethargic hydrocephalus, shunt preop. R. PcoA aneurysm treated 1968	IIIa	2 m	Pterion Clip/clip Clip	Recovery	Good

Posterior Cerebral Artery Aneurysms (P$_1$ Segment)

Anatomical Relationships

In 5 patients, an aneurysm took origin from the P$_1$ segment of the posterior cerebral artery. Each of these aneurysms was large, sclerotic and partially thrombosed. Aneurysms at this location are within the interpeduncular cistern. Thalamoperforating arteries and the posteromedial choroidal artery are often attached to the aneurysm, and the oculomotor nerve is usually involved. In one case, the aneurysm fundus compressed the adjacent superior cerebellar artery and this was seen to be thrombosed at operation. The aneurysm was on the right posterior cerebral artery in 4 cases and on the left side in one. There were no cases of multiple aneurysms in this group.

Operative Technique

These aneurysms were approached through a pterional craniotomy (Fig **128A–C**). In only one case (No. 3) was it possible to place a clip across the neck of the aneurysm, and even in this case, temporary clips to the P$_1$ segment were required to open the aneurysm and shrink it with bipolar coagulation. 2 thalamoperforating arteries were lost with this maneuver, however. In 3 cases, the aneurysm was trapped between clips placed proximal and distal on the P$_1$ segment. The following case is representative of the difficulties in performing such a procedure:

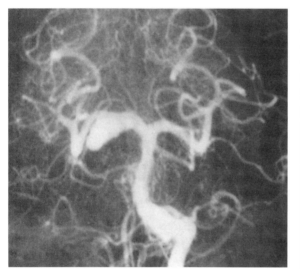
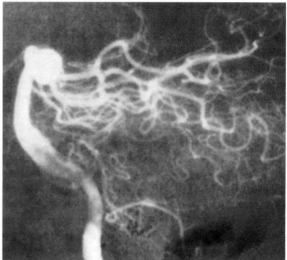
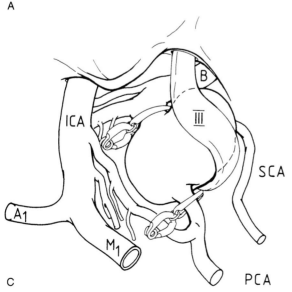

Fig **128A–C** Large partially thrombosed aneurysm of the right P$_1$ segment (**A** and **B**) that was trapped (**C**) (Case 4, Table **113**).

Aa, a 13 year old boy, suffered a subarachnoid hemorrhage in June, 1976, which went unrecognized. He then developed progressive headache, diplopia, and right hemiparesis over the next several months, and was ultimately transferred in December 1977. Angiography demonstrated a large aneurysm of the left posterior cerebral artery. He did not demonstrate a visual field defect. At operation, on 14 December, 1977, the aneurysm was approached through a left pterional craniotomy. Through the small gap between the internal carotid artery and the left optic nerve, the aneurysm was seen to be a large, fusiform lesion, beginning 2 mm from the basilar artery bifurcation and extending to the junction of the posterior communicating artery. A group of thalamoperforating arteries issued from the wall of the aneurysm. With considerable effort and difficulty, a space could be created on the P_1 segment just distal to the basilar artery bifurcation and a clip placed there. Temporary clips were placed on the P_2 segment and the posterior communicating artery and the aneurysm opened and emptied of thrombus and atheroma. It was then possible to move a clip to the P_1 segment, just before the junction of the posterior communicating artery to preserve flow between the internal carotid artery and the posterior cerebral artery. The patient tolerated the operation well and went on to a complete recovery. 5 years later he is a successful student and an active sportsman (Fig **129A–H**).

A similar procedure was carried out in 2 other cases, although in 1 case a small part of the aneurysm next to the junction of the posterior communicating and posterior cerebral arteries had to be left. In the fifth patient (No. 4) the aneurysm was sclerotic and broad based, with the fundus indenting the cerebral peduncle. Application of a clip produced severe torsion of the basilar artery bifurcation compromising perforating arteries. Because the aneurysm was 90 per cent thrombosed, it was wrapped with muscle and covered with acrylic.

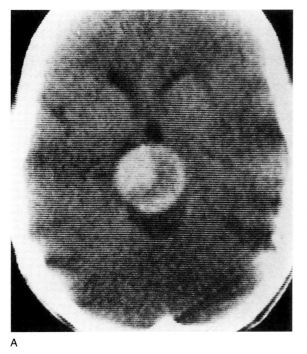

A

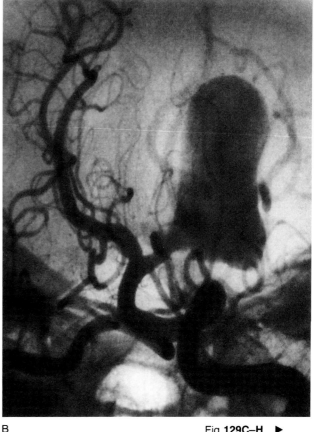

B

Fig **129A–H** CT scan (**A**) showing a giant aneurysm in a 13 year old patient with a progressive right hemiparesis. Vertebral angiography demonstrated a giant left P_1 fusiform aneurysm (**B**) (Case 2, Table **113**).

Fig **129C–H** ▶

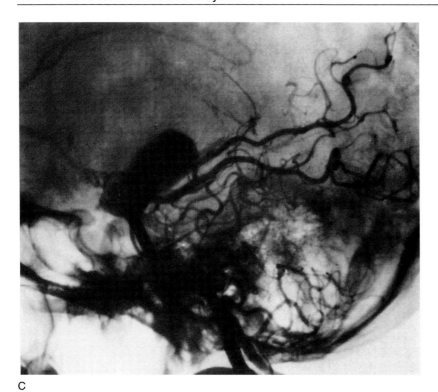

Fig 129 C Lateral view of vertebral angiogram. The left P_1 was trapped and the aneurysm decompressed.

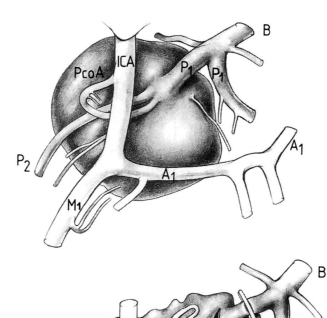

Fig 129 D The operative procedure is shown diagrammatically. The main problem was not in placing a clip on the proximal right P_1 segment but in advancing the clip to the distal P_1 segment without compromising the posterior communicating artery.

Operative Technique 263

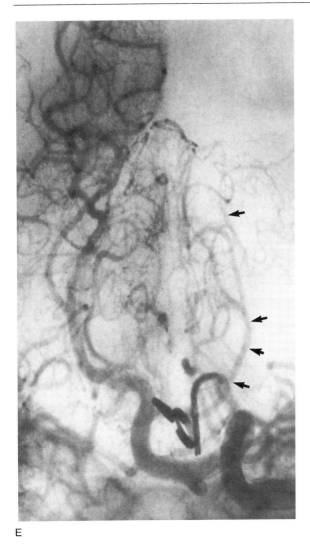

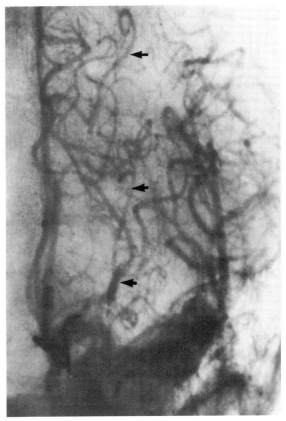

Fig 129 E–G Postoperative angiography showed complete obliteration of the aneurysm with no filling of the left posterior cerebral artery on the vertebral angiogram (arrows indicating the left superior cerebellar artery) (**E**). However, there was good collateral flow from the left internal carotid artery (arrows) (**F, G**) because the connection between posterior communicating artery and P_2 was saved.

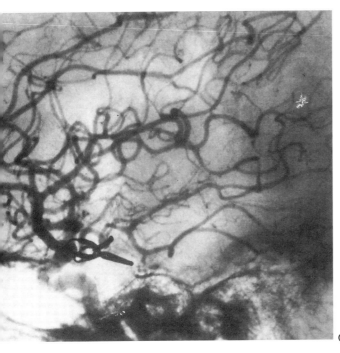

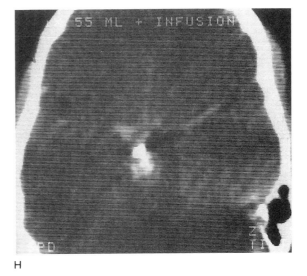

Fig 129 H Five years later the CT scan showed impressive shrinkage of the aneurysm (Case 2, Table **113**).

Clinical Presentation and Operative Results

3 of these patients were males and 2 females. Ages ranged from 13 to 59 years old. 3 of the patients sustained subarachnoid hemorrhage. One of these had 3 subarachnoid hemorrhages over a 10 year period, and another had a hemorrhage 18 months earlier and then a progressive brain stem syndrome. All 3 of these patients had oculomotor findings, and 2 had hemiparesis. 2 patients presented without subarachnoid hemorrhage, but with progressive oculomotor palsy, hemiparesis, ataxia, and sensory disturbances that had led to a diagnosis of brain tumor or multiple sclerosis. Clinical features are summarized in Table 113.

4 of these patients have made good recoveries. In 3 of the cases the aneurysm was trapped and patients showed increased neurological impairment in the postoperative period. They then went on to full recovery. One patient remains in a poor condition. He underwent operation in grade IIb, and his postoperative course was uncomplicated until about 3 weeks later, when he had a cardiac arrest secondary to pulmonary emboli. He was resuscitated, but remained in an akinetic state. A ventricular shunt was inserted with no real improvement. He lives with a left hemiparesis, seizure disorder and a peculiar Parkinsonian appearance with bradykinesia and rigidity.

Table 113 Clinical features in 5 patients with aneurysms on the P_1 segment of the posterior cerebral artery

Name	Age	Sex	Year	SAH	Side	Preoperative deficits	Grade	Timing	Operation	Postoperative course	Result
1. Bä	21	M	1972	2	R	R CN III palsy Drowsy L mild hpr.	IIb	2 weeks	Trapping large	Full recovery	Good
2. Aa	13	M	1972	0	L	R hemiparesis L CN III palsy Tremor	0a	–	Trapping giant	Full recovery	Good
3. Be	29	M	1973	0	R	L hemiparesis R CN III palsy Ataxia	IIb	–	Clip medium	Pulmonary emboli, Akinetic	Poor
4. Gö	39	F	1973	1	R	L hemiparesis R CN III palsy Emotional lab.	IIb	6 weeks	Muscle. Large thrombosed aneurysm	Full recovery	Good
5. Rö	59	F	1975	3	R	R CN III palsy L mild hpr.	Ib	3 years	Trapping medium	Full recovery	Good

Posterior Cerebral Artery Aneurysms (P_1/P_2 Junction)

Anatomical Relationships

In 3 patients an aneurysm was found at the junction of the P_1 and P_2 segments of the posterior cerebral artery. One of these cases was a typical saccular aneurysm which presented on the inferior side of the junction of the posterior communicating artery and the posterior cerebral artery (No. 1, Table 114). In the second case, the posterior communicating artery and the P_2 segment were joined by a fusiform aneurysm (Fig 130A–B). In the third case (No. 3, Table 114) there was a complex anomaly present wherein the right internal carotid artery was completely absent. The right posterior cerebral artery gave rise to the right middle cerebral artery at which point there was an aneurysm. The A_1 segment of the right anterior cerebral artery was also missing, and there was a small aneurysm on the left side of the anterior communicating artery, where the left A_1 supplied both distal anterior cerebral arteries (see Vol. I, Fig 38A–F). Aneurysms in these patients were all on the right side.

Table 114 Clinical features in 3 patients with aneurysms of the posterior cerebral artery (P_1/P_2 junction)

Name	Age	Sex	Year	Side	SAH	Preoperative deficits	Grade	Timing	Operation	Postoperative course	Result
1. Z.	30	F	1971	R Large	1	L hemiparesis Mild POS	Ib	8 months	Subtemp. Trapping	Improvement No HA	Good
2. P.	20	F	1974	R	1	L hemiparesis R CN III palsy Somnolent, Aplasia R ICA	IIIb	4 weeks	Pterion Clip	Improvement	Good
3. F.	28	F	1979	R	1	Recovered	Ia	2 months	Pterion Clip	Full recovery	Good

HA = Hemianopsia

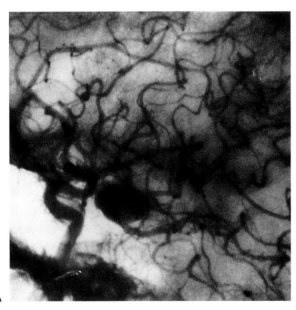

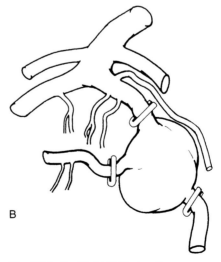

Fig 130A–B Right P_1/P_2 junction aneurysm which could be eliminated using a trapping technique (Case 1, Table 114).

Operative Technique

One of these cases (No. 1) earlier in the series was approached subtemporally, but the other 2 could be satisfactorily handled through a standard pterional craniotomy. The oculomotor nerve was attached to the aneurysm in each case, and had to be dissected free. With the smaller saccular aneurysm it was possible to prepare the posterior cerebral and posterior communicating arteries and their perforators without great difficulty, and following coagulation of the neck, a clip could then be applied. In the case with multiple anomalies it was, of course, mandatory that circulation to the right middle cerebral artery through the posterior cerebral artery be preserved. This large aneurysm could be progressively shrunk with bipolar coagulation until a clip could be satisfactorily placed across the neck. The corner of the aneurysm ruptured, however, and a temporary clip to the posterior cerebral artery was required before a clip could be applied. In the case (No. 1) of the fusiform aneurysm, the lesion was trapped by clipping the P_1 segment and the posterior communicating artery.

Clinical Presentation and Operative Results

All 3 patients were women aged 20 to 30 years old (Table **114**). The woman with a smaller aneurysm was in grade Ia, and has done very well. The patient with a fusiform aneurysm had sustained a subarachnoid hemorrhage 8 months prior to operation and presented with a right oculomotor palsy and a left hemiparesis. She did well from operation and no visual field deficit was noted after trapping the posterior cerebral artery owing to well developed collaterals from the middle and anterior cerebral arteries. The third patient with an anomalous carotid circulation presented in grade IIIb, somnolent with a dense left hemiparesis, and a right oculomotor palsy. Postoperatively, she showed full recovery of the oculomotor deficit and of the hemiparesis.

Posterior Cerebral Artery Aneurysms (P_2 Segment)

Anatomical Relationships

3 patients presented with aneurysms arising from the P_2 segment of the posterior cerebral artery between the junction of the posterior communicating artery and the entrance of the posterior cerebral artery into the quadrigeminal cistern. Aneurysms at this location are contained within the ambient cistern. All 3 aneurysms arose from the left posterior cerebral artery. 2 of the aneurysms were medium size and one of these was partially thrombosed. The third (No. 1) was a giant multilobular aneurysm about 60 mm in diameter, which was subtotally thrombosed (see Vol. I, Fig **232 A–D**). In one case there was an associated small aneurysm at the origin of the posterior communicating artery.

Operative Technique

Aneurysms at this location are approached subtemporally. A quadrilateral temporal bone flap is turned and the dura opened to give access to the floor of the middle fossa. There is often more than one small bridging vein on the undersurface of the temporal lobe, which must be coagulated and divided. The posterior cerebral artery is identified above the oculomotor nerve as it courses around the cerebral peduncle.

Each of these 3 aneurysms required a different method of treatment. The aneurysm (No. 2) which did not contain thrombus could be clipped following coagulation of the neck. The medium sized aneurysm (No. 3) which was partially thrombosed was also sclerotic and broad based. Temporary clips were applied to the posterior cerebral artery and the aneurysm was opened. Following removal of thrombus and calcified plaque from the walls of the aneurysm and artery, the artery was repaired with 8–0 sutures. The giant aneurysm (No. 1) extended both supratentorially into the temporal lobe and infratentorially along the mesencephalon. With removal of thrombus it could be seen that there was a general dilatation of the posterior cerebral artery at the base of the aneurysm. This segment of posterior cerebral artery, with the aneurysm was excised. Consideration was given to placing a bridge graft between the two ends of the posterior cerebral artery, but brisk back-bleeding from the distal end made this seem unnecessary.

Clinical Presentation and Operative Results

2 of these patients were men, a 29 year old with a medium sized aneurysm and a 36 year old with a giant aneurysm. The third patient was a 40 year old woman. 2 of the patients presented with subarachnoid hemorrhage and the patient with the giant aneurysm had had several episodes in previous years which were almost certainly subarachnoid hemorrhages, although his presenting history was that of a 3 year progressive right hemiparesis associated with a right homonymous hemianopia, epilepsy, and mental slowing. The clinical features of these patients are summarized in Table 115.

The 2 patients with smaller aneurysms have made complete recoveries and both have returned to their former activities. The man with a giant aneurysm is in a fair condition. He is able to care for himself, but not to work. He has a right hemiparesis and hemianopia as before. Another giant subtotally thrombosed aneurysm of the right P_2 segment was treated in a 20 year old female student in 1980 by clipping of the P_2 segment just proximal to the aneurysm-sac, thus saving the posterolateral choroidal artery (Fig **231A–C**, Vol. I, p. 293). This procedure could be contemplated because the carotid angiogram showed an excellent collateral circulation from the MCA and ACA to the PCA. The patient made a full recovery. The CT scan one year later showed almost total disappearance of the former giant aneurysm (Fig **231D–E**, Vol. I, p. 293).

Table 115 Clinical features in patients with aneurysms of the posterior cerebral artery (P_2 segment)

Name	Age	Sex	Year	SAH	Side	Preoperative deficits	Grade	Timing	Operation	Postoperative course	Result
1. Wy	35	M	1973	1	L	R hemiparesis R hemianopia Mild POS, Epilepsy	IIb	6 years	Trapping giant	Improvement	Fair
2. Be	39	F	1974	1	L	None	Ia	2 months	Clip	Full recovery	Good
3. Me	29	M	1975	2	L	Meningism Poor memory	IIa	7 days	Microsuture	Full recovery	Good

Posterior Cerebral Artery Aneurysms (P₃ Segment)

Anatomical Relationships

Included in this group are 3 patients whose aneurysms arose from the P₃ segment of the posterior cerebral artery within the quadrigeminal cistern at or near the primary division of the artery into calcarine and parieto-occipital branches (Table 116). This is just beneath the splenium of the corpus callosum and adjacent to the gyrus isthmus fornicati joining the hippocampal gyrus to the cingulate gyrus. 2 aneurysms were on the right side and 1 on the left; 2 were large aneurysms, and 1 small (see Fig 175A–B, Vol. I, p. 189). One aneurysm (No. 3) was completely thrombosed (see Fig 256A–F, Vol. I). One patient (No. 1) had undergone a previous exploration at another hospital through a subtemporal approach which was unsuccessful (Fig 131A–E). There were no additional aneurysms in these 3 patients.

Operative Technique

Aneurysms at this location are approached through an occipital craniotomy with the patient in the sitting position with a lumbar tape drain. The medial limb of the craniotomy should be just on the midline, so the retraction of the dura does not compress the superior sagittal sinus. The quadrilateral free bone flap is removed and the dura opened about 2 cm off midline, to create a rectangular flap which can be retracted across the midline. It is usually not necessary to open the more lateral dura over the occipital lobe which will protect the brain beneath the retractor, (although this may be opened in a stellate manner if required). Arachnoid bands holding the occipital pole to the falx are divided as are small bridging veins if necessary and the occipital lobe is retracted laterally a few millimeters after drainage of 20–30 cc cerebrospinal fluid. This should create the necessary space for the surgeon to visualize the quadrigeminal cistern beneath the splenium of the corpus callosum (Fig 131A–E).

The calcarine or parieto-occipital artery on the medial surface of the occipital lobe may be followed forward to identify the bifurcation of the posterior cerebral artery. The posterior cerebral artery can be prepared more laterally in the ambient cistern, just as it enters the quadrigeminal cistern. This gives proximal control should the aneurysm rupture during dissection. Attention is then turned to the preparation of the aneurysm neck. This was straightforward with the smaller aneurysm, but with the subtotally thrombosed aneurysm a clip could not be placed. A temporary clip had to be applied to the P₃ segment for 12 minutes to evacuate the aneurysm and to prepare a neck for clipping. The totally thrombosed aneurysm began to bleed from the base during dissection and was simply excised between 2 clips.

Clinical Presentation and Operative Results

All 3 patients were men, ages 44 to 46. 2 patients presented with subarachnoid hemorrhage, and the third (No. 3) was thought to have a pineal or thalamic tumor. The non-filling of the right PCA on vertebral angiogram and a well developed collateral circulation from the MCA and ACA to the area of the right PCA, seen on the carotid angiogram, was essential for the differential diagnosis and in predicting the outcome of operation. The 3 patients have done well. 2 made prompt recoveries, and the third who required temporary

Table 116 Clinical features in patients with aneurysms of the posterior cerebral artery (P₃ segment)

Name	Age	Sex	Year	SAH	Side	Preoperative deficits	Grade	Timing	Operation	Postoperative course	Result
1. Bu	45	M	1977	2	R	R hemianopia	IIb	4 months	Clip, large Temp. clip to PCA 12 min.	Improvement	Good
2. So	46	M	1978	1	L	Confusion Hydrocephalus	IIa	4 weeks	Clip small	Improvement	Good
3. St	44	M	1979	–	R	Somnolent L hemiparesis Ataxia	0b	–	Clip large	Improvement	Good

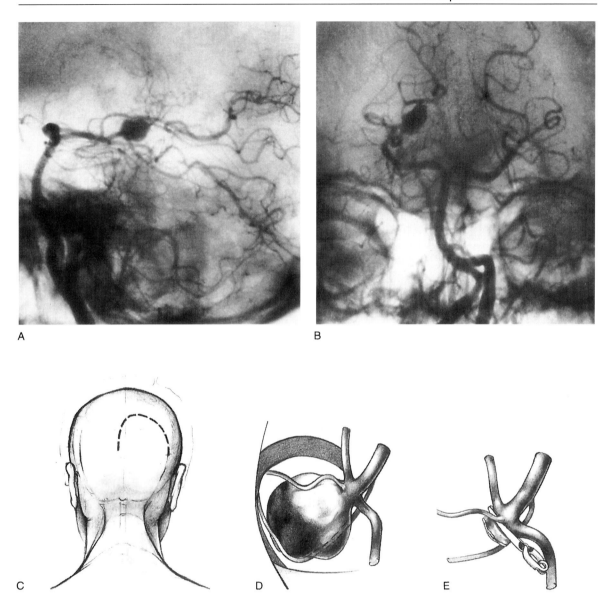

Fig 131A–E Right P_3–P_4 aneurysm (arrow) on angiography (**A** and **B**) that was clipped through an occipital craniotomy (**C**) with exposure of the aneurysm at the junction of the ambient and quadrigeminal cisterns (**D–E**) (Case 1, Table **116**).

clipping of the posterior cerebral artery had a transient homonymous hemianopia, but is now fully employed. The clinical features of these 3 patients are summarized in Table **116**. The important point with these aneurysms is that they must be approached by an occipital, interhemispheric route as they are not accessible by the subtemporal approach.

Saccular Aneurysms of the Lower Basilar Artery

Anatomical Relationships

There were 3 patients in the present series who presented with aneurysms arising from the lower basilar artery near the mid-portion of the artery (2 cases) or near the junction of the vertebral arteries (1 case). These aneurysms were large in 2 cases, and giant in one. In the 2 cases with smaller aneurysms, the fundus was directed anteriorly and was adherent to the dura over the clivus in each case. The giant aneurysm was directed posteriorly and had indented and expanded the pons. One of the 3 aneurysms involved the origin of an anterior inferior cerebellar artery, and in 1 case the trochlear nerve was compressed by the aneurysm.

Operative Technique

2 of these patients, a 51 year old man and a 23 year old woman had their aneurysms approached through a transoral clivectomy. The operative technique of transoral clivectomy for basilar artery aneurysm was discussed in detail in an earlier book (Yaşargil 1969a, pp. 132–139) and will not be elaborated upon here. Basically, under the foramen magnum using a high speed drill and the operating microscope, a trough about 25 mm by 8 mm is made in the clivus from the vomer to the foramen magnum, using a high speed drill and the dura opened to expose the basilar artery. While technically feasible, this procedure is fraught with complications and has not been used in the present series since 1968.

In the third case, a 34 year old woman was operated upon in 1975. The aneurysm was approached through a left lateral suboccipital craniotomy with the patient in the sitting position. Dissection had to be carried out between the left cranial nerves IX and X above and cranial nerve XI below, over the top of the hypoglossal rootlets. Vision was further hindered by an endostosis of the jugular foramen which was removed with the high speed drill. The anterior inferior cerebellar artery could be identified on the right side, but was absent on the left. When the arachnoid at the junction of the cerebellomedullary and prepontine cisterns had been dissected from the neck of the aneurysm, a clip could be slid beneath the left vertebral artery over cranial nerve VI to occlude the neck of the lesion. It was recognized at operation that if the aneurysm had ruptured during dissection, control of bleeding would have been exceedingly difficult as both vertebral arteries were supplying the aneurysm. Nevertheless, the case went well and at the present time these difficult aneurysms should be approached by the suboccipital route, rather than the transclival route (Fig **132A–C**). Completing this monograph (1982) a 34 year old female patient with a saccular aneurysm at the upper basilar trunk was operated through a right sided pterional craniotomy and the aneurysm clipped. The patient made a good recovery (Fig **133A–C**).

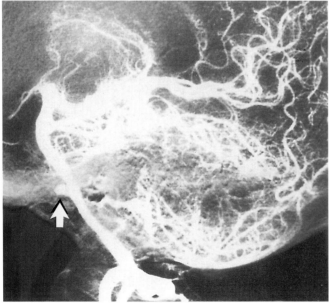

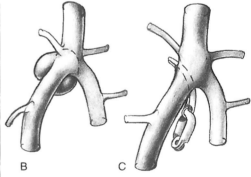

Fig **132A–C** Lower basilar trunk aneurysm (arrow) (**A** and **B**) with anteriorly directed fundus could be successfully clipped through a left sided lateral suboccipital approach (**C**).

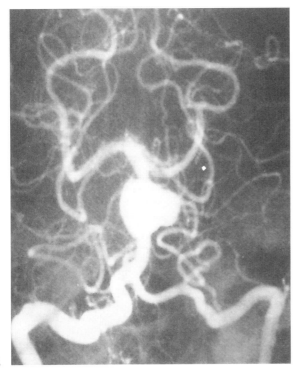
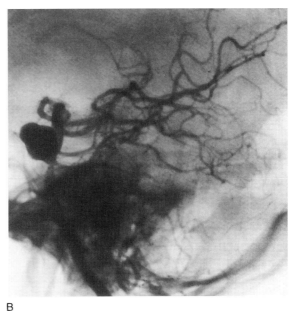
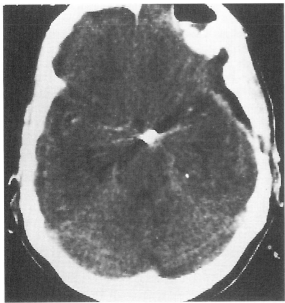

Fig 133A–C A saccular aneurysm of the upper third of the basilar trunk (**A** and **B**) could be clipped through a right sided pterional approach. Post-operative CT scan (**C**).

Clinical Presentation and Operative Results

These 3 patients each presented with subarachnoid hemorrhage. The 2 earlier patients both presented in grade IIIa and the more recent case was in grade IIa. The only focal abnormalities seen in these patients were a left abducens paresis in the male patient, and a partial loss of sensation in the face in the 23 year old lady.

The first 2 patients treated by the transoral clivectomy approach both died. A man who had only a mild left hemiparesis after surgery, ruptured a duodenal artery aneurysm and died from gastrointestinal hemorrhage 17 days after surgery. A young woman developed quadriparesis 12 hours after operation and subsequently required a ventricular shunt. This became infected and she died of meningitis 1 month after operation. Another 2 patients operated upon in 1975 and 1982 have returned to full activity.

Fusiform Aneurysms of the Lower Basilar Artery

Anatomical Relationships

5 patients have been seen in the last 6 years with giant fusiform aneurysms of the mid- and lower portions of the basilar artery. These aneurysms presented in younger patients, 5 to 25 years old. All were giant aneurysms which compressed the brain stem and cranial nerves, but also gave rise to subarachnoid hemorrhage. The aneurysms seemed to be inoperable when first evaluated.

The 5 aneurysms were similar in appearance. 4 began above the origin of the anterior inferior cerebellar arteries and ended below the origins of the superior cerebellar arteries. The segment of basilar artery giving rise to the aneurysm is between perforating arteries, such that even with large aneurysms, the perforating arteries arise from a short segment of normal appearing basilar artery just below the superior cerebellar arteries. The fifth began below the anterior inferior cerebellar arteries. These aneurysms are partially or subtotally thrombosed, and must expand slowly since despite marked displacement of brain stem and cranial nerves, symptoms were surprisingly minimal until just before the patients presented.

Operative Technique and Results

Because of the unique character of these aneurysms and the considerable operative difficulties encountered, the cases will be discussed individually:

Case 1: A. U., a 5 year old girl, complained of left retromastoid pain and disequilibrium in the summer of 1975. She was treated for anemia. In October 1975 she again complained of severe retromastoid pain and fell unconscious. Lumbar puncture revealed bloody cerebrospinal fluid. Vertebral angiography revealed a giant basilar artery aneurysm, and she was transferred 2 weeks later. Prior to operation she was somnolent with bilateral papilledema, absent left corneal reflex, paralysis of the motor branch of cranial nerve V, left facial weakness, a diminished gag reflex of the left, nasal speech, and a positive Babinski sign on the left (grade IIIb) (Fig **134A–C**).

The *first operation* was performed on 11 November, 1975. With the patient in the sitting position a suboccipital craniotomy was performed on the left side. The aneurysm ballooned into the left cerebellopontine angle. A clip was placed across the left vertebral above the origin of the posterior inferior cerebellar artery. A ventriculoperitoneal shunt was inserted. Postoperatively, the patient was alert and complained of lumbar pain. It was thought she might have vertebral tuberculosis because of an abnormal lumbar spine film, and she was transferred to a childrens hospital for treatment. On 15 December, 1975, 4 weeks after operation, she sustained a second subarachnoid hemorrhage. Angiography showed a greater contribution to the aneurysm from the right vertebral artery than had been present prior to the first operation (Fig **134D–E**).

At the *second operation* on 18 December, 1975, a right suboccipital craniotomy was performed and a clip placed on the right vertebral artery above the origin of the posterior inferior cerebellar artery. Postoperatively, she was mentally clear and moving all extremities. On 23 December, 1975, she suddenly became unresponsive with a right hemiparesis and left abducens palsy. Lumbar puncture showed fresh subarachnoid hemorrhage.

The *third operation* was performed on 24 December, 1975, as an emergency with the patient in grade IV. The upper basilar artery was exposed through a right pterional craniotomy. There was severe spasm of the right internal carotid artery and its branches, and the basal cisterns were full of hematoma. The lamina terminalis was bulging and was opened to release cerebrospinal fluid following which the brain immediately relaxed. Papaverine was applied to the carotid circulation and the temporal pole retracted laterally and posteriorly. The interpeduncular cistern was cleared of blood. Through a small gap lateral to the internal carotid artery and medial to the oculomotor nerve, the basilar artery was finally exposed. A clip could be brought across the basilar artery just below the origin of the anterior inferior cerebellar arteries. The aneurysm was opened and cleared of thrombus, but resection of the sac was not attempted (Fig **134F–H**).

The day following operation, the child was awake and active, and she recovered rapidly over the next several days. Carotid angiography showed good filling of the upper basilar artery through the posterior communicating arteries, and vertebral angiography showed filling of both vertebral arteries up to the posterior inferior cerebellar arteries. The patient showed mild bulbar symptomatology on discharge, but when seen 3 months later was free of symptoms. 7 years later she is in an excellent condition, physically and mentally.

Case 2: V. M., a 25 year old male sustained a subarachnoid hemorrhage on 24 August, 1976, associated with diplopia, dysarthria, tinnitus and a left hemiparesis. Angiography showed a giant fusiform aneurysm of the mid-basilar artery which was partially thrombosed. He was mentally slow with poor concentration span and recent memory (grade IIIb).

The *first operation* was performed on 23 November, 1976. The aneurysm was exposed through a right pterional craniotomy and the posterior clinoid process removed with the high speed drill. Nevertheless, it seemed impossible to clip this aneurysm and it was packed with muscle. He was discharged in good condition. In 1978, he complained of progressive ataxia,

Operative Technique and Results 273

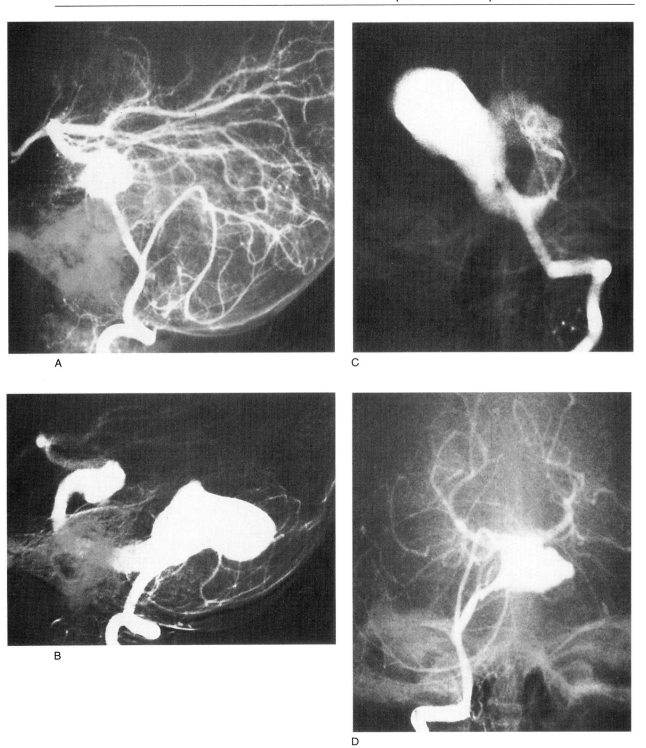

Fig 134 A–D Giant fusiform, partially thrombosed basilar trunk aneurysm in a 5 year old girl (**A, B, C** and **D**). It was trapped in 2 operations (see page 272, Case 1) with good recovery of the patient.

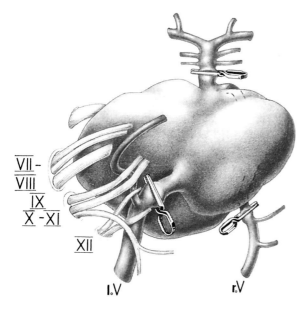

Fig 134 E   The operative procedure is shown diagrammatically.

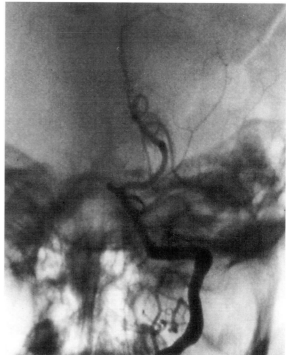

Fig 134 F   Postoperative left sided vertebral angiography demonstrated complete occlusion of the aneurysm.

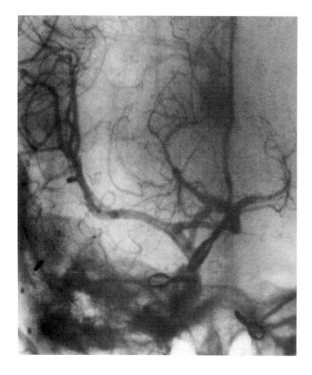

Fig 134 G   Right carotid angiography showed good collateralization of the upper basilar artery from the anterior circulation.

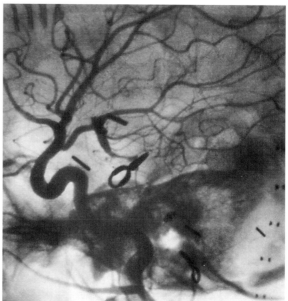

Fig 134 H   Lateral view of the right carotid angiogram.

Operative Technique and Results 275

dizziness, dysarthria, dysphagia and singultus. CT scan revealed the large basilar artery aneurysm. On examination he was slow, akinetic, ataxic, showed spasticity of all extremities and was unable to look to the left. Carotid angiography showed the right posterior communicating artery to be hypoplastic, but the left well developed.

At the *second operation* on 23 January, 1978, the aneurysm was approached through a left pterional craniotomy. A clip was placed across the basilar artery just above the anterior inferior cerebellar arteries and another across the basilar artery just below the superior cerebellar arteries. The aneurysm was opened and evacuated. Postoperatively, the patient's spasticity improved daily and his dysphagia and dysarthria disappeared within weeks. He returned to work and is in good condition.

Case 3: G. C., a 21 year old woman noted difficulty using her right limbs and paresthesia in the right hand in July, 1978. CT scan revealed a large prepontine tumor, which vertebral angiography demonstrated to be a large fusiform aneurysm of the basilar artery. She was first seen in Zurich on 25 August, 1978, at which time she was slow mentally with bilateral papilledema and a right hemiparesis and hemihypesthesia. CT scan showed the aneurysm to be 90 per cent thrombosed, and there was marked hydrocephalus. A shunt was inserted on 28 August, 1978, with general improvement. She persisted however, with a right hemiparesis and was often incontinent of urine (Fig **135A–C**).

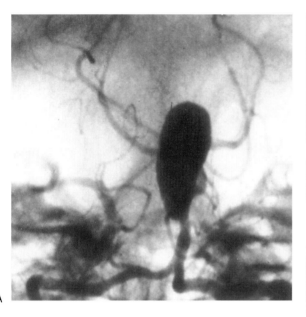

A

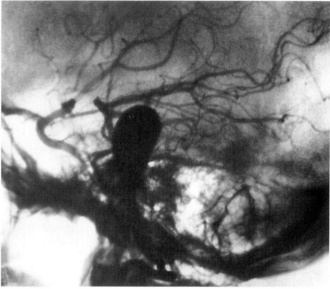

B

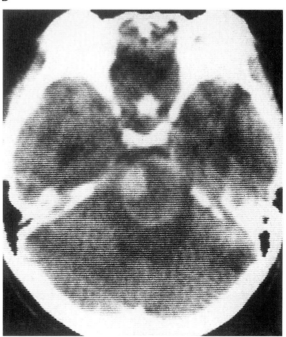

C

Fig **135A–F** Giant fusiform aneurysm of the distal basilar artery (**A** and **B**) that was partially thrombosed (**C**). The 21 year old patient underwent trapping and decompression of the aneurysm with good results.

Fig **135 D–F** ▶

Operation was performed on 7 September, 1978, with two consecutive craniotomies. The aneurysm was first approached through a left suboccipital craniotomy with the patient in the sitting position to introduce a clip across the basilar artery proximal to the aneurysm. The aneurysm completely filled the left cerebellopontine angle. The aneurysm was very close to the anterior inferior cerebellar arteries, and during tedious dissection to clear a space below the left artery, the aneurysm ruptured with torrential bleeding that was controlled only by introducing several pieces of muscle and oxycel into the aneurysm and closing the rent with cyanoacrylate. After a long battle, the left anterior inferior cerebellar artery finally had to be sacrificed to clip the basilar artery. The right anterior cerebellar artery had a more favorable proximal origin.

The patient was then turned to the supine position and the upper basilar artery exposed through a left pterional craniotomy. Angiography had shown that the right posterior communicating artery was the better collateral vessel. The basilar artery was clipped between the aneurysm and the origins of the superior cerebellar arteries, through a small gap between the internal carotid artery and oculomotor nerve.

Postoperatively, the patient was happily alert, but had respiratory difficulty and required a respirator for 9 days. By the end of a month she could speak and walk without assistance. The right hemiparesis cleared over the next several weeks and by 3 months she began to play the piano again. In April, 1979, she gave her first piano concert in over a year (Fig **135D–F**).

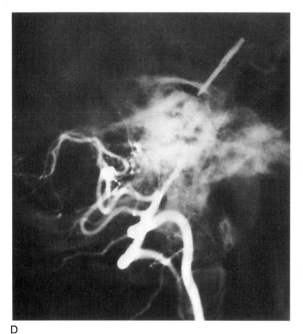

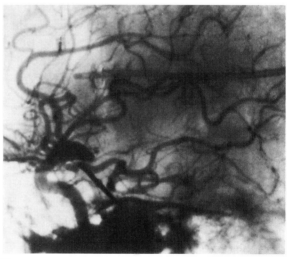

Fig **135D–F** Postoperative angiography (**D** and **E**) showed no filling of the aneurysm with good collateral flow from the carotids to the posterior cerebrals. On CT scan the aneurysm had disappeared (**F**) and the patient was able to complete her piano studies (Case 3, Table **117**).

Case 4: R. L., a 19 year old male sustained a subarachnoid hemorrhage on 25 March, 1978, without focal neurological deficit. Angiography showed a large basilar aneurysm. At the time of admission in April, 1978, he was somnolent and disorientated, with nuchal rigidity, papilledema, and dysdiachokinesis on the right side. CT scan showed hydrocephalus, but did not demonstrate the aneurysm. A ventriculo-atrial shunt was inserted on 17 April, 1978, with some improvement.

At *operation* on 5 May, 1978, the aneurysm was explored through a left suboccipital craniotomy. It was a large subtotally thrombosed lesion which could not be clipped, so it was partially covered with muscle on the exposed postero-inferior surface. The patient was discharged, but it was recommended that the patient undergo another attempt at a trapping procedure. The family wished to wait until summer. 6 weeks after discharge he re-bled and died (Fig **136A–B**).

Case 5: K. T., a 21 year old male noted onset of headache, vomiting, and difficulty with recent memory in June, 1978. CT scan showed a 30 mm prepontine tumor with hydrocephalus. A ventricular shunt was inserted on 3 August, 1978, with some improvement. Angiography on 25 October, 1978, showed a large fusiform basilar aneurysm. He was admitted to the University of Zurich on 2 November, 1978, and was noted to be mentally slowed with dysphagia, dysarthria, nystagmus on looking to the right, and a tetraparesis more pronounced on the right side. Following angiography, he became more somnolent and required respiratory assistance.

Operation was performed on 6 November, 1978. With the patient in the park bench position, a combined right sided temporo-occipital and suboccipital craniotomy was performed. The occipital artery had been damaged at the time of shunt insertion, and it was considered that the superficial temporal artery might be anastomosed to the superior cerebellar artery as the posterior communicating arteries were small bilaterally. The right vertebral artery was ligated above the origin of the posterior inferior cerebellar artery. The displacement of the brain stem from left to right by the aneurysm hindered application of clips to the left vertebral artery or upper basilar artery. This position and approach were much less satisfactory than if the patient had been in the sitting position using a suboccipital approach.

Immediately after operation, the patient was awake and breathing spontaneously. The following morning, he developed progressive respiratory insufficiency, and with the suspicion of tonsillar herniation he was returned to the operating theatre. In the sitting position, he was re-explored and no evidence of cerebellar edema found. He subsequently suffered a precipitious drop in blood pressure which led to cardiac arrest and he could not be resuscitated. The autopsy showed a partially thrombosed aneurysm at the lower basilar trunk. There was no sign of brain stem infarction (Fig **137A–D**).

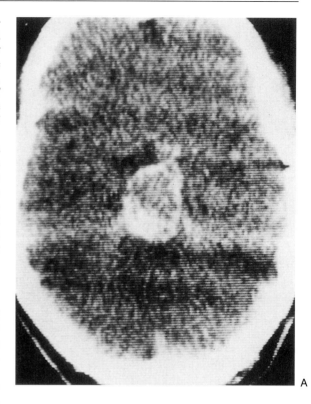

A

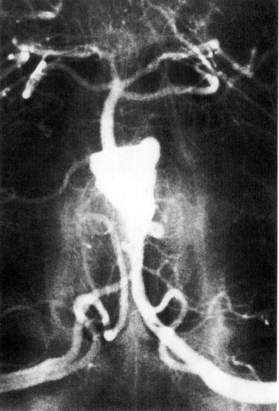

B

Fig **136A–B** Giant basilar aneurysm with no proper neck for clip application. The patient died before the scheduled trapping procedure could be performed (Case 4, Table **117**).

278 5 Vertebrobasilar Aneurysms

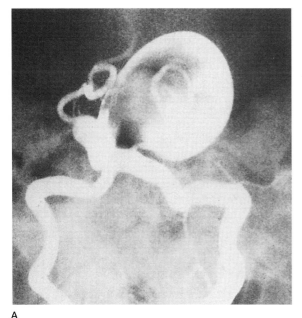

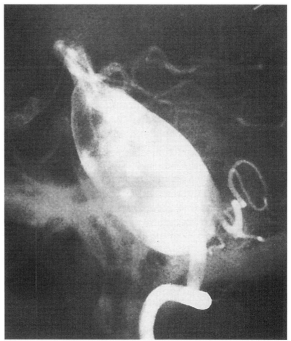

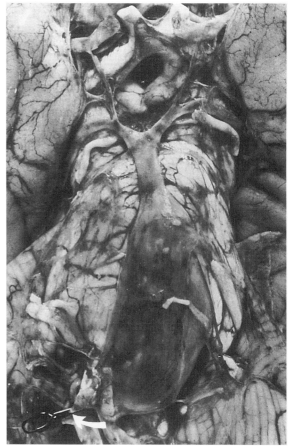

Fig 137A–D Giant fusiform aneurysm of the basilar artery (C) that produced bulbar symptoms and tetraparesis which deteriorated further after an angiogram (A and B). At operation the right vertebral artery was clipped with the patient in the lateral position. It was planned to attack the left vertebral artery at a second operation. The patient deteriorated progressively and died the next day. His autopsy showed a thrombosed basilar aneurysm (D) with no signs of brain stem infarction (Case 5, Table 117).

Table 117 Clinical features in 5 patients with giant fusiform aneurysms of the lower basilar artery

Name	Age	Sex	Year	SAH	Preoperative deficits	Grade	Timing	Operation	Postoperative course	Result
1. Ue	5	F	1975	3	Bulbar deficits L hemiparesis Somnolent	IIIb	3 weeks 3 days 1 day	Clip L Vert. A. Clip R Vert. A Clip Basilar A.	Full recovery	Good
2. Ma	25	M	1976	1	Bulbar deficits L hemiparesis	IIIb	4 weeks 3 months	Muscle Trap. basilar	Improvement	Good
3. Co	21	M	1978	0	Mentally slow Papilledema R hemiparesis	0b	6 weeks	Trapping Suboccipital Pterional	Full recovery	Good
4. Lo	19	M	1978	1	Somnolent R hemiparesis Preop shunt	IIIb	5 weeks	Muscle Trapping scheduled	Reruptured 2 months later	Death
5. Te	21	M	1978	0	Bulbar deficits Progressive parapar. Somnolent Impairment after angiography	0b	4 weeks	Lig. R. Vert. A.	Deterioration	Death

The clinical and operative features of these 5 patients are summarized in Table 117. 3 of the patients had good results and 2 died. Of those who died, one had only muscle wrapping of the aneurysm and while a trapping procedure had been planned, he reruptured and died. Trapping the mid-basilar artery has generally led to a rather stormy postoperative course, but with surprisingly good results after weeks to months. Untreated, these patients do very poorly. We assume that in case 3 ligation of the left vertebral artery would be a better course than partial muscle wrapping of the aneurysm sac. In case 5, an earlier exploration of the aneurysm and better scheduled surgery may have led to a good result.

Distal Superior Cerebellar Artery Aneurysms

Anatomical Relationships

In 2 cases aneurysms arose from the more distal portion of the superior cerebellar artery. Both aneurysms arose from the major division of the superior cerebellar artery into the superior vermian and hemispheric branches in the quadrigeminal cistern. The aneurysms were in close relation to the origin of the trochlear nerve. In 1 case the aneurysm was associated with an arteriovenous malformation on the anterior quadrangular lobule of the cerebellum draining to the quadrigeminal plate. One aneurysm arose from the left and 1 from the right. Both were large aneurysms and 1 was subtotally thrombosed with sclerotic walls. The aneurysms are shown in Fig **138A–D**.

Operative Technique and Results

These aneurysms were approached through a suboccipital retromastoid craniotomy. Dissection was carried out over the cerebellar hemisphere. Branches of the superior cerebellar artery were identified on the surface of the cerebellum and followed proximally into the cerebellopontine cistern where the aneurysm could be identified. In both cases it was indenting the trigeminal nerve. In addition to freeing the neck of the aneurysm from the parent arteries, it is important to dissect free the trochlear and trigeminal nerves. The superior petrosal vein is more lateral and can usually be preserved. One of these aneurysms was firmly adherent to the edge of the tentorial hiatus and had to be mobilized to some degree before a clip could be applied. In 1 case it was necessary to clip the superior cerebellar artery for 2 minutes in order to remove thrombus and atherosclerotic plaque (Fig **138A–D**).

These 2 patients were a 62 year old woman presenting in grade IIb and a 51 year old man undergoing operation in grade Ia. The first patient underwent operation 10 days after subarachnoid hemorrhage. Both patients have done well in the postoperative period and returned to their normal activities.

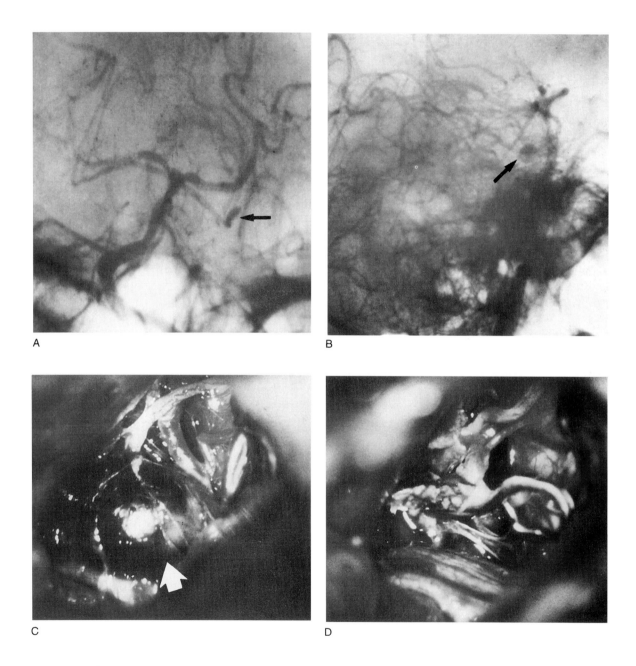

Fig **138A–D** Small left superior cerebellar bifurcation aneurysm (arrow) on angiography (**A** and **B**) and at operation before (arrow) (**C**) and after (**D**) clipping via a left suboccipital supracerebellar approach.

Saccular Aneurysms of the Vertebral Artery

Anatomical Relationships

In the present series, 10 patients presented with saccular aneurysms of the vertebral artery. In 9 cases the aneurysm arose at or just beyond the origin of the posterior inferior cerebellar artery. 7 of these aneurysms were medium to large lesions and 2 were giant aneurysms. In the tenth case, an aneurysm arose from the right vertebral artery just beyond its entrance into the subarachnoid space, and this was associated with a second small aneurysm arising in a fenestration of the vertebral artery, just distal to the origin of the posterior inferior cerebellar artery.

In 6 cases the aneurysm arose from the right side and in 4 cases from the left. In 2 cases there was marked hypoplasia of the vertebral artery, although in neither of these cases did the vertebral artery actually end as the posterior inferior cerebellar artery. One case had an associated large basilar bifurcation aneurysm, which was not explored. Aneurysms arising at the origin of the posterior inferior cerebellar artery are contained within the lateral cerebellomedullary cistern. They lie above or beneath the rootlets of the hypoglossal nerve in the neighborhood of cranial nerves X and XI. Hematoma was seen to dissect into the prepontine cistern in 2 cases and both these suffered abducens nerve pareses at the time of aneurysm rupture. These aneurysms are generally directed posteriorly elevating the hypoglossal nerve rootlets, but may be directed anteriorly, superiorly or laterally, and be attached to the dura.

Operative Technique

Small and medium sized aneurysms are best approached through a paramedian suboccipital craniotomy as described in detail in Vol. I, Chapter 3. The craniotomy may extend somewhat more medially than is routine, but it is generally not necessary to open into the foramen magnum. Orientation begins with identification of the spinal accessory nerve, which is followed to the jugular foramen. The bulbar nerves are then dissected in the lateral cerebellomedullary cistern to the brain stem. The vertebral artery is identified alongside the medulla as it enters the subarachnoid space. Almost invariably dissection must be performed between the rootlets of the hypoglossal nerve. Cranial nerve VII through XI, are more superior and dorsal and may be adherent to a large aneurysm. The neck of the aneurysm is developed by separating adhesions between the origin of the posterior inferior cerebellar artery and the aneurysm wall until a clip can be placed across the neck without compromising the adjacent artery (Fig **139A–D**).

It was possible in 7 cases to achieve good clip placement with coagulation and clip adjustments required in 4 cases. In one of these cases, there was some dilatation of the vertebral artery at the base of the aneurysm and a large anterior spinal artery exited at this point precluding the possibility of a trapping procedure. This portion of the artery was wrapped in muscle.

The 2 cases of giant aneurysm presented considerable operative difficulty and these will be presented in more detail.

H., a 61 year old lady experienced spontaneous dilatation of the left pupil at age 25, which resolved without sequelae. A year prior to admission she began to complain of paresthesia of the left toes and heaviness in the lower extremity. This came to be associated with dysphagia and drooping of the right corner of the mouth. 6 months prior to admission she began to complain of burning dysesthesia of the left index finger. At the time of admission on 6 July, 1970, she was alert, but demonstrated nystagmus on looking to the left, paralysis of the left trapezius and sternocleidomastoid muscles, left hemiparesis with a positive Babinski sign, and ataxia (grade 0b). Angiography revealed a large aneurysm of the right vertebral artery.

At operation on 10 July, 1970, the aneurysm was approached from the right side through a lateral suboccipital craniotomy. The aneurysm filled the entire subarachnoid space on the right side, compressing all cranial nerves from V to XII, and extending beneath the ventrolateral aspect of the pons and medulla. The neck began 3 to 4 mm distal to the origin of the posterior inferior cerebellar artery. Cranial nerves V, VII and VIII in the cerebellopontine cistern were draped superiorly over the fundus. Cranial nerve VI in the prepontine cistern was pushed anterolaterally and cranial nerves IX, X and XI in the lateral cerebello-medullary cistern were stretched over the inferior aspect of the fundus. The aneurysm was freed from surrounding structures and a silk ligature passed around the neck. The neck was partially occluded and a clip applied. The sac was then opened and thrombus removed. The wall of the aneurysm was coagulated and a second clip

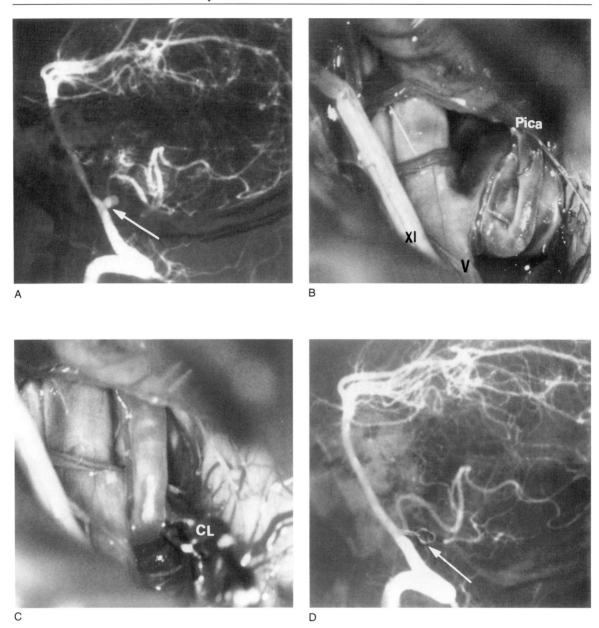

Fig 139A–D Case 10, Table 118. Small left vertebral artery aneurysm (arrow) at the origin of the posterior inferior cerebellar artery (A) before (B) and after (C) clipping. Postoperative angiogram (D) showing obliteration of the aneurysm with patency of PICA (arrow).

applied. The ligature could then be removed. Thrombus and plaque were removed from the aneurysm, but the fundus was too adherent to the brain stem to be safely removed (Fig **140A–C**).

The postoperative course was difficult. She required nasogastric feeding, developed aspiration pneumonitis and subsequently required a tracheostomy. The nasogastric tube was removed on 6 August, 1970, and she was able to return to her home hospital on 27 August, 1970, 48 days after operation. When examined 2 years later she showed no difficulty with swallowing and no extremity weakness. She has now fully recovered and is working.

E. F., a 44 year old woman presented in 1958 with a subarachnoid hemorrhage and was found to have an aneurysm of the anterior cerebral artery, which was clipped. 2 months after that operation she began to complain of intermittent heaviness of the left extremities, which occurred 3 to 4 times per day. Complaints persisted in mild degree over the next 9 years during which time she went through a normal pregnancy. In 1968, she noted numbness of the left face and on 22 April, 1971,

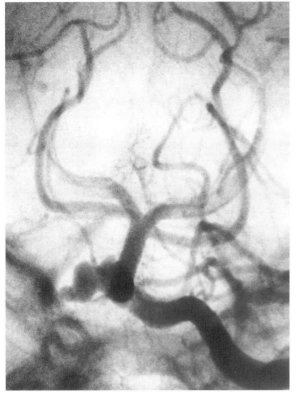
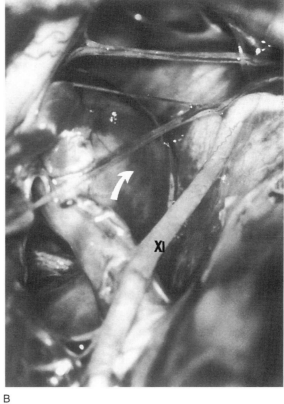
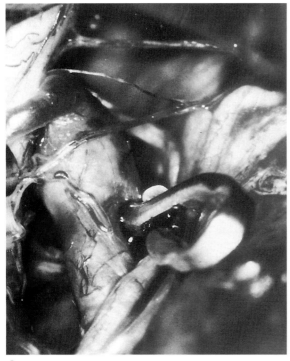

Fig 140A–C Case 2, Table 119. Partially thrombosed large right vertebral aneurysm at posterior inferior cerebellar artery (**A**), before (arrow) (**B**) and after clipping (**C**).

complained of sudden headache, diplopia, and dysphagia. A diagnosis of vertebrobasilar insufficiency was made. In November 1971 she exhibited nystagmus, anisocoria, weakness of the left face, left tongue and right side of the body. Vertebral angiography demonstrated a giant aneurysm arising from the left vertebral artery, which was 90 per cent thrombosed. On 30 November, 1971, she developed acute respiratory difficulty, and inability to swallow oral secretions and was taken to the operating room.

The aneurysm was approached through a left lateral suboccipital craniotomy with the patient in the sitting position. The large aneurysm compressed the pons and medulla on the left side and had displaced all the cranial nerves on that side. Despite the large size of the aneurysm, the neck was surprisingly small. Nevertheless, thrombus prevented application of a clip, which when placed on the neck would twist and strangulate the posterior inferior cerebellar artery. The wall of the aneurysm was partially calcified. An incision was made into the aneurysm without application of temporary clips and thrombus and plaque subtotally removed. A clip could then be applied to the aneurysm neck. No attempt was made to remove the adherent fundus from the brain stem.

In the immediate postoperative period, the patient required assisted ventilation and was quadriparetic. She was hypotensive and hypothermic and had large, sluggishly reactive pupils. Tracheostomy was performed on 2 December, 1971. A ventriculo-atrial shunt was performed on 15 February, 1972. She made a gradual, but progressive recovery and was discharged on 22 March, 1972, after the tracheostomy was removed. A year later, she was able to care for herself at home, 2 years later she was fully recovered and active.

Clinical Presentation and Operative Results

The ages of these 10 patients, of whom 8 were women, ranged from 14 years to 61 years. The 8 patients with medium to large aneurysms all presented with subarachnoid hemorrhage. 4 of these showed only symptoms of subarachnoid hemorrhage, and 1 other had conjugate deviation of the eyes for several hours as the only localizing finding. The other 3 patients had typical posterior fossa symptomatology, including unilateral hypoglossal palsy, ataxia, nystagmus, and hearing loss. The 2 patients with giant aneurysms each presented with a long history of progressive brain stem and cranial nerve dysfunction, although one had had a previous subarachnoid hemorrhage from another aneurysm. Clinical features of these patients are summarized in Table **118**.

8 patients (80%) made a good recovery, although in the case of the lady with a giant right vertebral artery aneurysm recovery was prolonged. One patient is fair. This patient was in grade IIa at the time of operation and required ventricular shunting postoperatively. She has remained somewhat slow with an insecure gait, but is able to care for herself at home.

Treatment of aneurysms of the vertebral artery is reasonably straightforward. Giant aneurysms acting like tumors, however, damage the brain stem and cranial nerves and a protracted postoperative course can be expected.

Table 118 Clinical features in 10 patients with saccular aneurysms of the vertebral artery

Name	Age	Sex	Year	SAH	Side	Preoperative deficits	Grade	Timing	Operation	Postoperative course	Result
1. Hy	61	F	1970	0	R	L hemiparesis Nystagmus R CN XI palsy	0b	–	Clip	Thrombosed giant L. CPA-aneurysm aspiration pneumonitis improved	Good
2. Fi	44	F	1971	0	L	AcoA An. 13 years before R hemiparesis Bulbar deficits	0b	–	Clip	Thrombosed giant L. PcoA aneurysm recovery	Good
3. Bi	42	M	1974	1	R	Drowsy	IIa	4 weeks	Clip	Full recovery	Good
4. He	49	F	1974	1	R	Confusion Ataxia	IIIa	5 weeks	Clip	Full recovery	Good
5. Ac	31	F	1974	2	L	Confusion Bil. CN VI pal.	IIIa	2 weeks	Clip	Full recovery	Good
6. Mi	40	F	1975	1	R	Drowsy Bil. CN VI pal.	IIa	II days	Clip	Full recovery	Good
7. Br	50	F	1975	2	R	Somnolent R CN XII palsy	IIa	3 weeks	Clip	Hydrocephalus, shunt mentally slow ataxia	Fair
8. Kl	14	M	1978	2	L	Neck pain	Ia	7 months	Clip	Full recovery	Good
9. Ri	33	F	1979	1	R	Meningism, Add. R. vert. aneurysm + Fenestration of VA and aneurysm	IIa	7 days	Clip	Full recovery	Good
10. Br	60	F	1979	1	L	Drowsy add. Bas. Bif. aneurysm	IIa	2 weeks	Clip	Full recovery	Good

Fusiform Aneurysms of the Vertebral Artery

Anatomical Relationships

3 patients presented with giant aneurysmal dilatations of one vertebral artery. In one case, the aneurysm began above the posterior inferior cerebellar artery, in a second the origin of this artery was thrombosed over a 5 mm segment and in the third the entire intracranial left vertebral artery had undergone dilatation, so that the posterior inferior cerebellar artery, the anterior spinal artery and the arteries to the medulla originated from the aneurysm.

In 2 of the cases, the aneurysm filled most of the ipsilateral cerebellomedullary and cerebellopontine cisterns.

In the larger of these, cranial nerve V was draped over the superior pole of the aneurysm, cranial nerves VII and VIII were stretched over the midportion and cranial nerves IX, X and XI were laid over the inferior pole. The hypoglossal rootlets could not be seen. The aneurysm extended partially beneath the medulla and had twisted the brain stem about 30 degrees to the left.

In the third case, the left vertebral artery which was grossly dilated coursed to the right side of the posterior fossa beneath the brain stem invading the prepontine and premedullary cisterns, and adhering partially to the clivus. The entire lower brain stem was displaced posteriorly, but the cranial nerves were, surprisingly, not involved with the aneurysm. In none of the 3 cases was the contralateral vertebral artery involved in the aneurysmal dilatation.

Operative Technique and Surgical Results

The first patient was a 39 year old man who presented with bulbar symptomatology and dysfunction of cranial nerves V to XII on the left. He first underwent operation from the left side. The aneurysm was seen to be a moderate dilatation of the entire intracranial vertebral artery, giving origin to the posterior inferior cerebellar artery, the anterior spinal artery, and several smaller medullary arteries. The medulla was compressed and displaced to the right by the very sclerotic dilated left vertebral artery. There was no place to put a clip without compromising these arteries, and the lesion was covered with muscle. Postoperatively, the patient was unchanged but over the next 6 months developed progressive

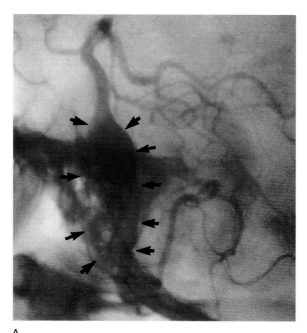

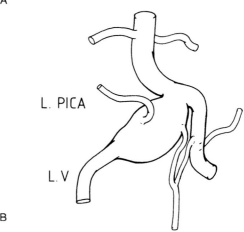

Fig **141A–B** Fusiform aneurysm of the left vertebral artery, which compressed and displaced the medulla to the right. Clip application was not possible (Case 1, Table **119**).

bulbar symptomatology and died (Fig **141A–B**) (No. 1, Table **119**).

The second patient, a 35 year old lady (No. 2, Table **119**), presented with subarachnoid hemorrhage and posterior fossa signs and left vertebral angiography disclosed a giant subtotally thrombosed aneurysm of the right distal vertebral artery and right vertebral angiography demonstrated only the PICA. Operation was performed through a generous midline suboccipital craniotomy. The bulk of the aneurysm on the right vertebral artery

Table 119 Clinical features in 3 patients with fusiform aneurysms of the vertebral artery

Name	Age	Sex	Year	Side	SAH	Preoperative deficits	Grade	Timing		Operation	Result
1. Ro	39	M	1970	L	–	Dysesthesia R. side of body CNs V–XII lesion L. since 3 m	0b	3 m	Fusiform L. VA aneurysm up to basilar junction	Muscle wrapping	6 m Death
2. Ha	35	F	1972	R	1	Headache, Vomiting L. hpr. after SAH, bulbar symptomatology Tracheostomy	IIIb	4 w	Subtotally thromb. R. VA aneurysm visualized by L. vert. angiography	Trapping and removal of giant aneurysm	Good
3. Pr	15	M	1975	R	1	Headache 3 y. Diplopia, Meningitis 4 w after SAH	IIa	2 w	Subtotally thromb. middle sized R. VA aneurysm visualized by L. vert. angiogr. in proximal part near basilar junction	Clip from L. side inferior to bulbus, to R. VA	Good

prevented any real progress in dissection, so the aneurysm was incised and thrombus removed until brisk bleeding was encountered. A temporary clip could then be placed across the right vertebral artery, just distal to the aneurysm. Following this all bleeding stopped, so it was traded for a permanent clip. A second clip was placed across the vertebral artery, just below the origin of the thrombosed posterior inferior cerebellar artery. Consideration was given to reimplanting the posterior inferior cerebellar artery into the vertebral artery, but with division of the posterior inferior cerebellar artery there was brisk backbleeding and it was decided simply to ligate the artery. The patient demonstrated marked bulbar symptomatology postoperatively, and required endotracheal intubation for 7 days. She nevertheless went on to make a complete recovery within 3 months. She is in an excellent condition in 1982.

The third case was that of a 15 year old boy who also presented with subarachnoid hemorrhage and lower cranial nerve dysfunction. Vertebral angiography suggested a left vertebral artery aneurysm, and the right vertebral artery was seen to end in the posterior inferior cerebellar artery. Operation was thus undertaken through a left suboccipital craniotomy. At operation, however, the aneurysm was, in fact, a large subtotally thrombosed aneurysm arising from the right vertebral artery, which covered, but did not directly involve the left vertebral artery. Working beneath the medulla it was possible to create enough space on the right vertebral artery at the vertebral artery junction to place a clip across it, thereby excluding flow from the left vertebral artery into the aneurysm. The lower portion of the aneurysm on the right side could not be seen, but this was felt to be thrombosed on the basis of the angiogram, and postoperative angiography indeed confirmed this. He made a rapid recovery, and is in an excellent condition in 1982 (Fig 142A–D).

Clinical features are summarized in Table 119.

Trapping of large fusiform aneurysms of the vertebral artery can be an effective treatment when collateral circulation in the posterior fossa is good. Both patients in whom the aneurysm could be trapped have done well, while the one patient (No. 1) who could not be treated showed progressive deterioration. There were no operative opportunities for repairing the whole left vertebral artery.

Completing this monograph, another patient (33 years old male) was admitted for treatment in extremis, after developing progressive deterioration on his pontobulbar symptoms. Ligation of the left vertebral artery in his home-hospital remained ineffective. Operative exploration showed that the left vertebral artery could be trapped and the subtotally thrombosed sac, which displaced the ponto-bulbar region massively from the left to the right, could be removed. The origin of the anterior spinal artery was saved. The postoperative course of the respiratory-dependent patient was dramatic as he recovered within a short time (Fig 143A–E).

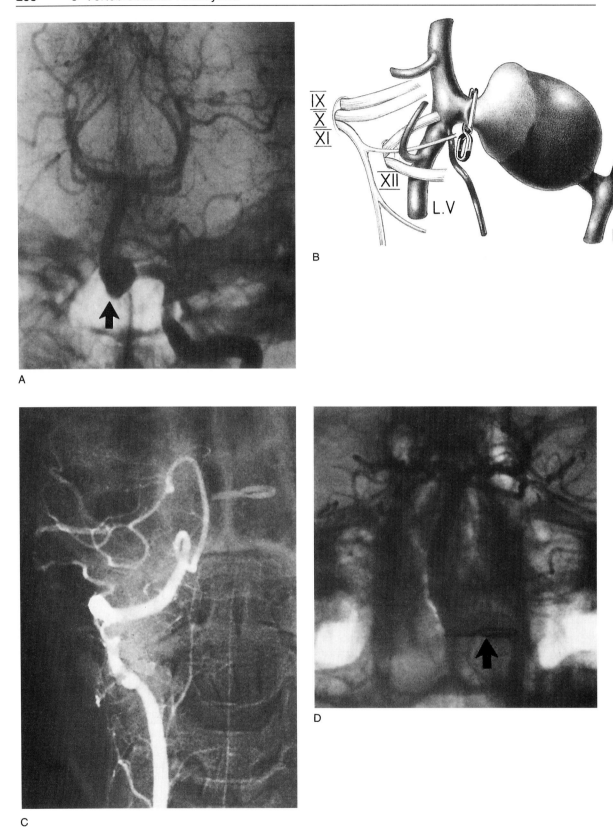

Fig 142A–D Partially thrombosed vertebral aneurysm (arrow) at its termination seen only on left vertebral angiography (**A**). It was explored via a left sided approach and clipped under the pons, sparing the anterior spinal artery (**B**). The patient made an uneventful recovery as evidenced by his normal postoperative angiography; right vertebral artery is ending as PICA (**C**). Left vertebral angiography (**D**) (Case 3, Table **119**).

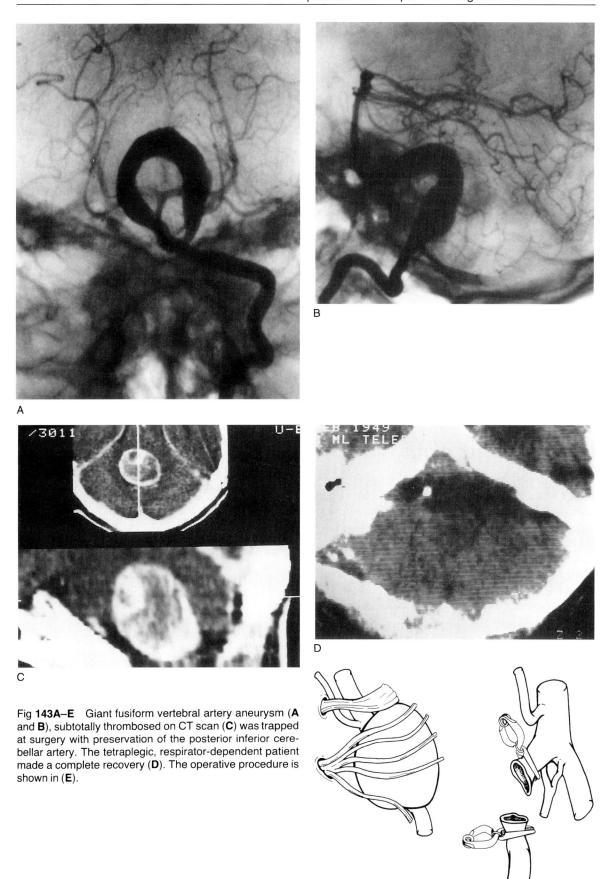

Fig 143A–E Giant fusiform vertebral artery aneurysm (**A** and **B**), subtotally thrombosed on CT scan (**C**) was trapped at surgery with preservation of the posterior inferior cerebellar artery. The tetraplegic, respirator-dependent patient made a complete recovery (**D**). The operative procedure is shown in (**E**).

Distal Posterior Inferior Cerebellar Artery Aneurysms

Anatomical Relationships

5 patients presented with aneurysms on the distal portion of the posterior inferior cerebellar artery. This segment of the artery lies in the vallecular portion of the cisterna magna on the dorsal surface of the lower cerebellar vermis and between the cerebellar tonsils. These aneurysms are in close proximity to the inferior cerebellar peduncle (restiform body) which accounts for the frequent findings of ataxia and nystagmus in these patients. In 1 of these cases there were 3 asymptomatic aneurysms on the right posterior inferior cerebellar artery associated with a ruptured arteriovenous malformation in the ipsilateral cerebellar hemisphere. In 2 other cases, there was a symmetrical small aneurysm on the opposite posterior inferior cerebellar artery, a situation reminiscent of that seen with aneurysms of the distal anterior cerebral artery.

Operative Technique

These 5 patients each underwent operation in the sitting position through a midline suboccipital craniotomy. The dorsal midline position of these aneurysms favors this over the usual paramedian suboccipital craniotomy employed for other aneurysms in the posterior fossa. The cisterna magna is opened in the midline and the cerebellar tonsils retracted. Hematoma is commonly present in the cisterna magna and in one of these cases this extended into the fourth ventricle and into the vermis and biventer lobule of the cerebellum. Hematoma is removed leaving a small amount in the immediate vicinity of the aneurysm until control of the posterior inferior cerebellar artery has been gained. Preparation of this artery is generally not difficult and arachnoid adhesions are separated until the neck of the aneurysm is delineated. The primary difficulty with clip application is that the neck may be broad such that the clip kinks the posterior inferior cerebellar artery. In 1 case it was necessary to use 2 clips to avoid this. A trapping procedure was not required in any of these 4 cases, although with adequate collateral circulation this may be feasible, especially when the aneurysm is quite distal on the artery, beyond the major supply to the lateral medulla and restiform body.

Clinical Presentation and Operative Results

Of these 5 cases, 3 were women and 2 men. All presented with at least one subarachnoid hemorrhage, and 3 of the 5 presented with focal neurological deficits, indicative of a posterior fossa lesion. Clinical features of the 5 patients are summarized in Table **120** (Figs **144A-B, 145A-B**). Good operative results were obtained in 4 patients. Of these, one patient (No. 2, Table **120**) had angiographic demonstration of her aneurysm only after a second subarachnoid hemorrhage, because the right vertebral artery was not injected at the initial angiography. The same situation was encountered in another case in 1981. These cases highlight the importance of complete angiography in cases of subarachnoid hemorrhage. In case No. 3 (Table **120**), the preoperative diagnosis (1975) was a cerebellar tumor, as at that time no CT was available. Vertebral angiography did not demonstrate the aneurysm and by operative exploration a bilobular aneurysm was found at the choroidal point of the left PICA within a hematoma. A second small aneurysm at the same level on the right PICA was also found.

Table 120 Clinical features in 5 patients with aneurysms of the distal posterior inferior cerebellar artery

Name	Age	Sex	Year	Side	SAH	Preoperative deficits	Grade	Timing	Operation	Postoperative course	Result
1. Fa	50	M	1971	R	3	Drowsy, ataxia, hearing loss, Addit. 3 aneurysms on the same PICA and associated AVM	IIb	18 d	3 aneurysms Clip/clip/clip Excision AVM	Full recovery	Good
2. Bu	30	F	1971	R	2	Somnolent R CN VII par.	IIIa	13 d	Clip	Full recovery	Good
3. Bo	15	F	1975	L	2	Drowsy Meningism Add. aneurysm of PICA R. Somnolent	IIa	12 d	Clip	Full recovery	Good
4. Ma	46	M	1978	L	1	Somnolent Meningism Add. aneurysm on other PICA	IIa	12 d	Clip	Full recovery	Good
5. Fr	56	F	1978	L	1	Somnolent, Bulbocerebellar def.	IIb	3 m	Clip	Slow recovery	Fair

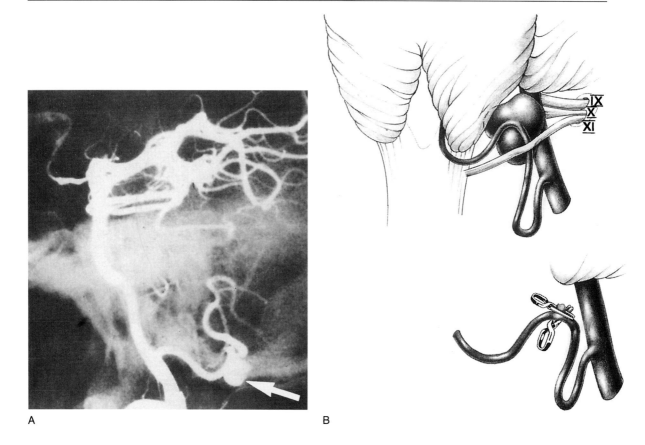

Fig 144 A–B Right distal posterior inferior cerebellar artery aneurysm (arrow) (bilobular) on angiography (**A**) and at exploration (**B**) (Case 2, Table **120**). After her first subarachnoid hemorrhage this 30 year old female patient was studied with bilateral carotid and left sided vertebral angiography which showed neither aneurysm nor AVM. Two years later she rebled and was comatose for several days, developing hydrocephalus which required a shunt. The previously neglected right vertebral angiogram was performed demonstrating a PICA aneurysm.

Fig **145A–B** Displacement of the infratentorial arteries due to a large hematoma (arrow). Bilobular choroidal point posterior inferior cerebellar artery aneurysm hidden on angiography (**A**) was discovered at surgery and clipped (**B**) (Case 3, Table **120**).

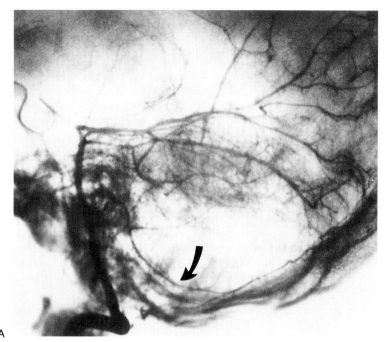

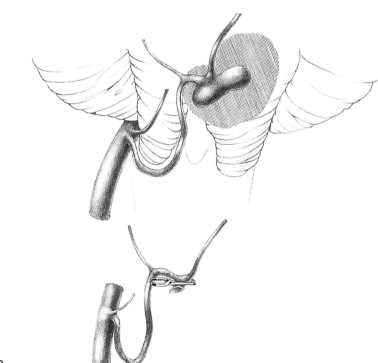

Summary

In the present series, 97 patients underwent operation for aneurysm of the vertebro-basilar circulation. Overall results are related to preoperative grade in Table **121**. Over half of the patients presented with aneurysms of the basilar artery bifurcation. Treatment of these aneurysms has success comparable to aneurysms of the anterior circulation when the aneurysm is directed away from the mesencephalon. However, for the more common posteriorly directed aneurysms, which are often large and filled with thrombus, operative treatment has been less successful in this series of patients. Timing of surgery and results are presented in Table **122a** and **b**.

Approaches to aneurysms on the vertebro-basilar circulation are summarized in Table **123**. Aneurysms present at distinct locations along the posterior cerebral artery. The exact location of these aneurysms is important, as aneurysms of the P_1 segment should be approached through a pterional craniotomy, aneurysms of the P_2 segment subtemporally, and those of the P_3 segment through an occipital, interhemispheric approach.

2 special types of fusiform aneurysm were encountered in this group of patients. 5 patients all under 25 years old had giant fusiform aneurysms of the middle and lower portions of the basilar artery. 3 of these could be successfully treated by trapping. 3 other patients had giant fusiform aneurysms of one vertebral artery and in two of these trapping was successful.

Treatment of saccular aneurysms of the vertebral arteries and lower basilar artery is best accomplished through a lateral paramedian suboccipital craniotomy in the sitting position. Experience with transoral clivectomy in 2 patients early in the series was unsatisfactory, and suboccipital craniotomy should be tried first in cases of lower basilar artery aneurysm. Aneurysms distal on the posterior inferior cerebellar artery are in the midline and are approached through a midline craniotomy. Brain stem, cranial nerve, and cerebellar symptomatology may alert the physician to the presence of an aneurysm in the posterior fossa, but the importance of complete angiography including vertebral artery injections in cases of subarachnoid hemorrhage is clear. Successful management of these aneurysms requires the use of varied therapeutic and operative modalities.

Table **121** Operative results related to preoperative grade in 97 patients with aneurysms of the vertebro-basilar arteries and their branches

Aneurysms	Total	Good	Clipped Fair	Poor	Death	Total	Good	Muscle Fair	Poor	Death
Bbi	40	32	2	4	2	10	5	2	1	2
PCA+SCA	4	3	–	–	1	1	1	–	–	–
P_1	4	3	–	1	–	1	1	–	–	–
P_1/P_2	3	3	–	–	–	–	–	–	–	–
P_2	3	2	1	–	–	–	–	–	–	–
P_3	3	3	–	–	–	–	–	–	–	–
SCA	2	2	–	–	–	–	–	–	–	–
Btr, sacc.	3	1	–	–	2	–	–	–	–	–
fusif.	4	3	–	–	1	1	–	–	–	1
VA PICA orig.	10	9	1	–	–	–	–	–	–	–
Vtr, sacc.	2	2	–	–	–	–	–	–	–	–
fusif.	–	–	–	–	–	1	–	–	–	1*
PICA distal	5	5	–	–	–	–	–	–	–	–
	83 (85.6%)	68 (81.9%)	4 (4.8%)	5 (6.0%)	6 (7.2%)	14 (14.4%)	7 (50%)	2 (14.3%)	1 (7.1%)	4 (28.6%)

* muscle wrapped

Summary 295

Table 122a Timing of surgery and results in 15 patients with ruptured aneurysm of the vertebral artery and its branches

	Good					Fair		
	Ia	IIa	IIb	IIIa	IIIb	IIa	IIb	
1–3 d	–	–	–	–	–	–	–	
4–7 d	–	1	–	–	–	–	–	
1–2 w	–	3	–	1	–	–	–	
2–4 w	–	3	1	1	1	–	–	
1–3 m	–	–	–	1	–	1	–	
> 3 m	1	–	–	–	–	–	1	
	1	7	1	3	1	1	1	= 15

Table 122b Timing of surgery and results in 24 patients with ruptured aneurysm of the basilar trunk and basilar branches

	Good					Fair		Death		
	Ia	Ib	IIa	IIb	IIIa	IIIb		IIa	IIIb	
1–3 d	–	–	–	–	–	–	–	–	–	
4–7 d	–	–	1	–	–	–	–	–	–	
1–2 w	–	–	–	1	–	–	–	1	1	
2–4 w	3	1	1	–	1	1	–	2	–	
1–3 m	3	1	–	1	1	1	–	–	–	
> 3 m	–	2	1	–	–	–	1	–	–	
	6	4	3	2	2	2	1	3	1	= 24

Table 123 Surgical approach to basilar aneurysms

	Approach	Total	Trapping	Clip	Muscle
1) Basilar trunk (giant)	Combined 1) Subocc. + pterional 2) Suboccip.	3 2	4	–	1
2) Basilar trunk (saccular)	1) Transclival 2) Subocc.	2 1	– –	2 1	– –
3) Superior cerebellar A.	Infratent. supracerebellar	2	–	2	–
4) Posterior cerebral A. P$_2$	Subtemp.	3	1	2	–
5) Posterior cerebral A. P$_3$	Parietooccipital	3	1	2	–
6) Superior cerebellar A. Posterior cerebral A.	Pterional	5	1	3	1
Basilar bifurcation	Pterional	50	2	38	10
Posterior cerebral A. P$_1$	Pterional	5	3	1	1
Posterior cerebral A. P$_1$/P$_2$	Pterional	3	1	2	–
		79	13	53	13

6 Giant Intracranial Aneurysms

Aneurysms larger than 2.5 cm in diameter have been defined as giant aneurysms (Morley and Barr 1969; Sahs et al. 1969). Most larger aneurysms are anatomically quite irregular and asymmetrical, thus making any size categorization both arbitrary and imprecise. In the present series, any aneurysm that measured more than 2.5 cm in any dimension was considered a giant aneurysm.

The incidence of giant aneurysms varies in the literature from 3–13 per cent of all intracranial aneurysms (Morley and Barr 1969; Sahs et al. 1969; Sonntag et al. 1977; Hosobuchi 1979; Onuma and Suzuki 1979; Sundt and Piepgras 1979; Pia 1980), but in large series averages 5 per cent (Locksley 1966). In most series these lesions have been reported in a female/male ratio of about 3:1 (Morley and Barr 1969; Sonntag et al. 1977; Hosobuchi 1979), but Onuma and Suzuki (1979) reported an equal sex prevalence in 32 cases. Creissard et al. (1980) reported that intracavernous and middle cerebral giant aneurysms predominate in males while internal carotid lesions are found more frequently in females. As with other smaller saccular intracranial aneurysms, giant aneurysms usually initially present in the 40–60 age group (Morley and Barr 1969; Hosobuchi 1979; Onuma and Suzuki 1979). Giant aneurysms may be one of multiple aneurysms in 10–30 per cent of cases (Morley and Barr 1969; Sonntag et al. 1977; Hosobuchi 1979).

When compared with smaller saccular aneurysms, giant intracranial aneurysms have been reported to present with subarachnoid hemorrhage in a much lower percentage of cases. Morley and Barr (1969), Bull (1969), Hosobuchi (1979), and Creissard et al. (1980) report subarachnoid hemorrhage as the presenting symptom in 27–47 per cent of cases, while Sonntag et al. (1977) and Onuma and Suzuki (1979) found this presentation in 70 of their cases. Due to their inherent bulk, giant aneurysms frequently present as an intracranial mass with headache, visual field deficits, cerebral hemispheric dysfunction, seizures, dementia, psycho-organic syndrome, or brainstem and cerebellar signs. Creissard et al. (1980) reported hemorrhage as a presenting symptom more often with anterior communicating and middle cerebral giant aneurysms and rarely with intracavernous and internal carotid artery lesions. Giant intracavernous carotid aneurysms usually present with dysfunction of cranial nerves III, IV, V or VI. They occasionally rupture to produce a C-C fistula, but very rarely present as an intracranial hemorrhage. Some giant carotid-paraophthalmic aneurysms project dorsally (instead of inferomedial like smaller carotid-ophthalmic aneurysms) and indent the optic nerves and chiasm to present with visual field deficits.

Giant internal carotid aneuryms, which are usually quite fusiform (global) present in a similar manner. Giant anterior communicating aneurysms frequently rupture or compress the optic chiasm, hypothalamus, and frontal lobes to present with visual field deficits, endocrine abnormalities, or the psycho-organic syndrome. Giant paraophthalmic, internal carotid, and anterior communicating aneurysms may present as a suprasellar or rarely, intrasellar mass. Giant middle cerebral aneurysms frequently rupture to produce an intracerebral hematoma or present with lateralizing hemispheric deficits. Giant vertebrobasilar aneurysms often grow to tremendous size and produce a variety of brainstem or cerebellar compressive syndromes.

The natural history of giant intracranial aneurysms has been debated in the literature. Sadik et al. (1965) supposed that the frequently seen laminated thrombus in their walls, protected these lesions from rupture. Multiple reports of giant aneurysms remaining static, decreasing in size, or even disappearing have been presented (Morley and Barr 1969; Scott and Ballantine 1972; Lukin et al. 1975; Carlson and Thomson 1976; Sonntag et al. 1977). Other investigators ascribe no relationship between the size of a saccular aneurysm and its likelihood of rupture (Williams et al. 1955), and several reports of giant aneurysms enlarging and rupturing have appeared (Gallagher et al. 1956; Jane 1961; Cuatico et al. 1967; Obrador et al. 1967; Polis et al. 1973; Garcia-Bengochea and Deland 1975; Sarwar et al. 1976; Sonntag et al. 1977). In general it is probable that most giant aneurysms will continue to enlarge with time and may rupture, and treatment plans should be based on this premise. The only exceptions are the intracavernous and thrombosed giant aneurysms which enlarge and rupture only on rare occasions (Cantu and LeMay 1966; Locksley 1966; Morley and Barr 1969; Terao and Muraoka 1972). Surgical and pathological observations indicate that giant aneurysms most commonly have sclerotic or calcified walls with visible vasa vasorum (see Fig **73A–G**) and adherent mural thrombus but without elastic or muscular components (Morley and Barr 1969; Sonntag et al. 1977; Terao and Muraoka 1972). These aneurysms usually thicken proximally and have a broad, sometimes fusiform base that makes surgical obliteration difficult.

The diagnosis of giant intracranial aneurysms rests on a combination of angiography and computed tomography. Plain skull radiographs may show mural calcification (see Fig **79A**) or bone erosion in up to 30 per cent of cases (Morley and Barr 1969). Unlike smaller saccular aneurysms in which angiography plays a major role and CT scanning a minor role in defining their topography, the surgical anatomy of giant aneurysms is adequately depicted only by a combination of angiography and CT scanning. In giant aneurysms, angiography often falls short in depicting the full extent of the aneurysmal fundus (due to the presence of thrombus) and in defining the aneurysmal orifice on the afferent vessel (due to the large, obscuring sac). The addition of CT scanning allows of a more reliable estimation of aneurysmal size and defines its precise anatomic location. Similarly it notes the presence of mural calcification and thrombus and in some situations may define the precise site of origin (Lavyne et al. 1978; Perrin et al. 1979; Thron and Bockenheimer 1979; Creissard et al. 1980) (Figs **146A–B, 147A–C, 148A–D**).

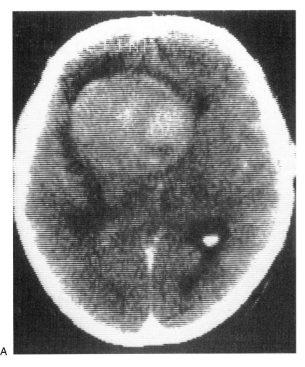

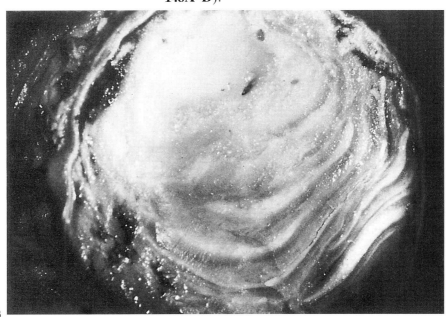

Fig **146A–B** Giant internal carotid artery bifurcation aneurysm on CT scan (**A**) in a 53 year old male patient with progressive headaches and then acute coma with fixed, dilatated pupils. The patient died within hours. The thrombosed aneurysm at autopsy (**B**).

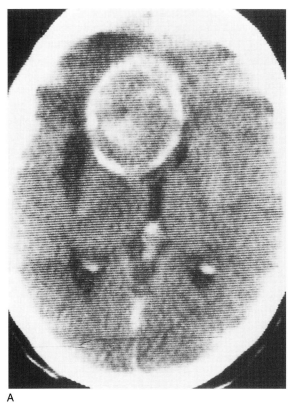
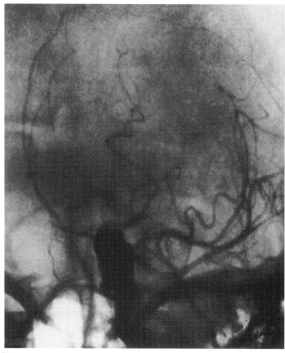

Fig 147A–C Giant subtotally thrombosed left ophthalmic aneurysm on CT scan (**A**) and angiography (**B** and **C**) in a patient with chiasmal syndrome and acute decompensation. At operation the aneurysm was too thick walled and sclerosed to eliminate, so a craniotomy was performed solely for decompression. Nonetheless the patient (71 years old) survived for 5 years in a good condition (Case 29, Table **14**).

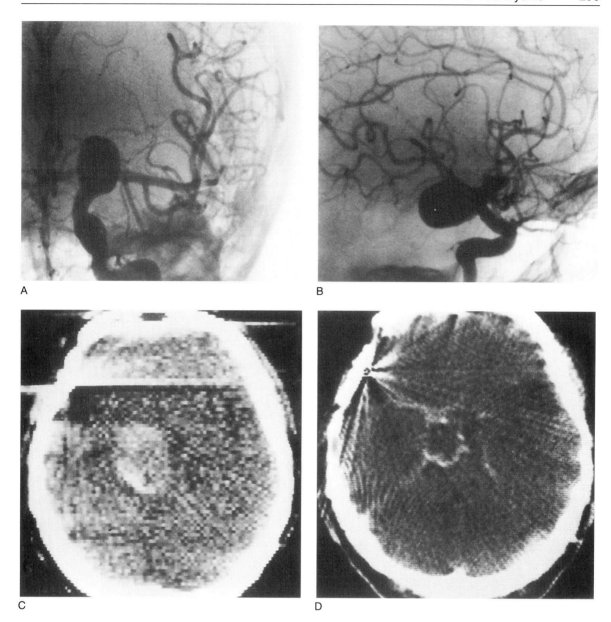

Fig 148A–D CT scan of a giant partially thrombosed aneurysm (C) that on left carotid angiography appeared to be arising at the carotid bifurcation on AP (A) but at the posterior communicating artery on the lateral (B). At operation the aneurysm originated from the inferior wall and could not be clipped. An EC-IC bypass was performed and the left carotid occluded in the neck. A postoperative CT scan (D) shows diminution in the size of the aneurysm. The 50 year old patient made an impressive recovery shortly after a shunt procedure (Case 12, Table 21).

Giant aneurysms, though found at any of the sites described for smaller intracranial saccular aneurysms, have a propensity to occur at certain locations. Creissard et al. (1980) analysed 253 giant aneurysms and found 28 intracavernous (11.0%), 26 carotid-paraophthalmic (10.2%), 3 carotid-posterior communicating (1.2%), 41 internal carotid (16.2%), 43 anterior communicating (17.0%), 59 middle cerebral (23.6%), 14 vertebral (5.4%), 4 PICA (1.6%), 31 basilar (12.2%), and 4 posterior cerebral (1.6%). A very similar series was reported by Sundt and Piepgras (1979). Morley and Barr (1969) reported a higher proportion of intracavernous giant aneurysms (25%) as did Pia (1980). Sahs et al. (1969) presented more internal carotid (39.3%) and anterior communicating (33.5%) giant aneurysms as did Hosobuchi (1979) and Onuma and Suzuki (1979). More frequent vertebrobasilar giant aneurysms have been reported by Drake (1975) – 61.5% and Pia (1980) – 21%. Overall, in comparison to smaller saccular aneurysms, the greater incidence of giant paraclinoid (intracavernous and paraophthalmic) and the rarity of internal carotid-posterior communicating giant aneurysms is noteworthy.

When compared to results obtainable with smaller saccular aneurysms, the surgical results for giant intracranial aneurysms remain less than satisfactory (see Table **125**). The early results of surgical intervention directed at these lesions were truly disappointing with between 60 and 80 per cent of patients dead within 1 year (Heiskanen and Nikki 1962; Bull 1969). The treatment of intracavernous giant aneurysms has generally involved carotid occlusion with or without EC-IC bypass. However in reviewing their results, Strenger (1966), Morley and Barr (1969), and Pia (1980) have concluded that in most instances, better results are obtainable with no treatment unless a carotid-cavernous fistula is present as many of these lesions will spontaneously thrombose. Recent reports by Borne et al. (1979), Gelber and Sundt (1980), and Spetzler et al. (1980) show good results using carotid occlusion with or without EC-IC bypass. Other techniques including direct intracavernous attack, intraluminal thrombosis, hypothermia with cardiac arrest, and balloon occlusion may be tried in isolated instances (Johnston 1979; Hosobuchi 1979; Taki et al. 1979b; Silverberg et al. 1980) (Figs **149A–C, 150A–C, 151A–D**).

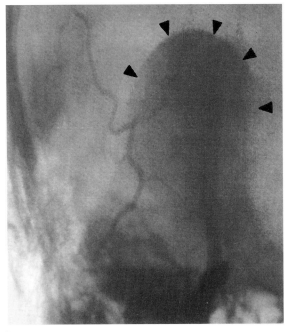

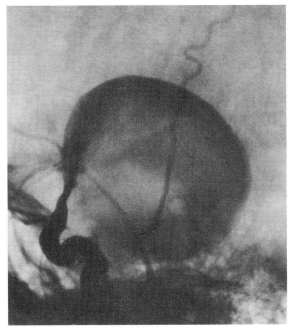

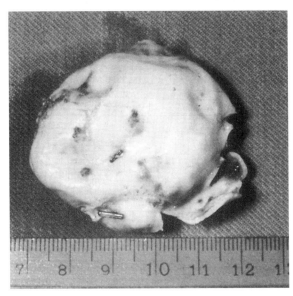

Fig **149A–C** Giant right carotid bifurcation aneurysm (**A** and **B**) presenting with a prgoressive left hemiparesis and seizures. The clipped and excised aneurysm (**C**) (Case 10, Table **45**).

6 Giant Intracranial Aneurysms   301

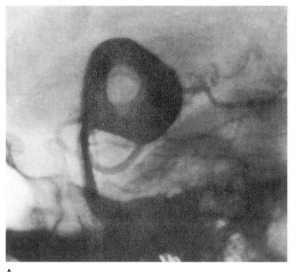

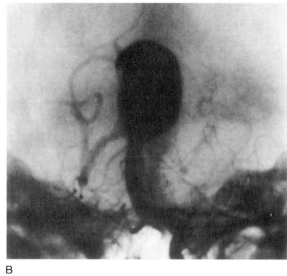

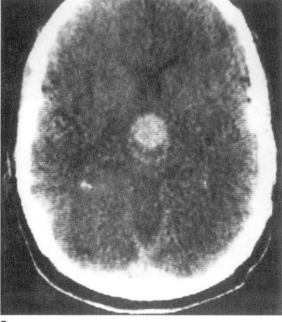

Fig **150A–C** Giant posteroinferiorly directed (for the surgeon) basilar bifurcation aneurysm on CT scan (**C**) and angiography (**A** and **B**) in a 52 year old male patient. No surgery could be performed because of the patient's grave condition, and the autopsy findings are shown in Fig **124**.

302   6 Giant Intracranial Aneurysms

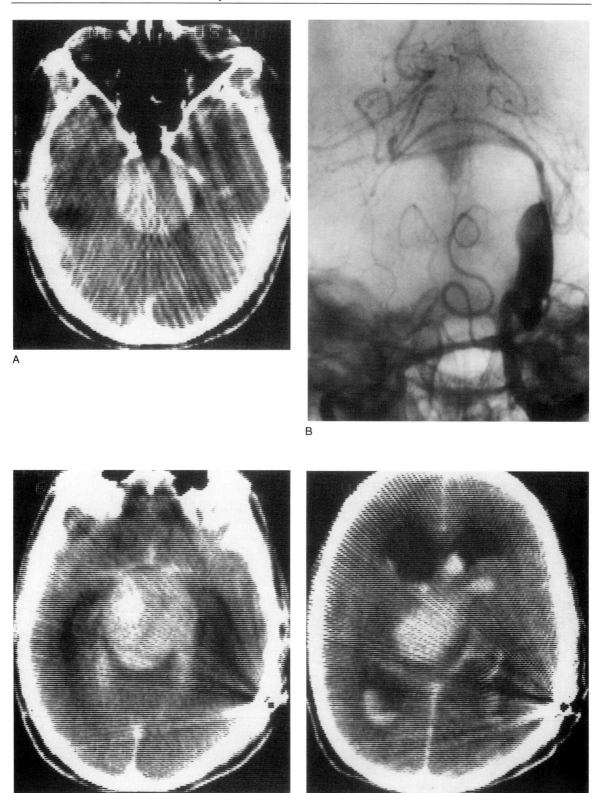

Fig **151A–D**   CT scan of a giant basilar aneurysm (**A**) presenting with tetraplegia and ponto-bulbar symptoms in a 32 year old patient. The day after angiography (**B**) the aneurysm ruptured (**C** and **D**) killing the patient before the scheduled operation could be performed.

The treatment of other giant aneurysms involves the selective application of a variety of obliterative techniques, including carotid or afferent vessel occlusion or trapping with or without EC-IC bypass, neck occlusion or aneurysmorrhaphy with or without hypothermia, wrapping, intraluminal thrombosis either directly or stereotactically and balloon occlusion (Taki et al. 1979b). Using a combination of carotid occlusion, wrapping, neck occlusion, resection, and EC-IC bypass, Sundt and Piepgras (1979) obtained favorable results in a group of 80 giant aneurysms with only a 4 per cent mortality and 14 per cent morbidity. Hosobuchi (1979) combined these techniques with intramural thrombosis in 40 patients and achieved good results in 80 per cent while 5 per cent had poor results and 15 per cent died. Onuma and Suzuki (1979) used primarily neck occlusion and resection in 24 patients with good results in 50 per cent, poor results in 18 per cent, and death in 21 per cent. Generally the poorest results (>50% mortality) have been seen in treating giant vertebrobasilar aneurysms. However, Drake (1978) using a combination of neck occlusion, afferent vessel occlusion, and wrapping in 82 cases achieved good results in 59 per cent, poor results in 23 per cent, and an 18 per cent mortality. The future application of balloon occlusion may improve the treatment of these lesions, but this needs further study. The following tables give comprehensive data concerning our experience with 30 patients (Tables **124** and **125**).

Table 124 Giant aneurysms. Site, age, sex, therapy, and results

	Age	Sex	Site	Therapy	Result
1. W.	57	M	L. CC	EIA and ligature (does not work)	Fair
2. W.	57	M	L. CC	Ligature	Good
3. C.	50	F	L. CC	EIA and ligature	Good
4. P.	67	F	L. Oph	Clip	Good
5. A.	37	F	R. Oph	Clip	Good
6. K.	29	F	L. Oph	Decompression	Good
7. W.	65	F	L. Oph	Clip	Good
8. B.	50	M	L. ICA inferior	EIA and ligature	Good
9. F.	42	M	L. ICA inferior	EIA and clip	Poor
10. G.	56	F	R. ICA inferior	Trapping	Good
11. H.	19	F	R. ICB	EIA	Good
12. R.	47	M	R. ICB	Clip	Fair
13. D.	19	F	R. ICB	Clip	Fair
14. W.	63	M	L. ICB	Clip	Good
15. L.	44	M	L. + R. MCA (bilat.)	EIA and clip	Fair
16. T.	57	M	R. MCA	Suture	Good
17. M.	62	F	L. MCA	Clip	Good
18. H.	61	F	L. Vertebr.	Clip	Good
19. F.	44	F	L. Vertebr.	Clip	Good
20. VA.	14	M	L. P$_1$	Trapping	Good
21. W.	36	M	L. P$_2$	Trapping	Fair
22. C.	24	F	M. Ba. trunk	Trapping	Good
23. L.	19	M	M. Ba. trunk	Muscle	Rerupture, death
24. T.	21	M	M. Ba. trunk	Trapping	Death
25. M.	25	M	M. Ba. trunk	Trapping	Good
26. U.	5	F	M. Ba. trunk	Trapping	Good
27. Z.	24	M	M. Ba. bifurcation	Muscle	Fair
28. E.	42	M	M. Ba. bifurcation	Muscle	Death (later)
29. C.	24	M	M. Ba. bifurcation	Trapping	Good
30. B.	16	M	L. A$_1$	Trapping	Good

6 Giant Intracranial Aneurysms

Table 125 Giant aneurysms. Summary of site and results

	Total No.	Good	Fair	Poor	Death
CC	3	2	1	–	–
Oph	4	4	–	–	–
ICA (inf.)	3	2	–	1	–
ICA (Bi)	4	2	2	–	–
MCA	3	2	1	–	–
VA	2	2	–	–	–
P_1–P_2	2	1	1	–	–
Ba.trunk	5	3	–	–	2
Ba-bifurcation	3	1	1	–	1
A_1	1	1	–	–	–
	30	20 (66.7%)	6	1	3 (10%)

7 Multiple Aneurysms

In a significant number of cases, a single saccular aneurysm is accompanied by one or more other saccular aneurysms, either ipsilaterally, contralaterally, supratentorially, infratentorially or even symmetrically (Table 126).

The incidence of multiple aneurysms varies depending on the method of investigation. Diagnostic studies including angiography are rarely able to identify aneurysms smaller than 3 mm, whilst operative and intentional post-mortem examinations can detect even the smallest lesions. Aneurysms less than 2–3 mm in size are only very rarely detected at angiography and these aneurysms are called microaneurysms. During exploration for other aneurysms, they are detected on a variety of vessels at the base of the brain (Fig 152A–P). In most instances (especially those that are 1 or 2 mm in size), these aneurysms are too small and broad based to accept a clip and must be coagulated and wrapped with muscle or sponge fiber. A review of the literature (Table 127) reveals a wide variation in the incidence of multiple aneurysms in both angiographic and post-mortem series, but cumulatively averages 12.9 per cent when studied angiographically and 22.7 per cent when examined at autopsy. Bilateral symmetrical aneurysms are seen in 4.2 per cent of cases. According to McKissock et al. (1964), Paterson and Bond (1973), Mount and Brisman (1971, 1974) and Suzuki and Sakurai (1979), female patients seem to predominate over males in multiple cases, and multiple aneurysms are most frequent in the 6th decade.

As discussed in Vol. I, Chapter 3 during the course of the usual pterional craniotomy, most of the major sites of aneurysmal eruption are explored. In the initial stages, the ipsilateral Sylvian cistern is opened and the middle cerebral bifurcation inspected. As the basal cisterns are entered, the entire supraclinoid internal carotid, the M_1 segment of the middle cerebral, and the A_1 segment of the anterior cerebral are immediately evident, and by dissecting above and beyond the optic chiasm, the anterior communicating artery and the contralateral A_1 segment, and supraclinoid carotid artery are seen. Finally, by entering the interpeduncular cistern, the distal basilar artery from superior cerebellar to bifurcation and the proximal posterior cerebrals are inspected. Thus all the common aneurysm sites are inspected with the exception of the contralateral middle cerebral, proximal basilar, and vertebral arteries. This means that the number of multiple aneurysms in our series is still not known precisely. This exploration is part of the paracisternal operative approach and there has been not a single case of operative morbidity from this procedure. There was no instance in which additional retraction or contralateral craniotomies were used to visualize these vessels.

The natural history of multiple intracranial saccular aneurysms parallels that of single unruptured lesions with a significant rate of subsequent rupture. In the past a few surgeons have recommended no treatment for asymptomatic aneurysms in

Table 126 Multiple aneurysms – observed locations

Multiple aneurysms at a single site:
2–3 or rarely 4 aneurysms arising separately but in close proximity at the same level (ICA, MCA, AcoA, basilar artery)

Multifocal multiple aneurysms:
1) Unilateral
   a) only ICA, or MCA, or ACA, or PCA, or VA, or BA
   b) combined ICA + MCA, ICA + ACA, MCA + ACA
   c) ICA + MCA + ACA
2) Bilateral
   a) *symmetrical* – ophthalmic artery, PcoA, bifurcation of ICA, MCA, pericallosal artery, PICA
   b) *asymmetrical* – both carotid arteries and branches, carotid and vertebrobasilar arteries and branches: e.g. R. ICA + L. MCA.

306   7 Multiple Aneurysms

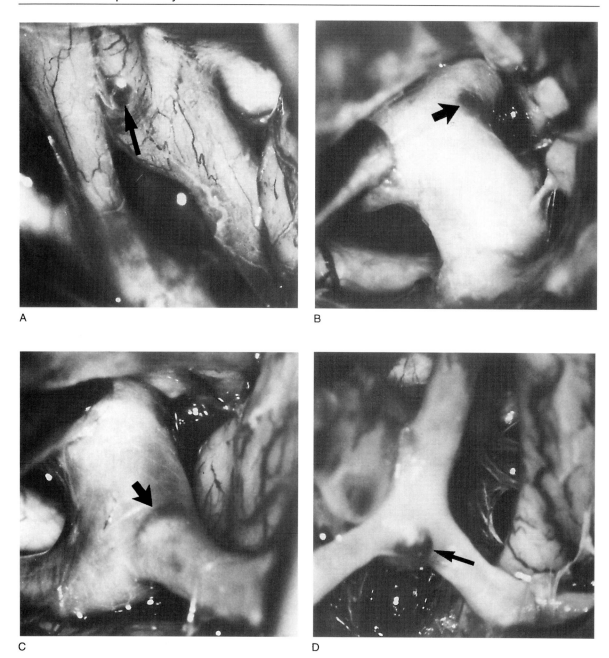

Fig **152A–P** Operative photographs of asymptomatic, incidental, angiographically unrecognized microaneurysms discovered during explorations for other ruptured aneurysms.
A Microaneurysm at the origin of the right ophthalmic artery (arrow).
B Microaneurysm at the origin of the right posterior communicating artery (arrow).
C Small bleb at the beginning of the right M$_1$ segment (arrow).
D Larger bleb at the right carotid bifurcation (arrow).

7 Multiple Aneurysms 307

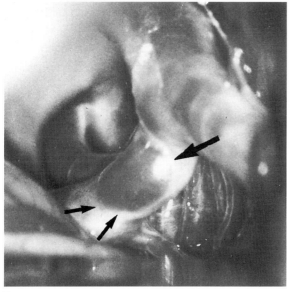
E

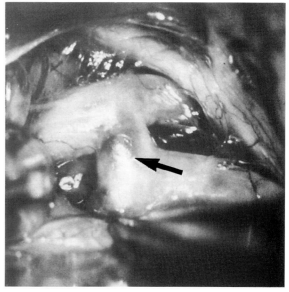
F

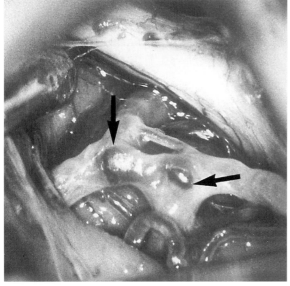
G

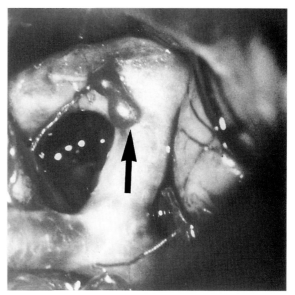
H

E Large bulge at the beginning of the right A_1 segment (arrow).
F Microaneurysm on the superior wall of the anterior communicating artery (arrow).
G Double microaneurysms of the anterior communicating artery (arrows).
H Double bulge at the A_1–A_2 segment (arrow).

Fig **152I–P** ▶

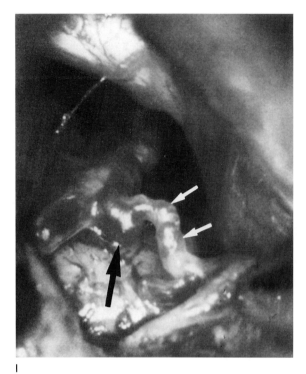
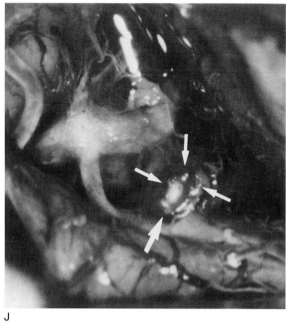
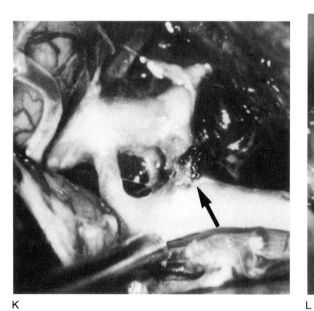
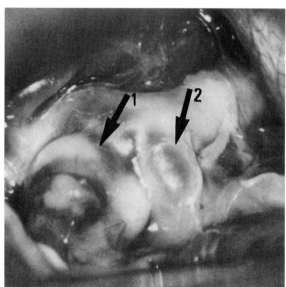

I Triple blebs along the anterior communicating artery (arrows).
J Ruptured microaneurysm at the anterior communicating artery (arrows).
K After coagulation of **J** (arrow).
L A microaneurysm of the anterior communicating artery (arrow 2) combined with a ruptured aneurysm (arrow 1).

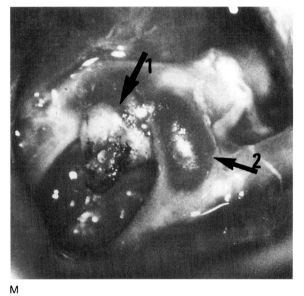
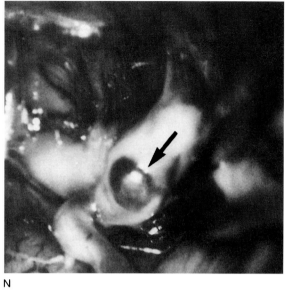
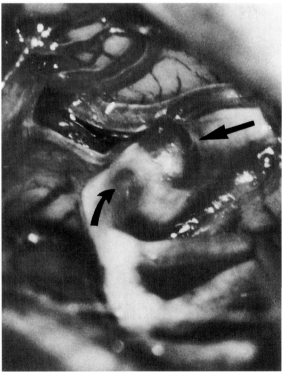
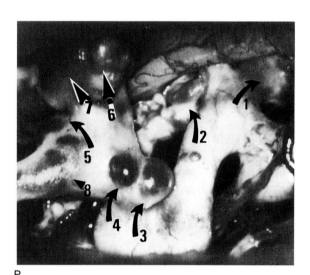

M After coagulation of the ruptured aneurysm (arrow 1), microaneurysm (arrow 2).
N Microaneurysm of the middle cerebral bifurcation (arrow).
O Similar middle cerebral bifurcation microaneurysms (arrows).
P 8 microaneurysms of the left P_1–P_2 segments (arrows).

Table 127 Multiple aneurysms

Author	Mode of examination	No. of cases	Bilateral symmetrical	Bilateral
Richardson and Hyland 1941	Autopsy	40		25%
Riggs and Rupp 1943	Autopsy	1400		21%
Magee 1943	–	–		15%
Dandy 1944	–	–		7%
Hamby 1952	–	–		9.3%
Basset et al. 1952	–	–		5.5%
Wilson et al. 1954	Autopsy	143		18.9%*
King et al. 1954	Angiography	18		33.3%
Norlén and Olivecrona 1953	–	–		5.4%
Bigelow 1955	Autopsy			23%
	Angiography	2237	2.7%*	15%
Williams et al. 1955	–	–		16.8%
Walton 1956	–	–		11.3%
McKissock and Walsh 1956	–	–		7.6%
Poppen and Fager 1959	–	312		8.8%
Hamby 1959	Autopsy			6.7%
	Angiography	189		4.1%
Crompton 1962	Autopsy	172		29.1%*
Taveras and Wood 1963	Autopsy	149		23.5%*
McKissock et al. 1964	Autopsy			28%
	Angiography	–		13.7%
Af Björkesten and Halonen 1965	Angiography	84		29.8%
Heiskanen 1965	Angiography	900		14.2%*
Locksley 1966	Autopsy	888		22.0%*
	Angiography	3321	5.0%*	18.9%
Suzuki et al. 1971	Angiography	3548		7.7%*
Moyes 1971	Angiography	241		10%
Paterson and Bond 1973	Angiography	1686		9.6%*
Mount and Brisman 1974	Angiography	637	7.1%*	19.0%
Karasawa et al. 1974	Angiography	196		13.6%
Suzuki and Sakurai 1979	Angiography	1080	3.1%*	15.4%*
			4.2%	Angiography 12.9%
				Autopsy 22.7%

* overall average

multiple aneurysm cases because of the high surgical morbidity and mortality incurred (McKissock et al. 1964; af Björkesten and Halonen 1965; Heiskanen and Marttila 1970; Paterson and Bond 1973). Others have recommended that all asymptomatic aneurysms be treated in either one or two stages to prevent the rupture of these aneurysms that seems to occur with increased frequency after the treatment of the symptomatic lesion (Hamby 1959; Poppen and Fager 1959; Pool and Potts 1965; Mount and Brisman 1971, 1974; Moyes 1971; and Heiskanen 1981) (Table **128, 129a** and **b**).

In the present series attempts were made to obliterate all accessible aneurysms in a single procedure and often operation was planned with this in mind.

In every instance multiple unilateral aneurysms arising from the internal carotid artery, the anterior cerebral and anterior communicating arteries, the middle cerebral artery, and the basilar bifurcation, and contralateral aneurysms arising from the anterior cerebral (A_1) and from the medial surface (ophthalmic) or bifurcation of the internal carotid artery were accessible from a unilateral approach.

7 Multiple Aneurysms

Table 128 Multiplicity: symmetrical – asymmetrical bilaterality

	C-C	Med	Sup	Oph	Inf	PcoA	AchoA	ICA-Bi	MCA	A₁	AcoA	PeA	Ba	Ba.Br	V	PICA
Single	11	2	–	17	20	122	10	37	125	11	330	11	32	26	3	10
Multifocal	2	–	1	16	1	51	11	18	59	3	45	12	18	3	–	5
unilateral	–	–	1	8	–	36	9	16	45	3	35	3	–	–	–	3
bilateral	2	–	–	8	1	15	2	2	14	–	10	9	–	–	–	2
symmetrical	2	–	–	6	–	9	1	1	8	–	8	8	–	–	–	1
asymmetrical	–	–	–	2	1	6	1	1	6	–	2	1	–	–	–	1

In most circumstances, operative planning is based on the results of angiography that delineates only about ½–⅓ of the total aneurysms present. Additional aneurysms discovered at surgery are generally obliterated as encountered. In most cases attempts are made to obliterate the ruptured aneurysm first. To assist in operative planning, this lesion can be identified by symptomatology (oculomotor palsy, hemisyndromes, etc.), angiography (spasm, size, lobulation, etc.) CT scanning (hematoma or EEG) in *almost* every case. The ruptured aneurysm is clipped first because of its greater propensity to rupture at surgery, while asymptomatic lesions, with much less likelihood of rupture, can wait. In some circumstances, placing a clip on the unruptured aneurysm impairs the approach to ruptured aneurysms, so in these cases, the asymptomatic lesion is coagulated and prepared for clipping, but not actually clipped until the ruptured aneurysm is obliterated. An example of this would be an incidental internal carotid-posterior communicating aneurysm and a ruptured basilar bifurcation aneurysm, in which case the posterior communicating artery is approached first and prepared for clipping with coagulation, but then left unclipped until after the basilar bifurcation aneurysm has been clipped (see Fig **161**).

The operative technique of obliterating additional aneurysms is the same as that used for ruptured lesions (see Chapter 3, p. 267, Vol. I). However, many of the incidentally discovered aneurysms are small (1–3 mm) and not amenable to clipping and are best obliterated with coagulation followed by application of muscle or sponge fiber together with acrylic adhesive, and not by clip application. On the average 2–3 separate aneurysms are encountered in multiple aneurysm cases, but as many as 8 or 9 aneurysms have been clipped in a single case at the same operation (Figs **152–160**). As previously described, the pterional craniotomy is used in most instances to obliterate multiple aneurysms at one sitting, but on occasion a different approach is necessary. In cases of bilateral pericallosal aneurysms, a single paramedian craniotomy will suffice. However, for pericallosal aneurysms associated with internal carotid, anterior communicating, middle cerebral, or basilar bifurcation aneurysms, a combined paramedian parasagittal and pterional craniotomy (see Vol. I, Chapter 3) is necessary to allow obliteration of all aneurysms at one sitting (Fig **162**).

Contralateral internal carotid lateral wall aneurysms (posterior communicating and anterior choroidal), and contralateral middle cerebral aneurysms ordinarily are not accessible. Thus in most instances bilateral internal carotid (posterior communicating or anterior choroidal), bilateral middle cerebral aneurysms, and basilar bifurcation aneurysms associated with proximal vertebrobasilar aneurysms require two separate operations (Figs **163** and **164A–C**).

On rare occasions, exceptional circumstances (such as severe medical problems) motivate attempts to obliterate additional aneurysms that are generally considered inaccessible from one approach. For instance, in the present series, bilateral posterior communicating and an anterior communicating (medioinferiorly directed fundus) aneurysm were clipped from one approach in an elderly patient with severe diabetes and heart disease (Fig **165A–G**). In another instance, bilateral middle cerebral aneurysms (contralateral proximal M₁) were obliterated from one side in a patient who had previously undergone kidney transplantation (Fig **166A–E**). In yet another instance, a patient with possible damage to both orbitofrontal and mesial temporal regions (sustained during a right sided approach to a ruptured ICA-PcoA aneurysm 10 years earlier) presented with both a basilar bifurcation and a left sided M₁ aneurysm. To minimize further injury to the areas of suspected damage both were clipped via a second right sided approach (see Fig **273A–E**, p. 298, Vol. I).

7 Multiple Aneurysms

Table 129a Multiplicity

		Single	Multiple	C-C	Oph	Inf	PcoA	AchoA	Ca-Bi	MCA	AcoA	PeA	Ba	PICA	Macro	Micro	Multiple total	Total No.
Ca-C 13	L	5	–	2	–	–	–	–	–	–	–	–	–	–	2	–	2	15
	R	6	2	–	–	–	–	–	–	–	–	–	–	–	–	–		
Ophthal. 33	L	6	8	–	5 (1)	–	2	1 (1)	2	2	–	–	–	–	10	2	22	55
	R	11	8	–	2 (1)	–	3 (1)	–	1	2 (1)	1	–	1	–	7	3		
Inferior 21	L	13	–	–	–	–	–	–	–	–	–	–	–	–	–	–	1	22
	R	7	1	–	–	–	1	–	–	–	1	–	–	–	1	–		
Medial 2	L	–	–	–	–	–	–	–	–	–	–	–	–	–	–	–	–	2
	R	2	–	–	–	–	–	–	–	–	–	–	–	–	–	–		
Superior 1	L	–	1	–	–	–	–	–	–	–	–	–	–	–	1	–	1	2
	R	–	1	–	–	–	–	–	–	–	–	–	1	–	–	–		
PcoA 173	L	52	21	1 (1)	3 (1)	–	3 (1)	9 (7)	8 (5)	10 (7)	11 (5)	1	–	–	19	27	97	270
	R	70	30	–	1 (1)	–	7 (1)	5 (3)	4 (4)	18 (11)	14 (8)	1	1	–	23	28		
AchoA 21	L	5	6	–	–	–	3 (1)	–	2	2 (1)	–	–	–	–	4	1	14	35
	R	5	5	–	–	–	1 (1)	1	3 (2)	–	–	–	1	–	4	5		
ICA-Bi 55	L	20	9	–	1	–	2 (1)	1 (1)	–	4 (2)	1	–	–	–	5	4	27	82
	R	17	9	–	–	–	3 (1)	2 (2)	2	6 (5)	5 (4)	–	–	–	6	12		
MCA 184	L	65	27	–	1	1	7 (4)	5 (4)	8 (4)	20 (14)	5 (1)	2 (1)	2	–	22	28	96	280
	R	60	32	–	1 (1)	–	6 (4)	5 (2)	2	22 (13)	8 (3)	–	1	–	23	23		
A₁ 14	L	7	3	–	–	–	–	–	1	–	–	–	–	–	1	–	4	18
	R	4	–	–	–	–	–	–	1	2	–	–	–	–	3	–		
AcoA 375	L	172	25	–	1	–	6 (1)	3	3	4	8 (2)	1	1 (1)	–	23	4	61	436
	M	66	4	–	–	–	–	–	–	–	5 (1)	–	–	–	4	1		
	R	92	16	–	1	–	6 (2)	2 (1)	4 (2)	7 (2)	6 (1)	2	2	–	21	8		
PeA 23	L	7	6	–	–	–	–	–	–	–	1	5 (5)	–	–	1	6	13	36
	R	4	6	–	1	–	1 (1)	–	–	1	–	5 (2)	1	–	5	2		
Ba-Bi 50		32	18	–	2 (1)	–	4 (2)	1 (1)	1 (1)	9 (6)	5 (1)	–	–	–	6	4	31	81
								1	2	1	3 (1)	–	–	–	11	10		
Ba-Br + Tr 29	L	9	3	–	–	–	1 (1)	–	–	1	–	–	–	–	1	1	4	33
	R	8	–	–	–	–	1	–	–	1	–	–	1	1 (1)	2	–		
	Tr	9	–	–	–	–	–	–	–	–	–	–	–	–	–	–		
Va 3	L	1	–	–	–	–	–	–	–	–	–	–	–	–	–	–	–	3
	R	2	–	–	–	–	–	–	–	–	–	–	–	–	–	–		
PICA orig. 10	L	3	1	–	–	–	–	–	–	–	–	–	1	–	1	–	2	12
	R	5	1	–	–	–	–	–	–	–	–	–	–	1 (1)	–	–		
PICA dist. 5	L	1	2	–	–	–	–	–	–	–	–	–	–	5 (3)	–	3	5	10
	R	1	1	–	–	–	–	–	–	–	–	–	–	–	2	–		
	L			3 (1)	12 (2)	–	25 (10)	20 (14)	25 (10)	42 (23)	31 (9)	9 (6)	4 (1)	–	95	76	⎫	
	M			–	–	–	–	–	–	–	5 (1)	–	–	–	4	1	⎬ 380	
	R			–	6 (4)	1	32 (12)	16 (8)	19 (8)	70 (39)	39 (18)	8 (2)	7	6 (4)	109	95	⎭	
1012		767 (76%)	245 (24%)	3 (1)	18 (6)	1	57 (22)	36 (22)	44 (18)	112 (62)	75 (28)	17 (8)	11 (1)	6 (4)	208	172		1392

( ) micro-aneurysm

7 Multiple Aneurysms

Table **129b** Multiplicity

Site of aneurysms	Total No.	Single	Multiple	Additional aneurysms 1	2	3	4	5	
Intracavernous	13	11	2	2	–	–	–	–	
Ophthalmic	33	17	16	11	4	1	–	–	
Medial wall	2	2	–	–	–	–	–	–	
Superior wall	1	–	1	1	–	–	–	–	
Inferior wall	21	20	1	1	–	–	–	–	
PcoA	173	122	51	29	8	6	6	2	
AchoA	21	10	11	9	1	1	–	–	
ICA-Bi	55	37	18	11	5	2	–	–	
MCA	184	125	59	41	6	6	5	1	
A_1	14	11	3	2	1	–	–	–	
AcoA	375	330	45	35	6	2	2	–	
PeA	23	11	12	11	1	–	–	–	
Ba-Bi	50	32	18	10	5	1	2	–	
Ba-Br	29	26	3	2	1		–	–	
VA	3	3	–	–	–	–	–	–	
PICA origin	10	8	2	2	–	–	–	–	
PICA distal	5	2	3	2	–	1	–	–	
	1012	767	245	169	38	20	15	3	
		75.8%	24.2%	16.7	3.8	2.0	1.5	0.3	% of 1012 cases
				69.0	15.5	8.2	2.0	1.2	% of 245 cases

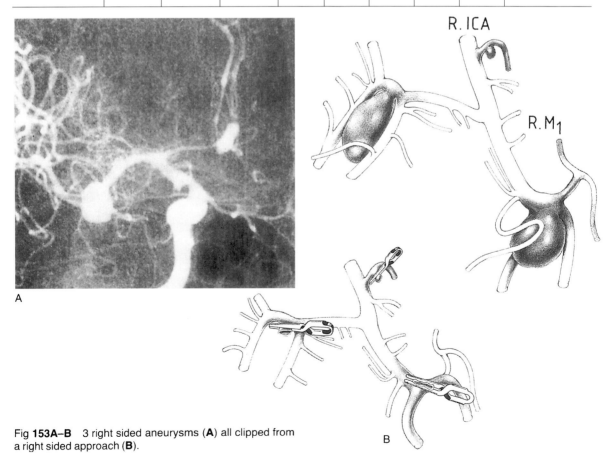

Fig **153A–B** 3 right sided aneurysms (**A**) all clipped from a right sided approach (**B**).

314   7 Multiple Aneurysms

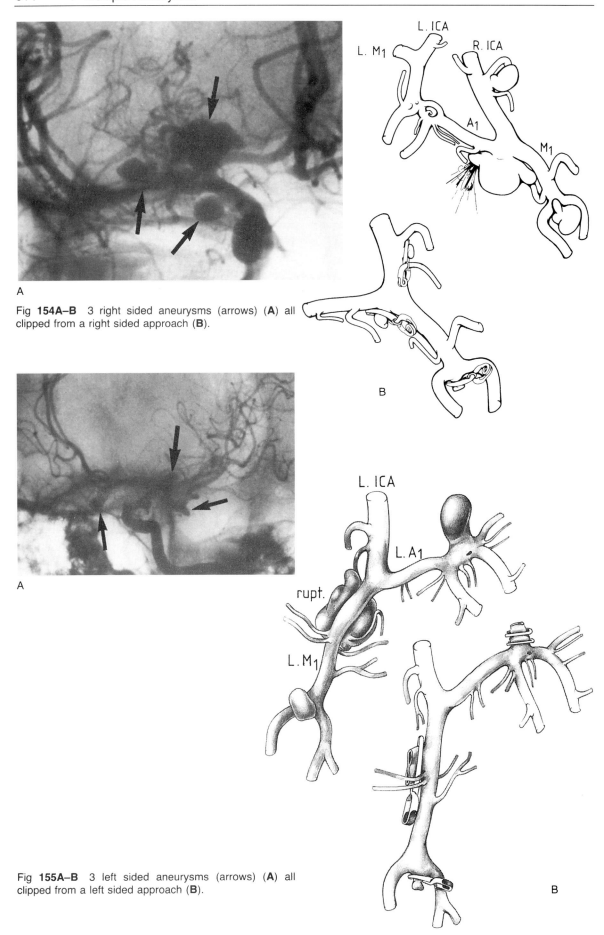

Fig **154A–B**   3 right sided aneurysms (arrows) (**A**) all clipped from a right sided approach (**B**).

Fig **155A–B**   3 left sided aneurysms (arrows) (**A**) all clipped from a left sided approach (**B**).

7 Multiple Aneurysms 315

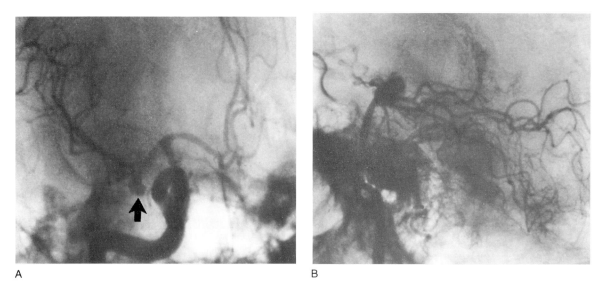

Fig 156A Combination of a ruptured basilar (**A**) and an unruptured right middle cerebral bifurcation aneurysm (arrow) (**B**) both clipped from a single pterional approach.

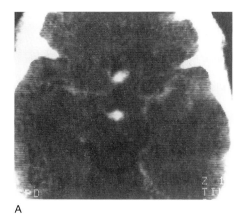

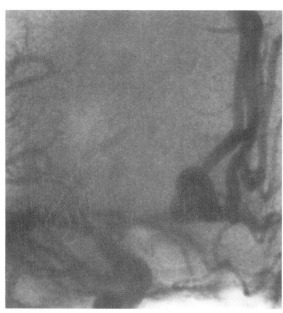

Fig 157A–E CT scan (**A**) shows anterior communicating and basilar aneurysms. Angiography (**B–D**) demonstrates an additional posterior communicating aneurysm.

Fig 157C–E ▶

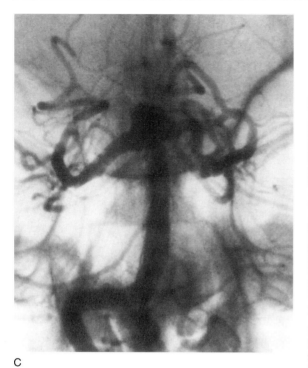

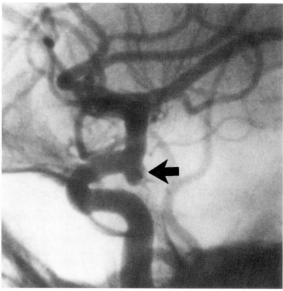

Fig 157 C–E Aneurysm at the basilar bifurcation on vertebral angiogram (**C**) and a further aneurysm at the origin of the right posterior communicating artery (arrow) (**D**). Exploration by right pterional approach allowed dissection and clipping of all these aneurysms as shown schematically in (**E**). The anterior communicating artery aneurysm had ruptured.

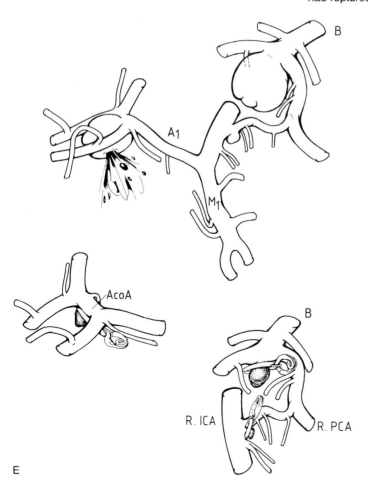

7 Multiple Aneurysms 317

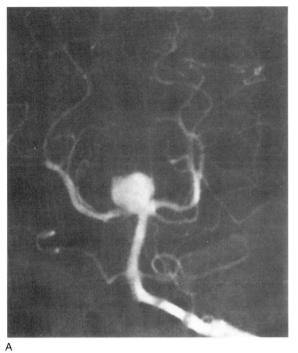

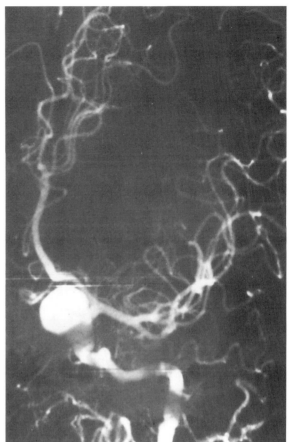

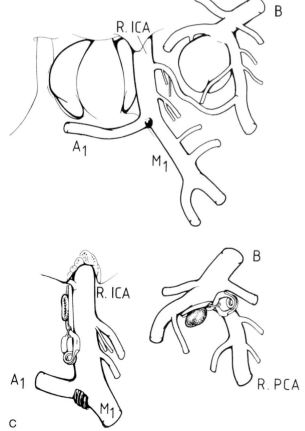

Fig 158A–C Ruptured basilar (**A**) and asymptomatic right ophthalmic aneurysms (**B**) both clipped via a single right pterional approach (**C**).

318   7 Multiple Aneurysms

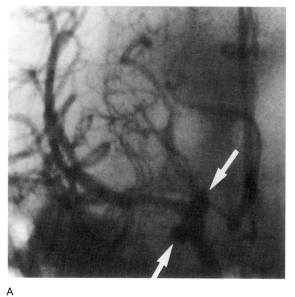
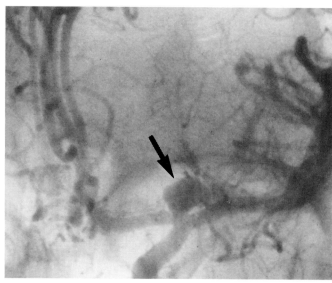
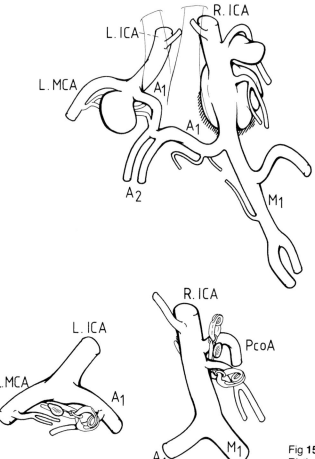

Fig 159A–F Multiple bilateral aneurysms (arrows) (**A** and **B**) that were clipped from a single one sided approach (**C**) with verification on plain x-ray (**D**). Postoperative CT scan (**E** and **F**) showed no evidence of infarction.

Fig **159D–F**

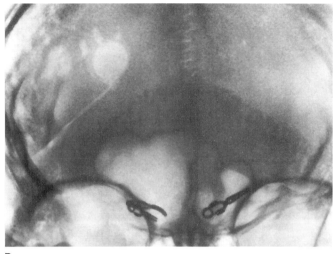

D

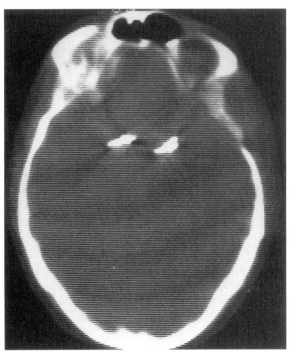

E

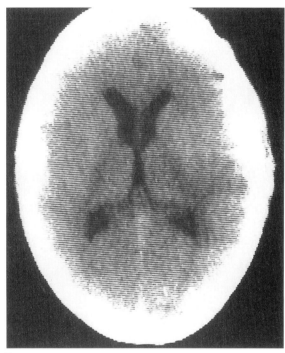

F

320 7 Multiple Aneurysms

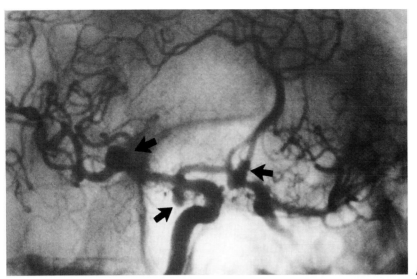

Fig 160A–D Multiple bilateral aneurysms (arrows) (A and B) all clipped from a single one sided approach (C).

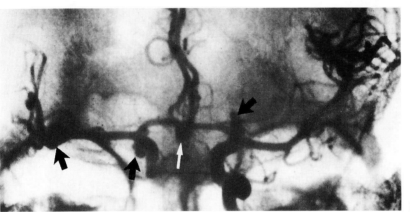

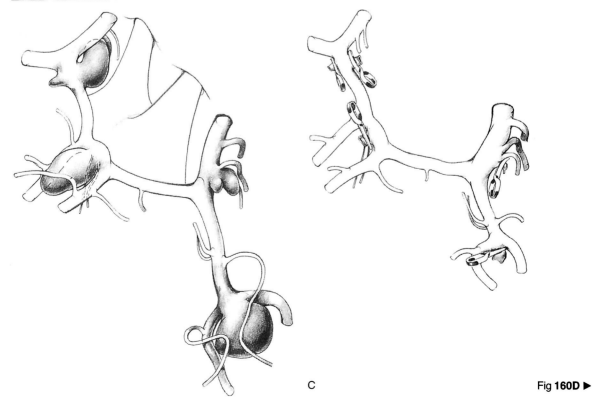

Fig 160D ▶

Fig **160D** Complete obliteration was verified on postoperative angiography. Arrow indicates the pterional approach.

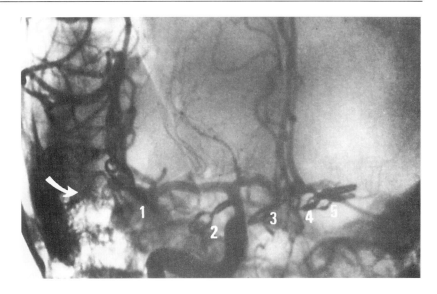

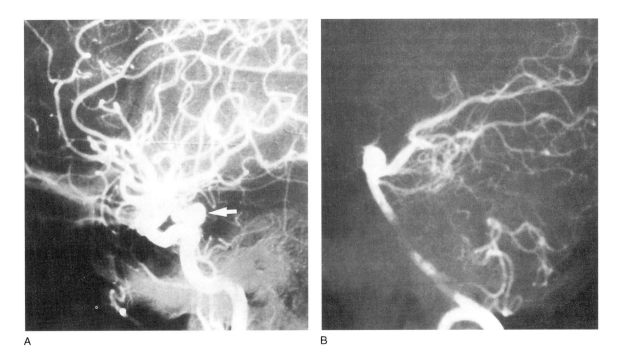

Fig **161A–B** Rare combination of an unruptured posterior communicating (arrow) (**A**) and a ruptured basilar aneurysm (**B**) both clipped from a single approach.

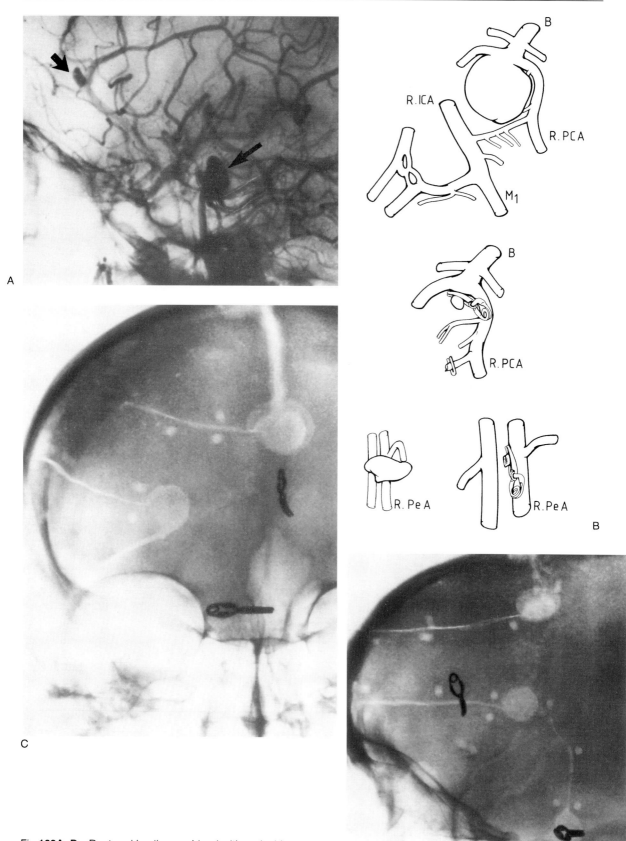

Fig **162A–D** Ruptured basilar combined with an incidental pericallosal aneurysm (arrows) (**A**) both clipped through one combined approach (**B**) with postoperative verification of the clips and craniotomy site (**C** and **D**).

Fig **163** The ruptured left sided posterior inferior cerebellar aneurysm (arrow) was clipped through a lateral suboccipital approach. The basilar bifurcation and left superior cerebellar artery aneurysms needed a pterional approach.

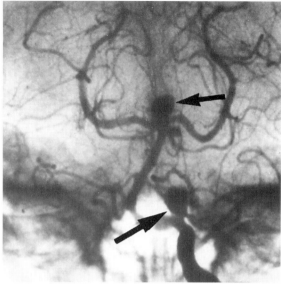

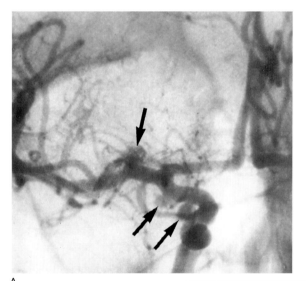

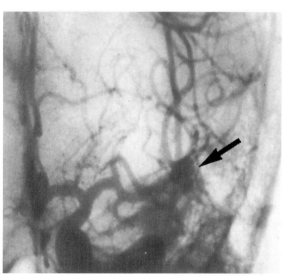

Fig **164A–C** Right sided posterior communicating, anterior choroidal and bilateral middle cerebral aneurysms (arrows) (**A** and **B**) requiring 2 separate approaches (**C**).

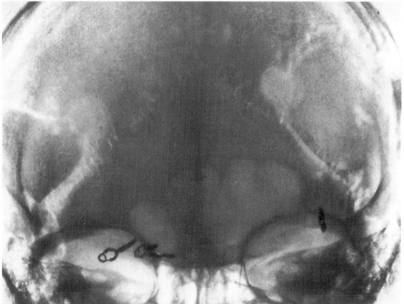

324   7 Multiple Aneurysms

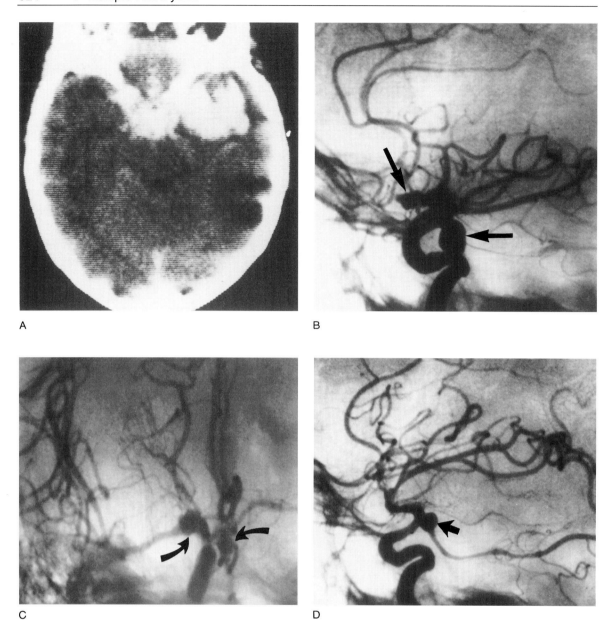

Fig 165A–G   Cisternal and intracerebral hematomas (**A**) from a ruptured right posterior communicating artery aneurysm (**B**) with multiple other aneurysms; anterior choroidal, anterior communicating and left posterior communicating artery aneurysms (arrows) (**C** and **D**). From a single right sided approach, all aneurysms were clipped.

Fig **165E–G** ▶

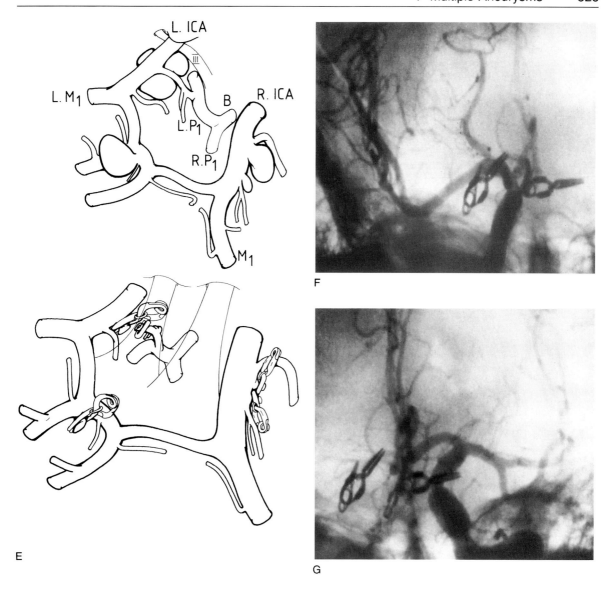

Fig 165 E–G The four aneurysms are shown diagrammatically before and after clipping (**E**). Right sided carotid angiography shows elimination of the posterior communicating artery, anterior choroidal artery and anterior communicating artery aneurysms (**F**). Left carotid angiography shows elimination of the left posterior communicating artery aneurysm (**G**).

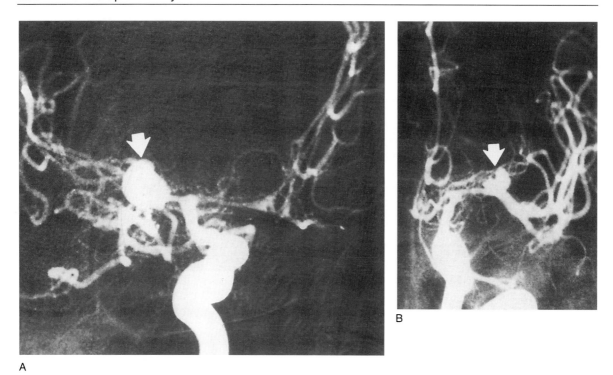

Fig 166 A–B Bilateral middle cerebral artery aneurysms (right sided aneurysm ruptured) on carotid angiogram (arrows). (A) right side, (B) left side.

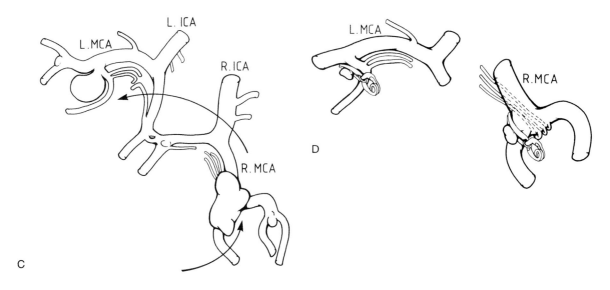

Fig 166 C–E Both aneurysms were clipped from a single right sided pterional approach in a patient undergoing renal dialysis. Arrows indicating the right sided pterional approach to the bilateral aneurysms.

Fig 166 E The postoperative course was uneventful, the patient making a full recovery. (The shunt was inserted preoperatively to treat a communicating hydrocephalus.)

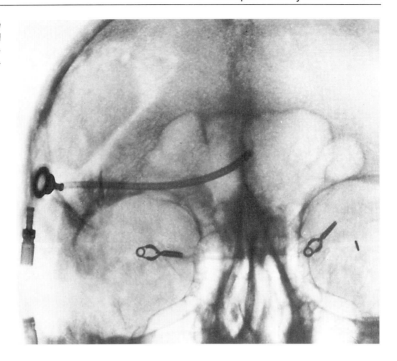

The results of surgery for multiple aneurysms have generally been slightly worse than those for single aneurysm cases (7.3% mortality multiple, 5.9% mortality single), but more recently the results have been identical (Suzuki and Sakurai 1979). In this present series, the postoperative results (Table 130) are the same for cases with multiple aneurysms and those with single aneurysms. The outcome following surgery depends more upon the preoperative condition of the patient than upon the number of aneurysms which are successfully occluded (Fig 167).

Table 130 Operative results in cases with multiple aneurysms

	Total No.	Good	Fair	Poor	Death
C-C	2	2	–	–	–
Ophthal.	16	16	–	–	–
Inf.	1	1	–	–	–
PcoA	51	45	6	–	–
AchoA	11	8	1	–	2
Ca-Bi	18	15	1	1	1
MCA	59	55	4	–	–
A_1	3	3	–	–	–
AcoA	45	40	1	3	1
PeA	12	10	1	1	–
Ba-Bi	18	14	1	2	1
Ba-Br	3	3	–	–	–
PICA	5	4	1	–	–
	244	216 (88.5%)	16 (6.5%)	7 (2.9%)	5 (2.0%)

328   7 Multiple Aneurysms

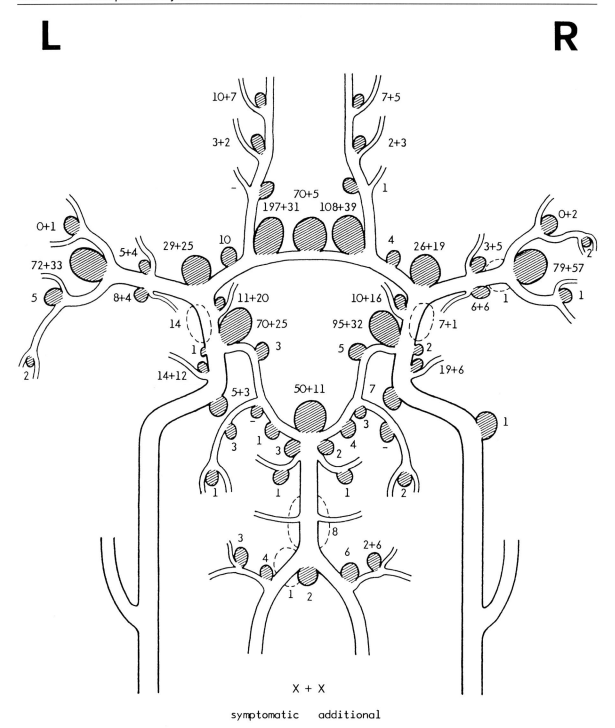

Fig 167   Schematic representation of the site of 1392 explored aneurysms (1967–1979) (see Table **129**).

8 Unoperated Cases

Of importance for a good understanding of the whole problem of subarachnoid hemorrhage from cerebral aneurysm is the examination of those cases that have not come to surgery. Between 1967–1979, the current series of 1012 patients comprising 349 (34.5%) patients from Zurich, 463 (45.7%) patients from elsewhere in Switzerland, and 200 (19.8%) patients from other countries underwent operation. In addition to these, a total of 105 patients were hospitalized at the University of Zurich for ruptured aneurysms, but not operated upon. In this group 27 (25.7%) refused surgery. The remaining 78 (74.3%) succumbed before surgery could be performed. The majority of these patients were grade IV or V upon admission (57%), but one third were grade III and one tenth were grade II. Of the 27 patients surviving but not undergoing surgery, 19 (70.4%) are known to be dead while 8 (29.6%) are known to be alive (see Vol. I, Chapter 5).

Our results show that for all grades (after ruptured aneurysm) the operative mortality was 5.5% and the overall management mortality was 13.3% with 78 patients dying before surgery could be carried out. These figures are very similar to those of Sundt et al. published in 1982 (operative mortality 5.1%, overall management mortality 17,1%, 78 patients died before operation (see also Shephard, 1983). At first sight an overall management mortality of about 13% seems quite low in view of the severity of the disease process but unfortunately this is a measure of the success achieved only with those patients actually reaching the neurosurgical unit.

A retrospective analysis of all cases of subarachnoid hemorrhage occurring only in the Canton Zurich during the same time period was performed. This region has a population of 1.1 million people, who are provided with a high standard of medical care through local hospitals and one major neurosurgical referral center, the University of Zurich. The Canton has an autopsy rate of over 40%. In this period there were a total of 624 cases of ruptured or symptomatic aneurysm in the area. Of these, 227 (36.4%) died before transfer to the University Hospital, 39 (6.3%) reached the University Hospital but died before operation could be performed, 9 (1.4%) arrived but refused surgery (5 died later), and 349 (55.9%) underwent aneurysm surgery (Table **131**).

An analysis of the 271 (227+39+5) patients dying from unoperated ruptured aneurysm in this area reveals that 142 (52.4%) suffered a severe subarachnoid hemorrhage and died immediately or within a few hours after hospital admission. 45 patients (16.6%) survived the initial hemorrhage but were not diagnosed due either to their failure to appreciate the seriousness of the situation (64.9%) or because of failure by the primary physician (26.2%) or neurosurgeon (6.3%) to make the correct diagnosis and these patients subsequently rebled and died. 7 patients (2.3%) had their symptoms interpreted correctly but the diagnosis was missed due to negative lumbar puncture or angiograms. In 9 cases (3.3%), the diagnosis was made but the patient (7) or his family (2) decided against surgery and of these 5 died during the next 2 years (55.5%). In 53 cases (19.6%), the diagnosis and decision to operate were made but there was a fatal delay in transferring the patient due to poor (15) or deteriorating condition (19), recurrent subarachnoid hemorrhage (8), intercurrent disease (7) or an arbitrary waiting period (4).

48 patients (17.8%) arrived at the university hospital but surgery was delayed due to progressive deterioration following LP (2), angiography (17)

or intubation (1), intercurrent disease such as myocardial infarction (2), breast cancer (1), hypernephroma (1), duodenal ulcer (1), sepsis (1), congestive heart failure (3), age over 65 (2), aspiration pneumonias (4), poor condition (IV–V) (9), recurrent subarachnoid hemorrhage (5), or weekend-holiday scheduling (2), and all of these patients rebled and died while awaiting surgery.

Overall, of 624 proven ruptured aneurysms in this area only 349 (55.9%) actually underwent operation and 5 died (1.4%). Of the other 275 (44.1%), only 4 (0.6%) survived, for a mortality in this nonoperated group of 98.5%.

This means that a ruptured cerebral aneurysm remains a highly fatal disease. In addition to greater education among our patients and fellow physicians, significant reductions in these figures will only be made through new techniques for earlier diagnosis, improved medical treatment after rupture and earlier, perhaps prophylactic surgery.

Recently an additional analysis was made of a group of 20 patients with ruptured intracranial aneurysms who died before surgery (Sept. 1979 – Dec. 1981). This group of patients was compared with a similar group of 193 patients who survived and underwent surgery, with 179 good results, 8 fair, 3 poor results, and 3 deaths (see Chapter 10). Comparisons were made of systolic and diastolic blood pressures taken at the time of the hemorrhage and before surgery. Those patients dying either before surgery or after surgery were found to have significantly higher systolic and diastolic blood pressures especially at the time of hemorrhage, but also during the period before surgery. This suggests that a patient's blood pressure may have some prognostic significance in terms of final outcome, and this possibility is continuing to undergo evaluation.

Table 131 1967–1979 (624 cases from Canton of Zurich)

Died before surgery		
At home	27 cases	
At other hospitals	200 cases	275 cases (44.1%)
At University Hospital Zurich	39 cases	
Refused surgery	9 cases	
died	5	
survived	4	
Operated cases		349 cases (55.9%)
survived	344 (98.6%)	
died	5 (1.4%)	
		624

9 Complications of Aneurysm Surgery

Introduction

Many of the complications of aneurysm surgery are difficult to delimit precisely. The usual presenting hemorrhage from an intracranial aneurysm sets into motion a complex pathophysiological process with inherent complications that will occur regardless of whether surgical intervention is attempted or not. A certain number of aneurysm patients suffering a subarachnoid hemorrhage will subsequently develop hydrocephalus or epilepsy (often prior to operation) and attempts to categorize these as direct complications of surgery are certainly incorrect. Of course, surgery may be the prime or contributing factor in the development and/or progression of a number of adversities befalling other aneurysm patients; relating these only to the disease process itself is equally incorrect.

To simplify the present discussion, the complications of aneurysm surgery in the group of patients under consideration include all those events which caused a patient's postoperative course to deviate from the expected ideal, whether the adversity was inherent in the disease process itself or was initiated and/or propagated by the surgeon. It must be kept in mind that the ideal postoperative course will differ among aneurysm patients depending on their condition at the time of operation. However the majority of complications listed in this section would have significantly affected a patient's course regardless of his preoperative status.

All postoperative situations which altered a patient's course unfavourably, delayed his discharge from the hospital, or resulted in physical impairment or death will be included in this discussion, while those complications occurring during surgery such as premature rupture of the aneurysm, injury to a cerebral vessel, inadequate clipping and postoperative rerupture, hypotension from blood loss, etc. have been thoroughly discussed in the previous sections and will not be repeated here. Also the problem of cerebral vasospasm as a complication of aneurysm surgery was discussed at length in Chapter 3, Vol. I, and Chapter 1, Vol. II, and this topic will not be reexamined.

Classification

A. *Central Nervous System Complications*
  1) Intracranial hematoma
  2) Surgical infection
  3) Ischemia
     a. Paresis
     b. Aphasia
     c. Psycho-organic syndrome (POS)
     d. Hypothalamic disorder
     e. Epilepsy
     f. Cranial nerve palsy
  4) Altered CSF circulation
     a. Subcutaneous CSF collection
     b. Malresorptive hydrocephalus
     c. Rhinorrhoea

B. *General Medical Complications*
  1) Circulatory
  2) Pulmonary
  3) Gastrointestinal
  4) Renal
  5) Hepatic
  6) Dermatologic.

Table 132 Complications

	CC	Opht	IC inf	PcoA	AchA	CaBi	MCA	A₁	AcoA	PeA	BaBi	BaBr	BaTr	V	Total
1a) Intracranial Hematoma															
Epidural	–	–	–	–	–	–	–	–	2	1	–	–	–	–	4
Subdural	–	–	–	–	–	–	1	–	3 (1)	–	–	–	–	–	4
Intracerebral	–	–	–	1	1	–	–	–	–	–	–	–	–	–	1
1b) Rerupture	–	–	–	1 (1)	–	1 (1)	–	–	7 (4)	1	1 (1)	1 (1)	–	–	11
1c) Edema	–	–	–	1	–	–	1	–	2	1	–	–	–	–	5
2) Infection															
Skin	1	–	–	2	–	–	–	–	3	–	–	–	–	–	6
Osteomyelitis	1	–	–	–	–	–	2	–	2	–	–	–	–	–	5
Epi- and subdural empyema	–	–	2	1	–	–	1	–	1	–	–	–	–	–	2
Bact. meningitis	–	–	2	1	–	–	–	–	2 (2)	1	1	–	–	–	6
Aseptic meningitis	–	–	1	4	–	1	4	–	6	1	1	–	–	–	16
3) Ischemia															
a) Hemiparesis															
transient (1–3 d)	1	2	2	13	4	3	14	1	16	2	1	2	–	1	62 (6.1%)
delayed (up to 3 m)	–	1	2	1	1	–	2	–	6	1	2	2	–	–	18 (1.8%)
permanent															
partial	1	–	–	6	–	2	4	–	4	1	–	1	–	–	18 (1.8%)
total	–	–	3 (2)	5 (5)	2 (1)	1 (1)	2 (1)	–	5 (5)	2	2 (1)	–	3 (3)	–	25 (2.5%)
b) Aphasia															
transient	1	–	1	14	4	2	15	–	13	–	–	–	–	1	51 (5.1%)
delayed	1	–	1	3	1	–	3	–	1	1	–	–	–	–	11 (1.1%)
permanent	–	–	2 (1)	2	–	–	2 (1)	–	–	2	3 (3)	–	2 (2)	–	13 (1.3%)
c) POS															
transient	–	–	2	8	2	4	6	2	62	–	2	–	–	–	88
delayed	–	–	1	5	2	2	6	–	9	–	4	–	–	–	29
permanent	1	–	1	1	1	1	2	–	5	2	2	1	–	–	17
Steroid psychosis	–	–	–	1	–	–	1	–	2	–	1	–	–	–	5
d) Hypothalamic															
transient	–	1	–	4 (2)	–	–	–	–	27	–	4	–	–	–	32
permanent	–	–	1	2	–	–	–	–	4	–	–	–	–	–	4 (0.4%)
e) Epilepsy															
transient	–	–	–	12	–	1	3	–	8	–	1	1	–	–	17
permanent	–	1	1	–	–	5	8	–	8	1	1	1	–	–	28 (2.8%)
f) III-Palsy															
transient	–	1	–	12	–	1	–	–	–	–	12	2	–	–	17
permanent	–	–	–	–	–	–	–	–	–	–	4	1	–	–	28 (2.8%)
4) Hydrocephalus															
liquid collec.	–	3	2	12	2	3	9	1	22	2	3	1	–	1	60
shunt	–	–	3	12	3	1	10	–	46	1	9	1	–	1	87
Rhinorrhea	–	1	1	–	–	–	–	–	2	1	–	1	–	–	4

( ) subsequently died

Central Nervous System Complications

Intracranial Hematoma

Of the 1012 patients in this series, 9 (0.9%) developed some form of intracranial hematoma postoperatively that required treatment. The distribution of hematomas into epidural, subdural and intracerebral is given in Table **132**. Presenting signs and symptoms included headache, changes in level of consciousness, hemiparesis, etc., beginning as a rule during the first several hours after surgery.

Despite the occurrence of these mass lesions, good results were still obtained in 4 patients. The development of symptoms suggesting intracranial hematoma formation anytime in the postoperative period demands evaluation by computerized tomography or angiography before other etiologies (such as vasospasm) are entertained. In this series intracranial hematomas contributed to fair results in 2 patients, poor results in 1 patient and death in 2 patients. The importance of early diagnosis and prompt evacuation of these intracranial masses cannot be over emphasized.

Significant subgaleal hematomas were seen in 10 (1.0%) patients, despite the routine insertion of subgaleal drains at operation. Treatment was generally conservative, and when unaccompanied by infection, this complication had no affect on the patient's outcome.

Infection

All patients undergoing microscopic neurosurgical procedures in Zurich are given prophylactic broad spectrum antibiotics (Chloroamphenicol 2 gm 1 day before and 1 day after surgery). However, infection of the soft tissue, bone, or intracranial structures was still seen in 19 patients (1.9%). The distribution according to location is given in Table **133**. Examination of the CSF was carried out as soon as the possibility of intracranial infection was raised. Intracranial infection was related to the presence of a shunting device in 2 cases.

With appropriate treatment the superficial infections such as osteomyelitis had no affect on the patient's final outcome, while the presence of intracranial infection (especially meningitis) contributed to a poor outcome in 1 patient and death in another patient. Good surgical technique and prophylactic antibiotics remain the critical factors in preventing these dreaded complications.

Some degree of sterile meningitis accompanies almost every subarachnoid hemorrhage, but significant, symptomatic aseptic meningitis was seen in 16 (1.5%) patients. In most instances this responded to conservative measures and had no affect on outcome.

Ischemia

The data regarding the occurrence of ischemic complications including hemiparesis, dysphasia, POS, hypothalamic disorders, cranial nerve palsies, and epilepsy are given in Table **137** and need little elaboration. Most of the severe complications occur in the higher grades, notably grades III, IV and V. However, 2 points are worthy of note. First, there seems to be a considerable difference between the outcome at all grade levels between the a and b groupings (see Table **1a**

Table **133** Postoperative complications related to site of aneurysm

	ICA	MCA	AcoA	PeA	Ba-Bi	Ba-Br + Tr	Total
Hematoma							
Edema	1.6%	1.1%	3.7%	8.7%	2.0%	3.4%	25/980 = 2.6%
Rupture							
Infection	3.8%	3.8%	4.8%	–	4.0%	–	35/980 = 3.6%
Ischemia							
Permanent Hpr.	6.2%	3.2%	2.4%	8.7%	4.0%	13.8%	= 3.2%
Permanent Aphasia	1.3%	1.1%	0.0%	8.7%	4.0%	6.8%	= 1.3%
Permanent POS	1.6%	1.1%	1.3%	8.6%	4.0%	3.4%	= 1.8%
Hydrocephalus	5.9%	5.4%	12.1%	4.3%	18.0%	3.4%	= 8.8%

and **b**). A "good" outcome was achieved in 95.6% of "*a*" subgroups of all grades against 67.2% in group "*b*". A "fair" result was seen in 1.5% "*a*" and 13.2% "*b*"; poor in 0.3% "*a*" and 8.1% "*b*"; and death in 2.5% "*a*" and 11.4% "*b*". This trend was seen in both the better grades 0, I and II and the poorer grades III, IV and V.

Secondly there is a fairly clear cut-off point in terms of a good outcome between grades IIa and IIIa with only 34.9% of grade IIIa patients making a smooth recovery compared with 75.8% of those in grade IIa. ("Good" outcome rates being 95.6% and 84.0% respectively).

These facts are of importance in determining whether or not individual patients should be scheduled for early operation. It would certainly seem safer to delay surgery in stable, alert patients with fixed lateralizing deficits and in those who exhibit profound drowsiness or a fluctuating level of consciousness until improvement to a better grade/group has occurred. In such cases the CT scan may be of little value in making a decision about the timing of operation but it is to be hoped that the PET scan will prove to be of value in the future.

The brain, like many other body tissues, reacts to injury or to surgical interference by swelling. Associated changes in cerebral vascular permeability may compound this normal reaction. The swelling may be minimal or of massive degree but, in general, the less retraction and manipulation of the brain at operation, the smaller the amount of swelling.

Postoperative swelling whether it be due to excessive handling or ischemia can lead to a deterioration in conscious level and progressive neurological deficits. Much can be done to avoid this by precise and careful operative technique as described in previous chapters.

However, some patients despite very careful and perfectly straightforward surgery are found to deteriorate with a progressive hemiparesis (sometimes without an impaired conscious level) sometimes several days after operation, having initially made a good recovery.

In the absence of any evidence of an intracranial hematoma or hydrocephalus one is often forced to assume that the deterioration must represent some form of ischemic deficit so that any subsequent brain swelling which could compound the deficit must be kept to a minimum. The methods employed in this clinic to achieve this aim are really extensions of the general treatment in the postoperative phase of all patients with aneurysmal subarachnoid hemorrhage which has already been described.

Virtually all patients (except those who may have had significant operative blood loss) receive only 1 litre of fluid as dextrose saline in the first 24 hours after operation and are kept on a carefully fluid restricted regime for 3–4 days thereafter. Blood electrolytes are monitored regularly and if the serum sodium exceeds 142 mmol/l without concomitant changes in urea and creatinine then intravenous 5% glucose solution is given rather than saline.

If the patient then shows evidence of developing a delayed neurological deficit, he is scanned to exclude hematoma or hydrocephalus and is given intravenous frusemide. Mannitol is not given as it can lead to more severe electrolyte inbalances and to fluid overload in children.

Those patients who fail to respond are given 500 ml Rheomacrodex over 24 hours and up to 24 mg papaverine intravenously. Steroid administration is continued according to the normal postoperative regime described earlier. Decompressive craniotomy has not been used for any patient in this series.

A few patients with drowsiness as well as a progressive hemiparesis in whom the CT scan has shown a little shift but no hematoma have been re-explored. About 5 unsuspected extradural or subdural hematomas have been thus discovered. One patient was found to have cerebrospinal fluid loculated in the basal cisterns by old hematoma and made a good recovery when the CSF was drained.

This method involving fluid depletion and measures aimed at reducing brain swelling in patients with delayed deterioration is in contrast to the regimes of intensive blood volume expansion with rigid control of blood pressure advocated in the treatment of postoperative vasospasm (in early operated cases) by several recent workers.

No claims are made that the method described above is in any way better or more rational than that of trying to increase cerebral blood flow to the ischemic brain by volume expansion and hypertension. The latter method simply has not been tried in Zurich and we have no experience of it. One has to accept a lack of understanding of the underlying cause for the deterioration and while this ignorance exists, many more methods of treatment will doubtless come to trial.

Whichever method is used, it requires careful handling of the patient in the intensive care unit and close cooperation between surgeon, anesthetist and intensivist.

Personality and Mental Changes

Many factors are responsible for the psycho-organic syndrome that occurs not infrequently in aneurysm patients postoperatively. These include the psychosis-producing effects of the ICU, metabolic derangements, and the use of steroids (decadron 16 mg/day is given beginning 2 days before operation, then for 5–7 days postoperatively). Appropriate preventive measures include early mobilization, metabolic balance, and the limited use of steroids. 88 out of 785 patients (11.2%) from the group 0–IIb showed transient POS, 29 patients (3.7%) from the same group showed a delayed POS and 17 patients a permanent POS (2.2%).

Epilepsy

6 patients with large and giant aneurysms, but without subarachnoid hemorrhage, and 14 patients with and 1 patient without neurologic symptoms after a subarachnoid hemorrhage suffered epileptic sizures before operation. Therefore 20 patients out of 21 cases belonged to group "b" with ischemic lesions. Postoperatively all these patients needed long-term anticonvulsant therapy. Each of our patients was also treated with prophylactic anticonvulsants (most commonly hydantoin for a total of 2–4 weeks beginning 1–2 days before surgery). Postoperatively, 17 patients had transient seizures (immediately after the operation or within 24 hours).

It should be added that in 1975 the technique of administering anesthesia in this series of patients changed. Formerly fentanyl alone had been used throughout the surgical procedure, necessitating reversal with lethidron at the end. Ethrane was then added to the fentanyl towards the later stage of the operation, obviating the need for lethidron reversal. Since this change over 7 years ago, not a single patient in this series has suffered an epileptic sizure in the immediate postoperative period. 7 patients developed seizures for the first time after surgery and required long-term anticonvulsant therapy to control this problem (Table **134**). Altogether 45 patients had epileptic seizures. Interestingly, 37 patients out of 45 belonged to the "b" group, in other words those who have had symptoms of an ischemic lesion due to a giant aneurysm (6 cases) or caused by the subarachnoid hemorrhage.

Of those patients who had seizures, 24 (55.8%) had good results, while 16 (37.2%) had fair, 1 (2.3%) poor results, and 2 (4.7%) died.

Table 134 Epilepsy

Site of aneurysm	Pre- and postop. Condition	No. of cases	For the first time postop. Transient Condition	No. of cases	Permanent Condition	No. of cases
Ophthalmic	0b	1	–		–	
ICA inferior	0b	1	–		–	
PcoA		–	IIb	2	IIa	1
					IIb	1
					IIIb	2
ICA Bifurcation	0b	4	–		–	
	IIb	1	–			
MCA	0b	1	IIb	2	0b	1
	IIb	2	IV	1	IIb	1
	IIIa	1				
	IIIb	1				
	IV	1				
AcoA	IIIb }	7	I-IIIa	4	IIIb	1
	IV }		II-IIIb	4		
Pe A		–		–	IIIb	1
Ba-Bi	IIIb	1	0b	1	–	
P$_2$	IIb	1	IIb	1	–	
	"b" group	21	"b" group	11	"b" group	7
	"a" group	1	"a" group	4	"a" group	1
		22		15		8 cases

Alterations of CSF Circulation

A variety of disturbances in the normal circulation of cerebrospinal fluid were encountered in this series of patients including hydrocephalus, cisternal loculation, CSF rhinorrhoea, subgaleal CSF collections with or without fistulae, and low intracranial pressure. These alterations are categorized in Table 135.

Following subarachnoid hemorrhage, hydrocephalus may occur acutely or after several weeks or months, and it may or may not resolve without treatment. The relationship of most cases of postoperative hydrocephalus to the surgical procedure is unclear although in some cases it is possible that the evacuation of blood clot from the basal cisterns may help retard its development (Fig 168A–B).

In the present series of 1012 patients with intracranial aneurysms, 97 (9.6%) showed progressive enlargement of the lateral and third ventricles as determined by angiography or pneumoencephalography (before 1976) or computerized tomography (since 1976). The usual manifestations of hydrocephalus are a decreased level of consciousness and slowly progressive hemiparesis with a neglecting syndrome of paretic limbs. In 88 (8.6%) patients, unrelenting symptomatology and a positive RHISA cisternogram indicated the need for a ventricular or subarachnoid shunting procedure. A ventriculo-atrial shunt was used in the majority of patients (Table 135).

The final outcome in these shunted patients was good in 42 (47.7%), fair in 15 (17%), poor in 16 (18.2%), while 15 (17.0%) died. The frequency of

Table 135 Pre- and postoperatively shunted cases with malresorptive hydrocephalus

Result	ICA	Pco	Acho	CA-Bi	MCA	AcoA	PeA	Ba-Bi	Ba-Br.	Vertebr.		Total
Good	3	6	1	–	3	27	–	1	1	–	=	42
Fair	–	5	1	–	3	2	–	3	–	1	=	15
Poor	–	–	1	–	1	10	1	3	–	–	=	16
Death	–	1	–	1	3	7	–	2	1	–	=	15
	3	12	3	1	10	46	1	9	2	1	=	88

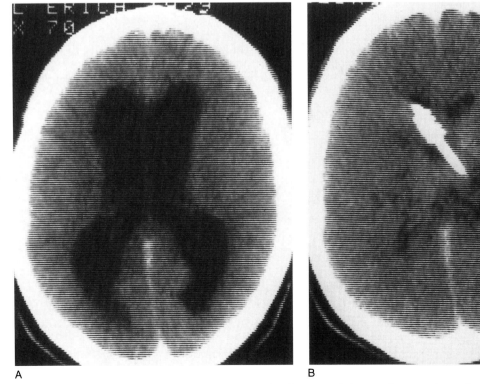

Fig 168A–B 52 year old patient with progressive development of the psycho-organic syndrome after clipping of an aneurysm of the anterior communicating artery showed enlarged ventricles (A) due to an absorptive defect. He showed rapid improvement to a normal condition following the insertion of a shunt (B).

shunted patients related to the site of the aneurysm is given in Table **129b**. Suffice it to say that the occurrence of hydrocephalus following subarachnoid hemorrhage in this group of patients was skewed toward those with anterior communicating, internal carotid artery and basilar bifurcation aneurysms, that is to say those bleeding directly into the basal cisterns.

Subgaleal CSF collections of significant size occurred in 60 patients (5.9%) despite the presence of a subgaleal drain in most instances. Since insisting on a water-tight dural closure (including patching small defects with muscle and acrylic), this problem has become much less frequent. A unique complication was observed in a 60 year old female patient. For a proper dissection of the proximal wall of an ophthalmic aneurysm the anterior clinoid was drilled off. The lateral recess of the sphenoid sinus was opened. Although this was locally repaired she developed bilateral frontal pneumocephalus (Fig **169A–D**).

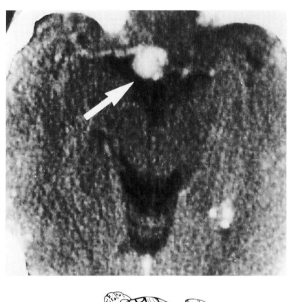

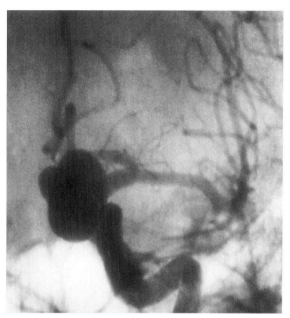

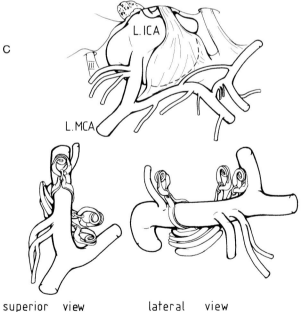

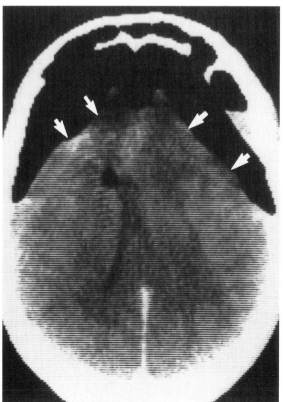

Fig **169A–D** Large left ophthalmic aneurysm (arrow) (**A** and **B**) necessitating removal of the anterior clinoid for clipping (**C**). Postoperativeley the patient developed progressive neurological deterioration and was found to have a tension pneumocephalus (**D**). The lateral recess of the sphenoid sinus in the anterior clinoid had been entered at surgery, requiring eventual ENT repair (**D**).

General Medical Complications

The general medical complications occurring in this series of patients and their relative frequencies are given in Table **136**. A detailed discussion of the pathophysiology, treatment, and prevention of the numerous medical complications that can follow aneurysm surgery is beyond the scope of this book. The more frequent problems include thrombophlebitis, pulmonary embolism, pneumonia, and gastric ulceration, all primarily affecting the poorer grade, immobilized patient. For the last 5 years, prophylactic low dose heparin has been administered (except on the day of operation) to all neurosurgical patients (5000 units subcut. every 12 hours) without any noticable increase in the frequency of perioperative bleeding. This has been combined with frequent leg physiotherapy and early mobilization, most patients getting out of bed the day after surgery, yet there has been no significant improvement in morbidity over the past 5 years.

Table **85**, page 214, shows the most frequent metabolic derangement, namely sodium imbalance, in the last 375 patients with aneurysms of the anterior communicating artery of this series. In this group 157 patients (42%) were found to be hyponatremic (serum sodium less than 135) on the first postoperative day, while 25 (7%) were hypernatremic (greater than 145). Of interest is the finding that a greater proportion of grade III and IV patients are hyponatremic than are grade I and II patients. Restoration of fluid balance was similar in all patients, so this may be a manifestation of hypothalamic dysfunction in the poorer grade patients. In any event, vigorous fluid administration to these patients postoperatively is hazardous and our policy of fluid restriction postoperatively in all aneurysm patients seems justified. This is, of course, modified in patients with elevated creatinine and BUN values.

Finally, we should note that a small number of patients, after entirely successful aneurysm obliteration, have continued to complain of frequent nonspecific headaches for months and sometimes years after surgery. These headaches were sometimes present before their subarachnoid hemorrhage and are not confined to the site of the operation. Clinical examination, EEG and CT scan appearances are normal and the patient can really only be treated by a combination of reassurance and suitable analgesics. We have made use of ergot alkaloids with some success in these cases on the grounds that the headaches may in some way be due to "a vascular reactivity" but the underlying etiology remains obscure.

Conclusions

In the present series of 1012 aneurysm patients operated upon by the senior author (MGY), a total of 377 (37.2%) suffered some type of postoperative adversity that deflected their course from the ideal. In Table **137**, these complications are divided into 4 categories: mild, moderate, severe and fatal, and these categories are related to the patient's condition immediately before operation. From this table it can be seen that relatively few complications, especially severe or fatal complications, occurred in grade I or II patients. The majority of these complications are grouped in the poorer grade (IIb, IIIa–b, IV +V) patients, possibly reflecting the inherent effects of the more severe disease processes in these patients.

Table **136** Medical complications

	ICA M	ICA F	MCA M	MCA F	ACA M	ACA F	Basilar M	Basilar F	Vertebr. M	Vertebr. F	Total M	Total F			%
Thrombophlebitis	4	9	2	4	5	12	1	1	–	–	12	26	=	38	3.8
Pulmonary embolism	2	4	1	4	7	10	1	1	–	2	11	21	=	32	3.2
Pneumonia	3	3	–	1	1	–	3	–	–	2	7	6	=	13	1.3
Gastrointestinal															
Stress ulcerat.	–	1	2	1	5	2	2	1	–	–	9	5	=	14	1.4
Resorption	–	–	–	–	1	–	1	–	–	–	2	–	=	2	0.2
Renal															
Urinary tract infection	1	5	2	3	3	6	1	2	2	2	9	18	=	27	2.7
Hepatitis	–	–	–	–	1	1	–	–	–	–	1	1	=	2	0.2

Table 137 Complications – transient

	Total No.	Number of complications				
		Smooth	Mild	Moderate	Severe	Fatal
0a	12	11 (91.7%)	–	–	–	1
0b	59	33 (55.9%)	12	6	3	5
Ia	242	196 (81.0%)	42	4	–	–
Ib	9	7 (77.8%)	1	–	–	1
IIa	314	238 (75.8%)	51	19	–	6
IIb	147	93 (63.3%)	34	16	2	2
IIIa	75	26 (34.7%)	29	10	1	9
IIIb	100	26 (26.0%)	38	16	10	10
IV	41	5 (12.2%)	5	6	12	13
V	13	–	–	–	2	11
	1012	635 (62.8%)	212 (20.9%)	77 (7.6%)	30 (3.0%)	58 (5.7%)

83.7%

377 (37.2%)

Mild	=	Subcutaneous CSF collecion, thrombophlebitis, urinary tract infection, transient electrolyte disturbance, transient POS, transient epileptic seizure, transient paresis, allergic rash.
Moderate	=	Delayed recovery from hemiparesis, aphasia, POS, rhinorrhea, epileptic seizures, subdural hematomas, pulmonary embolism, pneumonia, stress ulceration.
Severe	=	Permanent POS, paresis, aphasia, diabetes insipidus, permanent epilepsy.
Fatal	=	Rerupture, hematoma, ischemia, perforated ulcer, bacterial meningitis.

Thus, in this series a patient in grade Ia had only a 1.6% chance (and in grade IIa a 6.1% chance) of suffering a moderate complication. The fatal complication risk for these two grades was 0.0% and 1.9% respectively. However, a grade IIIa and b patient was much more at risk (14.8% moderate, 6.3% severe, and 10.9% fatal) and a grade IV severely at risk (14.6% moderate, 29.3% severe, and 31.7% fatal). Better grade patients are operated upon in a good overall condition that allows earlier mobilization, thereby preventing the development of many complications. On the other hand, poorer grade patients undergo surgery in a poor general state and often remain immobile for considerable periods of time, resulting in complications. Perhaps with further experience and improvements in technology, their high complication rate will be diminished, but the surgeon must recognize that the poor, unalterable preoperative condition of these patients will continue to foster postoperative adversity.

10 Addendum

The following account deals with those patients who presented during that part of the period of preparation of this book between August 1979 and December 1983. They have not been included in the larger series in the hope that further information might be gained by comparing the two series. The newer series is also part of a prospective study that may be reported at a later date.

In addition to the 1012 aneurysm patients described in this series, 355 patients with intracranial aneurysms have been operated upon at the University of Zurich between August 1, 1979 and December 31, 1983:

206 of these patients were women and 149 men; 106 were referred from the Canton of Zurich (29.8%), while 160 were transferred from other parts of Switzerland (45.1%) and 89 were from other countries (25.1%).

The age distribution of these patients (Table **138**) reveals that 274 (77.2%) were between the ages of 30 and 60. The presenting symptoms of all 355 patients were analyzed (Table **139**). 323 (91.0%) presented with a subarachnoid hemorrhage verified by either lumbar puncture or CT scan, 24 (6.7%) presented with symptoms such as epilepsy, vague headaches, visual loss, dizziness and paresis and were ultimately shown to have an aneurysm. Most of these latter symptoms on their own did not immediately suggest the diagnosis of an aneurysm. 6 patients (1.7%) from the previous series who had another ruptured aneurysm were operated upon again in the present series. Finally, of those patients presenting with subarachnoid hemorrhage, 62 (19.2%) had 2 hemorrhages prior to surgery, while 8 (2.5%) had 3 and 2 (0.6%) were asymptomatic with unruptured aneurysms.

347 patients had a CT scan prior to surgery. Of these 61 (17.6%) were completely normal and 260 (74.9%) pathological (see Table **140**). 133 (38.3%) showed a definite aneurysm on CT scan, while in 62 (17.9%) aneurysms were suspected.

Table **138** Age distribution

			%	
0 to 10 years	1	=	0.3	} 2.3%
11 to 20 years	7	=	2.0	
21 to 30 years	37	=	10.4	} 34.9%
31 to 40 years	87	=	24.5	
41 to 50 years	108	=	30.4	} 52.7%
51 to 60 years	79	=	22.3	
61 to 70 years	33	=	9.3	} 10.1%
71 and above years	3	=	0.8	

355 patients

Table **139** Reason for investigation for aneurysm in 355 patients

Number of cases			
323	=	91.0%	Proven SAH
251/323	=	77.7%	1 SAH
62/323	=	19.2%	2 SAH
8/323	=	2.5%	3 SAH
2/323	=	0.6%	4 SAH
6	=	1.7%	Repeated hemorrhages (previous surgery for another aneurysm)
24	=	6.7%	Other symptoms*
2	=	0.6%	Investigation for other pathology (tumor, AVM)

* Migraine	5 cases
Epilepsy	4 cases
Visual loss	7 cases
Hemiparesis	8 cases
	24 cases

Table 140 CT findings in patients with intracranial aneurysms (355 patients)

CT performed in	347 patients	(97.7%)
CT not performed in	8 patients	(2.3%)

Results of CT scan in 347 patients

	Ruptured aneurysms	Non-ruptured aneurysms	Total
CT normal	61 (17.6%)	2*	63 (18.2%)
CT pathological	260 (74.9%)	24	284 (81.8%)
	321	26	347

* Aneurysm invisible, but tumor or AVM visible

Pathological CT in 321 patients with ruptured aneurysms:

Hematomas:

	cases	
only cisternal	164/347	(47.3%)
cisternal + intracerebral	26	(7.5%)
cisternal + intracerebral + intraventricular	20	(5.8%)
cisternal + Infarction	17	(4.9%)
cisternal + Hydrocephalus	29	(8.3%)
No hematoma but aneurysm visible	65	(18.7%)

Visibility of aneurysms

	Ruptured aneurysms	Nonrupt./sympt.	Nonrupt./asympt.	Total
Visible	115 (35.8%)	17/23 = 73.9%	1/3 = 33.3%	133
Suspected	56 (17.4%)	6/23 = 26.1%	0/3 = 0%	62
Invisible	150 (46.7%)	0/23 = 0%	2/3 = 66.6%	152
Total	321	23	3	347

This data implies that the diagnosis of a subarachnoid hemorrhage can be made in about 70–75 per cent of cases based only on CT. The obvious need for a good quality CT scan in every patient suspected of having an intracranial aneurysm is emphasized. 29 of 321 patients (9.0%) with ruptured aneurysm showed hydrocephalus on CT scan.

The timing of operation as related to the latest subarachnoid hemorrhage is given in Tables 141 and 142. It can be seen that few patients (10.5%) were operated upon within the first 3 days, 26.4 per cent within 1 week, 56.2 per cent within 2 weeks, and 23.3 per cent later than the 4th week after the hemorrhage. This relates to the referral pattern of patients at this institution, with a majority arriving a week or more following their ictus.

Aneurysms at the anterior cerebral artery complex occurred most frequently (40.8%), followed by the internal carotid artery (32.7%), the middle cerebral artery (13.2%), and the vertebro-basilar system (13.2%). These figures are similar to those reported in the previous series with the exception of those for aneurysms of the middle cerebral

Table 141 Timing of operation in 352 cases (see Table 2)

						1976–1979	
Up to	3 days	in	37 cases	(10.5%)	}	4.5%	}
From	4th– 7th day	in	56 cases	(15.9%)	56.2%	13.6%	45.7%
	8th–14th day	in	105 cases	(29.8%)		27.6%	
	15th–28th day	in	72 cases	(20.5%)	}	30.3%	}
	29th day and later		82 cases	(23.3%)	43.8%	24.1%	54.4%
Total			352* cases				

* 3 asymptomatic cases excluded

Table 142 Timing of operation and results in 352 symptomatic cases

	Total No.	Good	Fair	Poor	Death
Before 3rd day:					
Ia	3	3	–	–	–
IIa	29	26	3	–	–
IIIa	2	2	–	–	–
IV	3	1	1	–	1[+]
	37	32 (86.5%)	4 (10.8%)	–	1 (2.7%)
4th–7th day:					
Ia	5	5	–	–	–
IIa	38	37	1	–	–
IIb	4	2	2	–	–
IIIa	7	6	1	–	–
IIIb	2	–	–	–	2
	56	50 (89.3%)	4 (7.1%)	–	2 (3.6%)
8th–14th day:					
0b	1	1	–	–	–
Ia	25	25	–	–	–
Ib	4	4	–	–	–
IIa	60	57	2	1*	–
IIb	10	6	2	2	–
IIIa	2	2	–	–	–
IIIb	3	–	1	2	–
	105	95 (90.5%)	5 (4.8%)	5 (4.8%)	–
15th–28th day:					
0b	2	2	–	–	–
Ia	23	23	–	–	–
Ib	13	13	–	–	–
IIa	18	17	–	–	1
IIb	12	11	–	–	1
IIIa	2	2	–	–	–
IIIb	2	–	2	–	–
	72	68 (94.4%)	2 (2.8%)	–	2 (2.8%)
After 29th day:					
0b	19	18	–	1	–
Ia	52	52	–	–	–
Ib	11	9	2	–	–
	82	79 (96.3%)	2 (2.4%)	1 (1.2%)	–
Total No.	352**	324 (92.0%)	17 (4.8%)	6 (1.7%)	5 (1.4%)

* Angiographic complication
** 3 asymptomatic excluded   [+] intracerebral hematoma

Table 143 Site of aneurysm and operative results

	Total No.	Good	Fair	Poor	Death
Internal carotid artery					
Cavernous	2	2	–	–	–
Carotid ophthalmic	12	11	–	1 (0b)	–
Carotid inferior	16	13	1 (IV)	2 (IIb, IIb)	–
PcoA	58	55	1 (IIa)	1 (IIIb)	1 (IIIb)
AchoA	9	9	–	–	–
Carotid bifurcation	19	16	1 (IIa)	1 (IIa)*	1 (IIa)
	116 (32.7%)	106	3	5	2
Middle cerebral artery					
M$_1$ segment	6	6	–	–	–
MCA-bifurcation	41	39	2 (Ib, Ib)	–	–
	47 (13.2%)	45	2	–	–
Anterior cerebral artery					
A$_1$ segment	5	4	1 (Ib)	–	–
AcoA	127	119	6 (Ib, IIa, IIa, IIb, IIIa, IIIb)	–	2 (IIa, IIb)
Pericallosal artery	13	12	–	–	1 (IIIb)
	145 (40.8%)	135	7	–	3
Vertebro-basilar arteries					
Basilar bifurcation	24	20 (1)	3 (IIb, IIIb, IIIb)	1 (IIb)	–
Basilar branch	10	8	2 (IIa, IIa)	–	–
Basilar trunk	4	4	–	–	–
Vertebral artery	3	3	–	–	–
PICA	6	6	–	–	–
	47 (13.2%)	41	5	1	–
Total	355	327	17	6	5

* Angiographic complication   () not clipped, muscle wrapped

artery (−5.0%) and the vertebro-basilar system (+3.6%) (see p. 299, Vol. I, Table 17). The site of aneurysms and the operative results are given in Table 143.

The preoperative status of the later group of patients is shown in Table 144. The results in this series (1979–1983) show an improvement over those in the earlier series of 1012 cases (1967–1979) with a 6.5 per cent increase in good results, a 4.3 per cent drop in mortality and a 0.9 per cent drop in fair and 1.4 per cent in poor categories (see Table 1a). Overall, good results were obtained in 327 (92.1%), fair results in 17 (4.8%), poor results in 6 (1.7%), and 5 patients (1.4%) died. The majority (75.8%) underwent surgery in grade 0a–Ia–IIa–IIIa (previous series 63.5%) and the remaining 24.2% were in grade 0b, Ib, IIb, IIIb or IV (previous series 35.2%). 93.5 per cent of patients were fully alert (previous series 77.3%) and only 6.4 per cent in grades III–IV (previous series 21.4%). The improved results achieved in the later series seem to be largely due to the fact that since 1979 fewer patients (0.8%) have been operated upon in grade IV (c.f. 4.1%, 1967–1979), and no patients in grade V.

A list of complications occurring in these patients is given in Table 145. The most frequently encountered problems included transient hemisyndromes with or without dysphasia (5.6%), permanent hemiparesis (2.0%), permanent psychoorganic syndrome (1.1%), transient oculomotor palsy (1.4%), deep venous thrombosis (4.2%), pulmonary embolus (3.1%), epilepsy (1.4%), hydro-

Table 144 Preoperative condition and results in 355 patients (August 1979–December 1983)

	Total No.	Good	Fair	Poor	Death
0a	3	3	–	–	–
0b	23	22 (95.6%)	–	1	–
Ia	108	108 (100%)	–	–	–
Ib	28	26 (92.9%)	2	–	–
IIa	145	137 (94.5%)	6	1°	1*
IIb	25	18 (72.0%)	4	2	1**
IIIa	13	12 (92.3%)	1	–	–
IIIb	7	– (0%)	3	2	2 {1***, 1****}
IV	3	1	1	–	1***
	355	327 (92.1%)	17 (4.8%)	6 (1.7%)	5 (1.4%)
Previous series (1967–1979)	1012	85.6%	5.6%	3.1%	5.7%

* Uneventful postoperative course; 2 weeks later bilateral ischemia. Autopsy showed bilateral thrombosis of the common carotid arteries, stenosis of the aorta
** Pulmonary emboli 2 weeks and 4 weeks respectively after uneventful postoperative course
*** Thrombosis of superior sagittal sinus
**** Bilateral infarction
° Angiographic complication (embolus in opposite MCA)

Table 145 Complications (see Table 132)

	Number of cases		1979–1983	1967–1979
A. *Central nervous system complications*				
Intracranial hematoma	2	=	0.6%	0.9%
Wound infection	3	=	0.8%	1.3%
Meningitis	1	=	0.3%	0.6%
Rerupture	2	=	0.6%	1.1%
Transient hemiparesis, with and without aphasia	20	=	5.6%	7.9%
Permanent hemiparesis	7	=	2.0%	4.3%
Transient POS	24	=	6.8%	11.6%
Permanent POS	4	=	1.1%	1.7%
Hypothalamic transient	7	=	2.0%	3.2%
permanent	–	=	0.0%	0.4%
Epilepsy, transient (postop.)	5	=	1.4%	1.7%
Transient III-palsy	5	=	1.4%	2.8%
Hydrocephalus	11	=	3.1%	8.6%
Rhinorrhea	1	=	0.3%	0.4%
B. *General medical complications*				
Superior sinus thrombosis	1	=	0.3%	0.0%
Deep venous thrombosis	15	=	4.2%	3.8%
Pulmonary embolus	11	=	3.1%	3.2%
Hepatitis	1	=	0.3%	0.2%

cephalus (3.1%), and intracranial hematoma (0.6%).

Compared with the earlier series there is a lower incidence of postoperative paresis, psychoorganic syndrome and epilepsy. The authors believe that this is mainly due to better patient selection for surgery (fewer grades III–V and fewer in subgroup b).

An interesting observation was made in 7 patients (in 1980 and 1981) each of whom had an uneventful course in the first 4–8 days postoperatively but who then developed over a 1–3 day period a stuttering hemiparesis. This resulted in a prolonged fixed deficit with only a modest improvement after weeks and months. The clinical deterioration was initially thought to be due to cerebral vasospasm and the patients were given intravenous papaverine and rheomacrodex but with no convincing effect.

Such effects of postoperative vasospasm simply had not been found to be a significant complication in the previous series. Two factors may have contributed toward this apparent difference. First, until 1979 only 4.5% of patients were operated upon with 3 days of their bleed. After 1979 this number rose to 10.5%. 3 of the 7 patients described above were operated upon within the first 3 days and the remaining 4 within 8 days. Although the numbers are small and the presence of vasospasm not confirmed by angiography these results provide some circumstantial evidence that early operation may predispose toward an increased risk of postoperative cerebral ischemic deficit.

Secondly, in an effort to reduce the risk of venous thrombosis and pulmonary embolism (a trial with anticoagulant therapy having been unsuccessful) patients have been mobilized early – usually the morning after surgery. It may be that this rapid mobilization is too premature in patients who have undergone early operation and one may provoke undesirable changes in cerebral perfusion in patients whose cerebro-vascular autoregulation is still impaired.

The personal view of the senior author is that patients undergoing early operation should be asked whether or not they feel comfortable in the upright position and should have their supine and erect blood pressure checked at regular intervals in the early stages of mobilization. Since these simple measures have been adapted there have been no further complications in 162 patients in a two year period (1982–1983).

In their recent paper, Ljunggren et al (1983) described their experience with early surgery for ruptured aneurysms and those factors which might predispose toward an unfavorable outcome. Our own figures show that up to 1979 4.5% of patients underwent surgery within 3 days of subarachnoid hemorrhage. Since then the figure has risen to about 10% with a total of 16% being operated upon within the first week. These numbers would undoubtedly be higher, if not for the diverse methods of referral to the Neurosurgical Department of Zurich.

Surgery within the first 48 hours should minimize the risk of early recurrence of hemorrhage and seems to be an ideal at which we should aim. It may, however, present its own peculiar problems even for the most experienced surgeon. Opening the basal cisterns and emptying them of fresh, sticky hematoma may be extremely difficult and dangerous. There may also be general metabolic and cardiovascular derangements in this acute phase which may make the added insults of surgery even more hazardous.

In the second series of 355 cases, 37 patients were operated upon within 3 days of subarachnoid hemorrhage with 86.5% good results, 10.8% fair results and 2.7% mortality. Between day 4–7, 56 patients underwent surgery with 89.3% good results, 7.1% fair results and 3.6% mortality. The further 105 cases were operated upon within 7 to 14 days (90.5% good results, 4.8% fair results, 4.8% poor results). Between 15 days and 4 weeks there were 72 patients (94.4% good results) and beyond 4 weeks 82 patients (96.3% good results), (see Table **142**).

Early surgery appears justified to prevent fatal early recurrent hemorrhage in grade I and grade II patients and to be occasionally life saving in the poor grade patients with significant mass effect from intracranial hematoma. Our results suggest that in experienced hands grade I and II patients may be safely operated upon at any time after subarachnoid hemorrhage. The timing of surgery in grade III patients with no space occupying hematoma is still in doubt. There is no generally acceptable method of determining clinically which patients in this grade may be suitable for early surgery. Overall, the choice of whether to perform early or delayed surgery must, as yet, remain the matter of personal preference based largely on the degree of experience of the individual surgeon.

The results of treatment of grade III to grade V patients remain most disappointing. Between August 1979 and the end of December 1983, 28 patients (19 female, 9 male, average age 50.2 years) were admitted in these grades (4 in condition IIa, one IIb, 9 IIIa, 9 IIIb, 4 IV and one V) of whom 23 deteriorated progressively and died before angiography. Of 4 cases admitted in grade

IIa and one in grade IIb all five showed deterioration after the angiography and died. Autopsy studies of the fatal cases revealed 3 PcoA aneurysms, 9 MCA aneurysms (one giant), 11 AcoA aneurysms, one pericallosal artery aneurysm, 2 basilar artery trunk (giant) aneurysms, one basilar bifurcation aneurysm and one vertebral artery aneurysm. Thus a total of 28 of 383 patients in the second series died before surgery (7.3%). These represent only those cases reaching the Neurosurgical Department and presumably only a fraction of those patients dying of ruptured aneurysm in the Zurich catchment area.

This once more highlights the need not only for progress in surgical and early medical treatment in subarachnoid hemorrhage, but also the need for a better understanding of the pathophysiology and epidemiology of these cases.

11 Final Comments

Although a few pioneering efforts preceded the introduction of angiography, the real establishment of aneurysm surgery as a discipline had to await the development of this essential diagnostic test. With the advent of angiography, not only the diagnosis but also the pathophysiology of cerebral aneurysms could be evaluated. In addition, effective treatment options could be conceived, developed, and implemented. As a result, with each passing year, more case and series reports were added to the existing knowledge, providing impetus for a large systematic study. This was undertaken in the United States and the results established a unified concept of the natural history and pathophysiology not only of aneurysms, but of all hemorrhagic cerebrovascular disease.

Once this concept was established, better methods for diagnosis and treatment of ruptured cerebral aneurysms began to evolve. The diagnosis and precise localization of ruptured aneurysms and the approach and timing of surgical intervention were improved with the addition of subtraction angiography, digital angiography, angiotomography, CT scanning, ICP monitoring, CBF studies, PET scanning, etc. New medical protocols including hypotensive drugs, antibiotics, and anticonvulsants were introduced, as were improved neuroanesthetic techniques and ICU care. Each successive innovation correspondingly improved our understanding and ability to treat ruptured cerebral aneurysms.

As the years passed, the surgical approaches to ruptured cerebral aneurysms were likewise improved, always attempting a greater degree of precision. Towards this end, the surgical microscope was applied to these lesions, transforming their obliteration into a highly refined process. With this technique, the importance of anatomical considerations including the basal cisterns and perforating vessels became evident. Precision instrumentation including the freely movable operating microscope, micro-instruments, bipolar coagulator and aneurysm clips were developed. As a result, the classical concept of quick aneurysm strangulation was revised to incorporate finesse, more perfect clip placement and complete elimination of the aneurysms.

The best current treatment of ruptured aneurysms is widely debated. Lists of contemporary reports could be drawn and compared to the present work, but the validity of any conclusions would be suspect. Each series encompasses an evolving spectrum of a surgeon's technical ability, the timing and extent of microscope use, the application of hypothermia, temporary vascular occlusion, different types of neuroanesthesia, the use of spinal drainage, etc. thereby making any meaningful comparison invalid. Likewise, no uniformity exists in preoperative classifications, operative timing, postoperative results, or follow-up periods, making these comparisons even more meaningless.

Finally, criticism of past performances based on present technical advantages seems unfair and unwarranted.

It is our hope that the revised preoperative classification introduced in this book will help in this regard. By separating a and b grade patients, preoperative deficits unrelated to surgery can be separated from surgically induced deficits. As a result real advantages of the microscopic technique will become evident for good results can be realized in nearly 95 per cent of grade 0a, Ia, and IIa patients. In many current reports this advantage is not evident due either to the confusing effects of preoperative deficits (0b, Ib, IIb, etc.) or to the inherent tenacity of the brain to survive and to camouflage operative intrusions through its vascular collateralization and neuronal plasticity.

Future improvements are needed in every aspect of ruptured aneurysm diagnosis and treatment. It is still impossible to predict before surgery the precise topography of perforating vessels and their relationship to an aneurysm, the state of the microvasculature, and the adequacy of vascular collateralization. Further neuroradiological advances are needed, including perhaps the use of refined ultrasonic techniques. With the surgical microscope, we can consistently improve the altered vascular anatomy of an aneurysm, yet reliable treatment for its associated pathophysiological alterations is not yet established. The best operative timing in grade III patients is still not clear. Perhaps CBF studies, positron emission tomography, and CSF flow studies will add insight in this important area.

The present two volumes have largely been dedicated to describing anatomical concepts, microsurgical techniques and technical advances developed by the senior author over the past 16 years. The hope is that they may bring about a better understanding by others of the problems involved in microneurosurgery for aneurysms thereby avoiding many of the pitfalls and leading to improved surgical results.

However, as can be seen by the figures in Table **131**, page 330, even experienced surgeons in a country providing high standards of general medical care currently help little more than 50% of patients with subarachnoid hemorrhage. Kassel and Drake (1983) and later Bucy (1983) emphasized the failure of overall management of patients with subarachnoid hemorrhage and put into perspective the modest improvements in mortality and morbidity brought about by surgical advances in the past two decades. They identified some potentially reversible causes for the still alarmingly high mortality rate from subarachnoid hemorrhage. Attention and investigation must be directed toward these and several other factors if we are to improve the numbers of patients who might safely be brought to curative surgery. Allowing for those patients who suffer catastrophic first bleeds and for the imperfections of surgery it should be possible to "cure" about 80% of subarachnoid hemorrhage patients without residual deficits.

Drake discussed the importance of recognizing the first "warning" bleed so frequently ignored by the patient and his relatives or missed by the family doctor and at the receiving hospital. Neurosurgeons must play their part in improving the education of the public and medical students and in reminding their medical colleagues of the need for earlier diagnosis, proper investigation, and prompt transfer to a neurosurgical centre.

Modern technology is moving rapidly forwards and some long-held principles of management must inevitably yield to such progress. As CT scanning facilities become more widely and more immediately available so the initial investigation in suspected subarachnoid hemorrhage must become that of scan prior to lumbar puncture. This should prevent inadvisable lumbar puncture in those cases with unsuspected raised intracranial pressure.

Further careful studies must be carried out into the pathophysiology of subarachnoid hemorrhage to try and improve the lot of those patients admitted in grades III–V and to enable them to be investigated and operated upon safely. The advent of PET and metabolic NMR scanning may lead to better understanding and treatment of the derangement of cerebral hemodynamics and metabolism in subarachnoid hemorrhage.

The recurring problems of preoperative rebleeding and of vasospasm have yet to be resolved and we await with interest the latest findings in terms of antifibrinolytic therapy and the calcium antagonists. Part of the answer must lie in safe early surgery and this remains an open topic in the mind of the senior author. If early surgery is undertaken in good grade patients attention must be focussed on the potential hazards of early mobilization in producing late cerebral ischemic deficits. Early surgery may allow a more aggressive hemodynamic and pharmacological approach to the treatment of postoperative vasospasm should it occur. At present, however, it is felt proper to advise a regime of careful postoperative fluid restriction in all cases, supplemented with thiazide diuretics if cerebral vasospasm or edema are suspected.

As for the surgeon himself increased experience will, up to a point, improve the results. This may be brought about by the acquisition of great technical skills by progressive reduction of operating time – and therefore brain retraction time – and by a greater ability to select the patients for save, effective and early surgery. The experience in Zurich reflects such a trend with about 10 per cent of patients now operated upon within the first three days, patients very rarely operated upon in grades IV and V, and operating time from about four hours at the beginning of the series to around one and a half hour at present.

The future artists of aneurysm surgery must paint pictures without any flaws. It is toward this goal that this book is dedicated; to all those patients that could not (and still cannot) be helped.

References

Chapter 1: Clinical Considerations

Allcock, J. M., C. G. Drake: Ruptured intracranial aneurysms. The role of arterial spasm. J. Neurosurg. 22: 21–29, 1965

Amacher A. L., G. G. Ferguson, C. G. Drake, J. P. Girvin, H. W. R. Barr: How old people tolerate intracranial surgery for aneurysm. Neurosurgery 1: 242–244, 1977

Appleton, D. B., P. J. Smith, W. J. S. Earwaker: Subarachnoid haemorrhage in children. Proc. Aust. Ass. Neurol. 11: 1–11, 1974

Artiola i Fortuny, L., L. Prieto-Valiente: Long-term prognosis in surgically treated intracranial aneurysms. Part 1: Mortality, Part 2: Morbidity. J. Neurosurg. 54: 26–43, 1981

Beck, O., J.: Preoperative treatment of intracranial aneurysms. In: Pia, H. W., C. Langmaid, J. Zierski: Cerebral Aneurysms, Advances in Diagnosis and Therapy. Springer, Berlin, 1979 (pp. 197–200)

Becker, D. H., G. D. Silverberg, D. H. Nelson: Saccular aneurysm of infancy and early childhood. Neurosurgery 2: 1–7, 1978

Botterell, E. H., W. M. Lougheed, J. W. Scott, S. L. Vanderwater: Hypothermia and interruption of carotid, or carotid and vertebral circulation, in the surgical management of intracranial aneurysms. J. Neurosurg. 13: 1–42, 1956

Boullin, D. J.: Cerebral Vasospasm. Wiley, Chichester, 1980

Bradford, F. K., P. C. Sharkey: Physiologic effects from introduction of blood and other substances into subarachnoid space of dogs. J. Neurosurg. 19: 1017–1022, 1962

Cannell, D. E., E. H. Botterell: Subarachnoid hemorrhage and pregnancy. Amer. J. Obstet. Gynec. 72: 844–855, 1956

Copelan, E. L., R. F. Maron: Spontaneous intracranial bleeding in pregnancy. Obstet. and Gynec. 20: 373–378, 1962

Daane, T. A., R. W. Tandy: Rupture of congenital aneurysm in pregnancy. Obstet. and Gynec. 15: 305, 1960

Drake, C. G.: Ruptured intracranial aneurysms. Proc. roy. Soc. Med. 64: 477–481, 1971

Ecker, A., P. A. Riemenschneider: Arteriographic demonstration of spasm of the intracranial arteries with special reference to saccular arterial aneurysms. J. Neurosurg. 8: 660–667, 1951

Ellington, E., T. Margolis: Block of arachnoid villus by subarachnoid hemorrhage. J. Neurosurg. 30: 651–657, 1969

Ferguson, G. G., A. M. Harper, W. Fitch, J. O. Rowan, B. Jennett: Cerebral blood flow measurements after spontaneous subarachnoid haemorrhage. Europ. Neurol. 8: 15–22, 1972

Flamm, E., J. Ransohoff: Subarachnoid hemorrhage and cerebral vasospasm. In: Pia, H. W., C. Langmaid, J. Zierski: Cerebral Aneurysms, Advances in Diagnosis and Therapy. Springer, Berlin 1979 (pp. 152–155)

Fodstad, H., B. Liliequist, M. Schannong, C.-A. Thulin: Tranexamic acid in the preoperative management of ruptured intracranial aneurysms. Surg. Neurol. 10: 9–15, 1978

Foltz, E. L., A. A. Ward Jr.: Communicating hydrocephalus from subarachnoid bleeding. J. Neurosurg. 13: 546–566, 1956

Gillingham, F. J., J. Barbera, U. M. Myint, V. S. Madan: Ruptured intracranial aneurysm. Factors influencing prognosis. In Gillingham, F. J., C. Mawdsley, A. E. Williams: Stroke. Proceedings of the Ninth Pfizer International Symposium. Churchill Livingston, London, Edinburgh 1976

Girvin, J.: Formal discussion of: Nibbelink, D. W. (1975), pp. 165–167

Graf, C. J.: Results of direct attack on nonfistulous intracranial aneurysms with remarks on statistics. J. Neurosurg. 12: 146–153, 1955

Graf, C. J., D. W. Nibbelink: Cooperative Study of Intracranial Aneurysms and Subarachnoid Hemorrhage. Report on a randomized treatment study. Stroke 5: 559–601, 1974

Grode, M. L., M. Saunders, C. A. Carton: Subarachnoid hemorrhage secondary to ruptured aneurysm in infants. Report of two cases. J. Neurosurg. 49: 898–902, 1978

Grubb, R. L., M. E. Reichle, J. O. Eichling, M. H. Gado: The effects of subarachnoid hemorrhage upon regional cerebral blood volume, blood flow and oxygen utilization in man. In: Harper, A. M., W. B. Jennett, J. D. Miller, J. C. Rowan: Blood Flow and Metabolism in Brain. Churchill Livingstone, Edinburgh, 1975 (13.12–13.16)

Hamby, W. B.: Intracranial Aneurysms. Thomas, Springfield/Ill. 1952

Hammes Jr., E. M.: The reactions of the meninges to blood. Arch. Neurol. Psychiat. 52: 505–514, 1944

Hase, U., H.-J. Reulen, A. Fenske, K. Schürmann: Intracranial pressure and pressure volume relation in patients with subarachnoid haemorrhage (SAH). Acta neurochir. (Wien) 44: 69–80, 1978

Hayashi, M., S. Marukawa, H. Fujii, T. Kitano. H. Kobayashi, S. Yamamoto: Intracranial hypertension in patients with ruptured intracranial aneurysms. J. Neurosurg. 46: 584–595, 1977

Hayashi, M., S. Marukawa, H. Fujii, T. Kitano, H. Kobayashi, S. Muneomote, S. Yamamoto: Intracranial pressure in patients with diffuse arterial spasm following ruptured intracranial aneurysms. Acta neurochir. (Wien) 44: 81–95, 1978

Heiskanen, O., I. Marttila: Risk of rupture of a second aneurysm in patients with multiple aneurysms. J. Neurosurg. 32: 295–299, 1970

Heiskanen, O., P. Nikki: Rupture of intracranial arterial aneurysms during pregnancy. Acta neurol. scand. 34: 202–208, 1963

Hungerford, G. D., J. M. Marzluff, L. G. Kempe, J. M. Powers: Cerebral arterial aneurysm in a neonate. Neuroradiology 21: 107–110, 1981

Hunt, H. B., B. S. Schifrin, K. Suzuki: Ruptured berry aneurysms and pregnancy. Obstet. and Gynec. 43: 827–837, 1974

Hunt, W. E., R. M. Hess: Surgical risk as related to time of intervention in the repair of intracranial aneurysms. J. Neurosurg. 28: 14–20, 1968

Hunt, W. E., E. J. Kosnik: Timing and perioperative cave in intracranial aneurysm surgery. Clin. Neurosurg. 21: 79–89, 1974

Jones, R. A. C.: Aneurysms in the elderly. Advance Neurol. 6: 144–147, 1978

Kagström, E., L. Palma: Influence of antifibrinolytic treatment on the morbidity in patients with subarachnoid haemorrhage. Acta neurol. scand. 48: 257–258, 1972

Kaste, M., M. Ramsay: Tranexamic acid in subarachnoid hemorrhage. A double-blind study. Stroke 10: 519–522, 1979

Kelly, P., R. J. Gorten, R. G. Grossman, H. M. Eisenberg: Cerebral perfusion, vascular spasm and outcome in patients with ruptured intracranial aneurysms. J. Neurosurg. 47: 44–49, 1977

Kibler, R. F., R. S. C. Couch, M. R. Crompton: Hydrocephalus in the adult following spontaneous subarachnoid hemorrhage. Brain 84: 45–61, 1961

Klafta Jr., L. A., W. B. Hamby: Significance of cerebrospinal fluid pressure in determining time for repair of intracranial aneurysms. J. Neurosurg. 31: 217–219, 1969

Knibestöl, M., A. Karadayi, D. Tovi: Echo-encephalographic study of ventricular dilatation after subarachnoid haemorrhage with special reference to the effect of antifibrinolytic treatment. Acta neurol. scand. 54: 57–70, 1976

Kohlmeyer, K.: Cerebral blood flow in subarachnoid hemorrhage. In Pia, H. W., C. Langmaid, J. Zierski: Cerebral Aneurysms, Advances in Diagnosis and Therapy. Springer, Berlin 1979 (pp. 144–152)

Lipper, S., D. Morgan, M. R. Krigman, E. V. Staab: Congenital saccular aneurysm in a 19 day old neonate. Surg. Neurol. 10: 161–165, 1978

Lougheed, W. M., B. M. Marshall: Management of aneurysms of the anterior circulation by intracranial procedures. In Youmans, J. R.: Neurological Surgery, Vol. II. Saunders, Philadelphia 1973 (pp. 731–767)

McCausland, A. M., F. Holmes: Spinal fluid pressure during labor. West. J. Surg. 65: 220–233, 1957

Matson, D. D.: Intracranial arterial aneurysms in childhood. J. Neurosurg. 23: 578–583, 1965

Meyer, J. S.: Noninvasive regional cerebral blood flow measurements in subarachnoid hemorrhage. In Pia, H. W., C. Langmaid, J. Zierski: Cerebral Aneurysms, Advances in Diagnosis and Therapy. Springer, Berlin 1979 (pp. 133–144)

Meyer, J. S., N. Ishihara, V. D. Desmukh, H. Naritomi et al.: An improved method for noninvasive measurement of regional cerebral blood flow and blood volume by ^{133}Xe inhalation. Description of the method and normal values obtained in healthy volonteers. Stroke 9: 195–205, 1978

Miller, J. H., C. M. Hinckley: Berry aneurysms in pregnancy: A ten year report. S. med. J. Bgham, Ala. 63: 279 and 285, 1970

Millikan, C. H.: Cerebral vasospasm and ruptured intracranial aneurysm. Arch. Neurol. (Chic.) 32: 433–449, 1975

Moyes, P. D.: Surgical treatment of multiple aneurysms and of incidentally discovered unruptured aneurysms. J. Neurosurg. 35: 291–295, 1971

Mullan, S.: Conservative management of the recently ruptured aneurysm. Surg. Neurol. 3: 27–32, 1975

Mullan, S., J. Dawley: Antifibrinolytic therapy of intracranial aneurysms. J. Neurosurg. 28: 21–23, 1968

Nibbelink, D. W.: Cooperative Aneurysm Study: Antihypertensive and antifibrinolytic therapy following subarachnoid hemorrhage from ruptured intracranial aneurysm. In Whisnant, J. P., B. A. Sandok: Cerebral Vascular Diseases, Ninth Conference. Grune & Stratton, New York 1975 (pp. 155–165)

Nibbelink, D. W., A. L. Sahs, L. A. Knowler: Antihypertensive and antifibrinolytic medications in subarachnoid hemorrhage and their relation to cerebral vasospasm. In Smith, R. R., J. T. Robertson: Subarachnoid Hemorrhage and Cerebrovascular Spasm. Thomas, Springfield/Ill. 1975 (pp. 177–205)

Nilsson, B. W.: Cerebral blood flow in patients with subarachnoid hemorrhage studied with an intravenous isotope technique. Its clinical significance in the timing of surgery of cerebral arterial aneurysms. Acta neurochir. (Wien) 37: 33–48, 1977

Norlén, G., H. Olivecrona: The treatment of aneurysms of the circle of Willis. J. Neurosurg. 10: 404–415, 1953

Nornes, H.: The role of intracranial pressure in the arrest of hemorrhage in patients with ruptured intracranial aneurysms. J. Neurosurg. 39: 226–234, 1973

Obrist, W. D., H. K. Thompson Jr., H. S. Wang, W. E. Wilkinson: Regional cerebral blood flow estimated by ^{133}Xe inhalation. Stroke 6: 245–256, 1975

Pakarinen, S.: Incidence, aetiology, and prognosis of primary subarachnoid haemorrhage. Acta neurol. scand., Suppl. 29, 1967 (128 p.)

Patel, A. N., A. E. Richardson: Ruptured intracranial aneurysms in the first two decades of life. A study of 58 patients. J. Neurosurg. 35: 571–576, 1971

Pedowitz, P., A. Perell: Aneurysms complicated by pregnancy. Part II. Aneurysms of the cerebral vessels. Amer. J. Obstet. Gynec. 73: 736, 1957

Perret, G., H. Nishioka: Cerebral angiography. J. Neurosurg. 25: 98–114, 1966

Pool, J. L.: Treatment of intracranial aneurysms during pregnancy. J. Amer. med. Ass. 192: 209–214, 1965

Pool, J. L., D. G. Potts: Aneurysms and Arteriovenous Malformations of the Brain. Diagnosis and Treatment. Harper & Row, New York 1965

Post, K. D., E. S. Flamm, A. Goodgold, J. Ransohoff: Ruptured intracranial aneurysms: Case morbidity and mortality. J. Neurosurg. 46: 296–303, 1977

Raimondi, A. J., H. Torres: Acute hydrocephalus as a complication of subarachnoid hemorrhage. Surg. Neurol. 1: 23–26, 1973

Richardson, A. E.: Aneurysms of childhood. In Pia, H. W., C. Langmaid, J. Zierski: Cerebral Aneurysms, Advances in Diagnosis and Therapy. Springer, Berlin 1979 (pp. 376–378)

Robinson, J. L., C. S. Hall, C. B. Sedzimir: Subarachnoid hemorrhage in pregnancy. J. Neurosurg. 36: 27–33, 1972

Robinson, J. L., C. S. Hall, C. B. Sedzimir: Arteriovenous malformations, aneurysms and pregnancy. J. Neurosurg. 41: 63–70, 1974

Rydin, E., P. O. Lundberg: Tranexamic acid and intracranial thrombosis. Lancet II: 49, 1976

Saito, I., Y. Ueda, K. Sano: Significance of vasospasm in the treatment of ruptured intracranial aneurysms. J. Neurosurg. 47: 412–429, 1977

Saito, I., T. Shigeno, K. Aritake, T. Tanishima, K. Sano: Vasospasm assessed by angiography and computerized tomography. J. Neurosurg. 51: 466–475, 1979

Sakamoto, T., T. Yoshimoto, A. Takaku, J. Suzuki: Occurrence and treatment of hydrocephalus following ruptured intracranial aneurysms. In Suzuki, J.: Cerebral Aneurysms. Neuron, Tokyo, 1979 (pp. 375–383)

Salazar, J. L.: Surgical treatment of asymptomatic and incidental intracranial aneurysms. J. Neurosurg. 53: 20–27, 1980

Samson, D. S., K. M. Hodosh, W. K. Clark: Surgical management of unruptured asymptomatic aneurysms. J. Neurosurg. 46: 731–734, 1977

Samson, D. S., R. H. Hodosh, W. R. Reid, C. W. Beyer, W. K. Clark: Risk of intracranial aneurysm surgery in the good grade patients: early versus late operation. Neurosurgery 5/4: 422–427, 1979

Sano, K., I. Saito: Timing and indication of surgery for ruptured intracranial aneurysms with regards to cerebral vasospasm. Acta neurochir. (Wien) 41: 49–60, 1978

Sano, K., I. Saito: Indication and timing of operation and vasospasm. In Pia, H. W., C. Langmaid, J. Zierski: Cerebral Aneurysms, Advances in Diagnosis and Therapy. Springer, Berlin 1979 (pp. 208–217)

Shulman, K., B. F. Martin, N. Popoff, J. Ransohoff: Recognition and treatment of hydrocephalus following spontaneous subarachnoid hemorrhage. J. Neurosurg. 20: 1040–1049, 1963

Slosberg, P.: Hypotensive therapy in acute intracranial bleeding. J. Mt Sinai Hosp. 23: 825–831, 1956

Slosberg, P.: Treatment of ruptured intracranial aneurysms by induced hypotension. Mt Sinai J. Med. (N.Y.) 40: 82–90, 1973

Smith, R. R., J. T. Robertson: Subarachnoid Hemorrhage and Cerebrovascular Spasm. Thomas, Springfield/Ill. 1975

Sonntag, V. K. H., B. M. Stein: Arteriopathic complications during treatment of subarachnoid hemorrhage with epsilon aminocaproic acid. J. Neurosurg. 40: 480–485, 1974

Steelman, H. F., G. J. Hayes, H. V. Rizzoli: Surgical treatment of saccular intracranial aneurysms. J. Neurosurg. 10: 564–570, 1953

Strain, R. E.: Progressive communicating hydrocephalus following subarachnoid hemorrhage – a neurosurgical emergency. Sth. med. J. (Bgham, Ala.) 56: 613–618, 1963

Suzuki, J.: Grading and timing of the operation on cerebral aneurysms. In Pia, H. W., C. Langmaid, J. Zierski: Cerebral Aneurysms, Advances in Diagnosis and Therapy. Springer, Berlin 1979 (pp. 203–208)

Symon, L.: Clinical assessment of regional cerebral perfusion and correlation of xenon clearance studies with anatomico-pathological data in subarachnoid haemorrhage. Fourth Europ. Congr. Neurosurg., Prag 1971

Theander, S., L. Granholm: Sequelae after spontaneous subarachnoid hemorrhage, with special reference to hydrocephalus and Korsakoff's syndrome. Acta neurol. scand. 43: 479–488, 1967

Thompson, J. R., D. C. Harwood-Nash, C. R. Fitz: Cerebral aneurysms in children. Amer. J. Roentgenol. 118: 163–175, 1973

Tomlinson, B. E.: Brain changes in ruptured intracranial aneurysms. J. clin. Path. 12: 391–399, 1959

Tovi, D., I. M. Nilson, C. A. Thulin: Fibrinolysis and subarachnoid hemorrhage. Inhibitory effect of tranexamic acid. A clinical study. Acta neurol. scand. 48: 393–402, 1972

Wilkins. R. H.: Aneurysm rupture during angiography: does acute vasospasm occur? Surg. Neurol. 5: 299–303, 1976
Wilkins, R. H.: Attempted prevention or treatment of intracranial arterial spasm: a survey. Neurosurgery 6: 198–210, 1980a
Wilkins, R. H.: Cerebral Arterial Spasm: Proceedings of Second International Workshop. Williams & Wilkins, Baltimore 1980b
Wilkins, R. H., J. A. Alexander, G. L. Odom: Intracranial arterial spasm: A clinical analysis. J. Neurosurg. 29: 121–134, 1968
Yaşargil, M. G., Y. Yonekawa, B. Zumstein et al.: Hydrocephalus following spontaneous subarachnoid hemorrhage. J. Neurosurg. 39: 474–479, 1973
Zingesser, L. H., M. M. Schechter, J. Dexter, R. Katzmann, L. C. Scheinberg: On the significance of spasm associated with rupture of a cerebral aneurysm: the relationship between spasm as noted angiographically and 71 regional blood flow determinations. Arch. Neurol. (Chic.) 18: 520–528, 1968

Chapter 2: Internal Carotid Artery Aneurysms
Chapter 3: Middle Cerebral Artery Aneurysms
Chapter 4: Anterior Cerebral and Anterior Communicating Artery Aneurysms
Chapter 5: Vertebrobasilar Artery Aneurysms
Chapter 8: Unoperated Cases
Chapter 9: Complications of Aneurysm Surgery
Chapter 10: Addendum

Acosta, C., P. E. Williams jr., K. Clark: Traumatic aneurysms of the cerebral vessels. J. Neurosurg. 36: 531–536, 1972
Adams, A. P.: Techniques of vascular control for deliberate hypotension during anaesthesia. Brit. J. Anaesth. 47: 777–792, 1975
Adams, H. P., N. F. Kassel, J. C. Torner, D. W. Nibbelink, A. L. Sahs: Early management of aneurysmal subarachnoid hemorrhage. A report of the Cooperative Aneurysm Study. J. Neurosurg. 54: 142–145, 1981
Adams, J. E.: Clinical experience with hypothermia. In Fields, W. S., A. L. Sahs: Intracranial Aneurysms and Subarachnoid Hemorrhage. Thomas, Springfield/Ill. 1965 (pp. 275–294)
Adams, J. E., J. Witt: The use of otologic microscope in the surgery of aneurysms. Presented at the Neurosurgical Society of America meeting on January 25, 1964
Adams, R. D., B. Castleman, E. P. Richardson jr.: Case records of Massachusetts General Hospital. Case 22, 1963. New Engl. J. Med. 268: 724–731, 1963
Adams, R. D., C. N. Fischer, S. Hakim, R. G. Ojemann, H. H. Sweet: Symptomatic occult hydrocephalus with normal "cerebro-spinal fluid pressure". A treatable syndrome. New Engl. J. Med. 273: 117–126, 1965
Adelman, L. S., F. D. Dole, H. B. Sarnat: Bilateral dissecting aneurysm of the internal carotid artery. Acta neuropathol. (Berl.) 29: 93–97, 1974
Af Björkesten, G.: Arterial aneurysms of the internal carotid artery and its bifurcation. An analysis of 69 aneurysms treated mainly by direct surgical attack. J. Neurosurg. 15: 400–410, 1958
Af Björkesten, G., V. Halonen: Incidence of intracranial vascular lesions in patients with subarachnoid hemorrhage investigated by four vessel angiography. J. Neurosurg. 23: 29–32, 1965
Af Björkesten, G., H. Troupp: Changes in the size of intracranial arterial aneurysms. J. Neurosurg. 19: 583–588, 1962
Agee, O. F.: The paraorbital oblique projection for the demonstration of posterior communicating area aneurysms. Radiology 90: 797–799, 1968
Ahmed, R. H., C. B. Sedzimir: Ruptured anterior communicating aneurysms. A comparison of medical and specific surgical treatment. J. Neurosurg. 26: 213–217, 1967
Aitken, R. R., C. G. Drake: A technique of anesthesia with induced hypotension for surgical correction of intracranial aneurysms. Clin. Neurosurg. 21: 107–114, 1974
Akerman, M., G. Arfel, J. De Pommery, C. Arrouvel, G. Sirvys, G. Vourc'h: Étude expérimentale des effects cérébro-vasculaires du nitroprussiate de soude chez le baboin Papio Papio. Son action sur le vasospasme expérimental. Neuro-chirurgie 22, No. 1: 43–57, 1976

Alexander, E., S. M. Wigser, C. H. Davis: Bilateral extracranial aneurysms of the internal carotid artery. Case report. J. Neurosurg. 25: 437–442, 1966
Alexander, S. C., P. J. Cohen, H. Wollman, T. C. Smith, M. Reivick, R. A. Van der Molen: Cerebral carbohydrate metabolism during hypocarbia in man: Studies during nitrous oxide anesthesia. Anesthesiology 26: 624–632, 1965
Alksne, J. F.: Magnetically controlled intravascular catheter. Surgery 64: 339–345, 1968
Alksne, J. F.: Stereotactic thrombosis of intracranial aneurysms using a magnetic probe. Confin. neurol. (Basel) 31: 95–98, 1969
Alksne, J. F.: Stereotactic thrombosis of intracranial aneurysms. New Engl. J. Med. 284: 171–174, 1971
Alksne, J. F., R. W. Rand: Current status of metallic thrombosis of intracranial aneurysms. Progr. neurol. Surg. 3: 212–229, 1969
Alksne, J. F., R. W. Smith: Iron-acrylic compound for stereotaxic aneurysm thrombosis. J. Neurosurg. 47: 137–141, 1977
Allcock, J. M.: Arterial spasm in subarachnoid hemorrhage. Acta radiol. Diagn. 5: 73–83, 1966
Allcock, J. M.: Angiotomography in detection of intracranial aneurysms. Invest. Radiol. 5: 200–205, 1970, cited by Decu et al. 1973
Allcock, J. M.: Aneurysms. In Newton, T. H., D. G. Potts: Radiology of the Skull and Brain. Angiography, Vol II Book 4 Mosby, St. Louis 1974 (pp. 2472–2473)
Allcock, J., P. B. Conham: Angiographic study of the growth of intracranial aneurysms. J. Neurosurg. 45: 617–621, 1976
Allcock, J. M., C. G. Drake: Postoperative angiography in cases of ruptured intracranial aneurysm. J. Neurosurg. 20: 752–759, 1963
Allcock, J. M., C. G. Drake: Ruptured intracranial aneurysms – The role of arterial spasm. J. Neurosurg. 22: 21–29, 1965
Allègre, G., R. Vigouroux: Traitement Chirurgical des Anéurysmes Intracrâniens du Système Carotidien. Anévrysmes Supraclinoïdiens, Vol. I. Masson, Paris 1957 (pp. 122)
Allègre, G., J. de Rougemont, A. Thierry: Spasme artériel de la carotide interne dû à un anévrysme rompu du système vertébro-basilaire. Neuro-chirurgie 9: 74–79, 1963
Allègre, G., G. Aimard, J. P. Dechaume, D. Michel: Une nouvelle observation d'anévrysme intra-pétreux de la carotide interne à sémiologie ectopique. Rev. neurol. 115: 1053–1055, 1966
Allen, G. S.: Cerebral arterial spasm – part 7. Surg. Neurol. 6: 63–70, 1976a
Allen, G. S.: Cerebral arterial spasm – part 8. Surg. Neurol. 6: 71–80, 1976b
Allen, G. W.: Angiography in Otolaryngology. Laryngoscope (St. Louis), 77: 1909–1961, 1967
Almeida, G. M., M. K. Shibata, E. Bianco: Carotid-ophthalmic aneurysms. Surg. Neurol. 5: 41–45, 1976
Alpers, B. J., R. G. Berry: Circle of Willis in cerebral vascular disorders. The anatomical structure. Arch. Neurol. (Chic.) 8: 398–402, 1963
Alpers, B. J., N. S. Schlezinger, I. M. Tassman: Bilateral internal carotid aneurysm involving cavernous sinus. Arch. Ophthal. 46: 403–407, 1951
Alvord, E. C. jr., J. D. Loeser, W. L. Bailey, M. K. Copass: Subarachnoid hemorrhage due to ruptured aneurysms. A simple method of estimating prognosis. Arch. Neurol. (Chic.) 27: 273–284, 1972
Amacher, A. L., C. G. Drake, G. G. Ferguson: Posterior circulation aneurysms in young people. Neurosurgery 8: 315–320, 1981
Amacher, L., J. Shillito Jr.: The syndromes and surgical treatment of aneurysms of the great vein of Galen. J. Neurosurg. 39: 89–98, 1973
Ambler, Z., M. Ulc, Q. Ledinsky: Aneurysma der A. Carotis int. im extrakraniellen Verlauf. Neurochirurgia (Stuttg.) 10: 169–175, 1967
Andersen, P. E.: Fibromuscular hyperplasia of the carotid arteries. Acta radiol. Diagn. 10: 90–96, 1970a
Andersen, P. E.: Fibromuscular hyperplasia in children. Acta radiol. Diagn. 10: 203–208, 1970b
Anderson, R. D., A. Liebeskind, M. M. Schechter, L. H. Zingesser: Aneurysms of the internal carotid artery in the carotid canal of the petrous temporal bone. Radiology 102: 639–642, 1972a
Anderson, R. D., A. Liebeskind, L. H. Zingesser, M. M. Schechter: Aneurysms of the cervical internal carotid artery. Amer. J. Roentgenol. 116: 31–36, 1972b

Anderson, R. G. G.: cAMP and calcium ions in mechanical and metabolic response of smooth muscles: Influence of some hormones and drugs. Acta physiol. scand. (Suppl.) 382 (1972)

Anderson, S., W. McKissock: Controlled hypotension with Arfonad in neurosurgery with special reference to vascular lesions. Lancet II: 754–759, 1953

Andrew, J., P. W. Nathan, N. C. Spanos: Disturbances of micturition and defaecation due to aneurysms of the anterior cerebral arteries. J. Neurosurg. 24: 1–10, 1966

Antunes, J. L., J. W. Correll: Cerebral emboli from intracranial aneurysms. Surg. Neurol. 6: 7–10, 1976

Araki, C., H. Handa, J. Handa, K. Yoshida: Traumatic aneurysm of the intracranial extradural portion of the internal carotid artery. J. Neurosurg. 23: 64–67, 1965

Armstrong, F. S., G. J. Hayes: Segmental cerebral arterial constriction associated with pheochromocytoma. J. Neurosurg. 18: 843–846, 1961

Arnould, G., P. Tridon, J. Y. Martin: Ophthalmoplégie par énorme anéurysme intra-caverneux. Rev. Otoneuroophthal. 29: 241–243, 1957

Arnulf, G.: Pathologie et Chirurgie des Carotides. Masson, Paris 1957

Aronson, H. A., J. H. Scattliff: Pseudothrombosis of internal carotid artery. J. Neurosurg. 19: 691–695, 1962

Arseni, C., S. Ionesco: Hemorragie nasale grave provoquée par la rupture d'un anévrysme carotidien post-traumatique. Rev. Oto-neuro-ophthal. 41: 149–154, 1969

Arutiunov, A. I., M. A. Baron, N. A. Majorova: The role of mechanical factors in the pathogenesis of short-term and prolonged spasm of the cerebral arteries. J. Neurosurg. 40: 459–472, 1974

Asenjo, A., P. Donoso: Aneurysmas de la arteria comunicante anterior. Neurocirurgia (Santiago) 15: 9–14, 1957

Askenasy, H. M., E. E. Herzberger, H. S. Wijsenbeek: Hydrocephalus with vascular malformations of the brain. A preliminary report. Neurology (Minneap.) 3: 213–220, 1953

Ask-Upmark, E., D. Ingvar: A follow-up examination of 138 cases of subarachnoid hemorrhage. Acta med. scand. 138: 15–31, 1950

Avman, N., R. G. Fisher: Exposure of middle cerebral aneurysm after the use of urea. Surgery 48: 491–494, 1960

Bader, D. C. H.: Microtechnical nursing in neurosurgery. J. neurosurg. Nursing 7: 22–24, 1975a

Bader, D. C. H.: Microsurgical treatment of intracranial aneurysms. J. neurosurg. Nursing 7: 25–27, 1975b

Bagley Jr., C.: Blood in the cerebrospinal fluid. Resultant functional and organic alterations in the Central Nervous System. A, experimental data. Arch. Surg. 17: 18–38, 1928a

Bagley Jr., C.: Blood in the cerebro-spinal fluid. Resultant functional and organic alterations in the Central Nervous System. B, clinical data. Arch. Surg. 17: 39–81, 1928b

Bakay, L., W. H. Sweet: Cervical and intracranial intra-arterial pressures with and without vascular occlusion. Surg. Gynec. Obstet. 95: 67–75, 1952

Baker, H. L.: The clinical usefulness of magnification cerebral angiography. Radiology 98: 587–591, 1971

Baptista, A. G.: Studies on the arteries of the brain. Neurology (Minneap.) 13: 825–835, 1963

Bär, H.-P.: Cyclic nucleotides and smooth muscle. Advance. Cyclic Nucleotide Res. 4: 195–237, 1974

Barley, W.-L., J. D. Loeser: Intracranial aneurysms. J. Amer. med. Ass. 216: 1993–1996, 1971

Barnett, H. J. M.: Some clinical features of intracranial aneurysms. Clin. Neurosurg. 16: 43–71, 1969

Barr, H. W. K., W. Blackwood, S. P. Meadows: Intracavernous carotid aneurysms, a clinical pathological report. Brain 94: 607–622, 1971

Barrett, J. H., L. van Lawrence: Aneurysm of the internal carotid artery as a complication of mastoidectomy. Arch. Otolaryng. 72: 366–368, 1960

Bassett, D. L.: A Stereoscopic Atlas of Human Anatomy. Williams & Wilkins, Baltimore 1954

Bassett, R. C.: Intracranial aneurysms. 1. Some clinical observations concerning their development. J. Neurosurg. 6: 216–221, 1949

Bassett, R. C.: Multiple cerebral aneurysms. Report of a case. J. Neurosurg. 8: 132–133, 1951

Battista, A. F., E. S. Flamm, M. Goldstein, L. S. Freedman: Effect of dopamine-beta-hydroxylase on cerebral vasospasm in the cat. J. Neurosurg. 44: 168–172, 1976

Baumann, C. H. H., P. C. Bucy: Aneurysms of the anterior cerebral artery. Evaluation of surgical and "conservative" treatments. J. Amer. med. Ass. 163: 1448–1454, 1957

Bayliss, W. M.: On the local reactions of the arterial wall to changes of internal pressure. J. Physiol. 28: 220–231, 1902

Beadles, C. F.: Aneurysms of the larger cerebral arteries. Brain 30: 285–336, 1907

Beall Jr., A. C., E. St. Crawford, D. A. Cooley, M. E. de Bakey: Extracranial aneurysms of the carotid artery, report of seven cases. Postgrad. Med. 32: 93–102, 1962

Beamer, Y. B., J. F. Corsino, R. G. Lynde: Rupture of an aneurysm of the internal carotid artery during arteriography with filling of the subarachnoid space and demonstration of a temporal lobe mass. J. Neurosurg. 31: 224–226, 1969

Beatty, R. A., A. E. Richardson: Predicting intolerance to common carotid artery ligation by carotid angiography. J. Neurosurg. 28: 9–13, 1968

Bebin, J., R. D. Currier: Cause of death in ruptured intracranial aneurysms. Arch. intern. Med. 99: 771–790, 1957

Beck, M. E.: Aneurysm of the middle meningeal artery. Brit. J. Radiol. 34: 667–668, 1961

Beck, O. J.: Indikation zur Aneurysmaoperation in Abhängigkeit vom Zeitpunkt zur SAB sowie vom Schweregrad der SAB. Int. Symp., Graz 29.–30.6.1973

Beck, O. J., Kh. R. Koczorek: Behandlung des Hirnödems nach schwerer Subarachnoidalblutung mit Vasospasmus durch hochdosierte Gaben von Aldactone (R)/Injektion und Aldocorten. Mitteilung erster Beobachtung. In Koczorek, Kh. R.: Die hepatische Encephalopathie und das Hirnödem. Primärer und sekundärer Aldosteronismus. Symposium der Ärztekammer Hamburg, 29.11.1970

Beck, O. J., H. X. Wieser: Die Bedeutung des Vasospasmus für die Prognose nach Aneurysmablutung. Zbl. Neurochir. 35: 21–34, 1974

Belber, C. J., R. B. Hoffmann: The syndrome of intracranial aneurysm associated with fibromuscular hyperplasia of the renal arteries. J. Neurosurg. 28: 556–559, 1968

Bell, W. E., C. Butler: Cerebral mycotic aneurysms in children. Two case reports. Neurology (Minneap.) 18: 81–86, 1968

Benedetti, A., D. Curri: Direct attack on carotid ophthalmic and large internal carotid aneurysms. Surg. Neurol. 81: 49–54, 1977

Benedetti, A., D. Curri, C. Carbonin, L. Rubini: On the radical treatment of a large carotid-ophthalmic aneurysm. J. neurosurg. Sci. 19: 176–180, 1975

Benoit, B. G., G. Wortzman: Traumatic cerebral aneurysms. Clinical features and natural history. J. Neurol. Neurosurg. Psychiat. 36: 127–138, 1973

Berger, E., M. Kyriazidou: Pre-operative angiography in cerebral aneurysms and angioma surgery. In Kitamura, K., T. H. Newton: Recent Advance in Diagnostic Neuroradiology. Igaku Shoin, Tokyo 1975 (pp. 124–136)

Berger, E., C. Duval, M. Kyriazidou: Pre-operative angiography in aneurysm and angioma surgery, using the microscope and deep-hypotension, acute fibrinolysis as a possible complication. In Handa, H.: Microneurosurgery. Igaku Shoin Tokyo, University Park Press, Baltimore 1975 (p. 27)

Bergvall, U., R. Galera: Time relationship between subarachnoid hemorrhage, arterial spasm, changes in cerebral circulation and posthaemorrhagic hydrocephalus. Acta radiol. Diagn. 9: 229–237, 1969

Berk, M. E.: Aneurysm of the middle meningeal artery. Brit. J. Radiol. 34: 667–668, 1961

Bernhard, W. F., A. S. Cummin, P. D. Harris, E. W. Kent: New flexible vascular adhesive for use in cardiovascular surgery. Circulation 27: 739–741, 1963

Beumont, P. J. V.: The familial occurrence of berry aneurysm. J. Neurol. Neurosurg. Psychiat. 31: 399–402, 1968

van Beusekom, G. T., W. Luyendijk, E. H. Huising: Severe epitaxis caused by rupture of a non-traumatic infraclinoid aneurysm of the internal carotid artery. Acta neurochir. (Wien) 15: 269–284, 1966

Bickerstaff, E. R.: Opthalmoplegic migraine. Rev. neurol. 110: 582–588, 1964

Bigelow, N. H.: The association of polycystic kidneys with intra-

cranial aneurysms and other related disorders. Amer. J. med. Sci. 225: 485–496, 1953
Bigelow, N. H.: Multiple intracranial arterial aneurysms. An analysis of their significance. Arch. Neurol. Psychiat. (Chic.) 73: 76–99, 1955a
Bigelow, N. H.: Congenital intracranial aneurysms. Arch. Neurol. (Chic.) 73: 76–84, 1955b
Bingham, W. G., G. I. Hayes: Persistent carotid basilar anastomosis. Report of two cases. J. Neurosurg. 18: 398–400, 1961
Birley, J. L.: Traumatic aneurysm of the intracranial portion of the internal carotid artery. With a note by Wilfred Trotter. Brain 51: 184, 1928
Birse, S. H., M. I. Tom: Incidence of cerebral infarction associated with ruptured intracranial aneurysms. A study of 8 unoperated cases of anterior cerebral aneurysm. Neurology (Minneap.) 10: 101–106, 1960
Biumi, F.: In: Sandifort: Thesaureus disserationem. Lugd. Bat., S. and J. Luchtmans (and others), Vol. III, p. 373, 1778
Black, S. P. W., W. J. German: The treatment of internal carotid artery aneurysms by proximal arterial ligation. J. Neurosurg. 10: 590–601, 1953
Black, S. P. W., W. J. German: Observations on the relationship between the volume and the size of the orifice of experimental aneurysms. J. Neurosurg. 17: 984–990, 1960
Blackall, L.: Observations on the Nature and Cure of Dropsies, 2. Ed. Longman, London 1814
Bloor, B. M., H. S. Majzoub, G. R. Nugent, C. A. Carrion: Cerebrovascular hemodynamics in intracranial hemorrhage. Excerpta med. (Amst.) No. 293: 46, 1973
Blümel, G., H. Frost, P. Maurer, F. Piza: Zur Lysierbarkeit chronischer arterieller Thromben. Fibrinolyse-autographische und raster-elektronenmikroskopische Untersuchungen. Langenbecks Arch. klin. Chir. 329: 1186–1187, 1971
Boatman, K. K., V. A. Bradford: Excision of an internal carotid aneurysm during pregnancy employing hypothermia and a vascular shunt. Ann. Surg. 148: 271–275, 1958
Boba, A.: Hypothermia. Appraisal of risk in 110 consecutive patients. J. Neurosurg. 19: 924–933, 1962
Boehm, E., R. Hugosson: Results of surgical treatment of 200 consecutive cerebral arterial aneurysms. Acta neurol. scand. 46: 43–52, 1970
Boehm, E., R. Hugosson: Experience of surgical treatment of 400 consecutive ruptured cerebral arterial aneurysms. Acta neurochir. (Wien) 40/1–2: 33–34, 1978
Bohmfalk, G. L., J. L. Story, J. P. Wissinger, W. E. Brown Jr.: Bacterial intracranial aneurysms. J. Neurosurg. 48: 369–382, 1978
Bonnal, J., A. Stevenaert: Thrombosis of intracranial aneurysms of the circle of Willis after incomplete obliteration by clip or ligature across the neck. J. Neurosurg. 30: 158–164, 1969
Bonnal, J., A. Stevenaert: Indications actuelles de l'abord direct des anévrysmes artériels du polygone de Willis. Acta neurol. belg. 70: 240–268, 1970
Bonnal, J., A. Stevenaert, J. Brotchi, J. C. Dethier: Bilan de neuf ans d'expérience de la chirurgie des anévrysmes arteriels intracrâniens. Acta neurol. belg. 74: 337–355, 1974
Bonnal, J., A. Thibaut, J. Brotchi, J. C. Dethier: Les anévrysmes méconnus du polygone de Willis, Neuro-chirurgie 21: 297–316, 1975
Bonnet, P.: Les Anévrismes Artériels Intra-crâniens. Masson, Paris 1955
Bonnet, P., I. Bonnet: Le syndrome du trou déchiré antérieur, symptomatique de l'anévrysme de la carotide intracrânienne. Rev. Oto-neuro-ophtalmol. 27: 22–27, 1955
Bossi, L., E. Caffaratti: On a case of aneurysm of the primitive trigeminal artery: clinical and radiological study. Minerva med. 54: 754–759, 1963
Botterell, E. H., W. M. Lougheed, T. P. Morley, S. L. Vanderwater: Hypothermia in the surgical treatment of ruptured intracranial aneurysms. J. Neurosurg. 15: 4–18, 1958
Botterell, E. H., W. M. Lougheed, J. W. Scott, S. L. Vanderwater: Hypothermia and interruption of carotid, or carotid and vertebral circulation, in the surgical management of intracranial aneurysms. J. Neurosurg. 13: 1–42, 1956
Boyd, R. J., J. E. Connolly: Tolerance of anoxia of the dog's brain at the various temperatures. Surg. Forum 12, 408–410 1961
Boyd-Wilson, J. S.: The association of cerebral angiomas with intracranial aneurysms. J. Neurol. Neurosurg. Psychiat. 22: 218–223, 1959a

Boyd-Wilson, J. S.: Oblique views: their place in the arteriographic diagnosis of intracranial aneurysms. J. Neurosurg. 16: 297–310, 1959b
Boysen, G.: Cerebral blood flow measurement as a safeguard during endarterectomy. Stroke 2: 1–10, 1971
Boysen, G., H. C. Engell, H. Henriksen: The effect of induced hypertension on internal carotid artery pressure and regional cerebral blood flow during temporary carotid clamping for endarterectomy. Neurology 22: 1133–1145, 1972
Boysen, G., H. G. Engell, G. R. Pistolese, P. Fiorani, A. Agnoli, N. A. Lassen: On the critical lower level of cerebral blood flow in man with particular reference to carotid surgery. Circulation 49: 1023–1025, 1974
Brackett, Ch. E.: The complications of carotid artery ligation in the neck. J. Neurosurg. 10: 91–106, 1953
Bradac, G. B., R. S. Simon, H. Heitzenberg: The clinical value of the magnification technique in cerebral angiography. Neurochirurgia 16: 179–183, 1973
Bramwell, E.: A note upon the aetiology of recurrent and periodic occular palsy and ophthalmoplegic migraine. Trans. opthal. Soc. 54: 205–221, 1934
Brawley, B. W., D. E. Strandness Jr., W. A. Kelly: The biophysic response of cerebral vasospasm in experimental subarachnoid hemorrhage. J. Neurosurg. 28: 1–8, 1968
Brenner, H.: Frontale Schädelspaltung mit traumatischem Aneurysma der Arteria pericallosa. Acta neurochir. (Wien) 10: 145–152, 1962
Bremer, J. L.: Congenital aneurysms of cerebral arteries: embryologic study. Arch. Path. 35: 819–831, 1943
Brihaye, J.: Aneurysms of the cervical internal carotid artery. In Pia, H. W., C. Langmaid, J. Zierski: Cerebral Aneurysms, Advances in Diagnosis and Therapy. Springer, Berlin 1979a (pp. 45–55)
Brihaye, J.: Internal carotid aneurysms arising in the carotid canal. In Pia, H. W., C. Langmaid, J. Zierski: Cerebral Aneurysms, Advances in Diagnosis and Therapy. Springer, Berlin 1979b (pp. 55–62)
Brihaye, J.: Intracavernous carotid aneurysms. In Pia, H. W., C. Langmaid, J. Zierski: Cerebral Aneurysms, Advances in Diagnosis and Therapy. Springer, Berlin 1979c (pp. 67–88)
Brihaye, J., J. Mage, G. Verriest: Anévrysme traumatique de la carotide interne dans sa portion supraclinoïdienne. Acta neurol. belg. 54: 411–438, 1954
Brihaye, J., E. Mouawad, L. Jeanmart: L'anévrysme de la bifurcation carotidienne intracrânienne. Acta neurol. belg. 76: 129–141, 1976
von Brockhoff, V., Th. Tiwisina: Aneurysma der A. primitiva trigemina persistens als seltene Ursache der spontanen Subarachnoidalblutung. Zbl. Neurochir. 26: 295–302, 1965
Brolin, S. B., O. Hassler: Minute aneurysms, detected by microdissection of basal cerebral arteries. Acta path. microbiol. scand. 44: 59–63, 1958
Brooks, B.: The treatment of traumatic arteriovenous fistula. Sth. med. J. (Bgham, Ala.) 23: 100–106, 1930
Bross, W., S. Koczorowski, A. Aronski: Problems in the surgical treatment of aneurysm of the internal carotid artery. Bull. Soc. int. Chir. 19: 219–224, 1960
Browder, J., A. J. Krieger, H. A. Kaplan: Cerebral veins in the surgical exposure of the middle cerebral artery. Surg. Neurol. 2: 359–363, 1974
Brown, A. S., A. A. Donaldson: Effects of angiography on cerebral blood flow. In Meyer, J. S., H. Lechner, M. Reivich: Cerebral Vascular Disease. 7th International Conference Salzburg. Thieme, Stuttgart 1976 (pp. 136–139)
Browne, L.: Hypertensive anaesthesia for direct attack of intracranial aneurysms. J. Irish med. Ass. 66: 65–72, 1973
Bruetman, M. E., W. S. Fields: Persistent hypoglossal artery (arteria hypoglossica primitiva). Arch. Neurol. (Chic.) 8: 368–372, 1963
Bull, J. W. D.: Use and limitations of angiography in the diagnosis of vascular lesions of the brain. Neurology (Minneap.) 11: 80–85, 1961
Bull, J. W. D.: Contribution of radiology to the study of intracranial aneurysms. Brit. med. J. II: 1701–1708, 1962
Bull, J. W. D.: Massive aneurysms at the base of the brain. Brain 92: 535–570, 1969
Bull, J. W. D., R. S. C. Couch, D. Joyce, J. Marshall, D. G. Potts, D. A. Shaw: Observer variation in cerebral angiography: An

assessment of the value of minor angiographic changes in the radiological diagnosis of cerebrovascular disease. Brit. J. Radiol. 33: 165–170, 1960

Buncke, H. J., D. E. Murray: Small vessel reconstruction. In Rand, R. W.: Microneurosurgery. Mosby, St. Louis 1969 (pp. 183–192)

Buncke, H. J., W. P. Schulz: Total ear reimplantation in the rabbit utilizing microminiature vascular anastomoses. Brit. J. plast. Surg. 19: 15–22, 1966

Buncke, H. J., W. P. Schulz: The suture repair of one millimeter vessels. In Donaghy, R. M. P., M. G. Yaşargil: Micro-Vascular Surgery. Mosby, St. Louis 1967 (pp. 24–35)

Buncke, H. J., N. L. Chater, Z. Szabo: The complete teaching manual of microvascular surgery. Unpublished work. Microvascular Research Laboratory, R. K. Davies Medical Center, San Francisco, California, October 1974

Buncke, H. J., J. R. Cobbett, J. W. Smith, S. Tamai: Techniques of Microsurgery. Pamphlet, Ethicon, Somerville/New Jersey

Burmester, K., A. Stender: Zwei Fälle von einseitiger Aplasie der A. carotis interna bei gleichzeitiger Aneurysmabildung im vorderen Anteil des Circulus arteriosus Willisi. Acta neurochir. (Wien) 9: 367–378, 1961

Burton, Ch., F. Velasco, J. Dorman: Traumatic aneurysm of a peripheral cerebral artery. J. Neurosurg. 28: 468–474, 1968

Busby, D. R., D. H. Slemmons, Th. F. Miller Jr.: Fatal epistaxis via aneurysm and Eustachian tube. Arch. Otolaryng. 87: 93–96, 1968

Busse, O.: Aneurysmen und Bildungsfehler der Arteria communicans anterior. Virchows Arch. path. Anat. 229: 178–206, 1921

Buxton, J. T., T. B. Stevenson, J. M. Stallworth: Arteriosclerotic aneurysm of the extracranial internal carotid artery treated by excision and primary reanastomosis under controlled hypertension. Ann. Surg. 159: 222–226, 1964

Cabanis, E. A.: Contribution à l'étude des anévrysmes intrapétreux de la carotide interne. (à propos de deux observations). Thèse Doct. Med., Paris 1970

Cabiesas, F. M., R. Landa: Problemas quirurgicos en los aneurismas de la cerebral media. Acta neurol. lat.-amer. 2: 159–164, 1956

Cahn, H. L.: The control of epistaxis by arterial ligation. Arch. Otolaryngl. 61: 641–644, 1955

Campbell, E., C. W. Burklund: Aneurysms of the middle cerebral artery. Ann. Surg. 137: 18–28, 1953

Campell, R. L., M. L. Dyken: Four cases of carotid-basilar anastomosis associated with central nervous system dysfunction. J. Neurol. Neurosurg. Psychiat. 24: 250–253, 1961

Campiche, R., E. Zander: Anévrysme de la carotide interne dans son trajet extracranien formant une tumeur pharyngienne. Neuro-chirurgie 8: 79–83, 1962

Cantu, R. C., A. Ames III.: Experimental prevention of cerebral vascular obstruction produced by ischemia. J. Neurosurg. 30: 50–54, 1969

Cantu, R. C., M. Le May, H. A. Wilkinson: The importance of repeated angiography in the treatment of mycotic-embolic intracranial aneurysms. J. Neurosurg. 25: 189–193, 1966

Cantu, R. C., Th. Sounders, R. S. Hepler: Effects of carotid ligation on aneurysm-induced oculomotor palsy. J. Neurosurg. 31: 528–532, 1969

Caram, P. C., P. C. Sharkey, E. C. Alvord: Thalamic angioma and aneurysm of the choroidal artery with intraventricular hematoma. J. Neurosurg. 17: 347–352, 1960

Carlson, D. H., D. Thomson: Spontaneous thrombosis of a giant cerebral aneurysm in five days. Report of a case. Neurology (Minneap.) 26: 334–336, 1976

Carmichael, B.: The pathogenesis of non-inflammatory cerebral aneurysms. J. Path. 35: 347–368, 1950a

Carmichael, R.: The pathogenesis of non-inflammatory cerebral aneurysms. J. Path. Bact. 62: 1–19, 1950b

Carton, C. A., M. D. Heifetz, L. A. Kessler: Patching of intracranial internal carotid artery in man using a plastic adhesive (Eastman 910 adhesive). J. Neurosurg. 19: 887–895, 1962

Carton, C. A., J. C. Kennady, M. D. Heifetz, J. K. Ross-Duggan: The use of a plastic adhesive (Methyl-2-cyanoacrylate monomer) in the management of intracranial aneurysms and leaking cerebral vessels: a report of 15 cases. In Fields, W. S., A. L. Sahs: Intracranial Aneurysms and Subarachnoid Hemorrhage. Thomas, Springfield/Ill. 1965 (pp. 372–440)

Castaigne, P., J. Cambier, B. Pertuiset, P. Brunet: Anévrysmes de l'artère auditive interne révéle par une paralysie faciale récidivante. Cure radicale. Presse méd. 49: 2493–2496, 1967a

Castaigne, P., B. Pertuiset, J. Cambier, P. Brunet: Anévrysmes de l'artère auditive interne révelé par une paralysie faciale récidivante. Cure radicale. Rev. neurol. 116: 443, 1967b

Cawthorne, T.: A Review of surgery of otosclerosis. Proc. roy. Soc. Med. 40: 320, 1947

Chadduck, W. M.: Traumatic cerebral aneurysm due to speargun injury. J. Neurosurg. 31: 77–79, 1969

Chang, V., N. B. Rewcastle, D. C. F. Harwood-Nash, M. G. Norman: Bilateral dissecting aneurysms of the intracranial internal carotid arteries in an 8-year-old boy. Neurology (Minneap.) 25: 573–579, 1975

Chason, J. L., W. M. Hindeman: Berry aneurysms of the circle of Willis. Neurology (Minneap.) 8: 41–52, 1958

Chater, N. L.: Anatomic localization of optimal middle cerebral branch for STA anastomosis. Presentation before the First International Symposium on Microneurosurgical Anastomosis for Cerebral Ischemia. Loma Linda, Calif., June 1973

Chater, N. L., N. Peters: Neurosurgical microvascular bypass for stroke. West J. Med. 124: 1–5, 1976

Chokyu, M.: An experimental study of cerebral vasospasm, especially on spasmogenic factors in red blood cells. Osaka Cy med. J. 24: 211–221, 1975

Chou, S. N., J. I. Ausman, D. L. Erickson, E. L. Seljeskog, C. L. Rockswold: Microneurosurgery at the University of Minnesota Hospitals. Minn. Med. 57: 580–586, 1974

Christensen, J. C.: Epitaxis por aneurismas carotideo infraclinoideos. Acta neurol. lat.-amer. 1: 60–70, 1955

Ciric, I.: Application of microneurosurgery in the treatment of cerebral aneurysm. Proc. Inst. Med. Chicago 29: 319, 1973

Cogan, D. G., H. T. J. Mount: Intracranial aneurysms causing ophthalmoplegia. Arch. Ophthal. 70: 757–771, 1963

Cole, F. M., P. O. Yates: Intracerebral microaneurysms and small cerebrovascular lesions. Brain 90: 759–768, 1967

Collet, M., P. Descuns, F. Legent, A. Charbonnel, F. Resche: Anévrysme intra-pétreux "en sablier" développé aux dépens de la carotide interne. Rev. Oto-neuro-ophtalm. 43: 167–173, 1971

Collier, J.: Cerebral haemorrhage due to causes other than arteriosclerosis. Brit. med. J. II: 519–521, 1931

Conley, J., V. Hildyard: Aneurysm of the internal carotid artery presenting in the middle ear. Arch. Otolaryng. 90: 61–64, 1969

Connolly, C.: Aneurysms of the middle cerebral artery. J. Neurol. Neurosurg. Psychiat. 22: 77–78, 1959

Constans, J. P., D. Dilenge, B. Jolivet: Un cas de persistance d'une artère hypoglosse embryonnaire. Neuro-chirurgie 10: 297–301, 1964

Conway, L. W., L. W. McDonald: Structural changes of the intradural arteries following subarachnoid hemorrhage. J. Neurosurg. 37: 715–723, 1972

Cook, A. W., D. M. Dooley, E. J. Browder: Anterior communicating aneurysms: treatment by ligation of an anterior cerebral artery. J. Neurosurg. 23: 371–374, 1965

Cooper, A.: Account of the first successful operation, performed on the common carotid artery, for aneurysm, in the year 1808; with the post-mortem examination, in 1821. Guy's Hosp. Rep. 1: 53–58, 1836

Cophignon, J., A. Rey, C. Thurel, R. Houdart: Microchirurgie des anévrysmes artériels de la partie antérieure du polygone de Willis. Étude d'une série consécutive de 48 cas. Neuro-chirurgie 19: 519–530, 1973

Cophignon, J., A. Rey, C. Thurel, F. Launay, R. Houdart: Microchirurgie des anérvysmes intracrâniens. Étude d'une série consécutive de 50 cas. Nouv. Presse med. 2: 2919–2990, 1973

Corday, E., S. F. Rothenberg, D. W. Irving: Cerebral angiospasm. A case of the cerebral stroke. Amer. J. Cardiol. 11: 66–71, 1963

Corkill, G., M. J. H. Hodgson: Hypotension with sodium nitroprusside in the surgery of cerebral aneurysms. Anaesthesia 28: 191–194, 1973

Cornelis, G., A. Bellet, P. van Eygen, P. Roisin, E. Libon: Rotational multiple sequence roentgenography of intracranial aneurysms. Acta radiol. Diagn. 13: 74–76, 1972

Cornelius, G.: Die Tomographie der intracraniellen Aneurysmen. Röntgen-Bl. 26: 177–181, 1973

Corradi, M., B. Guidetti, A. Riccio: Disturbi oculari negli

aneurismi della carotide interna, tratto C.2 ad estrinsecazione intra e soprasellare. Riv. Neuropsichiat. 5: 345–360, 1959
Courville, C. B.: Traumatic aneurysm of an intracranial artery. Bull. Los Angeles neurol. Soc. 25: 48–54, 1960
Courville, C. B., C. W. Olsen: Miliary aneurysm of the anterior communicating artery. A clinical and pathological report of nineteen cases, eighteen with fatal hemorrhage. Bull. Los Angeles neurol. Soc. 3: 1–20, 1938
Crafoord, C.: Pulmonary ventilation and anaesthesia in major chest surgery. J. thorac. Surg. 9: 237, 1940
Crawford, T.: Some observations on the pathogenesis and natural history of intracranial aneurysms. J. Neurol. Neurosurg. Psychiat. 22: 259–266, 1959
Cressman, M. R., G. J. Hayes: Traumatic aneurysm of the anterior choroidal artery. Case report. J. Neurosurg. 24: 102–104, 1966
Crompton, M. R.: The pathology of ruptured middle cerebral aneurysms with special reference to the differences between sexes. Lancet II: 421–425, 1962
Crompton, M. R.: Hypothalamic lesions following rupture of cerebral berry aneurysms. Brain 86: 301–314, 1963
Crompton, M. R.: Cerebral infarction following the rupture of cerebral berry aneurysms. Brain 87: 263–279, 1964a
Crompton, M. R.: The pathogenesis of cerebral infarction following the rupture of cerebral berry aneurysms. Brain 87: 491–510, 1964b
Crompton, M. R.: Mechanism of growth and rupture in cerebral berry aneurysms. Brit. med. J. I: 1138–1142, 1966a
Crompton, M. R.: The comparative pathology of cerebral aneurysms. Brain 89: 789–795, 1966b
Crompton, M. R.: The pathogenesis of cerebral aneurysms. Brain 89: 797–814, 1966c
Crompton, M. R.: Recurrent haemorrhage from cerebral aneurysms and its prevention by surgery. J. Neurol. Neurosurg. Psychiat. 29: 164–170, 1966d
Cronqvist, S., F. Laroche: Transitory hyperaemia in focal cerebral vascular lesions studied by angiography and regional cerebral blood flow measurements. Brit. J. Radiol. 40: 270–274, 1967
Cronqvist, S., H. Troupp: Intracranial arteriovenous malformation and arterial aneurysm in the same patient. Acta neurol. scand. 42: 307–316, 1966
Crowell, R. M., Y. Olsson, I. Klatzo, A. Ommaya: Temporary occlusion of the middle cerebral artery in the monkey: clinical and pathological observations. Stroke 1: 439–448, 1970
Crutchfield, W. G.: Instrument for use in treatment of certain intracranial vascular lesions. J. Neurosurg. 16: 471–475, 1959
Cuatico, W., A. W. Cook, V. Tyshenko, R. Khatib: Massive enlargement of intracranial aneurysms following carotid ligation. Arch. Neurol. (Chic.) 17: 609–613, 1967
Cummins, B. H., H. B. Griffith, J. L. G. Thomson: Per-operative cerebral angiography. Brit. J. Radiol. 47: 257–260, 1974
Cushing, H.: The control of bleeding in operations for brain tumors. With the description of silver "clips" for the occlusion of vessels inaccessible to the ligature. Ann. Surg. 54: 1–19, 1911
Cushing, H.: Contributions to the study of intracranial aneurysms. Guy's Hosp. Rep. 73: 159–163, 1923
Cushing, H.: The chiasmal syndrome of primary optic atrophy and bitemporal field defects in adult patients with a normal sella turcica. XIII Concilium Ophthalmologicum (Hollandia) 13 (3): 97–184, 1929
Dandy, W. E.: The Brain. In Lewis, D.: Practice of Surgery, Vol. XII. Prior, Hagerstown/Maryland 1936 (pp. 145, 583–585)
Dandy, W. E.: Intracranial aneurysm of internal carotid artery. Cured by operation. Ann. Surg. 107: 654–659, 1938a
Dandy, W. E.: Hirnchirurgie. Barth, Leipzig 1938b
Dandy, W. E.: Aneurysms of the anterior cerebral artery. J. Amer. med. Ass. 119: 1253–1254, 1942a
Dandy, W. E.: Results following ligature of the internal carotid artery. Arch. Surg. 45: 521–533, 1942b
Dandy, W. E.: Intracranial Arterial Aneurysms, Vol. VII. Comstock, Ithaca 1944 (147 pp)
Dandy, W. E., R. H. Follis Jr.: On the pathology of carotid-cavernous aneurysms (pulsating exophthalmos). Amer. J. Ophthal. 24: 365–385, 1941
Da Pian, R., A. Pasqualin, R. Scienza: Direct microsurgical approach to aneurysms of the internal carotid bifurcation. Surg. Neurol. 13: 21–39, 1980

David, M., M. Sachs: Les anévrysmes de la bifurcation de la carotide interne. Neurochirurgia (Stuttg.) 10: 96–105, 1967
David, M., B. Pertuiset, J. F. Guyot: Considérations cliniques post-opératoires. La cure radicale des anévrysmes de la communicante antérieure sans résection cérébrale chez le malade conscient. Rev. neurol. 118: 150–151, 1968
Davidoff, L. M., C. G. Dyke: The Normal Encephalogram. Lea & Febiger, Philadelphia 1946
Davidson, P., D. M. Robertson: A true mycotic (Aspergillus) aneurysm leading to fatal subarachnoid hemorrhage in a patient with hereditary hemorrhagic teleangiectasia. J. Neurosurg. 35: 71–76, 1971
Davis, L., R. A. Davis: Principles of Neurological Surgery. Saunders, Philadelphia 1963 (pp. 184–208)
Davis, R. A., N. Wetzel, L. Davis: An analysis of the results of treatment of intracranial vascular lesions by carotid artery ligation. Ann. Surg. 143: 641–648, 1965
Davis, U. R., P. F. J. New, R. G. Ojemann, R. M. Crowell, R. B. Morawetz, G. H. Roberson: Computed tomographic evaluation of hemorrhage secondary to intracranial aneurysm. Amer. J. Roentgenol. 127: 143–153, 1976
Dawson, B. H.: The blood vessels of the human optic chiasm and their relation to those of the hypophysis and hypothalamus. Brain 81: 207–217, 1958
Debrun, G., A. Fox, C. Drake, S. Peerless, J. Girvin, G. Ferguson: Giant unclippable aneurysms: treatment with detachable balloons. AJNR, 2: 167–173, 1981
Debrun, G., P. Lacour, J. P. Caron et al.: Balloon arterial catheter techniques in the treatment of arterial intracranial diseases. In Krayenbühl, H. et al: Advances and Technical Standards in Neurosurgery. Springer, Wien, New York 1977 (pp. 131–145)
Debrun, G., P. Lacour, J. P. Caron, M. Hurth, J. Comoy, Y. Keravel: Experimental approach of carotid-cavernous fistula with an inflatable and isolated balloon. Application in man. Neuroradiology 9: 9–12, 1975a
Debrun, G., P. Lacour, J. P. Caron, M. Hurth, J. Comoy, Y. Keravel: Inflatable and released balloon technique – Experimentation in dog. Application in man. Neuroradiology 9: 267–271, 1975b
Debrun, G., P. Lacour, J. P. Caron, M. Hurth, J. Comoy, Y. Keravel: Traitement des lésions vasculaires carotido-caverneuses par ballonnet gonflable et largable. Nouv. Presse méd. 5: 1294–1296, 1976
Debrun, G., P. Lacour, J. P. Caron, M. Hurth, J. Comoy, Y. Keravel, D. Loisance: Traitement des fistules artério-veineuses et d'anévrysmes par ballon gonflable et largable. Bases expérimentales. Application à l'homme. Nouv. Presse méd. 4: 2315–2318, 1975c
Debrun, G., P. Lacour, J. P. Caron, M. Hurth, J. Comoy, Y. Keravel. G. Laborit: Technique endovasculaire de ballonnet gonflable et largable. Ann. Radiol. 3: 313–315, 1975d
Debrun, G., P. Lacour, J. P. Caron et al.: Detachable balloon and calibrated-leak balloon techniques in the treatment of cerebral vascular lesions. J. Neurosurg. 49: 635–649, 1978
Dechaume, J. P., G. Aimard, D. Michel, P. Bret, M. Desgeorges, C. Lapras, J. Lecuire: Les anévrysmes de l'artère péricalleuse. A propos d'une serie de 12 cas. Neuro-chirurgie 19: 135–150, 1973
Deck, M. D. F., C. B. Grossman, M. D. Moody, D. G. Potts: Clinical experience with circular angiotomography. Radiology 105: 591–595, 1972
De Klerk, D. J. J., J. C. De Villiers: Microsurgery for aneurysms on the circle of Willis. S. Afr. med. J. 48: 825–830, 1974
Denny-Brown, D.: Symposium on specific methods of treatment: Treatment of recurrent cerebro-vascular symptoms and the question of "vasospasm". Med. Clin. N. Amer. 35: 1457, 1951
De Rougement, J., M. Abada, M. Barge: Les anévrysmes carotidiens intra-caverneux. A propos de certains aspects particuliers. Neuro-chirurgie 12: 511–519, 1966
De Rougement, J., J. L. Nivelon, J. Lamit, A. Thierry: Anévrysme bactérien du segment intracaverneux de la carotide interne consécutif à des lésions endartéritiques observées au cours d'un thrombophlébite des sinus caverneux. Lyon med. 36: 341–349, 1963
De Saussure, R. L., S. E. Hunter, J. T. Robertson: Saccular aneurysms of the posterior fossa. J. Neurosurg. 15: 385–391, 1958
Devadiga, K. V., K. V. Mathai, J. Chardy: Spontaneous cure of

intracavernous aneurysm of internal carotid artery in a 14-month old child. J. Neurosurg. 30: 165–168, 1969

Dick, A. R., M. E. McCallum, J. A. Maxwell, S. R. Nelson: Effect of dexamethasone on experimental brain edema in cats. J. Neurosurg. 45: 141–147, 1976

Dilenge, D., R. Wuthrich: L'anévrysme traumatique de la méningée moyenne. Neurochirurgia (Stuttg.) 4: 202–206, 1961

Dimsdale, H., V. Logue: Ruptured posterior fossa aneurysms and their surgical treatment. J. Neurol. Neurosurg. Psychiat. 22: 202–217, 1959

Dimtza, A.: Aneurysms of the carotid arteries. Report of two cases. Angiology 7: 218–227, 1956

Dinning, T. A. R.: Timing of surgery for leaking cerebral aneurysms: clinical, radiological and radio-isotopic consideration. Proc. Aust. Ass. Neurol. 9: 219–226, 1973

Dinning, T. A. R., M. A. Falconer: Sudden or unexpected natural death due to ruptured intracranial aneurysms: survey of 250 forensic cases. Lancet II: 799–801, 1953

Di Tullio, M. V., R. W. Rand, E. Frisch: Detachable balloon catheter. Its application in experimental arterio-venous fistulae. J. Neurosurg. 48: 717–723, 1978

Djindjian, R.: L'angiographie de la Moelle Épinière. Masson, Paris 1970

Djindjian, R., L. Picard, C. Manelfe: Fistules artério-veineuses carotide interne-sinus caverneux. Neuro-chirurgie 19: 75–90, 1973

Djindjian, R., J. Cophignon, J. Rey, R. Houdart: Polymorphisme neuro-radiologique des fistules carotido-caverneuses. Neurochirurgie 14: 881–890, 1968

Djindjian, R., M. Hurth, J. Bories, P. Brunet: L'artère trigéminale primitive (aspects artériographiques et signification à propos de 12 cas). Presse méd. 73: 2905–2910, 1965

Donaghy, R. M. P.: Patch and by-pass in microangeional surgery. In Donaghy, R. M. P., M. G. Yaşargil: Micro-Vascular Surgery. St. Louis 1967 (pp. 75–86)

Donaghy, R. M. P.: Pitfalls in extra-intracranial blood flow diversion. In: Proc. of First Int. Symp. Microneurosurg. Anastomoses for Cerebral Ischemia, Loma Linda/Ca. June 1973a

Donaghy, R. M. P.: Extra-intracranial blood flow diversion – criteria for selection of patients and type of operation. Presented at Internal Symposium on Microneurosurgery, Kyoto, 1973b

Donaghy, R. M. P., M. G. Yaşargil: Micro-Vascular Surgery. Mosby, St. Louis, Thieme Stuttgart 1967

Dott, N. M.: Intracranial aneurysms: cerebral arterioradiography: surgical treatment. Edinb. med. J. 40: 219–240, 1933

Dott, N. M.: Brain, movement and time. Brit. med. J. II: 12–16, 1960

Dott, N. M.: Intracranial aneurysmal formations. Clin. Neurosurg. 16: 1–15, 1969

Drake, C. G.: Subdural hematoma from arterial rupture. J. Neurosurg. 18: 597–601, 1961a

Drake, C. G.: Bleeding aneurysms of the basilar artery. Direct surgical management in four cases. J. Neurosurg. 18: 230–238, 1961b

Drake, C. G.: Surgical treatment of ruptured aneurysms of the basilar artery: experience with 14 cases. J. Neurosurg. 23: 457–473, 1965

Drake, C. G.: On the surgical treatment of ruptured intracranial aneurysms. Clin. Neurosurg. 13: 122–155, 1966

Drake, C. G.: Discussion of the paper by Hunt and Hess. Risk related to time of surgery in intracranial aneurysms. J. Neurosurg. 28: 19–20, 1968a

Drake, C. G.: Further experience with surgical treatment of aneurysms of the basilar artery. J. Neurosurg. 29: 372–392, 1968b

Drake, C. G.: The surgical treatment of aneurysms of the basilar artery. J. Neurosurg. 29: 436–446, 1968c

Drake, C. G.: The surgical treatment of vertebral-basilar aneurysms. Clin. Neurosurg. 16: 114–169, 1969

Drake, C. G.: Management of aneurysms of posterior circulation. In Youmans, J. R.: Neurological Surgery, Vol. II. Saunders, Philadelphia 1973 (pp. 787–806)

Drake, C. G.: The surgical treatment of vertebral basilar aneurysms. In: Recent Progress in Neurological Surgery. Proceedings of the 5. Internat. Congr. of Neurol. Surgery. Excerpta Medica, Amsterdam 1974 (pp. 183–190)

Drake, C. G.: Ligation of the vertebral (unilateral or bilateral) or basilar artery in the treatment of large intracranial aneurysms. J. Neurosurg. 43: 255–274, 1975

Drake, C. G.: Cerebral aneurysm surgery – an update. Princeton Conference, Jan. 1976

Drake, C. G.: Treatment of aneurysms of the posterior cranial fossa. Progr. neurol. Surg. 9: 122–194, 1978

Drake, C. G.: Progress in cerebrovascular disease. Management of cerebral aneurysm. Stroke 12 (3): 273–283, 1981

Drake, C. G., J. M. Allcock: Postoperative angiography and the "slipped" clip. J. Neurosurg. 39: 683–689, 1973

Drake, C. G., A. L. Amacher: Aneurysms of the posterior cerebral artery. J. Neurosurg. 30: 468–474, 1969

Drake, C. G., R. G. Vanderlinden: The late consequences of incomplete surgical treatment of cerebral aneurysms. J. Neurosurg. 27: 226–238, 1967

Drake, C. G., R. G. Vanderlinden, A. L. Amacher: Carotid-choroidal aneurysms. J. Neurosurg. 29: 32–36, 1968a

Drake, C. G., R. G. Vanderlinden, A. L. Amacher: Carotid-ophthalmic aneurysms. J. Neurosurg. 29: 24–31, 1968b

Drake, C. G., H. W. K. Barr, J. C. Coles, N. F. Gergely: The use of extracorporeal circulation and profound hypothermia in treatment of ruptured intracranial aneurysms. J. Neurosurg. 21: 575–581, 1964

Driesen, W.: Engstellung (Spasmen?) von Großhirnarterien im Angiogramm bei Aneurysmen und anderen Schädigungen des Hirns. Med. Welt (Stuttg.) 38: 1987–1996, 1962

Du Boulay, G.: Distribution of spasm in the intracranial arteries after subarachnoid haemorrhage. Acta radiol. Diagn. 1: 257–266, 1963

Du Boulay, G., J. Edmonds-Seal, Th. Bostick: The effect of intermittent positive pressure ventilation upon the caliber of cerebral arteries in spasm following subarachnoid haemorrhage – a preliminary communication. Brit. J. Radiol. 41: 46–48, 1968

Du Boulay, G. H.: Some observations on the natural history of intracranial aneurysms. Brit. J. Radiol. 38: 721–757, 1965

Du Boulay, G. H., D. C. Jackson: Cranial angiotomography. Clin. Radiol. 16: 148–153, 1965

Dukes, H. T., G. L. Odom, B. Woodhall: The unilateral cerebral circulation. Its importance in the management of aneurysms of the anterior communicating artery. J. Neurosurg. 23: 40–46, 1965

Dunker, R. O., A. B. Harris: Surgical anatomy of the proximal anterior cerebral artery. J. Neurosurg. 44: 359–367, 1976

Duplay, J., R. Coromine, P. Cona: Anévrysmes multiples de la carotide interne dans son segment exocranien et dans son segment endocranien. Rev. neurol. 95: 400–402, 1956

Dupuy, J. P., J. Rousseau, J. P. Pompon, J. L. Pascaud, D. Douvion: Volumineux anévrysme vrai de la carotide interne chez un enfant. J. Radiol. Electrol. 55: 914, 1974

Durity, F., V. Logue: The effect of proximal anterior cerebral occlusion on anterior communicating artery aneurysms. Postoperative radiological survey of 43 cases. J. Neurosurg. 35: 16–19, 1971

Dutton, J.: Intracranial aneurysm. A new method of surgical treatment. Brit. med. J. 2: 585, 1956

Dutton, J.: Acrylic investment of intracranial aneurysms. A report of 12 years' experience. J. Neurosurg. 31: 652–657, 1969

Dutton, J. E. M.: Acrylic resin investment of intracranial aneurysms. Brit. med. J. 2: 597–602, 1956

Duvoisin, R. G., M. D. Yahr: Posterior fossa aneurysms. Neurology (Minneap.) 15: 231–241, 1965

Eadie, M. J., K. G. Jamieson, E. A. Lennon: Persistent carotid-basilar anastomosis. J. neurol. Sci. 1: 501–511, 1964

Echlin, F. A.: Spasm of basilar and vertebral arteries caused by experimental subarachnoid hemorrhage. J. Neurosurg. 23: 1–11, 1965

Echlin, F. A.: Current concepts in the etiology and treatment of vasospasm. Clin. Neurosurg. 15: 133–160, 1968

Ecker, A.: Spasm of internal carotid artery. J. Neurosurg. 2: 479–484, 1945

Ecker, A., P. A. Riemenschneider: Arteriographic demonstration of spasm of intracranial arteries: with special reference to saccular arterial aneurysms. J. Neurosurg. 8: 660–667, 1951

Ectors, L.: Anatomo- et physiopathologie des anévrysmes intracrâniens. Acta neurol. belg. 50: 403–423, 1950

Edelsohn, L., L. Caplan, A. E. Rosenbaum: Familial aneurysms

and infundibular widening. Neurology (Minneap.) 22: 1056–1060, 1972
Egger, F. M., T. A. Tomsick, A. A. Chambus, R. R. Lukin: Aneurysms of persistent trigeminal arteries. Neuroradiology 24: 65–66, 1982
Ehni, G., J. H. Barrett: Hemorrhage from the ear due to an aneurysm of the internal carotid artery. New Engl. J. Med. 262: 1323–1325, 1960
Eichler, A., J. L. Story, D. E. Bennett, M. V. Galo: Traumatic aneurysm of a cerebral artery. J. Neurosurg. 31: 72–76, 1969
Eisterer, H., W. T. Koos, G. Woeber: A new method of controlled hypotensive anesthesia in neursurgery. Excerpta med. (Amst.) No. 293: 95 1973
Elstrom-Jodal, B. E., E. J. Hoggendhal, L. E. Linder et al.: Cerebral blood flow autoregulation at high arterial pressures and different levels of carbon dioxide tension in dogs. Europ. Neurol. 6: 6–10, 1972
Elvidge, A. R., W. H. Feindel: Surgical treatment of aneurysm of the anterior cerebral and the anterior communicating arteries diagnosed by angiography and electroencephalography. J. Neurosurg. 7: 13–32, 1950
Endo, S., S. Sato, J. Suzuki: Experiemental cerebral vasospasm after subarachnoid hemorrhage. Time of development and neurogenic participation. Tenth International Congress of Angiology. Tokyo, Aug. 30, 1976
Epstein, B., S.: Roentgenographic aspects of the thrombosis of aneurysms of the anterior communicating and anterior cerebral arteries. Amer. J. Roentgenol. 70: 211–217, 1953
Epstein, F., J. Ransohoff, G. N. Budzilovich: The clinical significance of junctional dilatation of the posterior communicating artery. J. Neurosurg. 33: 529–531, 1970
Epstein, M. H., B. G. Udvarhelyi: An electropneumatic occluder for the instantaneous control of cerebral circulation. In Handa: Microneurosurgery. Univ. Park Press, Baltimore, 1975 (pp. 8–16)
Escourolle, R., J.-C. Gautier, A. Rosa, P. D. Agopian, F. Lhermitte: Anévrysme dissequant vertébro-basilaire. Rev. neurol. 128: 95–104, 1972
Esser, A.: Z. Neurol. 114: 208, 1928 cited by Hiller 1936
Ethier, R., D. Melancon, G. Scotti, C. Milner, S. Tchang: CT in the evaluation of intracranial aneurysms and subarachnoid hemorrhage. Paper read at the Intern. Symp. Computerized Tomography, San Juan/Puerto Rico, April 6, 1976
Falconer, M. A.: The surgical treatment of bleeding intracranial aneurysms. J. Neurol. Neurosurg. Psychiat. 14: 153–186, 1951
Falconer, M. A.: Surgical treatment of spontaneous intracranial haemorrhage. Brit. med. J. I: 790–792, 1958
Faleiro, L. C. M., P. A. Rodrigues, J. A. Rodrigues et al.: Tratamento microcirúrgico de aneurismas da artéria communicante anterior. Arch. Neuro-psiquiat. (S. Paulo) 31: 264–270, 1973
Fawcett, E., J. V. Blackford: The circle of Willis: an examination of 700 specimens. J. Anat. Physiol. 40: 63–70, 1905
Fearnsides, E. G.: Intracranial aneurysms. Brain 39: 224–296, 1916
Fein, J. M., R. L. Rovit: Interhemispheric subdural hematoma secondary to hemorrhage from a calloso-marginal artery aneurysm. Neuroradiology 1: 183–186, 1970
Fein, J. M., W. J. Fior, S. L. Cohan, J. Parkhurst: Sequential changes of vascular ultrastructure in experimental cerebral vasospasm. Myonecrosis of subarachnoid arteries. J. Neurosurg. 41: 49–58, 1974
Feldman, R. L., S. W. Gross, S. Wimpfheimer: Ruptured intracranial aneurysm during pregnancy. Amer. J. Obstet. Gynec. 70: 289–295, 1955
Ferguson, G. G.: Turbulence in human intracranial saccular aneurysms. J. Neurosurg. 33: 485–497, 1970
Ferguson, G. G.: Direct measurement of mean and pulsatile blood pressure at operation in human intracranial saccular aneurysms. J. Neurosurg. 36: 560–563, 1972a
Ferguson, G. G.: Physical factors in the initiation, growth, and rupture of human intracranial saccular aneurysms. J. Neurosurg. 37: 666–677, 1972b
Ferguson, G. G., A. M. Harper, W. Fitch et al.: Cerebral blood flow measurements after spontaneous subarachnoid hemorrhage. Europ. Neurol. 8: 15–22, 1972
Ferrari, G., M. Vio: Radiological demonstration of rupture of a carotid aneurysm during cerebral angiography. Case report. J. Neurosurg. 31: 462–464, 1969
Ferris, E. J., J. C. Rudikoff, J. H. Shapiro: Cerebral angiography of bacterial infection. Radiology 90: 727–734, 1968
Ferris, E. J., Ch. A. Athanasoulis, J. H. Shapiro, R. Duffield: Pharmacological aspects of intracerebral spasm secondary to cerebral hemorrhage. Radiology 95: 561–655, 1970
Ferry, D. J., L. G. Kempe: False aneurysm secondary to penetration of the brain through orbito-facial wounds. Report of two cases. J. Neurosurg. 36, 503–506, 1972
Fields, W. S.: The significance of persistent trigeminal artery: carotid-basilar anastomosis. Radiology 91: 1096–1101, 1968
Fincher, W. J.: An aneurysm of the intracranial carotid artery treated surgically. Yale J. Biol. Med. 11: 423, 1939
Finkemeyer, H.: Verletzungen der A. Carotis Interna in ihrem intra-kraniellen, extraduralen Abschnitt. Zbl. Neurochir. 2: 63–73, 1955a
Finkemeyer, H.: Ein sackförmiges Aneurysma der A. cerebri media als postoperative Komplikation. Zbl. Neurochir. 15: 302–304, 1955b
Finney, H. L.: Giant intracranial aneurysm associated with Marfan's syndrome. J. Neurosurg. 45: 342–347, 1976
Finney, H. L., S. Roberts, R. E. Anderson: Giant intracranial aneurysm associated with Marfan's syndrome. Case report. J. Neurosurg. 18: 698–699, 1961
Finney, L. A., N. J. David: Aneurysm of the extracranial internal carotid artery. Report of a case and discussion. Neurology (Minneap.) 14: 376–379, 1964
Fisher, C. M.: The circle of Willis: Anatomical variations. Vasc. Dis. 2: 99, 1965
Fisher, R. G., V. Ciminello: Pericallosal aneurysms. J. Neurosurg. 25: 512–515, 1966
Fisher, R. G., A. Goran: Thrombosis of an intracranial aneurysm and cervical portion of the internal carotid artery in a child. J. Neurosurg. 18: 698–699, 1961
Fishman, R. A.: Cerebrospinal fluid. In Baker, A. B.: Clinical Neurology, 2nd Ed., Vol. I. Harper & Row, New York, 1962 (pp. 350–388)
Flamm, E. S.: Parasurgical treatment of aneurysms. Clin. Neurosurg. 24: 240–247, 1976
Flamm, E. S., J. Ransohoff: Treatment of cerebral vasospasm by control of cyclic adenosine monophosphate. Surg. Neurol. 6: 223–226, 1976
Flamm, E. S., M. G. Yaşargil, J. Ransohoff: Alteration of experimental cerebral vasospasm by adrenergic blockade. J. Neurosurg. 37: 294–301, 1972a
Flamm, E. S., M. G. Yaşargil, J. Ransohoff: Control of cerebral vasospasm with parenteral phenoxybenzamine. Stroke 3: 421–426, 1972b
Flamm, E. S., J. Kim, J. Lin, J. Ransohoff: Phosphodiesterase inhibitors and cerebral vasospasm. Arch. Neurol. (Chic.) 33: 569–571, 1975
Flamm, E. S., A. T. Viau, J. Ransohoff, N. E. Naftchi: Alterations in cyclic adenosine monophosphate concentrations in cat basilar artery during spasm and after treatment with isoproterenol and aminophylline. Neurology (Minneap.) 26: 664–666, 1976
Fletcher, J., G. T. Tindall: Arterial erosion and hemorrhage during graded carotid ligation with the Crutchfield clamp. J. Neurosurg. 27: 52–55, 1967
Fletcher, T. M., J. M. Taveras, J. C. Pool: Cerebral vasospasm in angiography for intracranial aneurysms: incidence and significance in one hundred consecutive angiograms. Arch. Neurol. (Chic.) 1: 38–47, 1959
Florey, H.: Microscopal observations on the circulation of the blood in the cerebral cortex. Brain 48: 43–64, 1925
Fodstad, H., I. M. Nilsson: Coagulation and fibrinolysis in blood and CSF after aneurysmal subarachnoid hemorrhage: effect of tranexamic acid. Acta neurochir. (Wien) 56: 25–38, 1981
Fodstad, H., A. Forssell, B. Liliequist, M. Schannong: Antifibrinolysis with tranexamic acid in aneurysmal subarachnoid hemorrhages: A consecutive controlled clinical trial. Neurosurgery 8: 158–165, 1981
Fog, M.: The relationship between the blood pressure and the tonic regulation of the pial arteries. J. Neurol. Psychiat. I: 187–197, 1938
Fogarty, T. J., J. J. Granley, J. R. Krause et al.: A method for

extraction of arterial emboli and thrombi. Surg. Gynec. Obstet. 116: 241–244, 1963
Foltz, E. L., A. A. Ward Jr.: Communicating hydrocephalus from subarachnoid bleeding. J. Neurosurg. 13: 546–566, 1956
Forbes, H. S., H. G. Wolff: Cerebral circulation. III. The vasomotor control of cerebral vessels. Arch. Neurol. Psychiat. (Chic.) 19: 1057–1086, 1928
Forbus, W. D.: On the origin of miliary aneurysms of the superficial cerebral arteries. Bull. Johns Hopk. Hosp. 47: 239–284, 1930
Fox, J. L.: Use of methylprednisolone in intracranial surgery. Med. Ann. D. C. 34: 261–265, 1965
Fox, J. L.: Obliterations of midline vertebral artery aneurysms via basilar craniotomy. J. Neurosurg. 26: 406–412, 1967
Fox, J. L., Microvascular Anastomosis Techniques of the Carotid Artery. A Sparta Instrument Corp., Fairfield/NJ. 1976
Fox, J. L.: Vascular clips for the microsurgical treatment of stroke. Stroke 7: 489–500, 1976
Fox, J. L., C. T. Baiz, R. L. Kakoby: Differentiation from aneurysms from infundibulum of the posterior communicating artery. J. Neurosurg. 21: 135–138, 1964
Fraser, R. A., B. M. Stein, R. E. Barrett et al.: Noradrenergic mediation of experimental cerebrovascular spasm. Stroke 1: 356–362, 1970
French, L. A., J. H. Galicich: The use of steroids for control of cerebral edema. Clin. Neurosurg. 10: 212–223, 1964
French, L. A., S. N. Chou, D. M. Long: The direct approach to intracranial aneurysms. Clin. Neurosurg. 15: 117–128, 1968
French, L. A., M. E. Zarling, E. A. Schultz: Management of aneurysms of the anterior communicating artery. J. Neurosurg. 19: 870–876, 1962
French, L. A., S. N. Chou, J. L. Story, E. A. Schultz: Aneurysm of the anterior communicating artery. J. Neurosurg. 24: 1058–1062, 1966
Freytag, E.: Fatal rupture of intracranial aneurysms. Survey of 250 medicolegal cases. Arch. Path. 81: 418–424, 1966
Fromm, H., J. Habel: Angiographischer Nachweis eines sackförmigen Aneurysmas als Ursache einer spontanen carotidocavernösen Fistel und Spontanheilung dieser Fistel nach Angiographie. Nervenarzt 36: 170–172, 1965
Frugoni, P., P. Conforti: Aneurismi sacculari di insolite dimensioni della cerebrale anteriore e del complesso cerebrale anteriore-commicante anteriore. Minerva neurochir. 6: 120–125, 1962
Frugoni, P., G. Iraci, L. Peserico: Risultati immediati ed a distanza della legatura della carotide cervicale secondo la tecnica di Smith nel trattamento di alcuni aneurismi sacculari della carotide interna. Minerva neurochir. 11: 281–282, 1967
Gabor, I., A. Potondi: Hirnbasis-Aneurysmen. Topographie und morphologische Befunde. Münch. med. Wschr. 5: 224–226, 1967
Galbraith, J. G.: Monitoring of brain oxygenation during carotid ligation. J. Neurosurg. 27: 102–104, 1967
Galbraith, J. G., R. Clark: Role of carotid ligation in the management of intracranial carotid aneurysms. Clin. Neurosurg. 21: 171–180, 1974
Galera, K., I. Greitz: Hydrocephalus in the adult secondary to the rupture of intracranial aneurysms. J. Neurosurg. 32: 634–641, 1970
Galicich, J. H., L. A. French, J. C. Melby: Use of dexamethasone in treatment of cerebral edema associated with brain tumors. J. Lancet 81: 46–53, 1961
Gallagher, J. P.: A new method for obliterating dangerous aneurysms of the brain. Mammalian hairs "shot" into lesions with Navy developed gun. Nav. Res. Rev. 1–6, Aug. 1962
Gallagher, J. P.: Obliteration of intracranial aneurysms by pilojection. J. Amer. med. Ass. 183: 231–236, 1963
Gallagher, J. P.: Pilojection for intracranial aneurysms. Report of progress. J. Neurosurg. 21: 129–134, 1964
Gallagher, J. P.: The closure of intracranial aneurysms by pilojection. In Fields, W. S., A. L. Sahs: Intracranial Aneurysms and Subarachnoid Hemorrhage. Thomas, Springfield/Ill. 1965 (pp. 444–458)
Gallagher, P. Q., J. F. Dorsey, M. Stefanini: Large intracranial aneurysms producing panhypopituitarism and frontal lobe syndrome. Neurology (Minneap.) 6: 829–837, 1956
Gannon, W. E.: Malformation of the brain. Persistent trigeminal artery and arteriovenous malformation. Arch. Neurol. (Chic.) 6: 496–498, 1962

Garcia-Bengochea, F., F. H. Deland: Bilateral giant carotid-ophthalmic aneurysms. Case report. J. Neurosurg. 42: 589–595, 1975
Garcia-Chavez, C., J. Moossy: Cerebral arterial aneurysm in infancy: association with agenesis of corpus callosum. J. Neuropath. Exp. Neurol. 24: 492–501, 1965
Gardener, W.: Cerebral angiomas and aneurysms. Surg. Clin. N. Amer. 16: 1019–1030, 1936
Gass, H. H., J. F. McGuire, D. R. Simmons: Intracranial eradication of middle cerebral aneurysms. J. Neurosurg. 15: 223–233, 1958
Genest, A. S.: Experimental use of intraluminal plastics in the treatment of carotid aneurysms. Preliminary report. J. Neurosurg. 22: 136–141, 1965
George, A. E., J. P. Lint, R. A. Morantz: Intracranial aneurysms on a persistent primitive trigeminal artery. Case report. J. Neurosurg. 35: 601–604, 1971
Géraud, J., A. Rascol, A. Bès, L. Arbus, A. M. Bénazet: Anévrisme fusiforme vertébro-basilaire à symptomatologie pseudotumorale. Rev. neurol. 110: 66–72, 1964
Gerhard, L., G. Schmitz-Bauer: Hirnbasisarterienveränderungen bei Marfan-Syndrom und idiopathischer Medianekrose. Acta neuropath. (Berl.) 26: 176–184, 1973
Gerlach, J., H. Spuler, G. Viehweger: Über das Aneurysma der Orbita. Klin. Mbl. Augenheilk. 140: 344–356, 1962
Gerlach, J., H. P. Jensen, H. Spuler, G. Viehweger: Traumatic carotico-cavernous fistula combined with persisting primitive hypoglossal artery. J. Neurosurg. 20: 885–887, 1963
Gerlock, A. J.: Rupture of posterior inferior cerebellar artery aneurysms into the subarachnoid space during angiography. Case report. J. Neurosurg. 42: 469–472, 1975
German, W. J., S. P. W. Black: Intra-aneurysmal hemodynamics – jet action. Circulat. Res. 3: 463–468, 1955
German, W. J., S. P. W. Black: Cervical ligation for internal carotid aneurysms. An extended follow-up. J. Neurosurg. 23: 572–577, 1965
Gerstenbrand, F., K. Weingarten: Aneurysmen und hypophysäres Syndrom. Wien. Z. Nervenheilk. 20: 300–310, 1963
Gessini, L., P. Frugoni: Considerazioni sulla persistenza della anastomosi carotido-basilare. Riv. Neurol. 24: 338–348, 1954
Geyer, K.-H.: Strömungsverhältnisse im großen Karotisaneurysma. Fortschr. Röntgenstr. 103: 440–443, 1965
Gibbs, J. R.: Effects of carotid ligation on the size of internal carotid aneurysms. J. Neurol. Neurosurg. Psychiat. 28: 383–394, 1965
Gilbert, R. G. B., G. F. Brindle, A. Galindo: Anesthesia for Neurosurgery. Little, Brown, Bosten 1966
Gillingham, F. J.: The management of ruptured intracranial aneurysms. Ann. roy. Coll. Surg. 23: 89–117, 1958
Gillingham, F. J.: The management of ruptured intracranial aneurysms. Scot. med. J. 12: 377–383, 1967
Gillingham, F. J.: 25 years experience with middle cerebral aneurysms. J. Neurol. Neurosurg. Psychiat. 38: 404–413, 1975
Gillingham, F. J., J. Barbera, U. M. Myint, V. S. Madan: Ruptured intracranial aneurysm. Factors influencing prognosis. In Gillingham, F. J., C. Mawdsley, A. R. Williams: Stroke, Proceedings of the Ninth Pfizer International Symposium. Churchill Livingstone, Edinburgh 1976
Gillingham, F. J., A. A. Donaldson, A. S. Brown, J. J. Maccabe: Neurological Surgery. 2nd European Congress, Rome. (Abstracts). Excerpta 1963
Giroire, H., A. Charbonnel, P. Verceletto, H. Dano: Lacune de la base du crâne, paralysises unilat. des nerfs crâniens, symptomatiques d'un anévrysme carotidien. Rev. Oto-neuro-ophtal. 37: 273–277, 1965
Glasgold, A. I., W. D. Horrigan: The internal carotid artery presenting as middle ear tumor. Laryngoscope (St. Louis) 82: 2217–2221, 1972
Glickman, M. G., J. S. Gletne, F. Mainzer: Basal projection in cerebral angiography. Radiology 98: 611–618, 1971
Glynn, L. E.: Medial defects in the circle of Willis and their relation to aneurysm formation. J. Pathol. 51: 213–222, 1940
Goldberg, H. I.: Multisectional cerebral angio-tomography in diagnosis of deep cerebral lesions. IX Symp. Neuroradiol. Göteborg. 24–28 Aug. 1970
Goldberg, J. L.: In: Newton, T. H., D. G. Potts: Radiology of the Skull and Brain, Vol. II, Part 2, Mosby, St. Louis 1974 (p. 1628)

Goldman, N. C., G. T. Singleton, E. H. Holly: Aberrant internal carotid artery. Arch. Otolaryng. 94: 269–273, 1971
Goldstein, S. L.: Ventricular opacification secondary to rupture of intracranial aneurysm during angiography. J. Neurosurg. 27: 265–267, 1967
Gottschaldt, M., H. Schmidt, W. Walter, W. Schiefer: Histopathologische Befunde bei angiographisch nachweisbaren reversiblen cerebralen Gefäßeinengungen. Radiologe 11: 444–446, 1971
Govaert, J. C., A. E. Walker: Pathology of intracranial aneurysms. Progr. Brain Res. 30: 283–288, 1968
Graf, C. J.: Familial intracranial aneurysm. Report of four cases. J. Neurosurg. 25: 304–307, 1966
Graf, C. J., D. W. Nibbelink: Cooperative Study of Intracranial Aneurysms and Subarachnoid Hemorrhage. Report on a randomized treatment study. Stroke 5: 559–601, 1974
Gratzl, O., P. Schmiedek, H. Steinhoff: Extra-intracranial arterial bypass in patients with occlusion of cerebral arteries due to trauma and tumor. In Handa, H.: Microneurosurgery. Univ. Park Press, Baltimore 1975 (pp. 68–80)
Gratzl, O., P. Schmiedek, R. Spetzler, J. Steinhoff, F. Marguth: Clinical experience with extra-intracranial arterial anastomosis in 65 cases. J. Neurosurg. 44, 313–324, 1976
Greenhoot, J. H., D. D. Reichenbach: Cardiac injury and subarachnoid hemorrhage. A clinical, pathological and physiological correlation. J. Neurosurg. 30: 521–531, 1969
Greenwood Jr., J.: Two point coagulation. A new principle and instrument for applying coagulation current in neurosurgery. Amer. J. Surg. 50: 267–270, 1940
Greenwood Jr., J.: Two point coagulation. A follow-up report on a new technique and instrument for electrocoagulation in neurosurgery. Arch. phys. Ther. (Omaha) 23: 522–554, 1942
Greenwood Jr., J.: Two-point or interpolar coagulation. Review after a twelve-year period with notes on addition of sucker tip. J. Neurosurg. 12: 196–197, 1955
Greenwood Jr., J.: Electrocoagulation in neurosurgery. Surg. Neurol. 2: 4, 1974
Greitz, T., T. Hindmarsh: Computer assisted tomography of intracranial CSF circulation using a water soluble contrast medium. Acta radiol. Diagn. 15: 497–507, 1974
Griffith, H. B., B. H. Cummins, J. L. G. Thomson: Cerebral arterial spasm and hydrocephalus in leaking arterial aneurysms. Neuroradiology 4: 212–214, 1972
Gros, C., B. Vlahovitch, R. Auteroche: Réflexions sur une série de 46 anévrysmes supraclinoïdiens rompus; évaluation du traitement chirurgical. Neuro-chirurgie 3: 253–258, 1957
Gros, C., B. Vlahovitch, R. Labauge, A. Thevenet, A. Kuhner, Ph. Frèrebeau: Les anévrysmes extra-crâniens de la carotide interne. Neuro-chirurgie 16: 367–382, 1970
Grote, W., P. Röttgen, J. Wappenschmidt: Erfahrungen mit Aneurysmen der A. communicans anterior. Neuro-chirurgie 6: 63–71, 1960
Grubb, R. L., M. E. Raichle, J. O. Eichling, M. H. Gado: The effects of subarachnoid hemorrhage upon regional cerebral blood volume, blood flow and oxygen utilization in man. In Harper, A. M., W. B. Jennett, J. D. Miller, J. C. Rowan: Blood Flow and Metabolism in Brain. Churchill Livingstone, Edinburgh 1975 (pp. 13.12–13.16)
Guidetti, B.: Surgical treatment of aneurysms of the anterior communicating artery. Progr. Brain Res. 30: 303–307, 1968
Guidetti, B.: Results of 98 intracranial aneurysm operations performed with the aid of operating microscope. Acta neurochir. (Wien) 29: 65–71, 1973
Guidetti, B., A. Spallone: The role of antifibrinolytic therapy in the pre-operative management of recently ruptured intracranial aneurysms. Surg. Neurol. 15: 239–248, 1981
Guidetti, B., E. La Torre: Carotid ophthalmic aneurysms. Acta neurochir. (Wien) 22: 289–304, 1970
Guidetti, B., E. La Torre: Management of carotid-ophthalmic aneurysms. J. Neurosurg. 42: 438–442, 1975
Guillaume, J., G. Mazars, A. Pansini: Essais de coagulation intracavitaire des anévrysmes endocrâniens. Neuro-chirurgie 3: 220, 1957
Guirguis, S., F. W. Tadros: An internal carotid aneurysm in the petrous temporal bone. J. Neurol. Neurosurg. Psychiat. 24: 84–85, 1961

Gull, W.: Cases of aneurysm of the cerebral vessels. Guy's Hosp. Rep. 3: 281, 1859
Gurdjian, E. S., L. M. Thomas: Operative Neurosurgery, 3rd Ed. Williams & Wilkins, Baltimore 1970 (pp. 324–333)
Gurdjian, E. S., J. E. Webster: Head Injuries – Mechanism, Diagnosis and Treatment, 2nd Ed. Little, Brown, Boston 1958
Gurdjian, E. S., D. W. Lindner, L. M. Thomas: Experiences with ligation of the common carotid artery for treatment of aneurysms of the internal carotid artery. J. Neurosurg. 23: 311–318, 1965
Gurdjian, E. S., L. M. Thomas, G. P. Scratch, W. R. Darmody: Cerebral vasospasm. In Fields, W. S., A. L. Sahs: Intracranial Aneurysms and Subarachnoid Hemorrhage. Thomas, Springfield/Ill. 1965
Guthkelch, A. N.: Large saccular aneurysm of the intracranial part of the vertebral artery. Brit. J. Surg. 37: 107, 1949
Hacker, H.: Detailangiographie – die direkte Röntgenvergrößerung bei der Serienangiographie. Electromedica 6: 347–349, 1970
Halasz, N. A., J. C. Kennedy: Excision of arteriosclerotic aneurysms of the cervical internal carotid artery. J. Neurosurg. 21: 352–357, 1964
Hallac, I., W. B. Hamby: A metallic fastener for intracranial vascular ligation. J. Neurosurg. 18: 261–262, 1961
Hamby, W. B.: Intracranial Aneurysms. Thomas, Springfield/Ill. 1952a
Hamby, W. B.: The modern treatment of intracranial aneurysms. N. Y. St. J. Med. 52: 2497–2502, 1952b
Hamby, W. B.: Multiple intracranial aneurysms. J. Neurosurg. 16: 558–563, 1959
Hamby, W. B.: Intracranial surgery for aneurysm. Effect of hypothermia upon survival. J. Neurosurg. 20: 41–45, 1963
Hamby, W. B.: Intracranial surgery for aneurysms. Prog. neurol. Surg. 3: 1–65, 1969
Hamby, W. B.: Remarks concerning intracranial aneurysm surgery. Clin. Neurosurg. 17: 1–17, 1970
Hamer, I., B. Gotte: Incidence and neurological significance of post-operative cerebral vasospasm. A study of 80 consecutive cases with clipped saccular aneurysms. Neurochirurgia (Stuttg.) 24: 118–130, 1981
Hammon, W. M.: Intracranial aneurysm encasement. J. Neurol. Neurosurg. Psychiat. 31: 524–527, 1968
Hammon, W. M., L. G. Kempe: The posterior fossa approach to aneurysms of the vertebral and basilar arteries. J. Neurosurg. 37: 339–347, 1972
Hanafee, W., P. J. Jannetta: Aneurysm as a cause of stroke. Amer. J. Roentgenol. 98: 647–652, 1966
Hanau, J., J. F. Foncin, J. Le Beau: On the role of cerebral ischemia in the fatal course of ruptured supratentorial aneurysms. Neuro-chirurgie 15: 353–368, 1969
Hancock, D. O.: A case of complete bilateral ophthalmoplegia due to an intrasellar aneurysm. J. Neurol. Neurosurg. Psychiat. 26: 81–82, 1963
Handa, H.: The neurosurgical treatment of intracranial vascular malformations, particularly with the use of plastics and polarographic measurements. Clin. Neurosurg. 9: 223–244, 1963
Handa, H., T. Ohta, Y. Kamijyo: Encasement of intracranial aneurysms with plastic compounds. Progr. neurol. Surg. 3: 149–192, 1969
Handa, H., T. Ohta, S. Ishikawa, J. Handa, I. Misawa: Coating and reinforcing of experimental cervical aneurysms with synthetic resins and rubbers. Neurologia medico-chirurgica (Tokyo): 158–186, 1960
Handa, J., H. Handa: Severe epistaxis caused by traumatic aneurysm of cavernous carotid injuries. Surg. Neurol. 5: 241–243, 1976
Handa, J., Y. Kamijyo, H. Handa: Posttraumatisches Aneurysma der leptomeningealen Arterien. Arch. Psychiat. Nervenkr. 211: 347–364, 1968
Handa, J., Y. Kamijyo, H. Handa: Intracranial aneurysm associated with fibromuscular hyperplasia of renal and internal carotid arteries. Brit. J. Radiol. 43: 483–485, 1970
Handa, J., Y. Kamijyo, H. Handa: Association of brain tumor and intracranial aneurysm. Surg. Neurol. 6: 25–30, 1976
Handa, J., Y. Smimui, K. Sato, H. Handa: Traumatic aneurysm and arteriovenous fistula of the middle meningeal artery. Clin. Radiol. 21: 39–41, 1970a
Handa, J., H. Kikuchi, K. Iwayama, T. Teraura, H. Handa:

Traumatic aneurysms of the internal carotid artery. Acta neurochir. (Wien) 17: 161–177, 1967
Handa, J. et al.: Traumatic aneurysm of the middle cerebral artery. Amer. J. Roentgenol. 109: 127–129, 1970b
Handler, F. P., H. T. Blumenthal: Inflammatory factor in pathogenesis of cerebrovascular aneurysms. J. Amer. med. Ass. 155: 1479–1483, 1954
Hardin, C. A.: Carotid body tumors and aneurysms. Angiology 12: 597–600, 1961a
Hardin, C. A.: Cervical aneurysms and tumors. Management of cases requiring resection and restoration of the carotid artery. Arch. Surg. 82: 435–439, 1961b
Hardy, J.: Lecture delivered as guest instructor, Theodore Gildred Microsurgical Education Center, University of Florida, Gainesville/Florida, November 1975
Hardy, W. G., L. M. Thomas, J. E. Webster, E. S. Gurdjian: Carotid ligation for intracranial aneurysm. J. Neurosurg. 15: 281–289, 1958
Harper, A.: Autoregulation of cerebral blood flow: influence of the arterial blood pressure on the blood flow through the cerebral cortex. J. Neurol. Neurosurg. Psychiat. 29: 398–403, 1966
Harrington, O. B., V. G. Crosby, L. Nicholas: Fibromuscular hyperplasia of the internal carotid artery. Ann. thorac. Surg. 9: 516–524, 1970
Harris, P., G. B. Udvarhelyi: Aneurysms arising at the internal carotid-posterior communicating artery junction. J. Neurosurg. 14: 180–191, 1957
Harrison, Th., G. L. Odom, E. C. Kunkle: Internal carotid aneurysm arising in carotid canal. Arch. Neurol. (Chic.) 8: 328–331, 1963
Harvey, F. H., J. L. Downer: Traumatic production of an intracranial berry-like aneurysm in a monkey. Acta neuropath. (Berl.) 31: 263–266, 1975
Hashi, K., S. Nishimura: The time course of cerebral vasospasm. In Meyer, J. S., H. Lechner, M. Reivich, E. O. Ott: Cerebral Vascular Disease. Proceedings of the Eight International Salzburg Conference 1976. Excerpta Medica New York, distributed by Elsevier, North Holland, 1977, 281 p.
Hashi, K., J. S. Meyer, S. Shinmaru, K. M. A. Welch, T. Teraura: Effect of glycerol and intracarotid phenobenzamine on cerebral hemodynamics and metabolism after experimental subarachnoid hemorrhage. J. Neurol. Sci. 17: 23–28, 1972
Hassler, O.: Morphological studies on the large cerebral arteries with reference to the aetiology of subarachnoid hemorrhage. Acta neurol. scand. (Suppl.) 154: 1–145, 1961
Hassler, O.: Medial defects in the meningeal arteries. J. Neurosurg. 19: 337–340, 1962
Hassler, O.: On the etiology of intracranial aneurysms. In Fields. W. S., A. L. Sahs: Intracranial Aneurysms and Subarachnoid Hemorrhage. Thomas, Springfield/Ill. 1965a
Hassler, O.: Intra-arterial bridges in the larger cerebral arteries. Acta radiol. Diagn. 3: 305–309, 1965b
Hassler, O.: Media defects in human arteries. Angiology 14: 368–371, 1968
Hassler, O.: A study of intracranial aneurysms with ultrasoft X-rays. J. Neurosurg. 34: 380–386, 1971
Hassler, O.: Scanning electron microscopy of saccular intracranial aneurysms. Amer. J. Path. 68: 511–520, 1972
Hassler, O., G. F. Saltzmann: Histologic changes in infundibular widening of the posterior communicating artery. Acta path. microbiol. scand. 46: 305–312, 1959
Hassler, O., G. F. Saltzmann: Angiographic and histological changes in infundibular widening of the posterior communicating artery. Acta radiol. Diagn. 1: 321–327, 1963
Haughton, V. M., A. E. Rosenbaum, H. A. Baker, R. L. Plaistowe: Lateral projection with inclined head for angiography of basal aneurysms. Radiology 116: 220–222, 1975
Hayashi, M., S. Marukawa, H. Fujii, T. Kitano et al.: Intracranial hypertension in patients with ruptured intracranial aneurysm. J. Neurosurg. 46: 584–590, 1977
Hayes, G. I.: Personal communication on the subject: Training in Neurosurgery with W. Dandy. Treatment of cerebral aneurysms prior to angiographic demonstration.
Hayes, G. J., R. C. Leaver: Methyl methacrylate investment of intracranial aneurysms. A report of seven years experience. J. Neurosurg. 25: 79–80, 1966
Hayes, G. J., H. C. Slocum: The achievement of optimal brain relaxation by hyperventilation technics of anesthesia. J. Neurosurg. 19: 65–69, 1962
Hayreh, S. S.: The ophthlamic artery. In Newton, T. H., D. G. Potts: Radiology of the Skull and Brain. Angiography, Vol. II, Book 2. Mosby, St. Louis 1974 (p. 1334)
Hayward, R. D., G. V. A. O'Reilly: Intracerebral haemorrhage. Accuracy of computerized transverse axial scanning in predicting the underlying aetiology. Lancet 1: 1–4, 1976
Heidelberger, K. P., W. M. Layton, R. G. Fisher: Multiple cerebral mycotic aneurysms complicating posttraumatic pseudomonas meningitis. J. Neurosurg. 29: 631–635, 1968
Heidrich, R.: Subarachnoid hemorrhage. In Vinken, P. J., G. W. Bruyn: Handbook of Clinical Neurology, Vol. XII. Elsevier-North Holland, Amsterdam 1972
Heifetz, M. D.: A new intracranial aneurysm clip. J. Neurosurg. 30: 753, 1969
Heilbrun, M. P., J. Olesen, N. A. Lassen: Regional cerebral blood flow studies in subarachnoid hemorrhage. J. Neurosurg. 37: 36–44, 1972
Heiskanen, O.: Multiple intracranial arterial aneurysms. Acta neurol. scand. 41: 356–362, 1965a
Heiskanen, O.: The identification of ruptured aneurysm in patient with multiple intra-cranial aneurysms. Neurochirurgia (Stuttg.) 8: 102–107, 1965b
Heiskanen, O., I. Marttila: Risk of rupture of a second aneurysm in patients with multiple aneurysms. J. Neurosurg. 32: 295–299, 1970
Heiskanen, O., P. Nikki: Large intracranial aneurysms. Acta neurol. scand. 38: 195–208, 1962
Henry, P., J. Guerin, J. M. Vallat: Extravasation per-angiographique du produit de contraste au cours de ruptures d'anévrismes (à propos de 2 cas). Neurochirurgia (Stuttg.) 14: 121–126, 1971
Henschen, C.: Operative Revascularisation des zirkulatorisch geschädigten Gehirns durch Auflage gestielter Muskellappen. Langenbecks Arch. klin. Chir. 264: 392–401, 1950
Heros, R. C., N. T. Zervas, M. Negoro: Cerebral vasospasm. Surg. Neurol. 5: 354–362, 1976
Heubner, O.: Zur Topographie der Ernährungsgebiete der einzelnen Hirnarterien. Zbl. Med. Wiss. 10: 817–821, 1872
Heuer, G. J.: The surgical approach and treatment of tumors and other lesions about the optic chiasm. Surg. Gynec. Obstet. 53: 489–518, 1931
Heuer, G. J., W. E. Dandy: Roentgenography in the localization of brain tumor. Based upon a series of one hundred consecutive cases. Bull. Johns Hopk. Hosp. 26: 311, 1916
Heyn, K., H. Noetzel: Über verschiedene Formen der Rupturblutungen intrakranieller Aneurysmen. Beitr. Path. 116: 61–70, 1956
Higazi, I., A. El-Banhawy, F. El-Nady: Importance of angiography in identifying false aneurysm of the middle meningeal artery as a cause of extradural hematoma. J. Neurosurg. 30: 172–176, 1969
Hilal, S. K., J. W. Michelsen, J. Driller et al: Magnetically guided devices for vascular exploration and treatment. Laboratory and clinical investigations. Radiology 113: 529–540, 1974
Hiller, F.: Die Zirkulationsstörungen des Rückenmarks und Gehirns. In: Handbuch der Neurologie, Vol. XI/1. Springer, Berlin 1936
Hinshaw, D. B., Ch. R. Simmons, W. Leech, J. Minkler, G. Austin: Loculated intracranial aneurysms: Angiography and possible etiology. Radiology 113: 101–106, 1974
Hiranandani, L. H., O. Chandra, N. K. Malpani, K. K. Ahuja: An internal carotid aneurysm in the petrous temporal bone. J. Laryng. 76: 703–706, 1962
Hirsch, J. F., M. David, M. Sachs: Les anévrysmes artériels traumatiques intracrâniens. Neuro-chirurgie 8: 189–201, 1962
Hockley, A. D.: Proximal occlusion of the anterior cerebral artery for anterior communicating aneurysm. J. Neurosurg. 43: 426–431, 1975
Hodgson, L.: A Treatise on the Diseases of Arteries and Veins. Underwood, London 1815
Høedt-Rasmussen, K. H., E. Skinhoj, O. B. Paulson, J. Ewald, J. K. Bjerrum, A. Fahrenkrug, N. A. Lassen: Regional cerebral blood flow in acute apoplexy. The "luxury perfusion" syndrome of brain tissue. Arch. Neurol. (Chic.) 17: 271–281, 1967
Hoff, J. T., D. G. Potts: Angiographic demonstration of hemor-

rhage into the fourth ventricle. Case report. J. Neurosurg. 30: 732–735, 1969
Hollin, S. A., R. E. Decker: Effectiveness of microsurgery for intracranial aneurysms. Postoperative angiographic study of 50 cases. J. Neurosurg. 39: 690–693, 1973a
Hollin, S. A., R. E. Decker: Microsurgical treatment of cerebral aneurysms. Mt Sinai J. Med. (N. Y.) 40: 91–103, 1973b
Hollin, S. A., R. E. Decker: Microsurgical treatment of internal carotid artery aneurysms. J. Neurosurg. 47: 142–149, 1977
Honjo, S., O. Tsujikawa, T. Sekitani, T. Yamada, K. Akisada: Aneurysms of the extracranial internal carotid artery. Bull. Yamaguchi med. Sch. 10: 67–70, 1963
Höök, O., G. Norlén: Aneurysms of the middle cerebral artery. A report of 80 cases. Acta chir. scand., Suppl. 235: 7–39, 1958
Höök, O., G. Norlén: Aneurysms of the internal carotid artery. Acta neurol. scand. 40: 200–218, 1964a
Höök, O., G. Norlén: Aneurysms of anterior communicating artery. Acta neurol. scand. 40: 219–240, 1964b
Höök, O., G. Norlén, J. Guzman: Saccular aneurysms of vertebral-basilar-arterial system: Report of 28 cases. Acta neurol. scand. 39: 271–304, 1963
Hori, S., J. Suzuki: Early intracranial operations for ruptured aneurysms. Acta neurochir. (Wien) 46: 93–104, 1979a
Hori, S., J. Suzuki: Early and late results of intracranial surgery of anterior communicating artery aneurysms. J. Neurosurg. 50: 433–440, 1979b
Horton, B. C., G. F. Abbott, R. S. Porro: True mycotic aneurysms of intracranial vessels. (Abstr.). J. Neuropath. exp. Neurol. 33: 565, 1974
Horten, B. C., G. F. Abbott, R. S. Porro: Fungal aneurysms of intracranial vessels. Arch. Neurol. (Chic.) 33: 577–579, 1976
Hosobuchi, Y.: Electrothrombosis of carotid-cavernous fistulas. J. Neurosurg. 41: 657, 1975
House, W. F.: Surgical exposure of the internal auditory canal and its contents through the middle, cranial fossa. Laryngoscope (St. Louis) 71: 1363–1385, 1961
House, W. F.: Monograph I: Transtemporal bone microsurgical removal of acoustic neuromas. Arch. Otolaryng. 80: 597–756, 1964
Housepian, E. M., J. L. Pool: A systematic analysis of intracranial aneurysms from the autopsy file of the Presbyterian Hospital. 1914–1956. J. Neuropath. exp. Neurol. 17: 409–423, 1958
Houser, O. W., H. L. Baker, B. A. Sandok, K. E. Holley: Cephalic arterial fibromuscular dysplasia. Radiology 101: 605–611, 1971
Howe, J. F., A. B. Harris, G. W. Sypert: Giant aneurysm of the middle cerebral artery. Surg. Neurol. 5: 231–233, 1976
Huber, P.: Kombinationen von sackförmigen Aneurysmen der A. pericallosa mit Anomalien des Circulus Willisi im Carotisangiogramm. Fortschr. Röntgenstr. 93: 178–184, 1960
Huber, P.: Angiographische Schichtungseffekte in den sackförmigen Aneurysmen der Hirngefäße. Fortschr. Röntgenstr. 94: 355–362, 1961
Huber, P.: Angiographische Darstellung der Zirkulationsverhältnisse in großen sackförmigen Aneurysmen. Fortschr. Röntgenstr. 105: 773–776, 1966
Huber, P.: Gefäßmißbildungen und Gefäßtumoren der A. carotis externa und der Dura. Fortschr. Röntgenstr. 109: 325–335, 1968
Huber, P., R. Rivoir: Die Zirkulation in und distal von sehr großen Aneurysmen des Circulus Willisi. Fortschr. Röntgenstr. 114: 457–463, 1971
Huber, P., R. Rivoir: Aneurysms of a persistent left hypoglossal artery. Neuroradiology 6: 277–278, 1974
Huber, P., F. Robert: Veränderungen von sackförmigen Aneurysmen zerebraler Arterien. Angiographische Kontrolluntersuchung bei konservativ behandelten sackförmigen Aneurysmen. Fortschr. Röntgenstr. 111: 184–195, 1969
Hudson, C. H., J. Raaf: Timing of angiography and operation in patients with ruptured intracranial aneurysms. J. Neurosurg 29: 37–41, 1968
Hugenholtz, H., T. P. Morley: The results of proximal anterior cerebral artery occlusion for anterior communicating aneurysms. J. Neurosurg. 37: 65–70, 1972
Hughes, J. T., P. M. Schianchi: Cerebral artery spasm. A histological study at necropsy of the blood vessels in cases of subarachnoid hemorrhage. J. Neurosurg. 48: 515–525, 1978
Hughes, M. G., B. Lockard, L. G. Kempe. P. L. Perot: Mesoscopic anatomy of posterior fossa and upper cervical canal in man. Surg. Forum 26: 472–474, 1975
Hugosson, R., S. Högström: Factors disposing to morbidity in surgery of intracranial aneurysms with special regard to deep controlled hypotension. J. Neurosurg. 38: 561–567, 1973
Hunt, W. E.: Grading of risk in intracranial aneurysms. In Sano, K., S. Ishii: Recent Progress in Neurological Surgery. Excerpta Medica, Amsterdam 1974 (pp. 169–175
Hunt, W. E., R. M. Hess: Surgical risk as related to time of intervention in the repair of intracranial aneurysms. J. Neurosurg. 28: 14–20, 1968
Hunt, W. E., E. J. Kosnik: Timing and perioperative care in intracranial aneurysm surgery. Clin. Neurosurg. 21: 79–89, 1974
Hunt, W. E., J. N. Meagher, J. E. Barnes: The management of intracranial aneurysms. J. Neurosurg. 19: 34–40, 1962
Hunter, A. R.: Neurosurgical Anesthesia. Davis, Philadelphia 1964
Ingvar, D. H., R. Cronqvist, J. Risberg, K. H. Rasmussen: Normal values of regional cerebral blood flow in man including flow and weight estimates of gray and white matter. Acta neurol. scand. 41 (Suppl. 14): 72–78, 1965
Isfort, A.: Traumatisches Hirnrindenaneurysma. Mschr. Unfallheilk. 64: 14–20, 1961
Isfort, A.: Zur prognostischen Bedeutung der Karotisstenosen im Angiogramm bei Aneurysmablutungen. Fortschr. Röntgenstr. 100: 130–137, 1964
Isfort, A., E. Nessel: Traumatisches Aneurysma der A. carotis interna nach Nebenhöhlenausräumung. Zentralbl. Chir. 90: 2150–2156, 1965
Isfort, A., P. Sunder-Plassman: Paradoxe Kreislaufreaktion bei Karotisligatur. Zbl. Neurochir. 28: 277–286, 1967
Isherwood, I., J. Dutton: Unusual anomaly of the anterior cerebral artery. Acta radiol. Diagn. 9: 345–351, 1969
Ishikawa, M., S. Waga, K. Moritake, H. Handa: Cerebral bacterial aneurysms: report of three cases. Surg. Neurol. 2: 257–261, 1974
Iwabuchi, T., Y. Kurushima, O. Fukawa, J. Suzuki: Multiple mycotic cerebral aneurysms. In Suzuki, J.: Cerebral Aneurysms. Neuron, Tokyo 1979 (pp. 690–696)
Iwabuchi, T., S. Suzuki, E. Sobota: Intracranial direct operation for carotid-ophthalmic aneurysm by unroofing of the optic canal. Acta neurochir. (Wien), 43: 163–169, 1978.
Jackson, F. E., J. R. W. Gleave, E. Janon: The traumatic cranial and intracranial aneurysm. Handbook of Clinical Neurology, Vol. XXIV. In Vinken, P. J., G. W. Bruyn: Elsevier-North Holland, Amsterdam – New York 1976 (pp. 381–398)
Jackson, I. J., R. Garza Mercado: Persistent carotid-basilar artery anastomosis: occasionally a possible cause of tic douloureux. Angiology 11: 103–107, 1960
Jackson, J. R., G. T. Tindall, B. S. Nashold Jr.: Rupture of an intracranial aneurysm during carotid arteriography, a case report. J. Neurosurg. 17: 333–336, 1960
Jacobson, J. H.: The development of microsurgical technique. In Donaghy, R. M. P., M. G. Yaşargil: Micro-Vascular Surgery. Mosby, St. Louis 1967 (p. 4–14)
Jacobson, J. H. II: Microsurgical technique. In Cooper, P.: The Craft of Surgery, Vol. I. Little, Brown, Boston 1964 (pp. 799–819)
Jacobson, J. H. II: Microsurgery. In: Current Problems in Surgery. Year Book Medical Publ., Chicago 1971a (pp. 1–56)
Jacobson, J. H. II: Microsurgical technique. In Cooper, P.: The Craft of Surgery, 2nd Ed. Little, Brown, Boston 1971b (pp. 826–847)
Jacobson, J. H. II, E. L. Suarez: Microsurgery in anastomosis of small vessels. Surg. Forum I1: 243–245, 1960
Jacobson, J. H. II, L. J. Wallman, C. A. Schumacher, M. Flanegan, E. L. Suarez, R. M. P. Donaghy: Microsurgery as an aid to middle cerebral artery endarterectomy. J. Neurosurg. 19: 108–114, 1962
Jaeger, R.: Aneurysm of the intracranial carotid artery. Syndrome of frontal headache with oculomotor nerve paralysis. J. Amer. med. Ass. 142: 304–309, 1950
Jain, K. K.: Mechanism of rupture of intracranial saccular aneurysms. Surgery 54: 347–350, 1963
Jain, K. K.: Some observations on the anatomy of the middle cerebral artery. Canad. J. Surg. 7: 134–139, 1964
Jain, K. K.: Surgery of the anterior communicating aneurysms:

experience with various techniques and evolution of a modified approach. Surg. Neurol. 2: 31–33, 1974
James, I. M.: Changes in cerebral blood flow and in systemic arterial pressure following spontaneous subarachnoid hemorrhage. Clin. Sci. 35: 11–22, 1968
Jamieson, K. G.: Rupture of an intracranial aneurysm during cerebral angiography. J. Neurosurg. 11: 625–628, 1954
Jamieson, K. G.: Aneurysms of the vertebrobasilar system. J. Neurosurg. 21: 781–797, 1964
Jamieson, K. G.: Aneurysms of the vertebro-basilar system: further experience with 9 cases. J. Neurosurg. 28: 544–555, 1968
Jane, J. A.: A large aneurysm of the posterior inferior cerebellar artery in a 1-year old child. J. Neurosurg. 18: 245–247, 1961
Javid, M.: Urea in intracranial surgery. A new method. J. Neurosurg. 18: 51–57, 1961
Jawad, K., J. D. Miller, D. J. Wyper, J. O. Rowan: Measurement of CBF and carotid artery pressure compared with cerebral angiography in assessing collateral blood flow supply after carotid ligation. J. Neurosurg. 46: 185–196, 1977
Jayaraman, A., M. Garofalo, R. A. Brinker, J. G. Chusid: Cerebral arteriovenous malformation and the primitive trigeminal artery. Arch. Neurol. (Chic.) 34: 96–98, 1977
Jeanmart, L., J. Noterman, J. Brihaye, D. Batériaux: Les anévrismes de la carotide intra-caverneuse. Neuro-chirurgie 19: 61–73, 1973
Jefferson, G.: Compression of the chiasma, optic nerves, and optic tracts by intracranial aneurysms. Brain 60: 444–497, 1937
Jefferson, G.: On the saccular aneurysm of the internal carotid artery in the cavernous sinus. Brit. Surg. 26: 267–302, 1938
Jefferson, G.: Further concerning compression of the optic pathways by intracranial aneurysms. Clin. Neurosurg. 1: 55–103, 1955
Jeffreys, R. V.: Early complications and results of surgery for ruptured intracranial aneurysms. Acta neurochir. (Wien) 56: 39–52, 1981
Jeffreys, R. V., A. E. Holmes: Common carotid ligation for the treatment of ruptured posterior communicating aneurysms. J. Neurol. Neurosurg. Psychiat. 34: 576–579, 1971
Jellinger, K.: Pathology of intracrebral haemorrhage. Zbl. Neurochir. 38: 25–42, 1977
Jellinger, K., K. Huber, G. Zervopoulos: Zur Pathologie und Klinik basaler Hirnschlagaderaneurysmen. Wien Z. Nervenheilk. 16: 35–58, 1959
Jenkinson, E. L., O. Sugar, H. Love: Rupture of an aneurysm of the internal carotid artery during cerebral angiography. Case report. Amer. J. Roentgenol. 71: 958–960, 1954
Jennett, N. B., J. Barker, W. Fitch et al.: Effect of anesthesia on intracranial pressure in patients with space-occupying lesions. Lancet 1: 61–64, 1969
Johnson, H. C.: Surgery of cerebrovascular anomalies. In Walker, A. E.: A History of Neurological Surgery, Vol. XII. Williams & Wilkins, Baltimore 1951 (pp. 250–269)
Johnson, R., J. M. Potter, R. G. Reid: Arterial spasm in subarachnoid hemorrhage mechanical considerations. J. Neurol. Neurosurg. Psychiat. 21: 68, 1958
Johnston, I.: Direct surgical treatment of bilateral intracavernous internal carotid artery aneurysms. Case report. J. Neurosurg. 51: 98–102, 1979
Joint Committee for Stroke Facilities: III, The laboratory evaluation of neurovascular disease (stroke). Stroke 3: 503–525, 1972
Joint Committee for Stroke Facilities: IV, Guidelines for the nursing care of stroke patients. Stroke 3: 631–681, 1972
Joint Committee for Stroke Facilities: VI, Special procedures and equipment in the diagnosis and management of stroke. Stroke 4: 11–137, 1973
Joint Committee For Stroke Facilities: VIII, Medical and surgical management of stroke. Stroke 4: 269–320, 1973
Jones, R. A. C.: Problems in the management of multiple intracranial aneurysms. J. Neurol. Neurosurg. Psychiat. 37: 281, 1974
Jones, R. K., E. W. Sherburn: Intracranial aneurysm in a four week old infant. J. Neurosurg. 18: 121–124, 1961
Kabot, H.: Recovery of function following arrest of the brain circulation. Amer. J. Physiol. 32: 737–747, 1941
Kahlau, G.: Über die traumatische Entstehung von Aneurysmen der Hirnarterien. Frankf. Z. Path. 51: 317–343, 1938
Kak, V. K., A. R. Taylor, D. S. Gordon: Proximal carotid ligation for internal carotid aneurysms. A long term follow-up study. J. Neurosurg. 39: 503–513, 1973
Kakkar, V. V., et al.: Prevention of fatal postoperative pulmonary embolism by low dose of heparin. An international multicentre trial. Lancet II: 45–51, 1975
Kamisasa, A.: Arteriography of the anterior communicating aneurysm. Neuroradiology 12: 227–232, 1977
Kaplan, H. A.: The lateral perforating branches of the anterior and middle cerebral arteries. J. Neurosurg. 23: 305–310, 1965
Kaplan, H. A., D. H. Ford: The Brain Vascular System. Elsevier, Amsterdam, New York 1966
Kapp, J., M. S. Mahaley, G. L. Odom: Cerebral arterial spasm. Part I: Evaluation of experimental variables affecting the diameter of the exposed basilar artery. Part 2: Experimental evaluation of mechanical and humoral factors in pathogenesis. J. Neurosurg. 29: 331–338, 1968a
Kapp, J., M. S. Mahaley Jr., G. L. Odom: Cerebral arterial spasm. Part 3: Partial purification and characterization of a spasmogenic substance in feline platelets. J. Neurosurg. 29: 350–356, 1968b
Karasawa, J., H. Kikuchi, S. Furuse, T. Manabe, T. Sakai: Surgery of multiple intracranial aneurysms. Neurol. Surg. 2: 763–769, 1974
Katsiotis, P. A., J. N. Taptas: Embolism and spasm following subarachnoid hemorrhage. Acta radiol. Diagn. 7: 140–144, 1968
Kaufmann, H. H.: Fibromuscular hyperplasia of the carotid artery in a case associated with an arteriovenous malformation. Arch. Neurol. (Chic.) 22: 299–304, 1970
Kazner, E., W. Lanksch, H. Steinhoff, J. Wilske: Die axiale Computer-Tomographie des Gehirnschädels – Anwendungsmöglichkeiten und klinische Ergebnisse. Fortschr. Neurol. Psychiat. 43: 487–574, 1975
Keane, J. R., A. Talalla: Posttraumatic intracavernous aneurysms. Epistaxis with monocular blindness preceded by chromatopsia. Arch. Ophthal. 87: 701–705, 1972
Keaney, N. P., V. W. Pickfrout, D. G. McDowall et al.: Cerebral circulatory and metabolic effects of hypotension produced by deep halothane anesthesia. J. Neurol. Neurosurg. Psychiat. 36: 898–905, 1973
Keen, W. W.: Intracranial lesion. Med. News (N. Y.) 57: 439–449, 1890
Kelly, P. J., R. J. Gorten, R. G. Grossman, H. M. Eisenberg: Cerebral perfusion, vascular spasm and outcome in patients with ruptured intracranial aneurysms. J. Neurosurg. 47: 44–49, 1977
Kempe, L. G.: Cranial, cerebral and intracranial vascular disease. In Kempe, L. G.: Operative Neurosurgery, Vol. I. Springer, Berlin 1968 (pp. 1–75)
Kempe, L. G.: Operative Neurosurgery, Vol. II. Springer, Berlin 1970 (pp. 67–71)
Kempe, L. G., D. R. Smith: Trigeminal neuralgia, facial spasm, intermedius and glossopharyngeal neuralgia with persistent carotid-basilar anastomosis. J. Neurosurg. 31, 445–451, 1969
Kempe, L. G., G. D. Vander Ark: Anterior communicating artery aneurysms. Gyrus rectus approach. Neurochirurgia (Stuttg.) 14: 63–70, 1971
Kendall, B. E., L. E. Claveria: The use of computerised axial tomography (C. A. T.) for the diagnosis and management of intracranial angiomas. In Du Boulay, G. H., J. F. Moseley: Computerised Axial Tomography in Clinical Practice. Springer, Berlin 1977 (pp. 261–271)
Kendall, B. E., C. P. Lee, E. Claveria: Computerized tomography and angiography in subarachnoid haemorrhage. Brit. J. Radiol. 49: 483–501, 1976
Kernohan, J. W., H. W. Walton: Postoperative, focal nonseptic necrosis of vertebral and cerebellar arteries. J. Amer. med. Ass. 122: 1173–1177, 1943
Kessler, L. A., M. H. Wholey: Internal carotid occlusion for treatment of intracranial aneurysms. Radiology 95: 581–583, 1970
Keucher, T. R., E. B. Solow, R. L. Campbell: Importance of monitoring antifibrinolytic therapy in spontaneous subarachnoid hemorrhage. Presented at the Annual Meeting of the Amer. Ass. Neurol. Surg., San Francisco/California, April 1976
Key, A., G. Retzius: Studien in der Anatomie des Nervensystems und des Bindegewebes. Norstad, Stockholm 1875
Khodadad, G.: Microvascular surgery. In Rand, R. W.: Microneurosurgery. Mosby, St. Louis, 1969 (pp. 170–182)
Kia-Noury, M.: Traumatisches intrakranielles Aneurysma der

Arteria meningica media nach Schädelbasisfraktur. Zbl. Neurochir. 21: 351–357, 1961

Kidron, D. P.: The electroencephalographic effects of carotid compression. E. E. G. Clin. Neurophys. 6: 469–472, 1954

Killian, H.: Aneurysmen des brachiocephalen Stromgebietes und weitere Erfahrungen mit der Mediastinotomia sternoclavicularis. Langenbecks. Arch. Chir. 269: 200–314, 1951

Kim, J., E. S. Flamm, J. Lin: Experimental cerebral vasospasm and cyclic adenosine monophosphate (c-AMP). Invest. Radiol. 10: 239–243, 1975

Kim, S. W., Kee Chan Lee: Bilateral carotid ligation. J. Neurosurg. 32: 103–107, 1970

Kimbel, F. D., R. C. Llewellyn, H. D. Kirgis: Surgical treatment of ruptured aneurysm with intracerebral and subarachnoid hemorrhages in a 16-month-old infant. J. Neurosurg. 17: 331–332, 1960

King, G., H. W. Slade, F. Campoy: Bilateral intracranial aneurysms. Arch. Neurol. Psychiat. 71: 326–336, 1954

Kirgis, H. D., W. L. Fisher, R. C. Llewellyn, E. McC. Peebles: Aneurysms of the anterior communicating artery and gross anomalies of the circle of Willis. J. Neurosurg. 25: 73–78, 1966

Klafta Jr. L. A., W. B. Hamby: Significance of cerebrospinal fluid pressure in determining time for repair of intracranial aneurysms. J. Neurosurg. 31: 217–219, 1969

Klausberger, E. M.: Fortschritte der Aneurysmadiagnostik durch den Bewegungsfilm. Wien. Z. Nervenheilk. 15: 148, 1958

Klemme, R. M., R. D. Woolsey: Suprasellar aneurysm. Report of a case with recovery. Arch. Neurol. Psychiat. (Chic.) 47: 662–666, 1942

Kloos, K.: Persistierende Karotis-Basilaris-Anastomose als Ursache einer Subarachnoidalblutung. Zbl. Neurochir. 13: 166–171, 1953

Klug, N.: Besonderheiten perforierender Schädelhirnverletzungen unter Friedensverhältnissen. Inaugural-Dissertation, Heidelberg 1968

Koczorek, Kh. R., W. Vogt, A. Kollmansberger, O. J. Beck, A. Beathmann, H. J. Reulen: Cerebroprotektive Effekte von Aldosteron und Aldosteronantagonisten. Colloque International sur l'action extra-renale de l'Aldosterone et de ses Antagonistes. V. Session, Nice, 29.9–1.10.1971

Kodama, N., T. Masumitsu, Y. Matsukado: Primitive hypoglossal artery associated with basilar artery aneurysm. Surg. Neurol. 6: 279–281, 1976a

Kodama, N., H. Ohara, J. Suzuki: Persistent hypoglossal artery associated with aneurysms. Report of two cases. J. Neurosurg. 45: 449–451, 1976b

Kodama, N., K. Koshu, K. Mineura, J. Suzuki: Surgical treatment of internal carotid bifurcation aneurysms. In Suzuki, J.: Cerebral Aneurysms. Neuron, Tokyo 1979 (pp. 261–267)

Kodama, N., K. Mineura, S. Fujiwara, J. Suzuki: Surgical treatment of carotid-ophthalmic aneurysms. In Suzuki, J.: Cerebral Aneurysms. Neuron, Tokyo 1979 (pp. 268–274)

Kodama, N., K. Koshu, K. Mineura et al.: Surgical treatment of internal carotid-posterior communicating artery aneurysms. From the experience of 213 cases. (Jpn.) Neurol. Surg. 1/2: 131–138, 1979

Koeppen, A. H. W., K. D. Barron: Superficial siderosis of the central nervous system. J. Neuropath. exp. Neurol. 30: 448–469, 1971

König, G. H., W. H. Marshall, J. Poole, R. A. Kramer: Rupture of intracranial aneurysms during cerebral angiography: Report of 10 cases and review of the literature. Neurosurgery 5: 314–323, 1979

Kothandaram, P., B. H. Dawson, R. C. Kruyt: Carotid-ophthalmic aneurysms. A study of 19 patients. J. Neurosurg. 34: 544–548, 1971

Kowada, M., A. Ames III., G. Majno, R. L. Wright: Cerebral ischemia I. an improved experimental method for study; cardiovascular effects and demonstration of an early vascular lesion in the rabbit. J. Neurosurg. 28: 150–157, 1968

Koyama, T., R. Yoshimoto, K. Uchida et al.: Intracranial saccular aneurysms. Surgical results based on 1000 consecutive cases. Tohoku J. exp. Med. 126: 112–124, 1978

Kramer: Hyperplasie fibromusculaire et anévrysme extracrânien de la carotide interne avec syndrome parapharyngien typique. Rev. neurol. 120: 239–244, 1969

Krauland, W.: Zur Entstehung traumatischer Aneurysmen der Schlagader am Hirngrund. Schweiz. Z. Path. 12: 113–127, 1949

Krauland, W.: Verletzungen der Schlagaderzweige an der Mantelfläche des Großhirns durch stumpfe Gewalt ohne Schädelbruch als Quelle tödlicher subduraler Blutungen. Dtsch. Z. Nervenheilk. 175: 54–65, 1956

Krauland, W.: Die Aneurysmen der Schlagadern am Hirn und Schädelgrund und der großen Rückenmarksadern. In Lubarsch, O., F. Henke, R. Rössle: Handbuch spez. path. Anat. Histol. Springer, Berlin 1957, Bd. 13/IB

Krause, F.: Chirurgie des Gehirns und Rückenmarks nach eigenen Erfahrungen, Vol. 1. Urban & Schwarzenberg, Berlin-Wien 1908 (pp. 76, plate XVII, fig. a)

Krayenbühl, H.: Das Hirnaneurysma. Schweiz. Arch. Neurol. Psychiat. 47: 155–236, 1941

Krayenbühl, H.: Beitrag zur Frage des cerebralen angiospastischen Insultes. Schweiz. med. Wschr. 90: 961–965, 1960

Krayenbühl, H.: Behandlung intracranieller Aneurysmen mit synthetischem Klebstoff. Münch. med. Wschr. 106: 1370–1376, 1962

Krayenbühl, H.: Klassifikation und klinische Symptomatologie der zerebralen Aneurysmen. Ophthalmologica (Basel) 167: 122–164, 1973

Krayenbühl, H., F. Lüthy: Hydrozephalus als Spätfolge geplatzter basaler Hirnaneurysmen. Schweiz. Arch. Neurol. Neurochir. Psychiat. 61: 7–21, 1948

Krayenbühl, H., M. G. Yaşargil: Die vaskulären Erkrankungen im Gebiet der Arteria vertebralis und Arteria basilaris. Thieme, Stuttgart 1957

Krayenbühl, H., M. G. Yaşargil: Das sackförmige Aneurysma der Hirnarterien. In: Das Hirnaneurysma. Documenta Geigy, Series Chirurgica, Nr. 4. Basel, Geigy 1958 (pp. 10–65)

Krayenbühl, H., M. G. Yaşargil: Étude clinique. In Krayenbühl, H., et al.: L'Anévrysme de l'Artère Communicante Antérieure. Masson, Paris 1959a (pp. 41–56)

Krayenbühl, H., M. G. Yaşargil: Radiologie. In Krayenbühl, H., et al.: L'Anévrysme de l'Artère Communicante Antérieure. Masson, Paris 1959b (pp. 57–70)

Krayenbühl, H., M. G. Yaşargil: Cerebral Angiography, 2nd Ed. Lippincott, Philadelphia 1968

Krayenbühl, H., M. G. Yaşargil: Diagnosis and therapy of intracranial aneurysms. In Cooper, P., L. M. Nyhus: Surgery Annual, Appleton-Century-Crofts, New York 1970 (pp. 327–343)

Krayenbühl, H., G. Weber, M. G. Yaşargil: Traitement chirurgical et pronostic. In Krayenbühl, H.: L'Anévrysme de l'Artère Communicante Antérieure. Masson, Paris 1959 (p. 100)

Krayenbühl, H., M. G. Yaşargil, E. S. Flamm, J. M. Tew: Microsurgical treatment of intracranial saccular aneurysms. J. Neurosurg. 37: 678–686, 1972

Krayenbühl, H., B. Hanhart, E. Laine, G. Lazorthes, F. Logue, E. Uehlinger, G. Weber, M. G. Yaşargil: L'Anévrysme de l'Artere Communicante Antérieure. Masson, Paris 1959

Kribs, R., P. Kleihues: The recurrent artery of Heubner. In Zülch, K. J.: Cerebral Circulation and Stroke. Springer, Berlin 1971 (pp. 40–56)

Kricheff, I. I., N. E. Chase, J. R. Ransohoff: The angiographic investigation of ruptured intracranial aneurysms. Radiology 83: 1016–1025, 1964

Kuhlendahl, H., K. Huse: Deep hypotension in the surgical treatment of intracranial saccular aneurysms. Joint meeting of German and Italian neurosurgical Societies, Taormina 12–14 June 1972

Kuhn, R. A., H. Kugler: False aneurysms of the middle meningeal artery. J. Neurosurg. 21: 92–96, 1964

Kukovetz, W. R., G. Pöch: Inhibition of cyclic-3',5'-nucleotidephosphodiesterase as possible mode of action of papaverine and similarly acting drugs. Naunyn-Schmiedeberg's Arch. Pharmak. 267: 189–194, 1970

Kunc, Z.: Aneurysms of carotid and posterior communicating artery. Progr. Brain Res. 30: 309–315, 1968

Kunst, H.: Die eindimensionale Echoenzephalographie bei neurologischen und psychiatrischen Krankheiten. Sammlung psychiatrischer und neurologischer Einzeldarstellungen. Thieme, Stuttgart 1974

Kurze, T.: Microtechniques in neurological Surgery. Clin. Neurosurg. 11: 128–137, 1964

Kurze, T., J. B. Doyle Jr.: Extradural intracranial (middle Fossa)

approach to the internal auditory canal. J. Neurosurg. 19: 1033–1037, 1962
Kusske, J. A., P. T. Turner, G. A. Ojemann, A. B. Harris: Ventriculostomy for the treatment of acute hydrocephalus following subarachnoid hemorrhage. J. Neurosurg. 38: 591–595, 1973
Kutzuzawa, T., S. Takahashi, C. Saito, T. Sato, T. Twabuchi: Studies of cerebral hemodynamics in subarachnoid hemorrhage. Tokohu J. exp. Med. 94: 407–415, 1968
Kuwayama, A., N. T. Zervas, R. Belson, A. Shintani, K. Pickren: A model for experimental cerebral arterial spasm. Stroke 3: 49–56, 1972
Kwak, R., H. Niizuma, M. Hatamaka, J. Suzuki: Anterior communicating artery aneurysms with associated anomalies. J. Neurosurg. 52: 162–164, 1980
Kwak, R., T. Ohi, H. Niizuma, J. Suzuki: Afferent artery and the site of neck of anterior communicating artery aneurysm. Surg. Neurol. 13: 221–223, 1980
Kwak, R., Y. Okudaira, J. Suzuki, Y. Watabe: Problems in hypothermic anesthesia for direct surgical treatment of intracranial aneurysms, with special reference to ventricular fibrillation. Brain Nerve (Tokyo, Japan) 24: 403–410, 1972
Labauge, R., A. Thevenet, C. Gros, B. Vlahovitch, C. Peguret, P. Frerebeau: Les anévrysmes du segment exocrânien de l'axe carotidien et leur traitement chirurgical. A propos de 13 observations personelles. Rev. neurol. 124: 512–525, 1971
Lafon, R., P. Betoulieres, S. P. Temple, M. Pelissier: Angiographie carotidienne et tomographie simultanée. Rev. neurol. 94: 263–267, 1956
Laine, E.: Traitement chirurgical des anévrysmes de l'artère communicante antérieure. In Krayenbühl, H., et al.: L'Anévrysme de l'Artère Communicante Antérieure. Masson, Paris 1959 (pp. 131–187)
Laine, E.: Arterial vertebro-basilar aneurysms. Progr. Brain Res. 30: 323–346, 1968
Laine, E., P. Galibert, J. M. Delandtsheer, P. Pruvot: Notre expérience du traitement chirurgical des anévrymes artériels intracrâniens; étude prognostique et indications opératoires. Neuro-chirurgie 3: 315–318, 1957
Laine, E., L. Andreussi, J.-M. Delandsheer, P. Galibert, J.-L. Christiaens, M. Gomin, J. Clarisse, J. Delcour: Anévrysmes de l'artère cérébrale moyenne. Étude anatomique, clinique et thérapeutique. A propos d'une série de 116 cas dont 100 ont été opérés. Neuro-chirurgie 16: 181–201, 1970
Laitinen, L., A. Servo: Embolization of cerebral vessels with inflatable and detachable balloons. J. Neurosurg. 48: 307–308, 1978
Laitinen, L., A. Snellman: Aneurysms of pericallosal artery; study of 14 cases verified angiographically and treated mainly by direct surgical attack. J. Neurosurg. 17: 447–458, 1960
Landolt, A. M., M. G. Yaşargil, H. A. Krayenbühl: Disturbance of serum electrolytes after surgery of intracranial arterial aneurysms. J. Neurosurg. 37: 210, 1972
Lang, E. F., J. L. Poppen: Aneurysms of the anterior communicating artery: results of surgical treatment. Surg. Clin. N. Amer. 42: 793–805, 1962
Lang, E. R., M. Kidd: Electron microscopy of human cerebral aneurysms. J. Neurosurg. 22: 554–562, 1965
Lapayowker, M. S., E. P. Liebman, M. L. Ronis, J. N. Safer: Presentation of the internal carotid artery as a tumor of the middle ear. Radiology 98: 293–297, 1971
Lapras, Cl., A. Goutelle, M. Brunat, J. P. Dechaume: Les anévrysmes intra-crâniens de l'enfant. A propos de 4 observations. Neuro-chirurgie 14: 891–900, 1968
Lapras, Cl., A. Thierry, D. Michel, J. P. Dechaume, L. Mansuy: Signes radiologique des anévrysmes intra-crâniens du système carotidien. Fortschr. Neurol. Psychiat., Suppl. 8: 172–187, 1965
Larson, A. G.: Deliberate hypotension. Anesthesiology 25: 682–706, 1964
Lasky, F. J., Multisectional cerebral angiotomography. Radiol. Technol. 44: 121–130, 1972
Lassen, H. C. A.: A preliminary report on the 1952 epidemic of polio in Copenhagen with specific reference to treatment of acute respiratory insufficiency. Lancet I: 37, 1953
Lassen, N. A.: Autoregulation of cerebral blood flow. Circulat. Res. 15 (Suppl.): 201–204, 1964
Lassen, N. A., D. H. Ingvar: Blood flow of cerebral cortex determined by radioactive Krypton[85]. Experientia (Basel) 17: 42–43, 1961
Lassman, L. P.: Internal carotid artery bifurcation aneurysms. In Pia, H. W., C. Langmaid, J. Zierski: Cerebral Aneurysms, Advances in Diagnosis and Therapy. Springer, Berlin 1979 (pp. 96–106)
Lassman, L. P., P. S. Ramani, R. P. Sengupta: Aneurysms of peripheral cerebral arteries due to surgical trauma. Vasc. Surg. 8: 1–5, 1974
Law, W. R., E. R. Nelson: Internal carotid aneurysm as a cause of Reader's paratrigeminal syndrome. Neurology (Minneap.) 18: 43–46, 1968
Lazarev, V. A., A. G. Lysachev: First experience of management of cerebral arterial aneurysms by means of the balloon catheter. In: XI Vsesojuznaja konf. molodykh neirokhirurgov, Moscow 1978, (pp. 156–157) (Rus.)
Lazorthes, G.: Les conséquences carotidiennes des lésions par projectiles du sinus caverneux. Neuro-chirurgie 5: 315–319, 1959
Lazorthes, G.: Vascularisation et Circulation Cérébrales. Masson, Paris 1961 (p. 323)
Lazorthes, G.: Etude anatomo-topographique de l'artère cérébrale antérieure et de l'artère communicante antérieure. In Krayenbühl, H. A.: L'Anévrysme de l'Artère Communicante Antérieure. Masson, Paris 1969 (pp. 5–21)
Lazorthes, G., J. Gaubert, J. Poulkes: The central and cortical distribution of the anterior cerebral artery. Neuro-chirurgie 2: 237–253, 1956
Le Beau, J.: Anévrismes de l'artère communicante antérieure. Ruptures et indications neurochirurgicales. Neurochirurgia (Stuttg.) 5: 38–57, 1962
Lechtape-Grüter, H., K. J. Zülch: Gibt es einen Spasmus der Hirngefäße? Radiologe 11: 429–435, 1971
Lecuire, J., J. Rougier, M. Bonnet, D. Laurent: Syndrome de la fente sphénoidale par volumineux anévrysme intra-caverneux. Bull. Soc. Ophthal. Fr. 64: 216–218, 1964
Lecuire, J., P. Buffard, A. Goutelle, J. P. Dechaume, D. Michel, G. Rambaud, J. P. Gentil, J. Verger: Considérations anatomiques, cliniques et radiologiques à propos d'une artère hypoglosse. J. Radiol. Électrol. 45: 217–222, 1965
Leeds, N. E., H. I. Goldberg: Angiographic manifestations in cerebral inflammatory disease. Radiology 98: 595–604, 1971
Lehrer, H. Z., L. A. Gross, T. P. Poon: Ruptured intracranial aneurysm. Contrast agent extravasation during brachial arteriography. Arch. Neurol. (Chic.) 27: 351–354, 1972
LeMay, M., C. A. Gooding: The clinical significance of the azygos anterior cerebral artery. Amer. J. Roentgenol. 98: 602–610, 1966
Lemesurier, A. B.: Erosion haemorrhage from the internal carotid artery. Canad. med. Ass. J. 25: 551–558, 1931
Lende, R. A.: Local spasm in cerebral arteries. J. Neurosurg. 17: 90–103, 1960
Lepoire, J., B. Coxam: Les anévrismes de la communicante antérieure. Aspects anatomique, modalités opératoires. Neuro-chirurgie 5: 162–182, 1959
Lepoire, J., J. Montaut, M. Renard, J. Grosdidier, P. Mathieu: Anévrysme sacculaire de la carotide cervicale, complication d'une angiographie carotidienne percutanée. Neuro-chirurgie 10: 275–281, 1964
Levy, A., B. Kellerhals, A. W. Nawaz: Foudroyante Epistaxis aus traumatischem Aneurysma des infraklionoidalen Teils der Arteria carotis interna. Acta neurochir. (Wien) 24: 37–53, 1971
Levy, L. F.: Subarachnoid hemorrhage without arteriographic vascular abnormality. J. Neurosurg. 17: 252–258, 1960
Lie, T. A.: Congenital Anomalies of the Carotid Arteries. Experta Med. Found., Amsterdam 1968
Liese, E. G. J.: Angiotomography: preliminary report. Radiology 75: 272–274, 1960
Liliequist, B.: The subarachnoid cisterns. An anatomic and roentgenologic study. Acta radiol. (Stockh.) Suppl, 185: 1–108, 1959
Liliequist, B., M. Lindqvist, F. Probst: Rupture of intracranial aneurysm during carotid angiography. Neuroradiology 11: 185–190, 1976
Liliequist, B., M. Lindqvist, E. Valdimarsson: Computed tomography and subarachnoid hemorrhage. Neuroradiology 14: 21–26, 1977
Lin, J. P., I. I. Krichoff: Angiographic investigation of cerebral aneurysms. Technical aspects. Radiology 105: 69–76, 1972

Lin, J. P., I. I. Kricheff, N. E. Chase: Blood pressure during retrograde brachial angiography. Radiology 83: 640–646, 1964

Lin, P. M., H. Javid, E. J. Doyle: Partial internal carotid artery occlusion treated by primary resection and vein graft: report of a case. J. Neurosurg. 13: 650–655, 1956

Lindemann, B. R.: Simultane Angiocardio-Tomographie. Fortschr. Röntgenstr. 73: 261–267, 1950

Lindqvist, G., G. Norlén: Korsakoff's syndrome after operation on ruptured aneurysm of the anterior communicating artery. Acta psychiat. scand. 42: 24–34, 1966

Lipovsek, M.: Ruptured aneurysms of the proximal middle cerebral artery. J. Neurosurg. 39: 498–502, 1973

List, C. F., F. J. Hodges: Intracranial angiography. I. The diagnosis of vascular lesions. J. Neurosurg. 3: 25–45, 1946

Litvak, J., M. D. Yahr, J. Ransohoff: Aneurysms of the great vein of Galen and midline cerebral arteriovenous anomalies. J. Neurosurg. 17: 945–954, 1960

Ljunggren, B., H. Säveland, L. Brandt: Causes of unfavorable outcome, after early aneurysm operation. Neurosurgery 13: 629–633, 1983

Loach, A. B., H. R. C. DeAzevedo: Some observations on the microneurosurgical treatment of intracranial aneurysms. Acta neurochir. (Wien) 35: 97–103, 1976

Locksley, H. B.: Report on the Cooperative Study of intracranial aneurysms and subarachnoid hemorrhage. Section V, Part I. Natural history of subarachnoid hemorrhage, intracranial aneurysms and arteriovenous malformations. Based on 6368 cases in the Cooperative Study. J. Neurosurg. 25: 219–239, 1966a

Locksley, H. B.: Report on the Cooperative Study of intracranial aneurysms and subarachnoid hemorrhage. Section V, Part II. Natural history of subarachnoid hemorrhage, intracranial aneurysms and arteriovenous malformations. J. Neurosurg. 25: 321–368, 1966b

Locksley, H. B., A. L. Sahs, L. Knowler: Report on the Cooperative Study of intracranial aneurysms and subarachnoid hemorrhage. Section II. General survey of cases in the central registry and characteristics of the sample population. J. Neurosurg. 24: 922–932, 1966a

Locksley, H. B., A. L. Sahs, R. Sandler: Report on the Cooperative Study of intracranial aneurysms and arteriovenous malformations. Section III. Subarachnoid hemorrhage unrelated to intracranial aneurysm and A-V malformation. J. Neurosurg. 24: 1034–1056, 1966b

Lodin, H.: Spontaneous thrombosis of cerebral aneurysms. Brit. J. Radiol. 39: 701–703, 1966

Loebell, G.: Das extrakranielle Aneurysma der Arteria carotis interna beim Kleinkind. HNO 10: 297–300, 1962

Löfstedt, St.: Intracranial arterial aneurysms. Acta radiol. (Stockh.) 34: 339–349, 1950

Logue, V.: Saccular aneurysms of the internal carotid artery in the cavernous sinus occurring bilaterally. Brit. J. Surg. 39: 181–182, 1951

Logue, V.: Surgery in spontaneous subarachnoid haemorrhage. Operative treatment of aneurysms on the anterior cerebral and anterior communicating artery. Brit. med. J. I.: 473–479, 1956

Logue, V.: Posterior fossa aneurysms. Clin. Neurosurg. 11: 183–219, 1964

Logue, V., M. Durward, R. T. C. Pratt, M. Piercy, W. L. B. Nixon: The quality of survival after rupture of an anterior cerebral aneurysm. Brit. J. Psychiat. 114: 137–160, 1968

Lombardi, G., A. Passerini, F. Migliavaca: Intracavernous aneurysms of the internal carotid artery. Amer. J. Roentgenol. 89: 361–271, 1963

Loop, J. W., E. L. Foltz: Applications of angiography during intracranial operation. Acta radiol. Diagn. 5: 363–367, 1966

Lougheed, W. M.: Selection, timing and technique of aneurysm surgery of the anterior circle of Willis. Clin. Neurosurg. 16: 95–113, 1969

Lougheed, W. M.: Personal communication, 1976

Lougheed, W. M., G. Khodadad: A new clip for surgery of intracranial and small blood vessels. J. Neurosurg. 22: 397–398, 1965

Lougheed, W. M., B. M. Marshall: The place of hypothermia in the treatment of intracranial aneurysms. Progr. neurol. Surg. 3: 115–148, 1969a

Lougheed, W. M., B. M. Marshall: The diploscope in intracranial aneurysm surgery: results in 40 patients. Canad. J. Surg. 12: 75–82, 1969b

Lougheed, W. M., B. M. Marshall: Management of aneurysms of the anterior circulation by intracranial procedures. In Youmans, J. R.: Neurological Surgery, Vol. II. Saunders, Philadelphia 1973 (pp. 731–767)

Lougheed, W. M., E. H. Botterell, T. P. Morley: Results of the direct attack in the surgical management of internal carotid and middle cerebral aneurysms. Clin. Neurosurg. 9: 193–200, 1963

Lougheed, W. M., B. Marshall, M. Hunter, E. Michel, H. Sandwith-Smith: Common carotid to intracranial internal carotid bypass venous graft. J. Neurosurg. 34: 114–118, 1971

Love, J. G., L. H. Dart: Results of carotid ligation with particular reference to intracranial aneurysms. J. Neurosurg. 27: 89–93, 1967

Lukin, R. R., A. A. Chambers, T. A. Tomsick: Cerebral vascular lesions: infarction, hemorrhage, aneurysms and arteriovenous malformations. Semin, Roentgenol. 12: 77–89, 1977

Lukin, R. R., A. A. Chambers, R. McLaurin, J. Tew Jr.: Thrombosed giant middle cerebral aneurysms. Neuroradiology 10: 125–129, 1975

McConnell, A. A.: Subchiasmal aneurysm treated by implantation of muscle. Zbl. Neurochir. 2: 269–274, 1937

McCormick, W. F., G. J. Acosta-Rua: The size of intracranial saccular aneurysms. An autopsy study. J. Neurosurg. 33: 422–427, 1970

McCormick, W. F., J. D. Beals: Severe epistaxis caused by ruptured aneurysm of the internal carotid artery. J. Neurosurg. 21: 678–686, 1964

McCormick, W. F., J. D. Nofzinger: Saccular intracranial aneurysms. An autopsy study. J. Neurosurg. 22: 155–159, 1965

McCormick, W. F., S. S. Schochet: Atlas of Cerebrovascular Disease. Saunders, Philadelphia 1976

McDonald, C. A., M. Korb: Intracranial aneurysms. Arch. Neurol. Psychiat. (Chic.) 42: 298–328, 1938

McDonald, C. A., M. Korb: The circle of Willis. Its angles and its aneurysms. R. I. med. J. 23: 145–149, 1940

McDowall, D. G.: The effects of clinical concentrations of halothane on the blood flow and oxygen uptake of the cerebral cortex. Brit. J. Anaesth. 39: 186–196, 1967

McDowell, F., H. Kutt: Complications of angiography. In Millikan, C. H., R. G. Siekert, J. P. Whisnant: Cerebral Vascular Diseases. Fourth Princeton Conference. Grune & Stratton, New York 1965 (pp. 18–25)

McFadden, J. T.: Metallurgical principles in neurosurgery. J. Neurosurg. 31: 373–385, 1969

McFadden, J. T.: The origin and evolutionary principles of spring forceps. Surg. Gynec. Obstet. 130: 356–368, 1970

McFadden, J. T.: Chocked-clip aneurysmorrhapy. Surg. Gynec. Obstet. 132: 898, 1971

McFadden, J. T.: Tissue reactions to standard neurosurgical metallic implants. J. Neurosurg. 36: 598–603, 1972

McKenzie, K. G.: Some minor modifications of Harvey Cushing's silver clip outfit. Surg. Gynec. Obstet. 45: 549–550, 1927

McKenzie, K. G.: Discussion of intracranial aneurysm: a surgical problem. Zbl. Neurochir. 3: 352, 1938

McKissock, W., K. W. Paine: Subarachnoid hemorrhage. Brain 82: 356–366, 1959

McKissock, W., L. Walsh: Subarachnoid hemorrhage due to intracranial aneurysms. Results of treatment of 249 verified cases. Brit. med. J. II: 559–565, 1956

McKissock, W., K. Paine, L. Walsh: The value of hypothermia in the surgical treatment of ruptured intracranial aneurysms. J. Neurosurg. 17: 700–707, 1960a

McKissock, W., K. W. Paine, L. S. Walsh: An analysis of the results of treatment of ruptured intracranial aneurysms. Report of 772 consecutive cases. J. Neurosurg. 17: 762–776, 1960b

McKissock, W., A. Richardson, L. Walsh: "Posterior communicating" aneurysms. Lancet I: 1203–1206, 1960

McKissock, W., A. Richardson, L. Walsh: Middle cerebral aneurysms: further results in the controlled trial of conservative and surgical treatment of ruptured intracranial aneurysms. Lancet II: 417–421, 1962

McKissock, W., A. Richardson, L. Walsh: Multiple intracranial aneurysms. Lancet I: 623–626, 1964

McKissock, W., A. Richardson, L. Walsh: Anterior communicat-

ing aneurysms. A trial of conservative and surgical treatment. Lancet I: 873–876, 1965
McMurty, J. G., E. M. Housepian, F. O. Bowman, R. S. Matteo: Surgical treatment of basilar artery aneurysms. Elective circulatory arrest with thoracotomy in 12 cases. J. Neurosurg. 40: 486–494, 1974
McMurty, J. G., J. L. Pool, H. R. Nova: The use of Rheomacrodex in the surgery of intracranial aneurysms. J. Neurosurg. 26: 218–222, 1967
McNeel, D., R. A. Evans, E. M. Ory: Angiography of cerebral mycotic aneurysms. Acta radiol. Diagn. 9: 407–412, 1969
McNichol, G. P., A. P. Fletcher, N. Alkjaersig et al.: The absorption distribution and excretion of ε-aminocaproic acid following oral or intravenous administration to man. J. Lab. clin. Med. 59: 15–24, 1962
Madonick, I. J., A. P. Ruskin: Recurrent oculomotor paresis. Paresis associated with a vascular anomaly, carotid-basilar anastomosis. Arch. Neurol. (Chic.) 6: 353–357, 1962
Magladery, J. W.: On subarachnoid bleeding – an appraisal of treatment. J. Neurosurg. 12: 437–449, 1955
Magnus, V.: Aneurysm of the internal carotid artery. J. Amer. med. Ass. 88: 1712–1713, 1927
Mahoudeau, D., S. Daum, George, Rosier: Ophtalmoplégie double révélatrice d'un anévrysme intra-crânien bilatéral de la carotide interne. Intérêt diagnostique de l'artériographie. Bull. Med. Soc. Chir. 289: 503–509, 1949
Malis, L. I.: Bipolar coagulation in microsurgery. In Donaghy, R. M. P., M. G. Yaşargil: Micro-Vascular Surgery, Mosby, St. Louis, Thieme, Stuttgart 1967 (pp. 126–130)
Mallett, B. L., N. Yeall: Measurement of regional clearance rate in man using ^{133}Xe inhalation and extracranial recording. Clin. Sci. 29: 179–191, 1965
Manelfe, C., J. Clarisse, D. Fredy, J. M. Andre, G. Crouzet: Dysplasie fibromusculaire des artères cervicocéphaliques. A propos de 70 cas. J. Neuroradiol. 1: 149–321, 1974
Marc, J. A., M. M. Schechter, B. Azar-Kia: Intraventricular bleeding from cerebral aneurysmal rupture. Neuroradiology 5: 184–186, 1973
Margolis, M. T., R. L. Stein, T. H. Newton: Extracranial aneurysms of the internal carotid artery. Neuroradiology 4: 78–89, 1972
Marguth, F., W. Schiefer: Spontanheilung eines intrakraniellen Aneurysmas. Acta neurochir. (Wien) 5: 38–45, 1957
Marino, R. Jr.: The anterior cerebral artery: I. Anatomoradiological study of its cortical territories. Surg. Neurol. 5: 81–87, 1976
Markwalder, H., P. Huber: Aneurysmen der Meningealarterien. Schweiz. med. Wschr. 45: 1344–1347, 1961
Marshall, B. M., Anesthesia for intracranial aneurysm surgery. Clin. Neurosurg. 9: 142–149, 1963
Marshall, W. H.: Delayed arterial spasm following subarachnoid hemorrhage. Radiology 106: 325–327, 1973
Martinez, S. N., C. Bertrand, A. Thierry: Les faux anévrysmes post-traumatiques. Canad. J. Surg. 9: 397–402, 1966
Masafumi, Y., M. Watanaba, Sh. Kuramoto: "True" posterior communicating artery aneurysm. Surg. Neurol. 11: 379–380, 1979
Maspes, P. E., G. Marini: Intracranial arterial spasm related to supraclinoid ruptured aneurysms. Acta neurochir. (Wien) 10: 630–638, 1962
Maspes, P. E., G. Marini: Aneurysms of the anterior communicating artery. Results of direct surgical treatment. Acta neurochir. (Wien) 11: 479–494, 1963
Matas, R., C. W. Allen: Occlusion of large surgical arteries with removable metallic bands to test the efficiency of the collateral circulation. Experimental and clinical observations. J. Amer. med. Ass. 56: 233, 1911
Matson, D. D.: Intracranial arterial aneurysms in childhood. J. Neurosurg. 23: 578–583, 1965
Mathew, N. T., J. S. Meyer, A. Hartmann: Diagnosis and treatment of factors complicating subarachnoid hemorrhage. Neuroradiology 6: 237–245, 1974
Mathew, N. T., J. S. Meyer, A. Hartmann, E. O. Ott: Abnormal cerebrospinal fluid-blood hydrocephalus. Arch. Neurol. (Chic.) 32: 657–664, 1975
Maurer, J. J., M. Mills, W. J. German: Triad of unilateral blindness, orbital fracture and massive epistaxis after head injury. J. Neurosurg. 18: 837–840, 1961
Mayfield, F. H., G. Kees Jr.: A brief history of the development of the Mayfield clip. Technical note. J. Neurosurg. 35: 97–100, 1971
Meadows, S. P.: Intracavernous aneurysms of internal carotid artery. Arch. Ophthal. 62: 566–574, 1959
Meese, W., A. Aulich, E. Kazner, R. Wüllenweber: CT findings in angiomas and aneurysms. In Lanksch, W., E. Kazner: Cranial Computerized Tomography. Springer, Berlin 1976 (pp. 291–297)
Menezes, A. H., et al.: True traumatic aneurysm of anterior cerebral artery. J. Neurosurg. 40: 544–548, 1974
Menschel: Ärzte Sachverst. Ztg. 1922, S. 13, cited by Krauland, 1949: Traum. Aneurysma der Art. vertebr. re.
Messer, H. B., L. Strenger, H. J. McVeety: Use of plastic adhesives for reinforcement of ruptured intracranial aneurysm. J. Neurosurg. 20: 360–362, 1963
Meyer, J. S.: Circulation changes following occlusion of the middle cerebral artery and their relation to function. J. Neurosurg. 15: 653–673, 1958
Meyer, J. S., R. B. Bauer: Medical treatment of spontaneous intracranial hemorrhage by the use of hypotensive drugs. Neurology (Minneap.) 12: 36–47, 1962
Meyer, J. S., G. Busch: Karotido-basilare Anastomose in Kombination mit multiplen Aneurysmen und weiteren Anomalien. Fortschr. Röntgenstr. 92: 690–693, 1960
Meyer, J. S., J. Z. Charney, V. M. Rivera, N. T. Mathew: Treatment with glycerol of cerebral edema due to acute cerebral infarction. Lancet II: 993–997, 1972
Meyer, J. S., Y. Fukuuchi, K. Shimazu, T. Ohuchi, A. D. Ericsson: Effect of intravenous infusion of glycerol on hemispheric blood flow and metabolism in patients with acute cerebral infarction. Stroke 3: 168–180, 1972
Meyer, J. S., N. Ishihara, V. D. Deshmukh, H. Naritomi, F. Sakai, M.-C. Hsu, P. Pollack: An improved method for noninvasive measurement of regional cerebral blood flow and blood volume by ^{133}Xe inhalation. Description of the method and normal values obtained in healthy volunteers. Stroke 9: 195–205, 1978
Meyer, J. S., V. D. Deshmukh, N. Ishihara, H. Naritomi, F. Sakai, M.-C. Hsu, P. Pollack, N. T. Mathew, F. I. Perez, J. L. Gedye: Noninvasive regional cerebral blood flow studies in cerebrovascular disorders. Proceedings of the Eisenhower Medical Center Symposium (1977) (in press)
Michael, W. F.:Posterior fossa aneurysms simulating tumors. J. Neurol. Neurosurg. Psychiat. 37: 218–223, 1974
Michallet, M., J. Natali, J. Wetterwald, R. Natali: A propos d'un cas d'anévrysme extracrânien de la carotide interne gauche, traité par ligature, et d'une dolicho-méga-carotide interne centro-latérale. Soc. Méd. milit. franç. Bull. 57: 179–182, 1963
Michallet, M., J. Wetterwald, J. Bourdial, J. Natali, R. Natali: Les anévrysmes de la carotide interne extra-crânienne. A propos de deux observations. Ann. Chir. Thorac. Cardiovasc. 3: 86–91, 1964
Michenfelder, J. D., J. W. Kirklin, A. Uihlein, H. J. Svein, C. S. MacCarty: Clinical experience with a closed-chest method of producing profound hypothermia and total circulatory arrest in neurosurgery. Ann. Surg. 159: 125–131, 1964
Miller, D. J., K. Jawad, B. Jennett: Safety of carotid ligation and its role in the management of intracranial aneurysm. J. Neurol. Neurosurg. Psychiat. 40: 64–72, 1977
Miller, H.: Un cas de rupture non traumatique d'anévrysme carotidien dans le sinus caverneux. Ann. Oculist. (Paris) 181: 410–413, 1948
Millikan, C. H.: Cerebral vasospasm and ruptured intracranial aneurysm. Arch. Neurol (Chic.) 32: 433–449, 1975
Misiuk, N. S.: A model of an angioblockader. Vop. nevropatol. i neirokhir. (Arkhangelsk) 3: 83–85, 1960 (Rus.)
von Mitterwallner, F.: Variationsstatistische Untersuchungen an den basalen Hirngefässen. Acta anat. (Basel) 24: 51–88, 1955
Miyaoka, M., T. Nonaka, H. Watanabe, H. Chigasaki, S. Ishii: Etiology and treatment of prolonged vasospasm. Experimental and clinical studies. Neurol. Med. Chir. (Tokyo) 16 (Part II): 103–114, 1976
Mizukami, M., H. Kin, G. Araki, H. Mihara, Y. Yoshida: Is angiographic spasm real spasm? Acta neurochir. (Wien) 34: 247–259, 1976
Mokri, B., D. G. Piepgras, T. M. Sundt, B. W. Pearson: Extracra-

nial internal carotid artery aneurysms. Mayo Clin. Proc. 57: 310–321, 1982
Molinari, G. F., L. Smith, M. N. Goldstein, R. Satran: Pathogenesis of cerebral mycotic aneurysms. Neurology (Minneap.) 23: 325–332, 1973
Moniz, E.: L'encephalographie artérielle son importance dans la localisation des tumeurs cérébrales. Rev. Neurol. 2: 72–90, 1927
Moniz, E.: Anévrysme intra-crânien de la carotide interne droite rendu visible par l'artériographie cérébrale. Rev. oto-neuroophtal. (B. Aires) 11: 746–748, 1933
Morantz, R. A., F. R. Kirchner, P. Kishore: Aneurysms of the petrous portion of the internal carotid artery. Surg. Neurol. 6: 313–318, 1976
Morello, A., E. Ponte: A case of intrasellar aneurysm simulating a pituitary adenoma. Acta neurochir. (Wien) 7: 391–402, 1959
Morgagni, J. B.: De sedibus er causis morborum per anatomia indagatis. Venetis ex typog. Remondiniana. 1791. (Cited in Walton, J. N.: Subarachnoid Haemorrhage. Livingstone, Edinburgh 1956
Morley, T. P., H. W. K. Barr: Giant intracranial aneurysms: diagnosis, course and management. Clin. Neurosurg. 16: 73–94, 1969
Morris, E. D., D. B. Moffat: Abnormal origin of the basilar artery from the cervical part of the internal carotid and its embryological significance. Anat. Rec. 12: 701–711, 1956
Morris, L.: Arteriographic studies in aneurysm of the internal carotid artery treated by carotid occlusion. Acta radiol. Diagn. 1: 367–372, 1963
Morrison, G., W. M. Hegarty, C. C. Brausch, T. J. Castelle, R. J. White: Direct surgical obliteration of a persistent trigeminal artery aneurysm. Case report. J. Neurosurg. 40: 249–251, 1974
Moskowitz, M. A., A. E. Rosenbaum: Angiographically monitored resolution of cerebral mycotic aneurysms. Neurology (Minneap.) 24: 1103–1108, 1974
Mount, L. A.: Results of treatment of intracranial aneurysms using the Selverston clamp. J. Neurosurg. 16: 611–618, 1959
Mount, L. A., J. L. Antunes: Results of treatment of intracranial aneurysms by wrapping and coating. J. Neurosurg. 42: 189–193, 1975
Mount, L. A., R. Brisman: Treatment of multiple intracranial aneurysms. J. Neurosurg. 35: 728–730, 1971
Mount, L. A., R. Brisman: Treatment of multiple aneurysms – symptomatic and asymptomatic. Clin. Neurosurg. 21: 166–170, 1974
Mount, L. A., J. M. Taveras: Cerebral angiographic studies following surgical treatment of intracranial aneurysms. Acta radiol. (Stockh.) 46: 333–341, 1956a
Mount, L. A., J. M. Taveras: The results of surgical treatment of intracranial aneurysms as demonstrated by progress arteriography. J. Neurosurg. 13: 618–626, 1956b
Mount, L. A., J. M. Taveras: Further observations of the significance of the collateral circulation of the brain as demonstrated arteriographically. Trans. Amer. neurol. Ass. 1960, p. 109
Mount, L. A., J. M. Taveras: Ligature of the basilar artery in treatment of an aneurysm of the basilar-artery bifurcation. J. Neurosurg. 19: 167–170, 1962
Moyes, P. D.: Basilar aneurysm associated with agenesis of the left internal carotid artery. Case report J. Neurosurg. 30: 608–611, 1969
Moyes, P. D.: Surgical treatment of multiple aneurysms and of incidentally-discovered unruptured aneurysms. J. Neurosurg. 35: 291–295, 1971
Mullan, S.: Experiences with surgical thrombosis of intracranial berry aneurysms and carotid cavernous fistulas. J. Neurosurg. 41: 657–670, 1974
Mullan, S.: Conservative management of the recently ruptured aneurysm. Surg. Neurol. 3: 27–32, 1975
Mullan, S., J. Dawley: Antifibrinolytic therapy for intracranial aneurysms. J. Neurosurg. 28: 21–23, 1968
Mullan, S., C. Reyes, J. Dawley, G. Dobsen: Stereotactic copper electric thrombosis of intracranial aneurysms. Progr. neurol. Surg. 3: 193–211, 1969
Mullan, S., T. Beckman, G. Vailati, E. Karasick, G. Dobson: Experimental approach to the problem of cerebral aneurysms. J. Neurosurg. 21: 838–846, 1964
Mullan, S., A. J. Raimondi, G. Dobson, G. Vailati, J. Hekmatopanah: Electrically induced thrombosis in intracranial aneurysms. J. Neurosurg. 22: 539–547, 1965
Murphy, D. J., R. J. Goldberg: Extravasation from an intracranial aneurysm during carotid angiography. Case report. J. Neurosurg. 27: 459–461, 1967
Murtagh, F., H. M. Stauffer, R. D. Harley: A case of persistent carotid basilar anastomosis associated with aneurysm of the homolateral middle cerebral artery manifested by oculomotor palsy. J. Neurosurg. 12: 46–49, 1955
Nacousz, J., R. Plante: Anévrysme exo-crânien de la carotide interne traité par résection et greffe. Un. méd. Can. 94: 1311–1315, 1965
Nadjmi, K. A., M. Bushe, M. R. Ratzka, G. Moissl: Angiotomographische Aspekte der zerebralen Aneurysmen und Angiome. Fortschr. Röntgenstr. 125: 427–428, 1976
Nadjmi, M., A. Pöschmann: Angiotomographie am Diagnost – N. Radiologe 12: 437–440, 1972
Nadjmi, M., A. Pöschmann: Über ein Gerät zur Serien-Angio-Tomographie. Fortschr. Röntgenstr. 123: 299–301, 1974
Nadjmi, M., G. Moissl, M. Ratzka, A. Pöschmann: Zerebrale Gefäße im Angiotomogramm. Thieme, Stuttgart 1977
Nagae, K., I. Goto, K. Ueda, Y. Morotomi: Familial occurrence of multiple intracranial aneurysms. J. Neurosurg. 37: 364–367, 1972
Nagai, H., Ts. Katsumata, M. Ohya, N. Kageyama: Subarachnoid hemorrhage on micro-circulation in hypothalamus and brain stem of dogs. Neurochirurgia (Stuttg.) 19: 135–144, 1976
Nakao, K.: Extrakranielle Aneurysmen der A. carotis interna. Med. Klin. 63: 58–60, 1968
Nakayama, N., J. P. Malin, M. Schwarz: Angiographische Untersuchungstechnik zum Nachweis von intrakraniellen Aneurysmen. Fortschr. Röntgenstr. 121: 141–145, 1974
Natali, J., A. Thevenet, J. P. Caron, A. Goutelle: Chirurgie des Artères Carotides et Vertébrales dans leur Segment Extra-Crânien. Masson, Paris 1973
Nedwich, A., H. Haft, M. Tellem, L. Kaufmann: Dissecting aneurysm of cerebral arteries. Arch. Neurol. (Chic.) 9: 477–484, 1963
New, P. F. J.: True aneurysm of the middle meningeal artery. Clin. Radiol. 16: 236–240, 1965
New, P. F. J.: True aneurysm of the middle meningeal artery. cranial Paget's disease and hypertension: a triad. Clin. Radiol. 18: 154–157, 1967
New, P. F. J., W. R. Scott: Computed Tomography of the Brain and Orbit. Williams & Wilkins, Baltimore 1975
Newbarr, F. D., C. B. Courville: Trauma as the possible significant factor in the rupture of congenital intracranial aneurysms. J. forens. Sci. 3: 174–200, 1958
Newton, T. H., D. G. Potts: Radiology of the Skull and Brain. Angiography, Vol. II, Books 2 and 3. Mosby, St. Louis 1974
Newton, T. H., J. E. Adams, E. J. Wylie: Arteriography of cerebrovascular disease. New Engl. J. Med. 270: 14–18, 1964
Nibbelink, D. W.: Cooperative Aneurysm Study: Antihypertensive and antifibrinolytic therapy following subarachnoid hemorrhage from ruptured intracranial aneurysm. In: Whisnant, J. P., B. A. Sandok: Cerebral Vascular Disease. Ninth Conference. Grune & Stratton, New York, 1975 (pp. 155–173)
Nibbelink, D. W., C. D. Jacobson: Antifibrinolytic activity during administration of Epsilon-aminocaproic-acid (EACA) in patients with SAH. Neurology (Minneap.) 22: 406, 1972
Nibbelink, D. W., A. L. Sahs, L. A. Knowler: Antihypertensive and antifibrinolytic medications in subarachnoid hemorrhage and their relation to cerebral vasospasm. In Smith, R. R., J. T. Robertson: Subarachnoid Hemorrhage and Cerebrovascular Spasm. Thomas, Springfield/Ill. 1975 (pp. 177–205)
Nibbelink, D. W., J. C. Torner, W. G. Henderson: Intracranial aneurysms and subarachnoid hemorrhage. A Cooperative Study. Antifibrinolytic therapy in recent onset subarachnoid hemorrhage. Stroke 6: 622–629, 1975
Niemeyer, P.: [Results of microsurgery in 54 intracranial aneurysms]. Arch. Neuro-psiquiat. (S. Paulo) 32: 175–186, 1974
Nishioka, H.: Report on the Cooperative Study of intracranial aneurysms and subarachnoid hemorrhage. Section VII, part I. Evaluation of the conservative management of ruptured intracranial aneurysms. J. Neurosurg. 25: 574–592, 1966a
Nishioka, H.: Report on the Cooperative Study of intracranial aneurysms and subarachnoid hemorrhage. Section VIII, part I. Results of the treatment of intracranial aneurysms by occlusion

of the carotid artery in the neck. J. Neurosurg. 25: 660–682, 1966b
Nishioka, H.: Evaluation of the conservative management of ruptured intracranial aneurysms. In Sahs, A. L., et al.: Intracranial Aneurysms and Subarachnoid Hemorrhage. A Cooperative Study. Lippincott, Philadelphia 1969 (pp. 125–142)
Nödinger, H.: Mykotisches Aneurysma und intracerebrale Massenblutung bei bakterieller Aortenklappenendokarditis. Inaug.-Diss., Tübingen, 1975
Norlén, G.: Some aspects of the surgical treatment of intracranial aneurysms. Clin. Neurosurg. 9: 214–221, 1963
Norlén, G.: Experiences with epsilon-amino-caproic acid in neurosurgery. A preliminary report. Neurochirurgia (Stuttg.) 10: 81, 1967
Norlén, G.: Aneurysm of the anterior communicating artery. Progr. Brain Res. 30: 295–302, 1968
Norlén, G.: A. S. Barnum: Surgical treatment of aneurysms of the anterior communicating artery. J. Neurosurg. 10: 634–650, 1953
Norlén, G., H. Olivecrona: The treatment of aneurysms of the circle of Willis. J. Neurosurg. 10: 404–415, 1953
Norlén, G., S. N. Paly: Aneurysms of the vertebral artery. Report of two operative cases. J. Neurosurg. 17: 830–835, 1960
Norlén, G., C. A. Thulin: The use of antifibrinolytic substances in ruptured intracranial aneurysms. Fourth Int. Congr. Neurol. Surg., New York 1969
Norman, R. M., H. Ulrich: Dissecting aneurysm of the middle cerebral artery as a cause of acute infantile hemiplegia. H. Path. Bact. 73: 580–583, 1957
Nornes, H.: The role of intracranial pressure in the arrest of hemorrhage in patients with ruptured intracranial aneurysms. J. Neurosurg. 39: 226–234, 1973a
Nornes, H.: The role of the circle of Willis in graded occlusion of the internal carotid artery in man. Acta neurochir. (Wien) 28: 165–178, 1973b
Nornes, H., P. Wikeby: Results of microsurgical management of intracranial aneurysms. J. Neurosurg. 51: 608–614, 1979
Northfield, D. W. C.: The Surgery of the Central Nervous System. Blackwell, Scientific Publication, Oxford 1973
Northfield, D. W. C.: Comment on Norlén, G.: The pathology, diagnosis and treatment of intracranial saccular aneurysms. Proc. roy. Soc. Med. 45: 302, 1952
Noterman, J., M. Warszawski, L. Jeanmart, J. Brihaye: Bilateral aneurysm of the internal carotid artery in the cavernous sinus: Case report. Neuroradiology 4: 63–65, 1972
Nukui, H., T. Aiba: Clinical features in cases with ruptured aneurysm of the distal anterior cerebral artery. (Jpn) Neurol. Med. Chir. 1811/1: 39–42, 1978
Nutik, S., D. Dilenge: Carotid-anterior cerebral artery anastomosis. Case report. J. Neurosurg. 44: 378–382, 1976
Nylen, C. O.: An oto-microscope. Acta oto-laryng. (Stockh.) 5: 414, 1924
Nyström, S. H. M.: Development of intracranial aneurysms as revealed by electron microscopy. J. Neurosurg. 20: 329–337, 1963
Nyström, S. H. M.: On factors related to spontaneous healing of ruptured intracranial aneurysms. Acta pathol. microbiol. scand. A 80: 566–572, 1972
Nyström, S., A. Snellman, T. Mäkelä: Sur le traitement des anévrysmes de la communicante antérieure. Neuro-chirurgie 8: 414–422, 1962
Obrador, S., G. Dierssen, J. R. Hernandez: Giant aneurysm of the posterior cerebral artery. Case report. J. Neurosurg. 26: 413–416, 1967
Obrador, S., J. Gomez-Bueno, J. Silvela: Spontaneous carotid-cavernous fistula produced by ruptured aneurysm of the meningohypophyseal branch of the internal carotid artery. Case report. J. Neurosurg. 40: 539–543, 1974
Obrist, W. D., H. K. Thompson Jr., C. H. King, H. S. Wang: Determination of regional cerebral blood flow by inhalation of Xenon[133]. Circulat. Res. 20: 124–135, 1967
Obrist, W. D., H. K. Thompson Jr., H. S. Wang, W. E. Wilkinson: Regional cerebral blood flow estimated by ^{133}Xe inhalation. Stroke 6: 245–256, 1975
Odom, G. L.: Cerebral vasospasm. Clin. Neurosurg. 22: 29–58, 1975
Odom, G. L., B. Woodhall, G. T. Tindall, J. R. Jackson: Change in distal intravascular pressure and size of intracranial aneurysm following common carotid ligation. J. Neurosurg. 19: 41–50, 1962
Ojemann, R. G.: Normal pressure hydrocephalus. Clin. Neurosurg. 18: 337–370, 1970
Ojemann, R. G., W. W. Montgomery, A. D. Weiss: Evaluation and surgical treatment of acoustic neuroma. New Engl. J. Med. 287: 895–899, 1972
Okawara, S., J. Hahn, J. Kimura: Cerebral circulation time and ruptured intracranial aneurysms. In Kitamura, K. T., H. Newton: Recent Advances in Diagnostic Neuroradiology. Igaku Shoin, Tokyo 1975 (pp. 137–141)
Osgood, C., L. G. Martin: Intraventricular contrast extravasation during carotid angiography. Surg. Neurol. 2: 49–50, 1974
Otomo, E.: The anterior choroidal artery. Arch. Neurol. (Chic.) 13: 656–658, 1965
Overgaard, J., J. Rieshede: Multiple cerebral saccular aneurysms. Acta neurol. scand. 41: 363–371, 1965
Overton III, M. C., T. H. Calvin Jr.: Iatrogenic cerebral cortical aneurysm. J. Neurosurg. 24: 672–675, 1966
Overton, S. B., F. N. Ritter: A high placed jugular bulb in the middle ear: a clinical and temporal bone study. Laryngoscope (St. Louis) 83: 1986–1991, 1973
Padget, D. H.: The circle of Willis. Its embryology and anatomy. In Dandy, W. E.: Intracranial Arterial Aneurysms. Hafner, New York, Comstock, Ithaca/N. Y. 1944, reprinted 1969 (pp. 67–90)
Paillas, J. E., J. Bonnal, J. Lavieille: Angiographic images of false aneurysmal sac caused by rupture of median meningeal artery in the course of traumatic extradural hematomata. Report of three cases. J. Neurosurg. 21: 667–671, 1964
Pakarinen, S.: Incidence, aetiology, and prognosis of primary subarachnoid haemorrhage. A study based on 589 cases diagnosed in a defined urban population during a defined period. Acta neurol. scand. 43 (Suppl. 29): 1–128, 1967
Palubinskas, A. J., D. Perloff, T. H. Newton: Fibromuscular hyperplasia: an arterial dysplasia of increasing clinical importance. Amer. J. Roentgenol. 98: 907–913, 1966
Palvolgyi, R.: Regional cerebral blood flow in patients with intracranial tumors. J. Neurosurg. 31: 149–163, 1969
Papo, I., G. Caruselli, U. Savolini: Epistaxis post-traumatique massive par rupture d'anévrysme infraclinoidien. Neuro-chirurgie 15: 283–290, 1969
Papo, I., U. Salvolini, G. Caruselli: Aneurysms of the anterior choroidal artery with intraventricular hematoma and hydrocephalus. case report. J. Neurosurg. 39: 225–260, 1973
Parkinson, D.: A surgical approach to the cavernous portion of the carotid artery. Anatomical studies and case report. J. Neurosurg. 23: 474–483, 1965
Parkinson, D.: Transcavernous repair of carotid cavernous fistula. J. Neurosurg. 26: 420–424, 1967
Parkinson, D.: Anatomy of the cavernous sinus. In Pia, H. W., C. Langmaid, J. Zierski: Cerebral Aneurysms, Advances in Diagnosis and Therapy. Springer, Berlin 1979a (pp. 62–66)
Parkinson, D.: Aneurysms of the "cavernous sinus". In Pia, H. W., C. Langmaid, J. Zierski: Cerebral Aneurysms, Advances in Diagnosis and Therapy. Springer, Berlin 1979b (pp. 79–81)
Parkinson, D.: Surgical approach to cavernous sinus aneurysms. In Pia, H. W., C. Langmaid, J. Zierski: Cerebral Aneurysms, Advances in Diagnosis and Therapy. Springer, Berlin 1979c (pp. 224–228)
Parkinson, D., K. K. Jain, J. B. Johnston: Saccular aneurysms of the ophthalmic artery: report of an unusual case. Canad. J. Surg. 4: 229–232, 1961
Passerini, A., E. de Donato: Su anastomosi carotido-basilari (10 casi). Radiol. med. (Torino) 48: 939–947, 1962
Passerini, A., G. Tagliabue: Gli aneurismi del sistema vertebr.-basilare. Riv. Pat. nerv. ment. 83: 86, 1962
Patel, A. N., A. E. Richardson: Ruptured intracranial aneurysms in first two decades of life: study of 58 patients. J. Neurosurg. 35: 571–576, 1976
Paterson, A.: Direct surgery in the treatment of posterior communicating aneurysms. Lancet II: 808–811, 1968
Paterson, A., M. R. Bond: Treatment of multiple intracranial arterial aneurysms. Lancet I: 1302–1304, 1973
Patterson, R. H. Jr.: Risk of carotid surgery with occlusion of the contralateral carotid artery. Arch. Neurol. (Chic.) 30: 188–189, 1974
Paul, R. L., J. G. Arnold Jr.: Operative factors influencing morta-

lity in intracranial aneurysm surgery: analysis of 186 consecutive cases. J. Neurosurg. 32: 289–294, 1970
Paulson, O. B.: Regional cerebral blood flow in apoplexy due to occlusion of the middle cerebral artery. Neurology (Minneap.) 20: 63–76, 1970
Paulson, O. B., N. A. Lossen, E. Skinhoj: Regional cerebral blood flow in apoplexy without arterial occlusion. Neurology (Minneap.) 20: 125–138, 1970
Paulson, O. B., S. Cronqvist, J. Risberg, F. I. Jeppesen: Regional cerebral blood flow: A comparison of 8 detector and 16 detector instrumentation. J. nucl. Med. 10: 169–173, 1968
Pechet, L.: Fibrinolysis. New Engl. J. Med. 273: 1024–1034, 1965
Pecker, J., A. Javalet: Le problème étiologique et chirurgical des hémorrhagies méningées spontanées d'adulte. Fortschr. Neurol. Psychiat., Suppl. 5: 74–91, 1962
Pecker, J., J. Hoel, A. Javalet, H. Fournier: Paralysie du moteur oculaire externe par anévrysme intra-pétreux traumatique de la carotide interne. Presse méd. 26: 1023–1024, 1960
Peerless, S. J.: The surgical approach to middle cerebral and posterior communicating aneurysms. Clin. Neurosurg. 21: 151–165, 1974
Peerless, S. J., M. J. Kendall: The innervation of the cerebral blood vessels. In Smith, R. R., J. T. Robertson: Subarachnoid Hemorrhage and Cerebrovascular Spasm. Thomas, Springfield/Ill. 1975 (pp. 38–54)
Peerless, S. J., M. G. Yaşargil: Adrenergic innervation of the cerebral blood vessels in the rabbit. J. Neurosurg. 35: 148–154, 1971
Peerless, S. J., M. G. Yaşargil, M. J. Kendall: The adrenergic and cholinergic innervation of the cerebral blood vessels. In Fusek, I., Z. Kunc: Present Limits of Neurosurgery. Avicenum Czechoslovak Medical Press, Prague, Excerpta Medica, Amsterdam 1972 (pp. 199–202)
Penfield, W.: Intracranial vascular nerves. Arch. Neurol. Psychiat. (Chic.) 27: 30–44, 1932
Perkins, J. J.: Principles and Methods of Sterilization in Health Sciences, Chapter 10, Thomas, Springfield/Ill. 1969
Perlmutter, D., A. L. Rhoton: Microsurgical anatomy of the anterior cerebral-anterior communicating-recurrent artery complex. J. Neurosurg. 45: 259–272, 1976
Perret, G., H. Nishioka: Report on the Cooperative Study on intracranial aneurysms and subarachnoid hemorrhage. Section IV. Cerebral angiography and analysis of the diagnostic value and complications of carotid and vertebral angiography in 5.484 patients. J. Neurosurg. 25: 98–114, 1966
Perret, L. V., J. W. D. Bull: The accuracy of radiology in demonstrating ruptured intracranial aneurysms. Brit. J. Radiol. 32: 85–92, 1959
Perria, L., G. L. Viale, C. Rivano: Anévrysmes de la jonction carotide interne-choroidienne antérieure: Etude clinique et radiologique. Acta neurochir. (Wien) 21: 153–166, 1969
Perria, L., G. L. Viale, C. Rivano: Further remarks on the surgical treatment of carotid-choroidal aneurysms. Acta neurochir. (Wien) 24: 253–262, 1971
Perria, L., C. Rivano, G. F. Rossi et al.: Aneurysms of the bifurcation of the internal carotid artery. Acta neurochir. (Wien) 19: 51–68, 1968
Pertuiset, B.: Les anévrismes sacculaires de la carotide interne supraclinoidienne. Neuro-chirurgie 5: 183–206, 1959
Pertuiset, B., D. Ancri: The effect of deep hypotension with sodium nitroprusside on cerebral blood volume computed by a radio isotopic technique. Ins. Neurol. Madras, Proc. 6: 235–238, 1976
Pertuiset, B., D. Ancri, J. Goutorbe: Variations du volume sanguin cérébral local en fonction de la pression artérielle moyenne chez l'homme. Rev. neurol. 132: 213–218, 1976a
Pertuiset, B., R. Van Effenterre, Y. Horn: Temporary external valve drainage in hydrocephalus with increased ventricular fluid pressure. Acta neurochir. (Wien) 33: 173–181, 1976b
Pertuiset, B., D. Aron, D. Dilenge, A. Mazalton: Les syndromes de l'artère choroïdienne antérieure. Étude clinique et radiologique. Rev. neurol. 106: 286–294, 1962
Pertuiset, B., J.-P. Houtteville, B. George, P. Margent: Dilatation ventriculaire précoce et hydrocéphalic secondaire aux ruptures des anévrysmes artériels sus tentoriels (diagnostic, mécanisme et traitement). Neurochirurgia (Stutt.) 15: 113–126, 1972
Pertuiset, B., J. Lepoire, G. Bodin, C. Cabezas: Les anévrismes de l'artère pericalleuse (Étude anatomo-clinique et thérapeutique à propos de 5 observations). Neuro-chirurgie 7: 321–338, 1961
Pertuiset, B., R. Van Effenterre, J. Goutorbe, N. Yoshimasu: Management of aneurysmal rupture during surgery, using bipolar coagulation, deep hypotension, and the operating microscope. Acta neurochir. (Wien) 30: 195–205, 1974a
Pertuiset, B., D. Vouyouklakis, J.-F. Guyot, O. Loeillet: Les résultats du traitement chirurgical des anévrysmes artériels sustentoriels rompus. D'après 81 cas personnels. Neurochirurgic 12: 421–437, 1966
Pertuiset, B., J. Goutorbe, N. Caruel, R. Van Effenterre, Y. E. Horn: L'hypotension préventive par Arfonad ou nitroprussiate de soude durant l'abord de 66 anévrysmes sacciformes sus tentoriels. Neuro-chirurgie 20: 555–564, 1974b
Pertuiset, B., J.-P. Houtteville, R. Van Effenterre, N. Caruel, J. Goutorbe: Chirurgie des anévrysmes artériels sus-tentoriels. Réduction par coagulation bipolaire sous hypotension profonde et exclusion par clip autobloquant: (52 cas opérés sous microscope). Nouv. Presse méd. 3: 1649–1652, 1974c
Pertuiset, B., R. Van Effenterre, N. Caruel, J. Goutorbe, B. Flandez: Les résultats de l'abord direct des anévrysmes intracrâniens sustentoriels en fonction de l'hypotension contrôlée, de la coagulation bipolaire et de la magnification optique. Rev. neurol. 129: 57–59, 1973
Petit-Dutaillis, D., H. W. Pittman: Aneurysm of the middle cerebral artery. Report of seven operative cases; review of literature; evaluation of surgical therapy. J. Neurosurg. 12: 1–12, 1955
Petruk, K. C., B. K. A. Weir, M. R. Marriott, Th. R. Overton: Clinical grade, regional cerebral blood flow and angiographical spasm in the monkey after subarachnoid and subdural hemorrhage. Stroke 4: 431–445, 1973
Petty, J. M.: Epistaxis from aneurysm of the internal carotid artery due to a gunshot wound. Case report. J. Neurosurg. 30: 741–743, 1969
Pevehouse, B.: Personal Communication, 1976
Philippides, D., F. Buchheit, A. Roth, E. Baldauf: Anévrysme post-traumatique de la carotide intra-caverneuse. Rev. Otoneuroophtal. 41: 345–349, 1969
Phillips, R. L.: Familial cerebral aneurysms. J. Neurosurg. 20: 701–703, 1963
Pia, H. W.: The microscope in neurosurgery. In Handa, H.: Microneurosurgery. University Park Press, Baltimore 1973a (pp. 3–7)
Pia, H. W.: Temporäre Drosselung der Hals-Carotiden. In: Chirurgie der intrakraniellen Aneurysmen. In Bier, A., H. Braun, H. Kümmell: Chirurgische Operationslehre. 8th. Ed.. Barth, Leipzig 1973b (pp. 138–140)
Pia, H. W.: Microsurgical treatment of intracerebral aneurysms. In Koos, W. Th., F. W. Böck, R. F. Spetzler: Clinical Microneurosurgery. Thieme, Stuttgart 1976
Pia, H. W.: Classification of aneurysms of the internal carotid system. Acta neurochir. (Wien) 40: 5, 1978a
Pia, H. W.: Microsurgical treatment of cerebral aneurysms. Neurosurg. Rev. 1: 35, 1978b
Pia, H. W.: Classification of vertebro-basilar aneurysms. Acta neurochir. (Wien) 47: 3–30, 1979a
Pia, H. W.: Classification and treatment of aneurysms of the vertebro-basilar system. Neurol. Med. Chir. (Tokyo) 19: 575–574, 1979b
Pia, H. W., H. Fontana: Aneurysms of the posterior cerebral artery. Acta neurochir. (Wien) 38: 13–35, 1977
Pia, H. W., S. Obrador, J. G. Martin: Association of brain tumours and arterial intracranial aneurysms. Acta neurochir. (Wien) 27: 189–204, 1972
Picard, L., J. Rebstock, A. L. Marchal, J. C. Mayer, A. Bertrand: Release of endovascular occlusion balloons using a thermoresistive technique. J. Neuroradiol. 7: 231–242, 1980
Pickering, G. W.: Vascular spasm. Lancet II: 845, 1951
Pickering, L., G. Hogan, E. Gilbert: Aneurysm of the posterior inferior cerebellar artery. Rupture in a newborn. Amer. J. Dis. Child. 119: 155–158, 1970
Piepgras, U., V. Kammerer: Die cerebrale Angiotomographie. Radiologe 12: 432–436, 1972
Piepgras, U., F. Pampus, F. Heuk: Der Wert der simultanen Angio-Tomographie für die Diagnostik von Hirngefäßaneurysmen. Fortschr. Röntgenstr. 108: 170–176, 1968
Pierini, E. A. A., A. Agra: Epistaxis como signo de hemorragia de

la carotida interna en su porcion timpanica. Probable aneurisma intrapetroso. Pren. méd. argent. 41: 945–948, 1954
Pilz, P., H. J. Hartjes: Fibromuscular dysplasia and multiple dissecting aneurysms of intracranial arteries. Further cause of moya-moya syndrome. Stroke 7: 393–398, 1976
Pirker, E.: Aneurysmaruptur während einer Karotisangiographie. Fortschr. Röntgenstr. 100: 415–416, 1964
Pirker, E., H. E. Diemath: Hämodynamik der sackförmigen arteriellen Aneurysmen. Acta radiol. Diagn. 9: 425–429, 1969
Poblete, R., A. Asenjo: Anastomosis carotide-basilar for persistencia de la arteria trigeminal primitiva. Neurocirurgia (Santiago) 11: 1–5, 1965
Polis, Z., J. Brzezinski, M. Chodak-Gajewicz: Giant intracranial aneurysm. Case report. J. Neurosurg. 39: 408–411, 1973
Pool, J. L.: Cerebral vasospasm. New Engl. J. Med. 259: 1259–1264, 1958
Pool, J. L.: Aneurysms of the anterior communicating artery. Bifrontal craniotomy and routine use of temporary clips. J. Neurosurg. 18: 98–111, 1961
Pool, J. L.: Timing and techniques in the intracranial surgery of ruptured aneurysms of the anterior communicating artery. J. Neurosurg. 19: 378–388, 1962
Pool, J. L.: A new dimension in aneurysm surgery. Columbia Univ. Phys. Surg. Q. 10: 18–20, 1965a
Pool, J. L.: Treatment of intracranial aneurysms during pregnancy. J. Amer. med. Ass. 192: 209–214, 1965b
Pool, J. L.: Surgery of anterior cerebral and anterior communicating aneurysms. In Logue, V., C. Rob, R. Smith: Operative Surgery, 2nd Ed., Vol. XIV: Neurosurgery, Lippincott, Philadelphia 1971 (pp. 159–166)
Pool, J. L.: Bifrontal craniotomy for anterior communicating artery aneurysms. J. Neurosurg. 36: 212–220, 1972
Pool, J. L.: Muslin gauze in intracranial vascular surgery. Technical note. J. Neurosurg. 44: 127–128, 1976
Pool, J. L., R. P. Colton: The dissecting microscope for intracranial vascular surgery. J. Neurosurg. 25: 315–318, 1966
Pool, J. L., D. G. Potts: Aneurysms and Arteriovenous Anomalies of the Brain. Diagnosis and Treatment. Harper & Row, New York 1965
Pool, J. L., S. Jacobson, T. A. Fletcher: Cerebral vasospasm – clinical and experimental evidence. J. Amer. med. Ass. 167: 1599–1601, 1958
Poppen, J. L.: An Atlas of Neurosurgical Techniques. Saunders, Philadelphia 1960
Poppen, J. L.: Operative treatment for aneurysms of the anterior communicating artery. Clin. Neurosurg. 11: 8–13, 1964
Poppen, J. L., C. Fager: Multiple intracranial aneurysms. J. Neurosurg. 16: 581–589, 1959
Poppen, J. L., C. Fager: Intracranial aneurysms. Results of surgical treatment. J. Neurosurg. 17: 283–296, 1960
Poppen, J. L., C. A. Fager: Anterior communicating aneurysms: improved surgical mortality and morbidity. Lahey Clin. Found. Bull. 19: 1–7, 1970
Porter, R. J., E. F. Eyster: Aneurysm in the anterior inferior cerebellar artery at the internal acustic meatus: report of a case. Surg. Neurol. 1: 27–28, 1973
Posner, M. A., F. L. Rodkey, R. E. Tobey: Nitroprusside induced cyanide poisoning. Antidotal effect of hydroxocobalamin. Anesthesiology 44: 330, 1976
Post, K. D., E. S. Flamm, A. Goodgold, J. Ransohoff: Ruptured intracranial aneurysms: Case morbidity and mortality. J. Neurosurg. 46: 296–303, 1977
Potter, J. M.: Carotid-Cavernous Fistula. Five cases with spontaneous recovery. Brit. med. J. II: 786–788, 1954
Pouyanne, H., A. Anayan, J. Guerin, V. Riemens: Les anévrysmes sacculaires multiples du système carotidien supra clinoidien. Étude anatomo-clinique et thérapeutique. Neuro-chirurgie 19, Suppl. 1, 1973
Pouyanne, H., P. Leman, M. Got, A. Gouaze: Anévrysme artériel traumatique de la méningée moyenne gauche. Neuro-chirurgie 5: 311–315, 1959
Preisker, R.: Über das gemeinsame Vorkommen von angeborenen (Forbusschen) Aneurysmen und Anomalien im Bereich des basalen Gefäßringes. Acta neurochir. (Wien) 12: 67–79, 1964
Pressman, B. D., G. E. Gilbert, D. O. Davis: Computerized transverse tomography of vascular lesions of the brain. Part II. Aneurysms. Amer. J. Roentgenol. 124: 215–219, 1975

Pribram, H. F. W., J. D. Hudson, R. J. Joynt: Posterior fossa aneurysms presenting as mass lesions. Amer. J. Roentgenol. 105: 334–340, 1969
Prolo, D. J., K. P. Burres, J. W. Hanberry: Balloon occlusion of carotid-cavernous fistula: Introduction of a new catheter. Surg. Neurol. 7: 209–214, 1977
Pudenz, R. H.: The use of tantalum clips for hemostasis in neurosurgery. Surgery 12: 791–797, 1942
Pudenz, R. H., C. H. Schelden: The lucite calvarium – A method for direct observation of the brain. J. Neurosurg. 3: 487–505, 1946
Punt, J.: Some observations on aneurysms of the proximal internal carotid artery. J. Neurosurg. 51: 151–154, 1979
Raimondi, A. J.: Intracranial false aneurysms. Neurochirurgia (Stuttg.) 11: 219–233, 1968
Raimondi, A. J., H. Torres: Acute hydrocephalus as complication of subarachnoid hemorrhage. Surg. Neurol. 1: 23–26, 1973
Raimondi, A. J., D. Yashon, C. Reyes, L. Yarzagaray: Intracranial false aneurysms. Neurochirurgia (Stuttg.) 11: 219–233, 1968
Ralston, B., T. Rasmussen, T. Kennedy: Occlusion of the middle cerebral artery under normotension, and anaemically induced and chemically induced hypotension. J. Neurosurg. 12: 26–33, 1955
Ramamurthi, B.: Incidence of intracranial aneurysms in India. J. Neurosurg. 30: 154–157, 1969
Ramella, G., M. Rosa: Angiotomographic study of the normal cerebral circulation. Neuroradiology 8: 15–23, 1974
Ramella, G., M. Rosa, G. F. Rossi: Angio-tomography for the study of endocranial aneurysms. Acta neurochir. (Wien) 21: 285–293, 1969
Rana, R. S.: Surgical management of internal carotid aneurysms. Neurol. India 13: 59–61, 1965
Rand, R. W.: Microneurosurgery instrumentation. In Rand, R. W.: Microneurosurgery. Mosby, St. Louis 1969a (pp. 21–37)
Rand, R. W.: Microneurosurgery. Mosby, St. Louis 1969b (pp. 198–209)
Rand, R. W., P. J. Jannetta: Micro-neurosurgery for aneurysms of the vertebral-basilar artery system. J. Neurosurg. 27: 330–335, 1967
Rand, R. W., P. J. Jannetta: Microneurosurgery: application of the binocular surgical microscope in brain tumors, intracranial aneurysms, spinal cord disease, and nerve reconstruction. Clin. Neurosurg. 15: 319–342, 1968
Rand, R. W., T. L. Kurze: Facial nerve preservation by posterior fossa transmeatal microdissection in total removal of acoustic tumors. J. Neurol. Neurosurg. Psychiat. 28: 311–316, 1965
Ransohoff, J., A. Goodgold, M. V. Benjamin: Preoperative management of patients with ruptured intracranial aneurysms. J. Neurosurg. 36: 525–530, 1972
Ransohoff, J., H. H. Guy, V. D. B. Mazzia: Deliberate hypotension in surgery of cerebral aneurysms and correlative animal studies. N.Y.J. Med. 69: 913–918, 1969
Raphael, H. A., P. E. Bernatz, J. A. Spitell, F. H. Ellis: Cervical carotid aneurysms: treatment by excision and restoration of arterial continuity. Amer. J. Surg. 105: 771–778, 1963
Raskind, R.: An intracranial arterial aneurysm associated with a recurrent meningioma. J. Neurosurg. 23: 622–625, 1965
Rath, S., K. V. Mathai, J. Chandy: Persistent trigeminal artery. Arch. Neurol. (Chic.) 19: 121–122, 1968
Rausch, F., W. Schiefer: Indirekte Röntgen-Kineatographie der Hirngefäße. Fortschr. Röntgenstr. 84: 88–99, 1956
Ravon, R., J. J. Bouquier, J. P. Dupuy, J. Bokor, P. Veiss, J. Vidal, A. Dany: Un cas d'anévrysme géant intra-pétreux et intracaverneux de la carotide interne chez l'enfant. Neuro-chirurgie 22: 621–626, 1976
Raynor, R. B., G. Ross: Arteriography and vasospasm. The effects of intracarotid contrast media on vasospasm. J. Neurosurg. 17: 1055–1061, 1960
Reichel, J., H. Intrau: Traumatisches intrakranielles Aneurysma. Zbl. Neurochir. 36: 199–202, 1975
Reigh, E. E., L. J. Lemman: Cerebral aneurysms with other intracranial pathology. J. Neurosurg. 17: 469–476, 1960
Repela, C. E., H. D. Green: Autoregulation of canine cerebral blood flow. Circulat. Res. 15 (Suppl.) 205–212, 1964
Rhonheimer, Ch.: Zur Symptomatologie der sellären Aneurysmen. Klin. Mbl. Augenheilk. 134: 1–34, 1959

Richardson, A. E.: The natural history of patients with intracranial aneurysms after rupture. Progr. Brain Res. 30: 269–273, 1968

Richardson, A. E., J. A. Jane, P. M. Payne: The prediction of morbidity and mortality in anterior communicating aneurysms treated by proximal anterior cerebral ligation. J. Neurosurg. 25: 280–383, 1966

Richardson, A. E., H. A. Jane, D. Yashon: Prognostic factors in the untreated course of posterior communicating aneurysms. Arch. Neurol. (Chic.) 14: 172–175, 1966

Richardson, J. C., H. H. Hyland: Intracranial aneurysms. A clinical and pathological study of subarachnoid and intracerebral hemorrhage caused by berry aneurysms. Medicine (Baltimore) 20: 1–83, 1941

Richardson, J. T. E.: Arterial spasm and recovery from subarachnoid haemorrhage. J. Neurol. Neurosurg. Psychiat. 39: 1134–1136, 1976

Riggs, H., C. Rupp: Miliary aneurysms; relation of anomalies of the circle of Willis to formation of aneurysms. Arch. Neurol. Psychiat. (Chic.) 49: 615–616, 1943

Riggs, H. E., C. Rupp: The pathologic anatomy of ruptured cerebral aneurysms. Atti I Congr. Int. Istopat. Sist. Nerv. Roma 3: 206, 1956

Riggs, H. E., C. Rupp: Variation in form of circle of Willis. Arch. Neurol. (Chic.) 8: 8–14, 1963

Risberg, J., D. Ancri, D. H. Ingvar: Correlation between cerebral blood volume and cerebral blood flow in the cat. Exp. Brain Res. 8: 321–326, 1969

Risberg, J., Z. Ali, E. M. Wilcox, E. L. Wells, J. Halsey: Regional cerebral blood flow by ^{133}Xenon inhalation. Stroke 6: 142–148, 1975

Rischbieth, R. H. C., J. W. D. Bull: The significance of enlargement of the superior orbital (sphenoidal) fissure. Brit. J. Radiol. 31: 125–135, 1958

Riser, M., G. Lazorthes, J. Géraud, H. Anduze: Deux cas de syndrome de Garcin par anévrysme carotidien intra-caverneux. Rev. neurol. 89: 373–374, 1953

Rizzoli, J.: Personal communication on the subject: A resident on the service of W. Dandy, exploring the Circle of Willis for ruptured aneurysms prior to the use of angiography.

Roach, M. R., C. G. Drake: Ruptured cerebral aneurysms caused by microorganisms. New Engl. J. Med. 273: 240–244, 1965

Robertson, E. G.: Cerebral lesions due to intracranial aneurysms. Brain 72: 150–185, 1949

Robin, P. E.: A case of upwardly situated jugular bulb in left middle ear. J. Laryng. 86: 1241–1245, 1972

Robinson, J. L., A. Roberts: Operative treatment of aneurysms and Coanda effect: a working hypothesis. J. Neurol. Neurosurg. Psychiat. 35: 804–809, 1972

Robinson, J. L., Ch. S. Hall, C. B. Sedzimir: Arteriovenous malformations, aneurysms and pregnancy. J. Neurosurg. 41: 63–69, 1974

Robinson, R. G.: Ruptured aneurysms of the middle cerebral artery. J. Neurosurg. 35: 25–33, 1971

Robinson, A. G., R. W. Butcher, E. W. Sutherland: Cyclic AMP. Academic Press, New York 1971

Rocca, P., G. Rosadini: Tecnica di angio-stratigrafica cerebrale. G. Psichiat. Neuropat. 88: 371–384, 1960

Rocca, P., G. Rosadini: Cerebral angiostratigraphy, first practical results. Radiology 77: 223–227, 1963a

Rocca, P., G. Rosadini: Simultane mehrschichtige Tomographie und ihre Anwendung in der Gehirnangiographie. Acta radiol. Diagn. 1: 385–388, 1963b

Rodbard, S.: Physical forces and the vascular lining. Ann. intern. Med. 50: 1339–1350, 1959

Rogers, L.: Ligature of arteries, with particular reference to carotid occlusion and the circle of Willis. Brit. J. Surg. 35: 43–50, 1947

Romodanov, A. P., V. I. Shcheglov: Endovascular method of excluding from the circulation saccular cerebral arterial aneurysms. Acta neurochir. (Wien), Suppl. 28: 312–315, 1979

Romodanov, A. P., V. I. Shcheglov: Intravascular occlusion of saccular aneurysms of the cerebral arteries by means of a detachable balloon catheter. In: Advances and Technical Standards in Neurosurgery. Vol. 9, Springer Wien, New York 1982

Romodanov, A. P., Yu. A. Zozulia, V. I. Shcheglov: Intravascular operations with balloon catheter in cerebrovascular disease and brain tumors. In: Mat. konf. posv. 100-letiu rozhd. L. M. Puuseppa. Tartu 1975, (pp. 120–123) (Rus.)

Romodanov, A. P., Yu. A. Zozulia, V. I. Shcheglov: Balloon catheter occlusion of the feeding vessels of arteriovenous malformations of the brain. Zbl. Neurochir. 40: 21–28, 1979

Romodanov, S. A., V. I. Shcheglov, V. V. Khoziainov: Cineangiography in intracranial aneurysms and carotid-cavernous fistulas. In: Klinika i khirurgicheskoie lechenie sosudistoi patologii mozga pri zabolevaniakh nervnoi sistemy, Leningrad 1979 (pp. 109–110) (Rus.)

Romy, M., A. Werner, E. Wildi: Sur la fréquence des anévrysmes intracrâniens et leur rupture. Neuro-chirurgie 19: 611–626, 1973

Rosa, M.: Value of angio-tomography in planning operative treatment of internal carotid artery aneurysms. Neuroradiology 3: 82–91, 1971

Rosadini, G., P. Rocca: Simultane mehrschichtige Tomographie und ihre Anwendung in der Gehirnangiographie. Acta radiol. Diagn. 1: 385–388, 1963

Ross, R. T.: Multiple and familial intracranial vascular lesions. Canad. med. Ass. J. 81: 477–479, 1959

Rosselet, E., E. Zander, P. Secretan: Migraine hémianopsique symptomatique d'un anévrisme occipital. Confin. neurol. (Basel) 21: 197–202, 1961

Rothenberg, S. F., E. J. Penka, L. W. Conway: Angiotractic surgery. Preliminary studies. J. Neurosurg. 19: 877–883, 1962

Rotter, W., M. J. Wellmer, G. Hinrichs, W. Müller: Zur Orthologie und Pathologie der Polsterarterien (sog. Verzweigungs- und Spornpolster) des Gehirns. Beitr. path. Anat. 115: 253–294, 1955

Roudaud, M., A. Gouaze, P. Vigneron, G. Jezegabee: Paralysies oculo-motrices et atteinte du trijumeau par volumineux anévrysme carotidien intracaverneux. Rev. neurol. 110: 155–158, 1964

Rubinstein, M. K., N. H. Cohen: Ehlers-Danlos syndrome associated with multiple intracranial aneurysms. Neurology (Minneap.) 14: 125–132, 1964

Rumbaugh, C. L., R. T. Bergeron, M. Tallala, Th. Kurze: Traumatic aneurysms of the cortical cerebral arteries. Radiology 96: 49–54, 1970

Russel, C. K.: Spontaneous subarachnoid hemorrhage following rupture of congenital aneurysm of the anterior communicating artery of the circle of Willis. Report of a case in which the aneurysm was excised. Trans. Amer. neurol. Ass. 65: 130–134, 1939

Russell, D. S.: Spontaneous intracranial haemorrhage. Proc. roy. Soc. Med. 47: 689–693, 1954

Russell, R. W. R.: Observations on intracerebral aneurysms. Brain 86: 425–442, 1963

Russell, W. W., T. H. Newton: Aneurysm of the vein of Galen: case report and review of the literature. Amer. J. Roentgenol. 92: 756–760, 1964

Sachs Jr., E.: The fate of muscle and cotton wrapped about intracranial carotid arteries and aneurysms. A laboratory and clinicopathologic study. Acta neurochir. (Wien) 26: 121–137, 1972

Sachs, M.: Les anévrysmes de l'artère sylvienne à propos de 75 observations. Ann. Chir. 15–18: 998–1019, 1966

Sachs, M., C. Cabezas, T. Posada, M. David: Recherches anatomiques sur les anévrysmes artériels intracraniens. J. neurol. Sci. 6: 83–103, 1968

Sadik, A. R., G. N. Budzilovich, K. Shulman: Giant aneurysm of middle cerebral artery. A case report. J. Neurosurg. 22: 177–181, 1965

Sahs, A. L.: Observations on the pathology of saccular aneurysms. J. Neurosurg. 24: 792–806, 1966

Sahs, A. L., G. E. Perret, H. B. Locksley, H. Nishioka: Intracranial Aneurysms and Subarachnoid Haemorrhage. A Cooperative Study. Lippincott, Philadelphia 1969

Sahs, A. L., G. Perret, H. B. Locksley, H. Nishioka, F. M. Skultety: Preliminary remarks on subarachnoid hemorrhage. J. Neurosurg. 24: 782–788, 1966

Saito, I., A. Tamura, K. Sano: Follow-up results of cases with anterior communicating aneurysms operated on in the acute stage, with special reference to the time course of morbidity of the operation. (Jpn.) Neurol. Med. Chir. 1911/3: 233–241, 1977

Sakai, N., K. Sakata, H. Yamada, M. Yamamoto, T. Aiba, F.

Takeda: Familial occurrence of intracranial aneurysms. Surg. Neurol. 2: 25–29, 1974
Salamon, G.: Atlas of the Arteries of the Brain. Sandoz, Basel 1971
Salazar, J. L.: Surgical treatment of asymptomatic and incidental intracranial aneurysms. J. Neurosurg. 53: 20–21, 1980
Saltzman, G. F.: Patent primitive trigeminal artery studies by cerebral angiography. Acta radiol. (Stockh.) 51: 329–334, 1959a
Saltzman, G. F.: Infundibular widening of the posterior communicating artery. Studies by carotid angiography. Acta radiol. (Stockh.) 51: 415–421, 1959b
Salvolini, U., A. Montesi: L'angio-tomografia cerebrale nello studi degli aneurismi intracraniali. Radiol. med. (Torino) 59: 217–222, 1973
Sano, K.: Surgery of intracranial aneurysms. (Jpn.) Brain Nerve (Tokyo) 23: 1252–1264, 1971
Sano, K., I. Saito: Follow-up results of microsurgery of intracranial aneurysms. (Jpn.) Brain Nerve (Tokyo) 29/9: 977–985, 1977
Sano, K., I. Saito: Timing and indication of surgery for ruptured intracranial aneurysms with regards to cerebral vasospasm. Acta neurochir. (Wien) 41: 49–60, 1978
Sano, K., M. Jimbo, I. Saito: Vertebro-basilar aneurysms with special reference to the transpharyngeal transclival approach to the basilar artery aneurysm. Brain Nerve (Tokyo) 18: 1197–1203, 1966
Sarasabharati, R.: An analysis of 213 intracranial aneurysms verified by autopsy. Amer. J. Path. 59: 473–481, 1970
Sartor, K.: Angiotomographische Detaildiagnostik bei Aneurysmen an der Hirnbasis. Fortschr. Röntgenstr. 122: 506–510, 1975
Sarwar, M.: Growing intracranial aneurysms. Radiology 120: 603–608, 1976
Sarwar, M., S. Banitzky, M. M. Schechter: Tumorous aneurysms. Neuroradiology 12: 79–97, 1976
Sato, O., H. Kamitani: Giant aneurysms of the middle cerebral artery: angiographic analysis of blood flow. Surg. Neurol. 4: 27–31, 1975
Sato, S., J. Suzuki: Anatomical mapping of the cerebral nervi vasorum in the human brain. J. Neurosurg. 43: 559–568, 1975
Sato, T., S. Sato, J. Suzuki: Ultrastructural changes of cerebral nervi vasorum after cervical sympathetic ganglionectomy. Tenth International Congress of Angiology. Tokyo, Sept. 3, 1976
Schaerer, J. P.: A case of carotid-basilar anastomosis with multiple associated cerebrovascular anomalies. J. Neurosurg. 12: 62–65, 1955
Scharfetter, F., H. J. Födisch, G. Menardi, K. Twerdy: Falsches Aneurysma der Art. gyri angularis durch Gefäßverletzung bei einer Ventrikelpunktion. Acta neurochir. (Wien) 33: 123–132, 1976
Schechter, D. C.: Cervical carotid aneurysms. N. Y. St. J. Med. 79: 892–901, 1979
Schechter, M. M., M. Elkin: Layering effect in cerebral angiography. Acta radiol. Diagn. 1: 427–435, 1963
Schiefer, W.: Zwischenfälle bei der Hirngefäßdarstellung. In Gänshirt, H.: Der Hirnkreislauf. Thieme, Stuttgart 1972 (pp. 781–796)
Schiefer, W., E. Kazner: Klinische Echo-Enzephalographie. Springer, Berlin 1967
Schiefer, W., F. Marguth: Intraselläre Aneurysmen. Acta neurochir. (Wien) 4: 344–354, 1956
Schiefer, W., W. Walter: Die Persistenz embryonaler Gefäße als Ursache von Blutungen des Hirns und seiner Häute. Acta neurochir. (Wien) 7: 53–65, 1959
Schlesinger, B.: The Upper Brain Stem in the Human, Its Nuclear Configuration and Vascular Supply. Springer, Berlin 1976
Schmid, K. O.: Zur Morphologie der posttraumatischen Anosmie und des intracerebralen posttraumatischen Aneurysmas. Fallbericht einer traumatischen Spätkomplexie. Virchows Arch. path. Anat. 334: 67–68, 1961
Schmiedek, P., J. Steinhoff, O. Gratzl, U. Steude, R. Enzenbach: rCBF measurements in patients treated for cerebral ischemia by extra-intracranial vascular anastomosis. Europ. Neurol. 6: 364–368, 1971–1972
Schmiedek, P., et al.: Selection of patients for extra-intracranial arterial bypass surgery based on rCBF measurements. J. Neurosurg. 44: 303–312, 1976

Schneck, St. A.: On the relationship between ruptured intracranial aneurysm and cerebral infarction. Neurology (Minneap.) 14: 691–702, 1964
Schneck, St. A., I. I. Kricheff: Intracranial aneurysm rupture, vasospasm, and infarction. Arch. Neurol. (Chic.) 11: 668–680, 1964
Schnider, B. I., N. J. Cotsonas: Embolic mycotic aneurysms, a complication of bacterial endocarditis. Amer. J. Med. 16: 246–255, 1954
Schreiber, D., W. Jänisch, R. Peschel: Rupturierte Hirnbasisaneurysmen, Zbl. allg. Pathol. 121: 11–21, 1977
Schottmüller, H.: Beitrag zur Artuntersuchung der pathogenen Streptokokken. Münch. med. Wschr. 57: 617–620, 1908
Schugk, P., M. Valpalahti, H. Troupp: Lokalisierte intrakranielle Gefäßschädigungen bei Schädel-Hirn-Trauma. Acta neurochir. (Wien) 22: 327–337, 1970
Schulze, A.: Seltene Verlaufsformen epiduraler Hämatome. Zbl. Neurochir. 17: 40–47, 1957
Schunk, H.: Spontaneous thrombosis of intracranial aneurysms. Amer. J. Roentgenol. 91: 1327–1338, 1964
Schwartz, H. G.: Arterial aneurysm of the posterior fossa. J. Neurosurg. 5: 312–316, 1948
Schwartz, M. J., I. D. Baronofsky: Ruptured intracranial aneurysm associated with coarctation of the aorta: a report of a patient treated by hypothermia and surgical repair of the coarctation. Amer. J. Cardiol. 6: 982–988, 1960
Scott, H. S.: Carotid basilar anastomosis-persistent hypoglossal artery. Brit. J. Radiol. 36: 847–851, 1963
Scott, M.: Ligation of an anterior cerebral artery for aneurysms of the anterior communicating artery complex. J. Neurosurg. 38: 481–487, 1973
Scott, R. M., H. Th. Ballantine: Spontaneous thrombosis in a giant middle cerebral artery aneurysm. J. Neurosurg. 37: 361–363, 1972
Scotti, G., A. Gattoni: Pneumoencephalographic presentation of a saccular aneurysm at the bifurcation of the basilar artery. Neuroradiology 7: 177–179, 1974
Scotti, G., D. Melançon, R. Ethier, K. Terbrugge: Diagnosis of subarachnoid haemorrhage by computerised tomography in intracranial aneurysms. In Du Boulay, G. H., J. F. Moseley: Computerised Axial Tomography in Clinical Practice. Springer, Berlin 1977 (pp. 255–260)
Scoville, W. B.: Miniature torsion bar spring aneurysm clip. Technical suggestion. J. Neurosurg. 25: 97, 1966
Sedzimir, C. B.: An angiographic test of collateral circulation through the anterior segment of the circle of Willis. J. Neurol. Neurosurg. Psychiat. 22: 64–88, 1959
Sedzimir, C. B., J. Robinson: Intracranial hemorrhage in children and adolescents. J. Neurosurg. 38: 269–281, 1973
Sedzimir, C. B., J. V. Occleshaw, P. H. Buxton: False cerebral aneurysm. Case report. J. Neurosurg. 29: 636–639, 1968
Seftel, D. M., H. Kolson, B. S. Gordon: Ruptured intracranial carotid artery aneurysm with fatal epistaxis. Arch. Otolaryng. 70: 62–70, 1959
Segal, H., R. L. Laurin: Giant serpentine aneurysm. J. Neurosurg. 46: 115–122, 1977
Selker, R. G., S. K. Wolfson Jr., J. C. Maroon, F. M. Steichen: Preferential cerebral hypothermia with elective cardiac arrest: resection of "giant" aneurysms. Surg. Neurol. 6: 173–179, 1976
Sellery, G. R., R. R. Aitken, C. G. Drake: Anesthesia for intracranial aneurysms with hypotension and spontaneous respiration. Canad. Anaesth. Soc. J. 20: 468–478, 1973
Seltzer, J., E. F. Hurteau: Bilateral symmetrical aneurysms of internal carotid artery within cavernous sinus: case report. J. Neurosurg. 14: 448–451, 1957
Selverstone, B.: Aneurysms at middle cerebral "trifurcation": treatment with adherent plastics. J. Neurosurg. 19: 884–886, 1962
Selverstone, B.: Treatment of intracranial aneurysms with adherent plastics. Clin. Neurosurg. 9: 201–213, 1963
Selverstone, B., N. Ronis: Coating and reinforcement of intracranial aneurysms with synthetic resins. Bull. Tufts-New Engl. med. Cent. 4: 8–12, 1958
Selverstone, B., J. C. White: A new technique for gradual occlusion of the carotid artery. Arch. Neurol. Psychiat. (Chic.) 66: 246, 1951

Sengupta, R. P.: Anatomical variations in the origin of the posterior cerebral artery demonstrated by carotid angiography and their significance in the direct surgical treatment of posterior communicating aneurysms. Neuro-chirurgie 18: 33–42, 1975

Sengupta, R. P., J. S. P. Chui, H. Brierley: Quality of survival following direct surgery for anterior communicating artery aneurysms. J. Neurosurg. 43: 58–64, 1975

Sengupta, R. P., S. C. So, F. J. Villarejo-Ortega: Use of epsilon-aminocaproic acid (EACA) in the preoperative management of ruptured intracranial aneurysms. J. Neurosurg. 44: 479–484, 1976

Sengupta, R. P., L. P. Lassman, A. A. Moraes, et al.: Treatment of internal carotid bifurcation aneurysms by direct surgery. J. Neurosurg. 43: 343–351, 1975

Serbinenko, F. A.: Catheterization and occlusion of cerebral major vessels and prospects for the development of vascular neurosurgery. Vop. Neirokhir. 35: 17–27, 1971 (Rus.)

Serbinenko, F. A.: Reconstruction of cavernous part of carotid artery in case of carotid-cavernous fistulae. Vop. Neirokhir. 36: 3–9, 1972 (Rus.)

Serbinenko, F. A.: Occlusion by ballooning of saccular aneurysms of the cerebral arteries. Vop. Neirokhir. 38: 8–15, 1974a (Rus.)

Serbinenko, F. A.: Balloon catheterization and occlusion of major cerebral vessels. J. Neurosurg. 41: 125–145, 1974b

Shcheglov, V. I.: Endovascular interventions in neurosurgical pathology. In: II Sjezd Neirokhirurgov SSSR, Moscow 1976 (pp. 558–559) (Rus.)

Shcheglov, V. I.: Current possibilities of intravascular operations by means of the detachable balloon catheter in the treatment of some vascular brain diseases. In: Klinika i khirurgicheskoie lechenie sosudistoi patologii mozga pri zabolevaniakh nervnoi sistemy, Leningrad 1979 (pp. 19–21) (Rus.)

Shelden, C. H., R. H. Pudenz, J. S. Restarski: A new position for frontal craniotomy. J. Neurosurg. 2: 546–550, 1945

Shelden, C. H., R. H. Pudenz, L. E. Brannon: Intracranial aneurysms. Arch. Surg. 61: 294–302, 1950

Shenkin, H. A., B. Goluboff, H. Haft: Use of mannitol for the reduction of intracranial pressure in intracranial surgery. J. Neurosurg. 19: 897–901, 1962

Shenkin, H. A., H. Pollack, F. Somach, S. Bijaisoradata: Value of routine urography during cerebral angiography. J. Amer. med. Ass. 187: 207–211, 1964

Shephard, R. H.: Ruptured cerebral aneurysms: early and late prognosis with surgical treatment. J. Neurosurg. 59: 6–15, 1983

Shepherd, A. P., C. C. Mao, E. D. Jacobson, et al.: The role of cyclic AMP in mesenteric vasodilatation. Microvasc. Res. 6: 332–341, 1973

Shibuya, S., S. Igarashi, T. Amo, H. Sato, T. Fukumitsu: Mycotic aneurysms of the internal carotid artery. J. Neurosurg. 44: 105–108, 1976

Shinebourne, E., R. White: Cyclic AMP and calcium uptake of the sarcoplasmic reticulum in relation to increased rate of relaxation under the influence of catecholamines. Cardiovasc. Res. 4: 194–200, 1970

Shintani, A., N. T. Zervas: Consequence of ligation of the vertebral artery. J. Neurol. 36: 447–450, 1972

Shiobara, R., S. Toya, S. Mikouchi, Z. Izumi: Surgery of posterior communicating artery that enlarge after common carotid ligation. J. Neurosurg. 52: 116–120, 1980

Shorstein, J.: Carotid ligation in saccular intracranial aneurysms. Brit. J. Surg. 28: 50, 1940

Shucart, W. A., S. M. Wolpert: Intracranial arterial aneurysms in childhood. Amer. J. Dis. Child. 127: 288–293, 1974

Shucart, W. A., S. K. Hussain, P. R. Cooper: Epsilon-aminocaproid acid and recurrent subarachnoid hemorrhage. J. Neurosurg. 53: 28:31, 1980

Shulman, K., B. F. Martin, N. Popoff, J. Ransohoff: Recognition and treatment of hydrocephalus following spontaneous subarachnoid hemorrhage. J. Neurosurg. 20: 1040–1047, 1963

Siegel, P., P. P. Moraca, J. R. Green: Sodium nitroprusside in the surgical treatment of cerebral aneurysms and arteriovenous malformations. Brit. J. Anaesth. 43: 790–795, 1971

Silcox, E., R. A. Updegrove: Extracranial aneurysm of the internal carotid artery. Arch. Otolaryng. 69: 329–333, 1959

Simeone, F. A., S. J. Peerless: Prolonged cerebral vasospasm without subarachnoid hemorrhage. In Smith, R. R., J. T. Robertson: Subarachnoid Hemorrhage and Cerebrovascular Spasm. Thomas, Springfield/Ill. 1975 (pp. 206–223)

Simeone, F. A., K. G. Ryan, J. R. Cotter: Prolonged experimental cerebral vasospasm. J. Neurosurg. 29: 357–366, 1968

Simmon, K. C., M. R. Sage, P. L. Reilly: CT of intracerebral hemorrhage due to mycotic aneurysms. Radiology 19: 215–217, 1980

Simpson, D. S., R. M. Hodosh, W. K. Clark: Surgical treatment of asymptomatic aneurysms. Presented at the American Assoc. of Neurolog. Surgeons, San Francisco, April 4–8, 1976

Skultety, F. M., H. Nishioka: Report on the Cooperative Study of intracranial aneurysms and subarachnoid hemorrhage. Section VIII, Part 2. The results of intracranial surgery in the treatment of aneurysms. J. Neurosurg. 25: 683–704, 1966

Skultety, F. M., H. Nishioka: The results of intracranial surgery in the treatment of aneurysms. In Sahs, A. L., et al.: Intracranial Aneurysms and Subarachnoid Hemorrhage. A Cooperative Study. Lippincott, Philadelphia 1969 (pp. 173–193)

Slosberg, P.: Hypotensive therapy in acute intracranial bleeding. J. Mt Sinai Hosp. 23: 825–831, 1956

Slosberg, P. S.: Treatment of ruptured aneurysms with induced hypotension. In Fields, W. S., A. L. Sahs: Intracranial Aneurysms and Subarachnoid Hemorrhage. Thomas, Springfield/Ill. 1965 (pp. 221–233)

Slosberg, P.: Treatment and prevention of stroke. Subarachnoid hemorrhage due to ruptured intracranial aneurysms. N. Y. St. J. Med. 73: 679, 1973

Slosberg, P. S.: Nonoperative management of ruptured intracranial aneurysms. Clin. Neurosurg. 21: 90–99, 1974

Smaltino, F., F.-P. Bernini, R. Elefante, G. Fucci: Les anévrysmes du système vertébro-basilaire. Ann. Radiol. 15: 725–731, 1972

Smith, A. L., et al.: Effect of arterial CO_2 tension on cerebral blood flow, mean transit time and vascular volume. J. appl. Physiol. 31: 701–707, 1971

Smith, B.: Cerebral pathology in subarachnoid hemorrhage. J. Neurol. Neurosurg. Psychiat. 26: 535–539, 1963

Smith, D. R., et al.: Cerebral false aneurysm formation in closed head trauma. J. Neurosurg. 32: 357–359, 1970

Smith, J. T., J. A. Goree, J. P. Jimenez, C. C. Harris: Cerebral angioautotomography. Amer. J. Roentgenol. 112: 315–323, 1971

Smith, K. R., J. A. Bardenheimer III.: Aneurysm of the pericallosal artery caused by closed cranial trauma. Case report. J. Neurosurg. 29: 551–554, 1968

Snyckers, F. D., C. G. Drake: Aneurysms of the distal anterior cerebral artery. A report of 24 verified cases. S. Afr. med. J. 47: 1787–1791, 1973

Somach, F. M., H. A. Shenkin: Angiographic end-results of carotid ligation in the treatment of carotid aneurysm. J. Neurosurg. 24: 966–974, 1966

Someda, K., N. Yasui, Y. Moriwaki, Y. Kawamura, H. Matsumura: Extravasation of contrast material into subdural space from internal carotid aneurysm during angiography. J. Neurosurg. 42: 473–477, 1975

Somlyo, A. P., A. V. Somlyo, V. Smiesko: Cyclic AMP and vascular smooth muscle. Advanc. Cyclic Nucleotide Res. 1: 175–194, 1972

Sonntag, V. K. H., R. H. Yuan, B. M. Stein: Giant intracranial aneurysms. A review of 13 cases. Surg. Neurol. 8: 81–84, 1977

Sonobe, M., A. Hori, J. Suzuki: Effect of spasmogenic substances on cerebral arteries. Tenth International Congress of Angiology. Tokyo, Aug. 31, 1976

Sosman, M. C., E. C. Vogt: Aneurysms of the internal carotid artery and the circle of Willis, from a roentgenological viewpoint. Amer. J. Roentgenol. 15: 122–134, 1926

Sparacio, R. R., T. H. Lin, A. W. Cook: Methylprednisolone sodium succinate in acute craniocerebral trauma. Surg. Gynec. Obstet. 121: 513–516, 1965

Spatz, E. L., J. W. D. Bull: Vertebral arteriography in the study of subarachnoid hemorrhage. J. Neurosurg. 14: 543–547, 1957

Speakman, T. J., J. L. Barlass: The bifrontal approach to aneurysms of the anterior communicating artery. Canad. J. Surg. 6: 237–243, 1963

Spencer, W. G., V. Horsley: Report on the control of haemorrhage from the middle cerebral artery and its branches by compression of the common carotid. Brit. med. J., March 2nd, 457, 1889

Sperling, M., G. Viehweger: Extrakranielle Aneurysmen der Arteria Carotis Interna und ihre Behandlung. Chirurg. 34: 369–373, 1963

Springer, Th., G. Fishbone, R. Shapiro: Persistent hypoglossal artery associated with superior cerebellar artery aneurysm. Case report. J. Neurosurg. 40: 397–399, 1974

Stallings, J. O., B. F. McCabe: Congenital middle ear aneurysm of internal carotid. Arch. Otolaryng. 90: 65–69, 1969

Steelman, H. F., G. J. Hayes, H. V. Rizzoli: Surgical treatment of saccular intracranial aneurysms. J. Neurosurg. 10: 564–576, 1953

Steffen, T. N.: Vascular anomalies of the middle ear. Laryngoscope (St. Louis) 78: 171–197, 1968

Stehbens, W. E.: Intracranial arterial aneurysms. Aust. Ann. Med. 3: 214–218, 1954a

Stehbens, W. E.: Medial defects of the cerebral arteries of man. J. Path. Bact. 78: 179–185, 1959b

Stehbens, W. E.: Hypertension and cerebral aneurysm. Med. J. Aust. 49: 8–10, 1962a

Stehbens, W. E.: Cerebral aneurysms and congenital abnormalities. Aust. Ann. Med. 11: 102–112, 1962b

Stehbens, W. E.: Histopathology of cerebral aneurysms. Arch. Neurol. (Chic.) 8: 272–285, 1963a

Stehbens, W. E.: Aneurysm and anatomical variation of the cerebral arteries. Arch. Path. 75: 45–64, 1963b

Stehbens, W. E.: Pathology of Cerebral Blood Vessels. Mosby, St. Louis 1972 (pp. 268–270)

Stehbens, W. E.: Ultrastructure of aneurysms. Arch. Neurol. (Chic.) 32: 798–807, 1975

Stengel, A., C. C. Wolferth: Mycotic (bacterial) aneurysms of intravascular origin. Arch. intern. Med. 31: 527–554, 1923

Stephens, R. B., D. I. Stilwell: Arteries and Veins of the Human Brain. Thomas, Springfield/Ill. 1969

Stepien, L.: Reinforcement of intracranial aneurysms with adherent plastics: Selverstone method. Progr. Brain Res. 30: 361–365, 1968

Stern, E., J. Brown, J. F. Alksne: The surgical challenge of carotid-cavernous fistula. The critical role of intracranial circulation. J. Neurosurg. 27: 298–308, 1967

Stern, W. E.: Carotid-cavernous fistula. In Vinken, P. J., G. W. Bruyn: Handbook of Clinical Neurology, Vol. XXIV. Elsevier-North Holland, Amsterdam–New York 1976 (pp. 399–439)

Steven, J. L.: Postoperative angiography in treatment of intracranial aneurysms. Acta radiol. Diagn. 5: 536–548, 1966

Stornelli, S. A., J. D. French: Subarachnoid hemorrhage – Factors in prognosis and management. J. Neurosurg. 21: 769–780, 1964

Strenger, L.: Neurological deficits following therapeutic collapse of intracavernous carotid aneurysms. J. Neurosurg. 25: 215–218, 1966

Stroobandt, G., J. M. Brucher, G. Cornellis, J. Vermonden: Traumatic carotido-cavernous fistula. Neuro-chirurgie 14: 855–868, 1968

Strully, K. J.: Successful removal of intraventricular aneurysm of the choroidal artery. J. Neurosurg. 12: 317–321, 1955

Stuntz, J. T., G. A. Ojemann, E. C. Alvord: Radiographic and histologic demonstration of an aneurysm developing on the infundibulum of the posterior communicating artery. J. Neurosurg. 33: 591–595, 1970

Sugai, M., M. Shoji: Pathogenesis of so-called congenital aneurysms of the brain. Acta path. jap. 18: 139–160, 1968

Sugar, O., M. Tinsley: Aneurysms of terminal portion of anterior cerebral artery. Arch. Neurol. Psychiat. (Chic.) 60: 81–85, 1948

Sugar, O., G. Tsuchiya: Plastic coating of intracranial aneurysms with "EDH-Adhesive." J. Neurosurg. 21: 114–117, 1964

Sugita, K., T. Hirota, R. Tsugane: Application of nasopharyngeal mirror for aneurysm operation – Technical note. J. Neurosurg. 43: 244–246, 1975

Sugita, K., R. Tsugane, N. Kageyama: Bipolar coagulator with automatic thermocontrol and some improvements of microsurgical instruments. In Handa, H.: Microneurosurgery. Univ. Park Press, Baltimore 1975 (p. 17)

Sugita, K., T. Hirota, I. Iguchi, T. Mizutani: Comparative study of the pressure of various aneurysm clips. J. Neurosurg. 44: 723–727, 1976

Sugita, K., S. Kobayashi, A. Shintani, N. Mutsuga: Microneurosurgery for aneurysms of the basilar artery. J. Neurosurg. 51: 615–620, 1979

Sundt, T. M.: Management of ischemic complications after subarachnoid hemorrhage. J. Neurosurg. 43: 418–425, 1975

Sundt, T. M., W. C. Grant, J. H. Carcia: Restoration of middle cerebral artery flow in experimental infarction. J. Neurosurg. 31: 311–322, 1969

Sundt, T. M., J. Szurszewski, F. W. Sharbrough: Physiological considerations important for the management of vasospasm. Surg. Neurol. 7: 259–268, 1977

Sundt, T. M., S. Kobayashi, N. C. Fode, J. P. Whisnant: Results and complications of surgical management of 809 intracranial aneurysms in 722 cases. J. Neurosurg. 56: 753–765, 1982

Sundt, T. M. Jr.: Clip-grafts for aneurysm and small vessel surgery. Part 4: Relative application to various aneurysms and repair of anterior communicating aneurysms using a right-angle clip holder. Technical note. J. Neurosurg. 37: 753–758, 1972

Sundt, T. M. Jr., F. Murphey: Clip-grafts for aneurysm and small vessel surgery. Part 3: Clinical experience in intracranial internal carotid artery aneurysm. J. Neurosurg. 31: 58–71, 1969

Sundt, T. M. Jr., B. M. Onofrio, J. Merideth: Treatment of cerebral vasospasm from subarachnoid hemorrhage with isoproterenol and lidocaine hydrochloride. J. Neurosurg. 38: 557–560, 1973

Sutton, D.: The vertebro-basilar system and its vascular lesions. Clin. Radiol. 22: 271–287, 1927

Sutton, D.: Anomalous carotid-basilar anastomosis. Brit. J. Radiol. 23: 617–619, 1950

Sutton, D., S. E. Trickey: Subarachnoid haemorrhage and total cerebral angiography. Clin. Radiol. 13: 297–303, 1962

Suwanwela, C., N. Suwanwela, S. Charuchinda, C. Hongsaprabhas: Intracranial mycotic aneurysms of extravascular origin. J. Neurosurg. 36: 552–559, 1972

Suzuki, J.: Direct intracranial operative approach to cerebral aneurysms. Brain Nerve (Tokyo) 18: 478–487, 1966

Suzuki, J.: Personal communication, 1975

Suzuki, J.: Direct surgery of intracranial aneurysms. Inst. Neurol. Madras, Proc. 6: 15–23, 1976

Suzuki, J.: Giant aneurysms. Results. In Pia, H. E., C. Langmaid, J. Zierski: Cerebral Aneurysms. Springer, Berlin 1979 (pp. 345–346)

Suzuki, J., S. Hori: Prediction of reattack following rupture of intracranial aneurysms. Neurol. Med. Chir. (Tokyo) 15 (Part 1): 35–39, 1975

Suzuki, J., M. Kowada: A method of temporal approach to chiasma region. Brain Nerve (Tokyo) 14: 165–167, 1962

Suzuki, J., Y. Miura: Surgery for multiple cerebral aneurysms. Shujutsu (Tokyo) 21: 67–76, 1967

Suzuki, J., T. Yoshimoto: Early operation for the ruptured intracranial aneurysm – Especially the cases operated within 48 hours after the last subarachnoid hemorrhage. Neurol. Surg. 4: 135–141, 1976

Suzuki, J., S. Hori, Y. Sakurai: Intracranial aneurysms in the neurosurgical clinics in Japan. J. Neurosurg. 35: 34–39, 1971

Suzuki, J., T. Iwabuchi, S. Hori: Cervical sympathectomy for cerebral vasospasm after aneurysm rupture. Neurol. Med. Chir. (Tokyo) 15 (Part 1): 41–50, 1975

Suzuki, J., H. Kaneko, M. Homma: A magnetic suture guide for ligation of intracranial aneurysms. J. Neurosurg. 25: 319–320, 1966a

Suzuki, J., N. Kodama, S. Fujiwara: Surgical treatment of internal carotid-posterior communicating aneurysms: From the experience of 213 cases. In Suzuki, J.: Cerebral Aneurysms. Neuron, Tokyo 1979 (pp. 256–262)

Suzuki, J., R. Kwak, R. Katakur: Review of incompletely occluded surgically treated cerebral aneurysms. Surg. Neurol. 13: 306–311, 1980

Suzuki, J., R. Kwak, Y. Okuradira: The safety time limit of temporary clamping of cerebral arteries in the direct surgical treatment of the intracranial aneurysm under moderate hypothermia. Brain Nerve (Tokyo) 25: 407–416, 1973

Suzuki, J., Shigeaki, Y. Sakurai: Intracranial aneurysms in the neurosurgical clinics in Japan. J. Neurosurg. 35: 34–39, 1971

Suzuki, J., A. Takaku, S. Hori: New surgical techniques for direct intracranial surgery of anterior communicating artery aneurysm. Excerpta med. (Amst.) Int. Congr. Series. No. 293: 96, 1973

Suzuki, J., A. Takaku, T. Yoshimoto: [Early operation of ruptured intracranial aneurysms.] Brain Nerve (Tokyo) 23: 1281–1286, 1971

Suzuki, J., T. Yoshimoto, S. Hori: Continuous ventricle drainage to lessen surgical risk in ruptured intracranial aneurysm. Surg. Neurol. 2: 87–90, 1974

Suzuki, J., A. Takaku, S. Hori, N. Harada: [Direct operation for aneurysm of the middle cerebral artery – a new approach.] Brain Nerve (Tokyo) 22: 445–454, 1970

Suzuki, J., A. Takaku, S. Hori, R. Kwak: "Keel form incision", a new approach to the cranial base. Shujutsu (Tokyo) 19: 595–604, 1965a

Suzuki, J., T. Iwabuchi, A. Takaku, S. Hori, N. Harada: [Management of intracranial aneurysms. Especially direct attack of 103 cases.] Brain Nerve (Tokyo) 19: 815–824, 1967

Suzuki, J., T. Iwabuchi, A. Takaku, S. Hori, R. Kwak: Aneurysm arising at the junction of internal carotid and posterior communicating artery. Brain and Nerve (Tokyo) 17: 1003–1008, 1965b

Suzuki, J., M. Kowada, H. Asahi, N. Harada, S. Takahashi, A. Takaku: [Surgical treatment of aneurysms of the anterior communicating artery.] Brain Nerve (Tokyo) 16: 391–397, 1964

Swain, R. D.: The surgical treatment of certain intracranial arterial aneurysms. Surg. Clin. N. Amer. 28: 396–404, 1948

Sweet, W. H., H. S. Bennett: Changes in internal carotid pressure during carotid and jugular occlusion and their clinical significance. J. Neurosurg. 5: 178–195, 1948

Sweet, W. H., S. J. Sarnoff, L. Bakay: A clinical method for recording internal carotid pressure. Significance of changes during carotid occlusion. Surg. Gynec. Obstet. 90: 327–334, 1950

Symon, L.: Clinical assessment of regional cerebral perfusion and correlation of xenon clearance studies with anatomico-pathological data in subarachnoid haemorrhage. Fourth Europ. Congr. Neurosurg., Prag 1971

Symon, L., R. Adlerman et al.: The use of the xenon clearance method in subarachnoid haemorrhage – postoperative studies with clinical and angiographic correlation. In: Cerebral Blood Flow and Intracranial Pressure, Proceedings of the Fifth International Symposium, Roma Siena, 1971

Symon, L., N. W. C. Dorsch, H. A. Crockard, N. M. Branston: Characteristics of vascular reactivity in chronic ischaemic lesions: An experimental study. In Meyer, J. S., H. Lechner, M. Reivich: Cerebral Vascular Disease. 7th International Conference, Salzburg 1974. Thieme, Stuttgart 1976 (pp. 140–146)

Symon, L., G. H. du Boulay, R. H. Ackerman, N. W. C. Dorsch, S. H. Shah: The time-course of blood induced spasm of cerebral arteries in baboons. Neuroradiology 5: 40–42, 1972

Symon, L., G. du Boulay, R. H. Ackerman, N. W. C. Dorsch, S. H. Shah: The reactivity of spastic arteries. Neuroradiology 5: 37–39, 1973

Symonds, C. P.: Clinical study of intra-cranial aneurysm. Guy's Hosp. Rep. 73: 139–158, 1923

Symonds, C. P.: Spontaneous subarachnoid hemorrhage. Quart. J. Med. 18: 93–122, 1924

Sypert, G. W., H. F. Young: Ruptured mycotic pericallosal aneurysm with meningitis due to neisseria meningitidis infection. J. Neurosurg. 37: 467–469, 1972

Takahashi, S., M. Sonobe, Y. Nagamine: Early operations for ruptured intracranial aneurysms. Comparative study with computed tomography. Acta neurochir. (Wien) 57: 23–31, 1981

Takaku, A., S. Tanaka, T. Mori et al.: Clinical analysis of postoperative complications in 1000 cases of intracranial saccular aneurysms. (Jpn.) Neurol. Med. Chir. 18111/3: 191–198, 1978

Taki, W., H. Handa, S. Yamagata, I. Matsuda, Y. Yonekawa, Y. Ikada, H. Iwata: Balloon embolization of a giant aneurysm using a newly developed catheter. Surg. Neurol. 12: 363–365, 1979

Tanabe, Y., K. Sakata, H. Yamada, T. Ito, M. Takasa: Cerebral vasospasm and ultrastructural changes in cerebral arterial wall. An experimental study. J. Neurosurg. 49: 229–238, 1978

Tanishima, T., K. Sano: Vasospasm assessed by angiography and computerized tomography. J. Neurosurg. 51: 466–506, 1979

Taptas, J. N.: Les anévrysmes artério-veineux carotido-caverneux. Neuro-chirurgie 8: 385–394, 1962

Taptas, J. N., P. A. Katsiotis: Arterial embolism as a cause of hemiplegia after subarachnoid hemorrhage from aneurysm. Progr. Brain Res. 30: 357–360, 1968

Taveras, J. M., E. H. Wood: Diagnostic Neuroradiology. Williams & Wilkins, Baltimore 1964 (pp. 17–27)

Taylor, P. E.: Delayed postoperative hemorrhage from intracranial aneurysm after craniotomy for tumor. Neurology (Minneap.) 11: 225–231, 1961

Taylor, T. H., M. Styles, A. J. Lamming: Sodium nitroprusside as a hypotensive agent in general anesthesia. Brit. J. Anaesth. 42: 859–864, 1970

Teal, J. S., R. Th. Bergeron, C. L. Rumbaugh, H. D. Segall: Aneurysms of the petrous or cavernous portions of the internal carotid artery associated with nonpenetrating head trauma. J. Neurosurg. 38: 568–574, 1973a

Teal, J. S., C. L. Rumbaugh, H. D. Segall, R. T. Bergeron: Anomalous branches of the internal carotid artery. Radiology 106: 567–573, 1973b

Teal, J. S., P. J. Wade, Th. R. Bergeron, C. L. Rumbaugh, H. D. Segall: Ventricular opacification during carotid angiography secondary to rupture of intracranial aneurysm. Case report. Radiology 106: 581–583, 1973c

Terao, H., I. Muraoka: Giant aneurysm of the middle cerebral artery containing blood channel. Case report. J. Neurosurg. 37: 352–356, 1972

Ter-Pogossian, M. M.: In vivo flow studies by means of excited X-ray characteristics radiation. In Ziefler, C. A.: Applications of Low Energy X- and Gamma-rays. Gordon and Breach Science Publishers, New York 1971 (pp. 241–248)

Thierry, A., J. Ballivet, D. Binnert, J. P. Mabille, E. Huot, J.-C. Foissac: Les anévrysmes sacciformes de l'artère cérébelleuse moyenne (Artère cérébelleuse antérieure et inférieure). Présentation d'un cas opéré avec succès et revue de la litérature. Neurochirurgie 17: 137–142, 1971

Thomas, D. G. T., A. Paterson: Results of surgical treatment of pericallosal aneurysms. J. Neurol. Neurosurg. Psychiat. 38: 826–827, 1975

Thomas, H., P. Tridon, M. Laxenaire, J. Montant: Anévrisme simulant tumeur hypophysaire avec hypopituitarism. Rev. Otoneuro-ophtal. 36: 128–135, 1964

Thompson, J. E., D. J. Austin: Surgical management of cervical carotid aneurysms. Arch. Surg. 74: 80–88, 1957

Thompson, J. R., D. C. Harwood-Nash, C. R. Fitz: Cerebral aneurysms in children. Amer. J. Roentgenol. 118: 163–175, 1973

Thurel, C., A. Rey, J. B. Thiebaut, N. Chai, R. Houdart: Anévrysmes carotido-ophtalmiques. Neuro-chirurgie 20: 25–39, 1974

Tindall, G. T., A. Goree, J. F. Lee, G. L. Odom: Effects of common carotid ligation on size of internal carotid aneurysms and distal intracarotid and retinal artery pressures. J. Neurosurg. 25: 503–511, 1966

Tindall, G. T., G. L. Odom: Treatment of intracranial aneurysms by proximal carotid ligation. Progr. neurol. Surg. 3: 66–114, 1969

Tindall, G. T., J. Kapp, G. L. Odom, S. C. Robinson: A combined technique for treating certain aneurysms of the anterior communicating artery. J. Neurosurg. 33: 41–47, 1970

Tinker, J. H., J. D. Michenfelder: Sodium nitroprusside: Pharmacology, toxicology and therapeutics. Anesthesiology 45: 340–354, 1976

Todd, E. M., B. L. Crue Jr.: The coating of aneurysms with plastic materials. In Fields, W. S., A. L. Sahs: Intracranial aneurysms and subarachnoid hemorrhage. Thomas, Springfield/Ill. 1965 (pp. 357–371)

Todd, E. M., C. H. Sheldon, B. L. Crue, R. H. Pudenz, W. F. Agnew: Plastic jackets for certain intracranial aneurysms. J. Amer. med. Ass. 179: 935–939, 1962

Todorow, S., K. H. Niessen: Bilaterales cervikales Aneurysma der A. carotis interna mit einseitiger intrakranieller Ausdehnung. Neuro-chirurgie 17: 58–62, 1974

Tomlinson, B. E.: Brain changes in ruptured intracranial aneurysm. J. Clin. Path. 12: 391–399, 1959

Tomono, Y., S. Shirai, Y. Maki: Aneurysm of the upper cervical portion of the internal carotid artery due to exogenous focal arteritis. Neuroradiology 10: 55–58, 1975

Tönnis, W.: Erfolgreiche Behandlung eines Aneurysmas der Arteria communicans anterior cerebri. Zbl. Neurochir. 1: 39–42, 1936

Tönnis, W.: Zur Behandlung intracranieller Aneurysmen. Langenbecks Arch. klin. Chir. 189: 474, 1937

Tönnis, W.: Die Behandlung der intracraniellen Aneurysmen. Dtsch. med. J. 3: 1, 1952

Tönnis, W., W. Walter: Ein neuer operativer Zugang zu den sackförmigen Aneurysmen der basalen Hirngefäße. Wien. med. Wschr. 110: 145–147, 1960

Tönnis, W., W. Walter: Die Behandlung der sackförmigen intrakraniellen Aneurysmen. In Olivecrona, H., W. Tönnis: Klinik und Behandlung der raumbeengenden intrakraniellen Prozesse. Handbuch der Neurochirurgie, Vol. IV. Springer, Berlin 1966

Toole, F. J., J. E. Bevilacqua: The carotid compression test. Evaluation of the diagnostic reliability and prognostic significance. Neurology (Minneap.) 13: 600–606, 1963

Tovi, D.: Studies on fibrinolysis in the central nervous system with special reference to intracranial hemorrhage and to the effect of antifibrinolytic drugs. Umea University Medical Dissertations No. 8. Centraltryckeriet, Umea/Sweden 1972

Tovi, D., I. M. Nilson, C. A. Thulin: Fibrinolysis and subarachnoid hemorrhage. Inhibitory effect of tranexamic acid. A clinical study. Acta neurol. scand. 48: 393–402, 1972

Trevani, E.: Ein als parasellärer Tumor operiertes Aneurysma der Arterie carotis interna. Dtsch. Z. Chir. 237: 534–535, 1932

Triner, L., G. G. Nahas, Y. Vulliemoz, N. I. A. Overweg, M. Verosky, D. V. Habif, S. H. Ngai: Cyclic AMP and smooth muscle function. Ann. N. Y. Acad. Sci. 185: 458–476, 1971

Triska, H.: Ein Fall von Kontrastmittelextravasat bei einem rupturierten Aneurysma der A. cerebri media. Zbl. Neurochir. 22: 291–295, 1962

Troupp, H.: Infraclinoid aneurysm of the internal carotid artery as a cause of nosebleed. Acta oto-laryng. (Stockh.) 55: 326–330, 1962

Troupp, H., G. af Björkesten: Results of a controlled trial of late surgical versus conservative treatment of intracranial aneurysms. J. Neurosurg. 35: 20–24, 1971

Troupp. H., S. Cronqvist: The combination of arterial aneurysm and arteriovenous malformation in the same patient. Acta neurol. scand. 40: 190–196, 1964

Trumpy, J. H.: Subarachnoid hemorrhage, time sequence of recurrences and their prognosis. Acta neurol. scand. 43: 48–60, 1967

Tsuchiya, G., O. Sugar, D. Yashon, J. Hubbard: Reactions of rabbit brain and peripheral vessels to plastics used in coating arterial aneurysms. J. Neurosurg. 28: 409–416, 1968

Turnbull, H. M.: Intracranial aneurysms. Brain 41: 50–56, 1918

Tuerk, K., N. E. Chase, I. I. Kricheff, J. P. Lin, J. Ransohoff: Relation of preoperative angiographic characteristics of the posterior communicating artery to the results of common carotid ligation. J. Neurosurg. 36: 564–568, 1972

Tyson, G. W., et al.: Intraventricular extension of a ruptured basilar artery aneurysm. Surg. Neurol. 13: 129–133, 1980

Tytus, J. S., E. Reifel, M. P. Spencer, L. L. Burnett, L. N. Hungerford: Common carotid ligation for intracranial aneurysms. Results in 26 cases. J. Neurosurg. 32: 63–73, 1970

Tytus, J. S., A. A. Ward Jr.: The effect of cervical carotid ligation on giant intracranial aneurysms. J. Neurosurg. 33: 184–190, 1970

Udvarhelyi, G. B., L. Maxwell, M. Lai: Subarachnoid haemorrhage due to rupture of aneurysm on a persistent left hypoglossal artery. Brit. J. Radiol. 36: 843–847, 1963

Uehlinger, E.: Anévrysmes artériels intracrâniens de la base. In Krayenbühl, H., et al.: L'Anévrysme de l'Artère Communicante Antérieure. Masson, Paris 1950 (pp. 22–40)

Uihlein, A., R. A. Huges: The surgical treatment of intracranial vestigial aneurysms. Surg. Clin. N. Amer. 35: 1071–1083, 1955

Uihlein, A., C. S. MacCarty, J. D. Michenfelder, H. R. Terry, E. F. Daw: Deep hypothermia and surgical treatment of intracranial aneurysms. A five-year survey. J. Amer. med. Ass. 195: 639–641, 1966

Ulric, D. P., O. Sugar: Familial cerebral aneurysm including one extracranial internal carotid aneurysm. Neurology (Minneap.) 10: 288–294, 1960

Umebayashi, Y. M., M. Kuwayama, J. Handa, K. Mori, H. Handa: Traumatic aneurysm of a peripheral cerebral artery. Case report. Clin. Radiol. 21: 36–38, 1970

Urban, J. C.: The surgical microscope, its use and care. In Rand, R. W.: Microneurosurgery. Mosby, St. Louis 1969 (pp. 9–20)

Valvassori, G. E., R. A. Buckingham: Middle ear masses mimicking glomus tumors: radiographic and otoscopic recognition. Ann. Otol. 83: 606–612, 1974

Vance, B. M.: Rutpures of surface blood vessels on cerebral hemispheres as a cause of subdural hemorrhage. Arch. Surg. 61: 992–1006, 1950

VanderArk, G. D., L. C. Kempe: Classification of anterior communicating aneurysms as a basis for surgical approach. J. Neurosurg. 32: 300–303, 1970

VanderArk, G. D., L. G. Kempe, A. Kobrine: Classification of internal carotid aneurisms as a basis for surgical approach. Neurochirurgia (Stuttg.) 15: 81–85, 1972

VanderArk, G. D., L. G. Kempe, D. R. Smith: Anterior communicating aneurysms. The gyrus rectus approach. Congr. Neurol. Surg. 21: 120–133, 1974

Van Effenterre, R.: Les anévrysmes artériels du système vertébrobasilaire. Etude diagnostique et thérapeutique. Thèse, Paris 1971

Vapalahti, P. A., P. Schugk, L. Tarkkanen, G. af Björkesten: Intracranial arterial aneursm in a three-month old infant. J. Neurosurg. 30: 169–171, 1969

Verbiest, H.: Extracranial and cervical arteriovenous aneurysms of the carotid and vertebral arteries. Report of a series of 12 personal cases. Johns Hopk. med. J. 122: 350–357, 1968

Viale, G. L., A. Pau: Carotid-choroidal aneurysms: Remarks on surgical treatment and outcome. Surg. Neurol. 11: 141–145, 1979

Viano, J., J. Metzger, B. Pertuiset: L'angio-tomographie cérébrale. Rev. neurol. 125: 155–164, 1971

Vicq d'Azyr, F.: Traité d'Anatomie et de Physiologie. Didot L'Aine, Paris 1786

Viets, H.: Unilateral ophthalmoplegia: report of a case due to carotid aneurysm. J. nerv. ment. Dis. 47: 249–253, 1918

Vines, F. S., D. O. Davis: Rutpure of intracranial aneurysm at angiography. Case report and comment on causative factors. Radiology 99: 353–354, 1971

Voris, H. C., J. X. R. Basile: Recurrent epistaxis from aneurysm of the internal carotid artery. Case report with cure by operation. J. Neurosurg. 18: 841–842, 1961.

Wada, J., T. Rasmussen: Intracarotid injection of sodium amytal for the lateralization of cerebral speech dominance. Experimental and clinical observations. J. Neurosurg. 17: 266–282, 1960

Waddington, M. M.: Atlas of Cerebral Angiography with Anatomic Correlation. Little, Brown, Boston 1974

Waga, S., M. Matsuda, H. Handa: Bilateral giant aneurysms of the internal carotid artery. Amer. J. Roentgenol. 116: 23–29, 1972

Waga, S., K. Ohtsubo, H. Handa: Warning signs in intracranial aneurysms. Surg. Neurol. 3: 15–20, 1975

Waga, S., A. Kondo, K. Moritake, H. Handa: Rupture of intracranial aneurysm during angiography. Neuroradiology 5: 169–173, 1973

Walker, A. E.: Clinical localization of intracranial aneurysms and vascular anomalies. Neurology (Minneap.) 6: 79–90, 1956

Walker, A. E., G. E. Allègre: Pathology and pathogenesis of cerebral aneurysms. J. Neuropath. exp. Neurol. 13: 248–259, 1954

Walsh, F. B.: Visual field defects due to aneurysm at circle of Willis. Arch. Ophthal. 71: 15–54, 1964

Walsh, L.: Experience in the conservative and surgical treatment of ruptured intracranial aneurysms. Res. Publ. Assoc. Res. nerv. ment. Dis. 41: 169–178, 1966

Walsh, L. S.: Results of Treatment of Spontaneous Subarachnoid Hemorrhage. Modern Trends in Neurology (Second Series). Butterworth, London 1957 (pp. 119–129)

Walsh, L. S.: Posterior communicating aneurysms. Neurology (Minneap.) 11: 158–161, 1961

Walter, W., W. Schütte: Über die Gefäßspasmen bei frisch rupturierten sackförmigen Aneurysmen der Hirnarterien. Acta neurochir. (Wien) 11: 631–652, 1964

Walton, J. N.: Subarachnoid Haemorrhage. Livingstone, Edinburgh 1956 (p. 208)

Weaver, D. F., E. M. Gates, A. E. Nielsen: Traumatic intracranial vascular lesions producing late massive nasal hemorrhage. Trans. Amer. Acad. Ophthal. Otolaryng. 65: 759–744, 1961

Weibel, J., W. S. Fields, R. J. Campos: Aneurysms of the posterior cervocranial circulation: clinical and angiographic considerations. J. Neurosurg. 26: 223–234, 1967

Weichmann, F., W. Buchholz: Aneurysma-Ligatur durch Plombierung statt Knüpfung des Fadens. Zbl. Neurochir. 27: 155–158, 1966

Weinstein, P. R., N. L. Chater, J. Ausman, R. Lamond: Extra intracranial arterial bypass for occlusive vertebro-basilar cerebro-vascular disease. Presented at the annual meeting. Amer. Ass. Neurol. Surg. Bal Harbor/Fl., April 6–10, 1975

Weir, B., K. Aronyk: Management mortality and timing of surgery for supratentorial aneurysms. J. Neurosurg. 54: 146–150, 1981

Wemple, J. B., G. W. Smith: Extracranial carotid aneurysm. report of 4 cases. J. Neurosurg. 24: 667–671, 1966

Wende, S., K. Schindler: Technique and use of X-ray magnification in cerebral arteriography. Neuroradiology 1: 117–120, 1970

Wende, S., K. Schindler, G. Moritz: Der diagnostische Wert der angiographischen Vergrößerungstechnik mit Flist-Fokus Röhren in 2 Ebenen. Radiologie II: 471–475, 1971

Wende, S., E. Zieler, N. Nakayama: Cerebral Magnification Angiography. Springer, Berlin 1974 (pp. 129–139)

Werner, S. C., A. H. Blakemore, B. G. King: Aneurysm of internal carotid artery within the skull: wiring and electrothermic coagulation. J. Amer. med. Ass. 116: 578–582, 1941

Weyer, K. H., H. van de Bühl: Multiple Hirnaneurysmen. Fortschr. Röntgenstr. 100: 119–122, 1964

White, J. C.: Aneurysms mistaken for hypophyseal tumors. Clin. Neurosurg. 10: 224–250, 1962

White, J. C., R. D. Adams: Combined supra- and infraclinoid aneurysm of internal carotid artery. J. Neurosurg. 12: 450–459, 1955

White, J. C., H. T. Ballantine: Intrasellar aneurysms simulating hypophyseal tumors. J. Neurosurg. 18: 34–49, 1961

White, J. C., G. P. Sayre, J. P. Whisnant: Experimental destruction of the media for the production of intracranial arterial aneurysms. J. Neurosurg. 18: 741–745, 1961

Wholey, M. H., L. A. Kessler, M. Boehnke: A percutaneous balloon catheter technique for the treatment of intracranial aneurysms. Acta radiol. Diagn. 13: 286–292, 1972

Wichern, H.: Klinische Beiträge zur Kenntnis der Hirnaneurysmen. Dtsch. Z. Nervenheilk. 44: 220–263, 1912

Wickbom, I., O. Bartley: Arterial spasm in peripheral arteriography using catheter method. Acta radiol. (Stockh.) 47: 433–448, 1957

Wiklund, P. E.: Controlled hypotension at intracranial operations. J. Neurosurg. 10: 617–623, 1953

Wilkins, R. H.: Hypothalamic dysfunction and intracranial arterial spasms. Surg. Neurol. 4: 472–480, 1975

Wilkins, R. H.: Aneurysm rupture during angiography: does acute vasospasm occur? Surg. Neurol. 5: 299–303, 1976

Wilkins, R. H., J. A. Alexander, G. L. Odom: Intracranial arterial spasm: a clinical analysis. J. Neurosurg. 29: 121–134, 1968

Wilkins, R. H., D. Silver, G. L. Odom: The role of circulating substance in intracranial arterial spasm. 1. Serotonin and histamin. Neurology (Minneap.) 16: 482–490, 1966

Wilkinson, H. A., R. L. Wright, W. H. Sweet: Correlation of reduction in pressure and angiographic cross-filling with tolerance of carotid occlusion. J. Neurosurg. 22: 241–245, 1965

Wilkinson, I. M. S., J. W. D. Bull, G. H. du Boulay, J. Marshall, R. W. Ross-Russell, L. Symon: Regional cerebral blood flow in normal cerebral circulation. J. Neurol. Neurosurg. Psychiat. 32: 367–378, 1967

Wilks, S.: Sanguineous meningeal effusion (apoplexy); spontaneous and from injury. Guy's Hosp. Rep. 5: 119–127, 1859 (Cited in Hamby, W. B.: Intracranial Aneurysms. Thomas, Springfield/Ill. 1952)

Williams, R. R., R. R. Bahn, G. P. Sayre: Congenital cerebral aneurysms. Proc. Mayo Clin. 30: 100–107, 1956

Williamson, W. P., C. E. Brackett Jr.: Management of intracranial aneurysms of the anterior communicating artery. Amer. Surg. 22: 100–107, 1956

Wilson, C. B., V. Hoisang: Surgical treatment for aneurysms of the upper basilar artery. J. Neurosurg. 44: 537–543, 1976

Wilson, C. B., F. K. Myers: Bilateral saccular aneurysms of the internal carotid artery in the cavernous sinus. J. Neurol. Neurosurg. Psychiat. 26: 174–177, 1963

Wilson, D. H.: Limited exposure in cerebral surgery. Technical note. J. Neurosurg. 34: 102–106, 1971

Wilson, G., H. E. Riggs, C. Rupp: The pathologic anatomy of ruptured cerebral aneurysms. J. Neurosurg. 11: 128–134, 1954

Wilson, J. R., P. H. Jordan: Excision of an internal carotid artery aneurysm: restitution of continuity by substitution of external for internal carotid artery. Ann. Surg. 154: 45–47, 1961

Windle, B. C. A.: On the arteries forming the circle of Willis. J. Anat. Physiol. 22: 289–293, 1888

Winn, H. R., A. E. Richardson, J. A. Jane: Late mortality and morbidity in cerebral aneurysms. A ten-year follow-up of 364 conservatively treated patients with a single cerebral aneurysm. Trans. Amer. neurol. Ass. 98: 148–150, 1973

Winn, H. R., A. E. Richardson, J. A. Jane: Late morbidity and mortality of common carotid ligation for posterior communicating artery aneurysms. A comparison to conservative treatment. J. Neurosurg. 47: 727–736, 1977

Winn, H. R., A. E. Richardson, J. A. Jane: The incidence of late hemorrhage in cerebral aneurysms. A ten-year evaluation of 364 patients. Ann. neurol. 1: 358–370, 1977

Winslow, N.: Extracranial aneurysm of the internal carotid artery: history and analysis of the cases registered up to Aug. 1, 1925. Arch. Surg. 13: 689–729, 1926

Wise, B. L., E. Boldrey, R. B. Aird: The value of electroencephalography in studying the effects of ligation of the carotid arteries. E.E.G. Clin. Neurophys. 6: 261–268, 1954

Wise, B. L., A. J. Palubinskas: Persistent trigeminal artery (carotid-basilar anastomosis). J. Neurosurg. 21: 199–206, 1964

Wise, G. R., T. W. Farmer: Bacterial cerebral vasculitis. Neurology (Minneap.) 21: 195–200, 1971

Wissinger, J. P., D. Danoff, E. S. Wisiol, L. A. French: Repair of an aneurysm of the basilar artery by a transclival approach: case report. J. Neurosurg. 26: 417–419, 1967

Wollman, H., S. C. Alexander, P. J. Cohen, P. E. Chose, E. Melman, M. G. Behar: Cerebral circulation of man during halothane anesthesia: Effects of hypocarbia and d-tubocurarine. Anesthesiology 25: 180–184, 1964

Wollschlaeger, G., P. B. Wollschlaeger: The primitive trigeminal artery as seen angiographically and at post mortem examination. Amer. J. Roentgenol. 92: 761–768, 1964

Wollschlaeger, G., P. B. Wollschlaeger: Postmortem angiography. In Newton, T. H., D. G. Potts: Radiology of the Skull and Brain, Vol. II, part 2. Mosby, St. Louis 1974 (pp. 1002–1019)

Wollschlaeger, P. B., G. Wollschlaeger, W. M. Hart, C. H. Ide: Eigene Beobachtungen zur Blutversorgung des Fasciculus opticus. Chiasma fasciculorum opticorum. Tractus opticus. Tuber cinereum und Infundibulum. Radiologe 10: 433–437, 1970

Wolpert, S. M.: The trigeminal artery and associated aneurysms. Neurology (Minneap.) 16: 610–614, 1966

Wood, E. H.: Angiographic identification of the ruptured lesion in patients with multiple cerebral aneurysms. J. Neurosurg. 21: 182–198, 1964

Wood, E. H.: Intracranial aneurysms. Radiol. Clin. N. Amer. 4: 217–233, 1966

Woolmer, R. S.: Symposium on pH and Blood Gas Measurement. Churchill, London 1959

Woringer, E., J. Kunlin: Anastomose entre la carotide primitive et la carotide intracrânienne de la sylvienne par greffon selon la technique de la suture suspendue. Neuro-chirurgie 9: 181, 1963

Wortzmann, G.: Roentgenologic aspects of extradural hematoma. Amer. J. Roentgenol. 90: 462–471, 1963

Wright, D. C., Ch. B. Wilson: Surgical treatment of basilar aneurysms. Neurosurgery 5: 325–333, 1979

Wright, R. L.: Pressure considerations in carotid compressions during angiography. J. Neurosurg. 19: 375–377, 1962

Yamaura, A., et al.: Posterior inferior cerebellar aneurysm in the fourth ventricle. Surg. Neurol. 13: 297–299, 1980

Yarborough, W. L., J. A. Harrill, E. Alexander: Traumatic internal carotid aneurysm rupture into sphenoid sinus with angiographic demonstration. Laryngoscope (St. Louis) 73: 1313–1325, 1963

Yaşargil, M. G.: Experimental small vessel surgery in the dog including patching and grafting of cerebral vessels and the formation of functional extra-intracranial shunts. In Donaghy, R. M. P., M. G. Yaşargil: Micro-Vascular Surgery. Mosby, St. Louis 1967 (pp. 87–126)

Yaşargil, M. G.: Microsurgery. Applied to Neurosurgery. Academic Press, New York, Thieme, Stuttgart, 1969a (pp. 132–139)

Yaşargil, M. G.: Experimental microsurgical operations in animals. In Yaşargil, M. G.: Microsurgery. Applied to Neurosurgery, Chapter 3. Academic Press, New York 1969b (pp. 60–79)

Yaşargil, M. G.: Suturing techniques. In Yaşargil, M. G.: Microsurgery. Applied to Neurosurgery, Chapter 2. Academic Press, New York 1969c (pp. 51–57)

Yaşargil, M. G.: Reconstructive and constructive surgery of the

cerebral arteries in man. In Yaşargil, M. G.: Microsurgery. Thieme, Stuttgart 1969d (pp. 82–119)
Yaşargil, M. G.: Intracranial microsurgery. Clin. Neurosurg. 17: 250–255, 1970a
Yaşargil, M. G.: Structure and reaction of cerebral arteries. In Meyer, J. S., M. Reivich, H. Lechner, O. Eichhorn: Research on the Cerebral Circulation. Fourth International Salzburg Conference. Thomas, Springfield/Ill. 1970b (pp. 275–278)
Yaşargil, M. G.: Microsurgical approach to the cerebrobascular diseases. In Fusek, I., Z. Kunc: Proceedings of the Fourth European Congress of Neurosurgery. Present Limits of Neurosurgery. Avicenum, Czechoslovak Medical Press, Prague, Excerpta Medica, Amsterdam 1972 (pp. 357–361)
Yaşargil, M. G., L. P. Carter: Saccular aneurysms of the distal anterior cerebral artery. J. Neurosurg. 39: 218–223, 1974
Yaşargil, M. G., J. L. Fox: The microsurgical approach to intracranial aneurysms. Surg. Neurol. 3: 7–14, 1975
Yaşargil, M. G., R. D. Smith: Association of middle cerebral artery with saccular aneurysms and Moyamoya disease. Surg. Neurol. 5: 39–43, 1976
Yaşargil, M. G., W. B. Boehm, R. E. Ho: Microsurgical treatment of cerebral aneurysms at the bifurcation of the internal carotid artery. Acta neurochir. (Wien) 41: 61–72, 1978
Yaşargil, M. G., J. L. Fox, W. M. Ray: The operative approach to aneurysms of the anterior communicating artery. In Krayenbühl, H.: Advances and Technical Standards in Neurosurgery, Vol. II. Springer, New York 1975 (pp. 113–170)
Yaşargil, M. G., H. A. Krayenbühl, J. H. Jacobson: Microneurosurgical arterial reconstruction. Surgery 67: 221–233, 1970
Yaşargil, M. G., R. D. Smith, J. L. Firth: Anterior communicating artery aneurysms. In: Operative Surgery, 3rd, Ed. Butterworths, London 1978 (pp. 233–251)
Yaşargil, M. G., R. D. Smith, C. Gasser: Microsurgery of the aneurysms of the internal carotid artery and its branches. Progr. neurol. Surg. 9: 58–121, 1978
Yaşargil, M. G., J. C. Gasser, R. M. Hodosh, T. V. Rankin: Carotid-ophthalmic aneurysms: direct microsurgical approach. Surg. Neurol. 8: 155–165, 1977
Yaşargil, M. G., K. Kasdaglis, K. K. Jain, H.-P. Weber: Anatomical observations of the subarachnoid cisterns of the brain during surgery. J. Neurosurg. 44: 298–302, 1976
Yaşargil, M. G., Y. Yonekawa, B. Zumstein, H.-J. Stahl: Hydrocephalus following subarachnoid hemorrhage. Clinical features and treatment. J. Neurosurg. 39: 474–479, 1973
Yaşargil, M. G., J. Antic, R. Laciga, K. K. Jain, R. M. Hodosh, R. D. Smith: Microsurgical pterional approach to aneurysms of the basilar bifurcation. Surg. Neurol. 6: 83–91, 1976
Yashon, D., J. A. Jane, M. C. Gordon, J. L. Hubbard, O. Sugar: Effects of methyl 2-cyanoacrylate adhesives on the somatic vessels and the central nervous system of animals. J. Neurosurg. 24: 883–888, 1966
Yashon, D., R. J. White, B. A. Arias, W. E. Hegarty: Cyanoacrylate encasement of intracranial aneurysms. Technical note. J. Neurosurg. 34: 709–713, 1971
Yaskin, H. E., B. Y. Alpers: Aneurysm of the vertebral artery. Report of a case in which the aneurysm simulated a tumor of the posterior fossa. Arch. Neurol. Psychiat. (Chic.) 51: 271–281, 1944
Yates, A. J.: Intra-arterial balloon tamponade. Surgery 66: 634–636, 1969
Yodh, S. B., N. T. Pierce, R. J. Weggel, D. B. Montgomery: A new magnetic system for intravascular navigation. Med. biol. Engin. 6: 143–147, 1968
Yoshimoto, T., J. Suzuki: Eight year documented study of an aneurysm growth at the origin of the posterior communicating artery. Neurol. Surg. 2: 571–573, 1974
Yoshimoto, T., J. Suzuki: Intracranial definitive aneurysm surgery under normothermia and normotension, utilizing temporary occlusion of brain artery and preoperative mannitol administration. Neurol. Surg. (Tokyo) 4: 775–783, 1976
Yoshimoto, T., A. Takaku, J. Suzuki: Bilateral symmetrical aneurysms at the middle cerebral artery: Report of two cases. Brain Nerve 23: 541–544, 1971
Yoshimoto, T., K. Uchida, J. Suzuki: Surgical treatment of distal anterior cerebral aneurysms. J. Neurosurg. 50: 40–44, 1979
Youmans, J. R., G. W. Kindt, O. C. Mitchell: Extended studies of direction of flow and pressure in the internal carotid artery following common carotid artery ligation. J. Neurosurg. 27: 250–254, 1967
Young, N.: Bleeding from the ear as a sign of leaking aneurysm of the extracranial portion of the internal carotid artery. J. Laryng. 56: 35–64, 1941
Young, R., W. F. Meacham, J. H. Allen: Documented enlargement and rupture of a small arterial sacculation. Case report. J. Neurosurg. 34: 814–817, 1971
Zakrzewski, A.: Spontaneous extracranial aneurysms of the internal carotid artery. J. Laryng. 77: 342–350, 1963
Zervas, N. T., A. Kuwayama, C. B. Rosoff, E. W. Saltzman: Cerebral arterial spasm. Modification by inhibition of platelet function. Arch. Neurol. (Chic.) 28: 400–404, 1973
Zingesser, L. H., M. M. Schechter, J. Dexter et al.: On the significance of spasm associated with rupture of a cerebral aneurysm: the relationship between spasm as noted angiographically and 71 regional blood flow determinations. Arch. Neurol. (Chic.) 18: 520–528, 1968
Zlotnik, E. I., S. P. Sekach: Treatment of carotid-cavernous fistulas and internal carotid aneurysms by the Serbinenko method. In: II Sjezd Neirokhirurgov SSSR. Moscow 1976 (pp. 401–402) (Rus.)
Zlotnik, E. I., F. V. Oleshkevich, J. Z. Stolkarts: Microsurgical technique in the treatment of intracranial aneurysms. J. Neurosurg. 46: 591–595, 1977
Zozulia, Yu. A., V. I. Shcheglov: Experience and employment of intravascular intervention with a balloon catheter in some type of cerebral pathology. Vop. Neĭrokhir. 1: 7–12, 1976
Zozulia, Yu. A., G. A. Pedachenko, V. I. Shcheglov: Intravascular reconstructive operations for some vascular brain lesions. In: 6th Int. Congr. Neurol. Surgery, Sao Paolo 1977 (p. 18)
Zubkov, Yu. N.: Intravascular surgery for intracranial internal carotid saccular aneurysms. In: Diagnostika i khir. lechenie sosud. zabol. golovnogo mozga. Leningrad 1974 (pp. 173–175) (Rus.)
Zubkov, Yu. N.: Intraarterial interventions from arterial cerebral aneurysms. In: Akt. vopr. neurol. psikhiat. i neirokhir. Riga 1979 (pp. 199–200) (Rus.)
Zuidema, G. D.: The SOSSUS report and its impact on neurosurgery. J. Neurosurg. 46: 135–144, 1977

Chapter 6: Giant Aneurysms

Alajouanine, T., J. Le Beau, R. Houdart: La symptomatologie tumorale des volumineux anévrysmes des artères vertebrales et basilaires. Rev. neurol. 80: 321–337, 1948
Alksne, J. F., A. G. Fingerhut, R. W. Rand: Magnetically controlled focal intravascular thrombosis in dogs. J. Neurosurg. 25: 516–525, 1966
Almeida, G. M., M. K. Shibatu, E. Bianco: Carotid ophthalmic aneurysms. Surg. Neurol. 5: 41–45, 1976
Anderson, R. E., T. M. Sundt Jr.: An automated cerebral blood flow analyzer: concise communication. J. nucl. Med. 18: 728–731, 1977
Azar-Kia, B., E. Palacios, M. Spak: The megadolichobasilar artery anomaly and expansion of the internal auditory meatus. Neuroradiology 11: 109–111, 1976
Beck, D. W., D. J. Boarini, N. F. Kassell: Surgical treatment of giant aneurysms of vertebral-basilar junction. Surg. Neurol. 12: 283–285, 1979
Bhushan, C., F. J. Hodges, J. Posey: Successful surgical treatment of giant aneurysm of the basilar artery. Case report. J. Neurosurg. 49: 124–128, 1978
Bird, A. C., B. Nolan, F. P. Garbano, et al.: Unruptured aneurysm of the supraclinoid carotid artery. Neurology (Minneap.) 20: 445–454, 1970
Black, S. P. W., W. J. German: Observations of the relationship between the volume and the size of the orifice of experimental aneurysms. J. Neurosurg. 17: 984–990, 1960
Bladin, P. F., M. G. F. Donnan: Cerebral arterial ectasia. Clin. Radiol. 14: 349–352, 1963
Bloor, B. M., G. G. Glista: Observations on simultaneous internal carotid artery and total cerebral blood flow measurements in man. Neurosurgery 1: 249–255, 1977

Boysen, G.: Cerebral hemodynamics in carotid surgery. Acta neurol. scand., Suppl. 52: 1–84, 1973

Bloor, B. M., G. I. Odom, B. Woodhall: Direct measurement of intravascular pressure in components of the circle of Willis. Arch. Surg. 63: 821–823, 1951

Boeri, R., A. Passerini: The megadolichobasilar anomaly. J. neurol. Sci. 1: 475–484, 1964

Borne, G., B. Arnoud, G. Bedou, et al.: Les anévrismes géants de la carotide interne, intracrânienne, infra-clinoidienne. Neuro-chirurgie 25: 101–107, 1979

Bull, J.: Massive aneurysms at the base of the brain. Brain 92: 535–570, 1969

Byrd, S. E., J. R. Bentson, J. Winter, G. H. Wilson, P. W. Joyce, L. O'Connor: Giant intracranial aneurysms simulating brain neoplasms on computed tomography. J. Comput. assist. Tomogr. 2: 303–307, 1978

Campbell, E., C. W. Burklund: Aneurysms of the middle cerebral artery. Ann. Surg. 137: 18–22, 1953

Cantu, R. C., M. LeMay: A large middle cerebral aneurysm presenting as a bizarre vascular malformation. Brit. J. Radiol. 39: 317–319, 1966

Carella, A., G. Caruso, P. Lamberti: Hemifacial spasm due to elongation and ectasia of the distal portion of the vertebral artery. Neuroradiology 6: 233–236, 1973

Carlson, D. H., D. Thomson: Spontaneous thrombosis of a giant cerebral aneurysm in five days. Report of a case. Neurology (Minneap.) 26: 334–336, 1976

Carmody, J. T. B.: Aneurysm of the internal carotid artery associated with hypothalamic fits. J. Neurosurg. 3: 81–86, 1946

Case records of the Massachusetts General Hospital: Case 22-1963. New Engl. J. Med. 268: 724–731, 1963

Chater, N.: Surgical results and measurements of intraoperative flow in microneurosurgical anastomoses. In Austin, G. M.: Microneurosurgical Anastomoses for Cerebral Ischemia. Thomas, Springfield/Ill. 1976 (pp. 295–304)

Chou, N. S., H. J. Ortiz-Suarez: Surgical treatment of arterial aneurysms of the vertebrobasilar circulation. J. Neurosurg. 41: 671–680, 1974

Columella, F., A. Beduschi, L. Papo: Un interessante caso de arteriosclerosi cerebrale. Chirurgia (Pavia) 10: 302–306, 1955

Courville, C. B.: Arteriosclerotic aneurysms of the circle of Willis. Some notes on their morphology and pathogenesis. Bull. Los Angeles neurol. Soc. 27: 1–13, 1962

Creissard, P., J. Godlewsky, M. Tadie, P. Freger, J. Thiebot, J. Tayot: Les anévrismes géants. Neuro-chirurgie 26: 309–353, 1980

Crockard, H. A., L. Symon, N. M. Branston et al.: Changes in regional cortical tissue oxygen tension and cerebral blood flow during temporary middle cerebral artery occlusion in baboons. J. neurol. Sci. 27: 29–44, 1976

Crompton, M. R.: Mechanism of growth and rupture in cerebral artery aneurysms. Brit. med. J. I: 1138–1142, 1966

Crutchfield, W. G.: Instruments for use in the treatment of certain intracranial vascular lesions. J. Neurosurg. 16: 471–474, 1959

Cuatico, W., A. W. Cook, V. Tyshchenko, R. Khatib: Massive enlargement of intracranial aneurysms following carotid ligation. Arch. Neurol. (Chic.) 17: 609–613, 1967

Dandy, W. E.: Results following ligation of the internal carotid artery. Arch. Surg. 45: 521–533, 1942

Dandy, W. E.: Intracranial Arterial Aneurysms. Comstock, Ithaca: 1945

Danziger, J., S. Bloch: Intracranial aneurysms presenting as mass lesions. Clin. Radiol. 26: 267–273, 1975

Dettori, P., G. Cristi, S. Dalbuono: Anomalia megadolichobasilare. Studio clinico-radiologico di 8 casi. Radiol. med. (Torino) 52: 1259–1273, 1966

Discussion on the treatment of giant aneurysms. In: Pia, H. W., C. Langmaid, J. Zierski: Cerebral Aneurysms. Springer, Berlin 1979 (pp. 350–351)

Donley, R. F., T. M. Sundt Jr., R. E. Anderson et al.: Blood flow measurements and the "look through" artifact in focal cerebral ischemia. Stroke 6: 121–131, 1975

Drake, C. G.: On the surgical treatment of ruptured intracranial aneurysms. Clin. Neurosurg. 13: 122–152, 1966

Drake, C. G.: Experience with direct surgical obliteration of "giant" intracranial aneurysms. Presented at the Annual Meeting of the American Association of Neurological Surgeons, Miami Beach, Florida, April 1975a (Paper No. 1)

Drake, C. G.: Ligation of the vertebral (unilateral or bilateral) or basilar artery in the treatment of large intracranial aneurysms. J. Neurosurg. 43: 255–274, 1975b

Drake, C. G.: Direct surgical treatment of "giant" intracranial aneurysms. AANS Annual Meeting, 1975c

Drake, C. G.: Cerebral aneurysm surgery: an update. In Scheinberg, P.: Cerebrovascular Diseases. Tenth Princeton Conference. Raven, New York 1976 (pp. 289–310)

Drake, C. G.: Advances in the neurosurgical treatment of aneurysms, arteriovenous malformations, and hematomas of the vertebral circulation. Green: Stroke. Advances in Neurology, Vol. 16. Raven, New York 1977 (pp. 211–255)

Drake, C. G.: Treatment of aneurysms of the posterior cranial fossa. In Krayenbühl, H., P. E. Maspes, W. H. Sweet: Progress in Neurological Surgery, Vol. 9. Karger, Basel 1978 (pp. 122–194)

Driesen, W.: Über zwei ungewöhnliche Operationsbefunde bei raumfordernden intrasellären Prozessen. Zbl. Neurochir. 19: 28–35, 1959

Duvoisin, R., M. D. Yahr: Posterior fossa aneurysms. Neurology (Minneap.) 15: 231–241, 1965

Dvorak, M., E. Klaus: Schwierigkeiten in der Röntgen-Diagnostik und in der Behandlung von großen intrakranialen sakkularen Aneurysmen. Acta neurochir. (Wien) 15: 182–193, 1966

Ehni, G.: Screw-clamp stenosis for internal carotid aneurysms. J. Neurosurg. 42: 616, 1975

Faria, M. A., A. S. Fleischer, R. H. Spector: Bilateral giant intracavernous carotid aneurysms treated by bilateral carotid ligation. Surg. Neurol. 14: 207–210, 1980

Ferguson, G. G.: Physical factors in the initiation, growth, and rupture of human intracerebral saccular aneurysms. J. Neurosurg. 37: 666–667, 1972

Fiore, D. L., et al.: The value and limitations of the CT scan in the diagnosis of giant intracranial aneurysms. Acta neurochir. (Wien) 53: 19–24, 1980

Fodstad, H., B. Liliequist: Serpigenous giant internal carotid artery aneurysm in a young female. In Pia, H. W., C. Langmaid, J. Zierski: Cerebral Aneurysms. Springer, Berlin 1979 (pp. 346–351)

Fodstad, H., B. Liliequist, S. Wirell, P. E. Nilsson, et al.: Giant serpentine intracranial aneurysm after carotid ligation. J. Neurosurg. 49: 903–909, 1978

Franck, G., M. Reznik, A. Thibaut: Étude clinique et anatomique d'un cas de clonies vélo-pharyngo-laryngées secondaires a un anévrysme fusiforme athéroscléreux du tronc vertébro-basilaire. Rev. neurol. 113: 56–67, 1965

Frasson, F., G. Ferrari, C. Fugazzola, A. Fiaschi: Megadolichobasilar anomaly causing a brainstem syndrome. Neuroradiology 13: 279–281, 1977

Fried, L. C., A. Ybalk: Rapid formation of giant aneurysm. Case report. J. Neurol. Neurosurg. Psychiat. 35: 527–530, 1972

Galbraith, J. G., R. M. Clark: Role of carotid ligation in the management of intracranial carotid aneurysms. Clin. Neurosurg. 21: 171–181, 1973

Gallagher, G. P., J. F. Dorsey, M. Stefanini, et al.: Large intracranial aneurysm producing panhypopituitarism and frontal lobe syndrome. Neurology (Minneap.) 6: 829–837, 1956

Garcia-Bengochea, F., F. H. Deland: Bilateral giant carotid-ophthalmic aneurysms. Case report. J. Neurosurg. 42: 589–592, 1975

Gelber, B. R., Th. M. Sundt: Treatment of intracavernous and giant carotid aneurysms by combined internal carotid ligation and extra- to intracranial bypass. J. Neurosurg. 52: 1–10, 1980

Géraud, J., A. Rascol, A. Bès, L. Arbus, A. M. Bénazet: Anévrysme fusiforme vertébro-basilaire à symptomatologie pseudotumorale (Étude clinique et radiologique). Rev. neurol. 110: 66–72, 1964

German, W. J., S. P. W. Black: Cervical ligation for internal carotid aneurysms. An extended follow-up. J. Neurosurg. 23: 572–577, 1965

Giannotta, S. I., J. E. McGillicuddy, G. W. Kindt: Gradual carotid artery occlusion in the treatment of inaccessible internal carotid artery aneurysms. Neurosurgery 5: 417–421, 1979

Givel, J. C., N. de Tribolet, E. Zander: Anévrismes extra-crâniens bilatéraux de la carotide interne. Neuro-chirurgie 25: 108–112, 1979

Greitz, T., S. Löfstedt: The third ventricle and the basilar artery. Acta radiol. (Stockh.) 42: 85–100, 1954

Greitz, T., K. Ekbom, E. Kugelberg, A. Breig: Occult hydrocephalus due to ectasia of the basilar artery. Acta radiol. Diagn. 9: 310–316, 1969

Grumme, T., H. Steinhoff, S. Wende: Diagnosis of supratentorial tumors with computerized tomography. In Lanksch, W., E. Kazner: Cranial Computerized Tomography. Springer, Berlin 1976 (pp. 80–85)

Guidetti, B.: Internal carotid-ophthalmic aneurysms. In Pia, H. W., C. Langmaid, J. Zierski: Cerebral Aneurysms. Springer, Berlin 1979 (pp. 83–89, 244–250)

Guidetti, B., E. LaTorre: Management of carotid-ophthalmic aneurysms. J. Neurosurg. 42: 438–442, 1975

Guillain, G., P. Schmitte, I. Bertrand: Anévrysme du tronc basilaire ayant determiné la symptomatologie d'une tumeur de l'angle ponto-cérébelleux. Rev. neurol. 1: 795–892, 1930

Handa, J., Y. Nakano, H. Aii, et al: Computed tomography with giant intracranial aneurysms. Surg. Neurol. 9: 257–263, 1978

Handa, J., H. Kikuchi, K. Iwayama, T. Teraura, H. Handa: Traumatic aneurysms of the internal carotid artery. Acta neurochir. (Wien) 17: 161–177, 1967

Hanson Jr., E. J., R. E. Anderson, T. M. Sundt Jr.: Comparison of ^{85}krypton and ^{133}xenon cerebral blood flow measurements before, during and following focal, incomplete ischemia in the squirrel monkey. Circulat. Res. 36: 18–26, 1975

Hardesty, W. H., B. Roberts, J. F. Toole, et al.: Studies of carotid artery blood flow in man. New Engl. J. Med. 263: 944–946, 1960

Harris, F. S., A. L. Rhoton Jr.: Anatomy of the cavernous sinus. A microsurgical study. J. Neurosurg. 45: 169–180, 1976

Heilbrun, M. P., O. H. Reichman, R. E. Anderson, et al.: Regional cerebral blood flow studies following superficial temporal-middle cerebral artery anastomosis. J. Neurosurg. 43: 706–716, 1975

Heiskanen, O., P. Nikki: Large intracranial aneurysms. Acta neurol. scand. 38: 195–208, 1962

Hilal, S. K., J. A. Resch, K. Amplatz: Determination of the carotid and regional cerebral blood flow by a radiographic technique. Acta radiol. Diagn. 5: 232–240, 1966

Hoff, J. T., L. H. Pitts, R. Spetzler, et al.: Barbiturates for protection from cerebral ischemia in aneurysm surgery. Acta neurol. scand. (Suppl.) 56 (64): 158–159, 1977

Hoff, J. T., A. I. Smith, H. L. Hankinson, et al.: Barbiturate protection from cerebral infarction in primates. Stroke 6: 28–33, 1975

Hoff, W. V., R. W. Hornabrook, V. Marks: Hypopituitarism associated with intracranial aneurysms. Brit. med. J. II: 1190–1193, 1961

Hosobuchi, Y.: Electrothrombosis of carotid-cavernous fistula. J. Neurosurg. 42: 76–85, 1975

Hosobuchi, Y.: Direct surgical treatment of giant intracranial aneurysms. J. Neurosurg. 51: 743–756, 1979

Howe, J. F., A. B. Harris, G. W. Sypert: Giant aneurysms of the middle cerebral artery. Surg. Neurol. 6: 231–233, 1976

Jain, K. K.: Surgery of intracranial berry aneurysms. A review. Canad. J. Surg. 8: 172–187, 1965

Jamieson, K. G.: Aneurysms of the vertebrobasilar system. J. Neurosurg. 21: 781–797, 1964

Jane, J. A.: A large aneurysm of the posterior inferior cerebellar artery in a one-year old child. J. Neurosurg. 18: 245–247, 1961

Jawad, K., J. D. Miller, D. J. Wyper, J. Q. Rowan: Measurement of CBF and carotid artery pressure compared with cerebral angiography in assessing collateral blood supply after carotid ligation. J. Neurosurg. 46: 185–196, 1977

Jefferson, G.: Compression of the chiasma, optic nerves and optic tracts by intracranial aneurysms. Brain 60: 444–497, 1937

Jefferson, G.: On the saccular aneurysms of the internal carotid artery in the cavernous sinus. Brit. J. Surg. 26: 267–302, 1938

Jefferson, G.: On the saccular aneurysms of the internal carotid artery in the cavernous sinus. In: Selected Papers. Pitman, London 1960 (p. 273)

Jennett, B., J. D. Miller, A. M. Harper: Effect of Carotid Artery Surgery on Cerebral Blood Flow. Excerpta Medica, Amsterdam 1976 (170 pp.)

Johnston, I.: Direct surgical treatment of bilateral intracavernous internal carotid artery aneurysms. Case report. J. Neurosurg. 51: 98–102, 1979

Judice, D., E. S. Connolly: Foramen magnum syndrome caused by a giant aneurysm of the posterior inferior cerebral artery. J. Neurosurg. 48: 639–641, 1978

Kak, V. K., A. R. Taylor, D. S. Gordon: Proximal carotid ligation for internal carotid aneurysms. A long term follow-up study. J. Neurosurg. 39: 503–513, 1973

Katakura, R., T. Yoshimoto, J. Suzuki: A case of a giant aneurysm of the basilar artery. Angiography and autopsy. In Suzuki, J.: Cerebral Aneurysms. Neuron, Tokyo 1979 (pp. 704–710)

Katf, N. Y., W. F. T. Tatlow: Two cases of vertebral-basilar aneurysm. Canad. med. Ass. J. 92: 471–474, 1965

Kazner, E., W. Klein, O. Stochdorph: Möglichkeiten und Aussagewert der Computertomographie bei nicht tumorbedingten raumfordernden intracraniellen Prozessen. Röntgen-Bl. 31: 181–198, 1978

Kazner, E., W. Lanksch, H. Steinhoff, J. Wilske: Die axiale Computer-Tomographie des Gehirnschädels. Thieme, Stuttgart 1975

Kempe. L. G.: Vertebral artery aneurysms. Operative treatment. In Pia, H. W., C. Langmaid, J. Zierski: Cerebral Aneurysms. Springer 1979 (pp. 297–306)

Kendall, B. E., L. E. Claveria, W. Quiroga: CAT in leukodystrophy and neuronal degenerations. In Du Boulay, G. H., J. F. Moseley: First European Seminar on Computerised Axial Tomography in Clinical Practice. Springer, Berlin 1977 (pp. 191–202)

Kety, S. S., C. F. Schmidt: The effects of altered arterial tensions of carbon dioxide and oxygen on the cerebral blood flow and cerebral oxygen consumption of normal young men. J. clin. Invest. 27: 484–492, 1948

Khatile, R.: Massive enlargement of intracranial aneurysm following carotid ligation. Arch. Neurol. (Chic.) 17: 609–613, 1967

Kindt, G. W.: Arterial clamp for more gradual blood flow reduction: Technical note. J. Neurosurg. 30: 508–510, 1969

Kindt, G. W., J. R. Youmans, O. Albrand: Factors influencing the autoregulation of the cerebral blood flow during hypotension and hypertension. J. Neurosurg. 26: 299–305, 1967

Kothandaram, P., B. H. Dawson, R. C. Kruyt: Carotid-ophthalmic aneurysms. A study of 19 patients. J. Neurosurg. 34: 544–548, 1971

Krayenbühl, H., M. G. Yaşargil: Die vaskulären Erkrankungen im Gebiet der Arteria vertebralis und Arteria basilaris. Thieme, Stuttgart 1957

Krayenbühl, H. A., M. G. Yaşargil, E. S. Flamm, et al.: Microsurgical treatment of intracranial saccular aneurysms. J. Neurosurg. 37: 678–686, 1972

Kretzschmar, K., T. Grumme, H. Steinhoff: Der Wert der Computer-Tomographie und Angiographie für die Diagnose supratentorieller Hirntumoren. Neuroradiology 16: 487–490, 1978

Kristiansen, K., J. Krog: Electromagnetic studies on the blood flow through the carotid system in man. Neurology (Minneap.) 12: 20–22, 1962

Kümmell, R.: Zur Kenntnis der Geschwülste der Hypophysengegend. Münch. med. Wschr. 58: 1293–1298, 1911

Landolt, A. M., C. H. Millikan: Pathogenesis of cerebral infarction secondary to mechanical carotid artery occlusion. Stroke 1: 52–62, 1970

Lavyne, M. H., J. Kleefield, K. R. Davis, R. G. Ojemann, R. M. Crowell: Giant intracranial aneurysms of the anterior circulation: Clinical characteristics and diagnosis by computed tomography. Neurosurgery 3: 356–363, 1978

Leech, P. J., J. D. Miller, W. Fitch, J. Barker: Cerebral blood flow, internal carotid artery pressure, and the EEG as a guide to the safety of carotid ligation. J. Neurol. Neurosurg. Psychiat. 37: 854–862, 1974

Little, J. R.: Modification of acute focal ischemia by treatment with mannitol and high-dose dexamethasone. J. Neurosurg. 49: 517–524, 1978

Little, J. R., Y. L. Yamamoto, W. Feindel, et al.: Superficial temporal artery to middle cerebral artery anastomosis. Intraoperative evaluation by fluorescein angiography and xenon-133 clearance. J. Neurosurg. 50: 560–569, 1979

Locksley, H. B.: Report on the Co-operative Study of intracranial aneurysms and subarachnoid hemorrhage. Section V, Part II. Natural history of subarachnoid hemorrhage, intracranial aneurysms and arteriovenous malformations. J. Neurosurg. 25: 321–368, 1966

Love, J. G., L. H. Dart: Results of carotid ligation with particular reference to intracranial aneurysms. J. Neurosurg. 27: 89–93, 1967

Lukin, R. R., A. A. Chambers, R. McLaurin, J. Tew Jr.: Thrombosed giant middle cerebral aneurysms. Neuroradiology 10: 125–129, 1975

McGillicuddy, J. E., S. L. Giannotta, P. S. Ostrowski, G. W. Kindt: Focal cerebral blood flow in induced vasospasm. Modification by intravascular volume expansion. Presented at a Meeting of the Association for Academic Surgery. Cleveland/Ohio, November 16, 1978

Marshall, L. F., F. Durity, R. Lounsbury, et al.: Experimental cerebral oligemia and ischemia produced by intracranial hypertension. Part I: Pathophysiology, electroencephalography, cerebral blood flow, blood-brain barrier, and neurological function. J. Neurosurg. 43: 308–317, 1975

Massachussetts General Hospital. Case records. New Eng. J. Med. 271: 260–264, 1964

Masson, M., J. Cambier: Les anévrysmes vertébro-basilaires. La dolichmégabasilaire. Rev. Prat. (Paris) 17: 2759–2769, 1967

Matson, D. D.: Intracranial arterial aneurysms in childhood. J. Neurosurg. 23: 578–583, 1965

Maxwell, R. E., S. N. Chou: Aneurysmal tumors of the basifrontal region. J. Neurosurg. 46: 438–445, 1977

Michael, W. F.: Posterior fossa aneurysms simulating tumours. J. Neurol. Neurosurg. Psychiat. 37: 218–223, 1974

Michenfelder, J. D., J. H. Milde, T. M. Sundt Jr.: Cerebral protection by barbiturate anesthesia. Use after middle cerebral artery occlusion in Java monkeys. Arch. Neurol. (Chic.) 33: 345–350, 1976

Miller, J. D., K. Jawad, B. Jennet: Safety of carotid ligation and its role in the management of intracranial aneurysms. J. Neurol. Neurosurg. Psychiat. 40: 64–72, 1977

Molinari, G. F., J. C. Oakley, J. P. Laurent: The pathophysiology of barbiturate protection in focal ischemia. Stroke 7: 3–4, 1976 (Abstract 11–9)

Morgnani 1761. Quoted without citation by Pribram et al. 1969 (q.v.)

Morley, T. P., H. W. K. Barr: Giant intracranial aneurysms: diagnosis, course, and management. Clin. Neurosurg. 16: 73–94, 1969

Mount, L. A.: Results of treatment of intracranial aneurysms using the Selverstone clamp. J. Neurosurg. 16: 611–618, 1959

Mourgues, G.: Aneurysmen der Arteria basilalis als extracerebrale Pseudotumoren. Ärztl. Wschr. 9: 417–420, 1954

Mullan, S.: Experiences with surgical thrombosis of intracranial berry aneurysms and carotid cavernous fistulas. J. Neurosurg. 41: 657–670, 1974

Mullan, S., C. Reyes, J. Dawley, et al.: Stereotactic copper electric thrombosis of intracranial aneurysms. Progr. neurol. Surg. 3: 193–211, 1969

Nadjmi, M., M. Ratzka, M. Wodartz: Giant aneurysms in CT and angiography. Neuroradiology 16: 284–286, 1978

Nijensohn, D. E., J. Ruben, J. Saez, T. J. Reagan: Clinical significance of basilar artery aneurysms. Neurology (Minneap.) 24: 301–305, 1974

Nishioka, H.: Report on the Cooperative Study of intracranial aneurysms and subarachnoid hemorrhage. Section VIII, Part I. Results of treatment of intracranial aneurysms by occlusion of the carotid artery in the neck. J. Neurosurg. 25: 660–682, 1966

Noda, S., N. Tamaki, M. Yamaguchi, S. Matsumoto: Giant suprasellar aneurysm with extravasation of contrast media. Surg. Neurol. 13: 208–210, 1980

Norlén, G.: Personal communications, 1979

Nornes, H.: The role of the circle of Willis in graded occlusion of the internal carotid artery in man. Acta neurochir. (Wien) 28: 165–177, 1973

Nutik, S.: Carotid paraclinoid aneurysms with intradural origin and intracavernous location. J. Neurosurg. 48: 526–533, 1978

Nyström, S. H. M.: Development of intracranial aneurysms as revealed by electron microscopy. J. Neurosurg. 20: 329–337, 1963

Obrador, S., G. Dierssen, J. R. Hernandez: Giant aneurysm of the posterior cerebral artery: case report. J. Neurosurg. 26: 413–416, 1967

Odom, G. L., G. T. Tindall: Carotid ligation in the treatment of certain intracranial aneurysms. Clin. Neurosurg. 15: 101–116, 1968

Odom, G. L., B. Woodhall, G. T. Tindall, J. R. Jackson: Changes in distal intravascular pressure and size of intracranial aneurysm following common carotid ligation. J. Neurosurg. 19: 41–50, 1962

Olesen, J., O. B. Paulson, N. A. Lassen: Regional cerebral blood flow in man determined by the initial slope of the clearance of intra-arterially injected ^{133}Xe. Stroke 2: 519–540, 1971

Onuma, T., J. Suzuki: Surgical treatment of giant intracranial aneurysms. In Suzuki, J.: Cerebral Aneurysms. Neuron, Tokyo 1979 (pp. 308–312)

Parkinson, D.: A surgical approach to the cavernous portion of the carotid artery. Anatomical studies and case report. J. Neurosurg. 23: 474–483, 1965

Paulson, G., B. S. Nashold, G. Margolis: Aneurysms of the vertebral artery. Report of 5 cases. Neurology (Minneap.) 9: 590–598, 1959

Perrin, D. P., et al.: CT findings in giant intracranial aneurysms. J. Neuroradiol. 6: 317–326, 1979

Peterson, N. T., P. M. Duchesneau, E. L. Westbrook, M. A. Weinstein: Basilar artery ectasia demonstrated by computer tomography. Radiology 122: 713–715, 1977

Pfeiffer, J., H. Haas, J. W. Boellaard: Basilaris-Vertebralis-Aneurysmen als Ursache scheinbarer Halswirbelsäulensyndrome. Dtsch. med. Wschr. 103: 331–335, 1978

Pia, H. W.: Classification of vertebro-basilar aneurysms. Acta neurochir. (Wien) 47: 3–30, 1979a

Pia, H. W.: Microsurgical treatment of vertebro-basilar aneurysms. In Pia, H. W., C. Langmaid, J. Zierski: Cerebral Aneurysms. Springer, Berlin 1979b (pp. 319–326)

Pia, H. W.: Classification and treatment of aneurysms of the vertebro-basilar system. Neurol. Med. Chir. (Tokyo) 19: 575–594, 1979c

Pia, H. W.: Large and giant aneurysms. Neurosurg. Rev. 3: 7–16, 1980

Pia, H. W., J. Zierski: Giant cerebral aneurysms. Problems in treatment. In Pia, H. W., C. Langmaid, J. Zierski: Cerebral Aneurysms. Springer, Berlin 1979 (pp. 336–342)

Pia, H. W., C. Langmaid, J. Zierski: Cerebral Aneurysms. Advances in Diagnosis and Therapy. Springer, Berlin 1979

Polis, Z., J. Brezezinski, M. Chodak-Gajewicz: Giant intracranial aneurysm. J. Neurosurg. 39: 408–411, 1973

Poppen, J. L., C. A. Fager: Intracranial aneurysms. Results of surgical treatment. J. Neurosurg. 17: 283–296, 1960

Pribram, H. F., J. D. Hudson, M. D. Joynt: Posterior fossa aneurysms presenting as mass lesions. Amer. J. Roentgenol. 105: 334–340, 1969

Pritz, M. B., S. L. Giannotta, G. W. Kindt, J. E. McGillicuddy, R. L. Prager: Treatment of patients with neurological deficits associated with cerebral vasospasm by intravascular volume expansion. Neurosurgery 3: 364–368, 1978

Rand, R. W.: Retinal arterial pressure studies associated with cervical carotid artery occlusion in the treatment of cerebral aneurysms. Bull. Los Angeles neurol. Soc. 21: 175–187, 1956

Raymond, L. A., J. Tew: Large suprasellar aneurysms simulating pituitary tumour. J. Neurol. Neurosurg. Psychiat. 41: 83–87, 1978

Richardson, A. E., J. A. Jane, D. Yashon: Prognostic factors in the untreated course of posterior communicating aneurysms. Arch. Neurol. (Chic.) 14: 172–176, 1966

Roach, M. R.: Changes in arterial distensibility as a cause of poststenotic dilatation. Amer. J. Cardiol. 12: 802–815, 1963

Roberts, R., W. H. Hardesty, H. E. Holling, et al.: Studies on extracranial cerebral blood flow. Surgery 56: 826–833, 1964

Rozario, R. A., H. L. Levine, R. M. Scott: Obstructive hydrocephalus secondary to an ectatic basilar artery. Surg. Neurol. 9: 31–34, 1978

Sadik, A. R., G. N. Budzilovich, K. Shulman: Giant aneurysm of middle cerebral artery. A case report. J. Neurosurg. 22: 177–181, 1965

Sahs, A. L., G. E. Perret, H. B. Locksley, H. Nishioka: Intracranial aneurysms and Subarachnoid Haemorrhage. A Cooperative Study. Lippincott, Philadelphia 1969

Sano, K.: Giant aneurysms. Management. In Pia, H. W., C. Langmaid, J. Zierski: Cerebral aneurysms. Springer, Berlin 1979 (pp. 342–344)

Sarwar, M., S. Batnitzky, M. M. Schechter: Tumorous aneurysms. Neuroradiology 12: 79–97, 1976
Sarwar, M., S. Batnitzky, M. M. Schechter, A. Liebeskind, A. E. Zimmer: Growing intracranial aneurysms. Radiology 120: 603–607, 1976
Schmiedek, P., O. Gratzl, R. Spetzler: Selection of patients for extra-intracranial arterial bypass surgery based on rCBF measurements. J. Neurosurg. 44: 303–312, 1976
Schunk, H.: Spontaneous thrombosis of intracranial aneurysms. Amer. J. Roentgenol. 41: 1327–1338, 1964
Scott, M., H. M. Stauffer: A case of aneurysmal malformation of the vertebral and basilar arteries causing cranial nerve involvement. Amer. J. Roentgenol. 92: 836–837, 1964
Scott, R. M., H. T. Ballantine Jr.: Spontaneous thrombosis in a giant middle cerebral artery aneurysm. Case report. J. Neurosurg. 37: 361–363, 1972
Scotti, G., C. De Grandi, A. Colombo: Ectasia of the intracranial arteries diagnosed by computed tomography. Megadolichobasilar artery: CT diagnosis. Neuroradiology 13: 183–184, 1978
Segal, H. D., R. L. McLaurin: Giant serpentine aneurysm. Report of two cases. J. Neurosurg. 46: 115–120, 1977
Selverstone, B., J. C. White: A new technique for gradual occlusion of the carotid artery. Arch. Neurol. Psychiat. (Chic.) 66: 246, 1951 (Abstracts)
Sengupta, D., M. Harper, B. Jennett: Effect of carotid ligation on cerebral blood flow in baboons: 2. Response to hypoxia and haemorrhagic hypertension. J. Neurol. Neurosurg. Psychiat. 37: 578–584, 1974
Sengupta, R. P., G. L. Gryspeerdt, J. Hankinson: Carotid-ophthalmic aneurysms. J. Neurol. Neurosurg. Psychiat. 39: 837–853, 1976
Serbinenko, F. A.: Balloon catheterization and occlusion of major cerebral vessels. J. Neurosurg. 41: 125–145, 1974
Sharbrough, F. W., J. M. Messick Jr., T. M. Sundt Jr.: Correlation of continuous electroencephalograms with cerebral blood flow measurements during carotid endarterectomy. Stroke 4: 674–683, 1973
Shucart, W. A., S. A. Wolpert: An aneurysm in infancy presenting with diabetes insipidus. Case report. J. Neurosurg. 37: 368–370, 1972
Silverberg, G. D., B. A. Reitz, A. K. Ream, G. Taylor, D. R. Enzmann: Operative treatment of giant cerebral artery aneurysm with hypothermia and circulatory arrest. Neurosurgery 6/3: 301–305, 1980
Smith, A. L., J. T. Hoff, S. L. Nielsen, et al.: Barbiturate protection in acute focal cerebral ischemia. Stroke 5: 1–7, 1974
Smith, R. W., J. F. Alksne: Stereotaxic thrombosis of inaccessible intracranial aneurysms. J. Neurosurg. 47: 833–839, 1977
Sonntag, V. K. H., R. H. Yuan, B. M. Stein: Giant intracranial aneurysms: a review of 13 cases. Surg. Neurol. 8: 81–84, 1977
Spetzler, R., N. Chater: Microvascular bypass surgery. Part 2: Physiological studies. J. Neurosurg. 45: 508–513, 1976
Spetzler, R. F., H. Schuster, R. A. Roski: Elective extracranial-intracranial arterial bypass in the treatment of inoperable giant aneurysms of the internal carotid artery. J. Neurosurg. 53: 22–27, 1980
Stehbens, W. E.: Intracranial arterial aneurysms. Aust. Ann. Med. 3: 214–220, 1954
Stern, W. E.: Circulatory adequacy attendant upon carotid artery occlusion. Arch. Neurol. (Chic.) 21: 455–465, 1969
Strenger, L.: Neurological deficits following therapeutic collapse of intracavernous carotid aneurysms. J. Neurosurg. 25: 215–218, 1966
Sundt, T. M. Jr., J. D. Michenfelder: Focal transient cerebral ischemia in the squirrel monkey: effect on brain adenosine triphosphate and lactate levels with electrocorticographic and pathologic correlation. Circulat. Res. 30: 703–712, 1972
Sundt, T. M. Jr., D. G. Piepgras: Surgical approach to giant intracranial aneurysms. Operative experience with 80 cases. J. Neurosurg. 51: 731–742, 1979
Sundt, T. M. Jr., J. P. Whisnant: Subarachnoid hemorrhage from intracranial aneurysms. Surgical management and natural history of disease. New Engl. J. Med. 299: 116–122, 1978
Sundt, T. M. Jr., J. R. Pluth, G. A. Gronert: Excision of giant basilar aneurysm under profound hypothermia. Report of case. Mayo Clin. Proc. 47: 631–634, 1972
Sundt, T. M. Jr., F. W. Sharbrough, R. E. Anderson, et al.: Cerebral blood flow measurements and electroencephalograms during carotid endarterectomy. J. Neurosurg. 41: 310–320, 1974
Sundt, T. M. Jr., R. G. Siekert, D. G. Piepgras, et al.: Bypass surgery for vascular disease of the carotid system. Mayo Clin. Proc. 51: 677–692, 1976
Sutton, D.: The vertebro-basilar system and its vascular lesions. Clin. Radiol. 22: 271–287, 1971
Suzuki, J.: [Surgery of intracranial aneurysm. A method of prolongation of temporary stopping of the cerebral blood flow.] Presented at the 33rd Annual Meeting of the Japan Neurosurgical Society, Sendai, Japan, October, 1974 (Presidential address) (Jpn)
Suzuki, J.: Giant aneurysms. Results. In Pia, H. W., C. Langmaid, J. Zierski: Cerebral Aneurysms. Springer, Berlin 1979a (pp. 345–346)
Suzuki, J.: Cerebral Aneurysms. Neuron, Tokyo 1979b
Symon, L., N. M. Branston, A. J. Strong: Autoregulation in acute focal ischemia. An experimental study. Stroke 7: 547–554, 1976
Symon, L., H. A. Crockard, N. W. C. Dorsch, et al.: Local cerebral blood flow and vascular reactivity in a chronic stable stroke in baboon. Stroke 6: 482–492, 1975
Taki, W., H. Handa, S. Yamagata, et al.: Embolization and superselective angiography by means of balloon catheters. Surg. Neurol. 12: 7–14, 1979a
Taki, W., H. Handa, S. Yamagata, I. Matsuda, Y. Yonekawa, et al.: Balloon embolization of a giant aneurysm, using a new developed catheter. Surg. Neurol. 12: 363–365, 1979b
Taveras, J. M., E. H. Wood: Diagnostic Neuroradiology, 2nd Ed. 2. Williams & Wilkins, Baltimore 1976
Terao, H., I. Muraoka: Giant aneurysm of the middle cerebral artery containing an important blood channel: Case report. J. Neurosurg. 37: 352–356, 1972
Terao, I., A. Ikeda, S. Kobayashi, A. Teraoka: A thrombosed giant aneurysm of the internal carotid artery with brain stem displacement. Surg. Neurol. 10: 157–160, 1978
Thron, A., S. Bockenheimer: Giant aneurysms of the posterior fossa suspected as neoplasms on computed tomography. Neuroradiology 19: 93–97, 1979
Tindall, G. T.: Management of aneurysms of anterior circulation by carotid artery occlusion. In Youmans, J. R.: Neurological Surgery, Vol. II. Saunders, Philadelphia 1973 (pp. 768–786)
Tindall, G. T., G. L. Odom: Treatment of intracranial aneurysms by proximal carotid ligation. Prog. neurol. Surg. 3: 66–114, 1969
Tindall, G. T., J. A. Goree, J. F. Lee, G. L. Odom: Effect of common carotid ligation on size of internal carotid aneurysms and distal intracarotid and retinal artery pressures. J. Neurosurg. 25: 503–511, 1966
Tindall, G. T., G. L. Odom, H. B. Cupp, Jr. et al.: Studies on carotid artery flow and pressure. Observations in 18 patients during graded occlusion of the proximal carotid artery. J. Neurosurg. 19: 917–923, 1962
Tomasello, F., V. Albanese, F. A. Gioffi: Giant serpentine aneurysms. A separate entity. Surg. Neurol. 12: 429–432, 1979
Tönnis, W.: Zur Behandlung intracranieller Aneurysmen. Arch. klin. Chir. 189: 474–476, 1937
Traquair, H. M.: An Introduction to Clinical Perimetry, 6th Ed. Mosby, St. Louis 1949
Tridon, P., M. Masingue, L. Picard, F. Briquel, J. Roland: Hémispasme facial et mégadolichobasilaire à symptomatologie pseudotumorale. Rev. Oto-neurophtal. 43: 279–286, 1971
Tytus, J. S., A. A. Ward Jr.: The effect of cervical carotid ligation on giant intracranial aneurysms. J. Neurosurg. 33: 184–190, 1970
Waltz, A. G., A. R. Wanek, R. E. Anderson: Comparison of analytic methods for calculation of cerebral blood flow after intracarotid injection of ^{133}Xe. J. nucl. Med. 13: 66–72, 1972
Weitbrecht, W.-U., M. Schumacher, U. Thoden, W. Kleine: Spindelförmiges Basilarisaneurysma mit Symptomen eines basalen Tumors. Nervenarzt 48: 688–691, 1977
Wende, S., A. Aulich, K. Kretzschmar, T. Grumme, W. Meese, S. Lange, H. Steinhoff, W. Lanksch, E. Kazner: Die Computer-Tomographie der Hirngeschwülste. Eine Sammelstudie über 1658 Tumoren. Radiologe 17: 149–156, 1977
White, J. C.: Aneurysms mistaken for hypophyseal tumors. In Clinical Neurosurgery (Proceedings of The Congress of Neurological Surgeons 1962), ed. by William H. Mosberg, Vol. 10, Ch. 13. Williams & Wilkins, Baltimore 1964
White, J. C., R. D. Adams: Combined supra- and infraclinoid

aneurysms of internal carotid artery. J. Neurosurg. 12: 450–459, 1955
White, J. C., H. T. Ballentine Jr.: Intrasellar aneurysms simulating hypophyseal tumours. J. Neurosurg. 18: 34–50, 1961
Wilkinson, H. A., R. L. Wright, W. H. Sweet: Correlation of reduction in pressure and angiographic cross-filling with tolerance of carotid occlusion. J. Neurosurg. 22: 241–245, 1965
Williams, R. R., R. C. Bahn, G. P. Sayre: Congenital cerebral aneurysms. Proc. Mayo Clin. 30: 161–168, 1955
Wilson, C. B., R. W. Rand, J. M. Grollmus, et al.: Surgical experience with a microscopic transsphenoidal approach to pituitary tumors and non-neoplastic parasellar conditions. Calif. Med. 117: 1–9, 1972
Winn, H. R., A. E. Richardson, J. A. Jane: Late morbidity and mortality of common carotid ligation for posterior communicating aneurysms. A comparison to conservative treatment. J. Neurosurg. 47: 727–736, 1977
Wood, E. H.: Angiographic identification of the ruptured lesion in patients with multiple cerebral aneurysms. J. Neurosurg. 21: 182–198, 1964
Yaşargil, M. G.: Microsurgery Applied to Neurosurgery. Academic Press, New York 1969 (pp. 105–117)
Yaşargil, M. G., R. D. Smith: Surgery on the carotid system in the treatment of hemorrhagic stroke. Advanc. Neurol. 16: 181–209, 1977
Yaşargil, M. G., H. A. Krayenbühl, J. H. Jacobson: Microneurosurgical arterial reconstruction. Surgery 67: 221–233, 1970
Yaşargil, M. G., J. C. Gasser, R. M. Hodosh, T. V. Rankin: Carotid-ophthalmic aneurysms: Direct microsurgical approach. Surg. Neurol. 8: 155–165, 1977
Yaskin, H. E., B. Alpers: Aneurysms of the vertebral artery. Report of case in which the aneurysm simulated a tumor of the posterior fossa. Arch. Neurol. Psychiat. (Chic.) 51: 271–281, 1944
Yatsu, F. M., I. Diamond, C. Graziano, et al.: Experimental brain ischemia: protection from irreversible damage with a rapid-acting barbiturate (methohexital). Stroke 3: 726–732, 1972
Yoshimoto, T., J. Suzuki: [Intracranial definitive aneurysm surgery under normothermia and normotension utilizing temporary occlusion of brain artery and preoperative mannitol administration.] Neurol. Surg. 8: 775–783, 1976 (Jpn)
Yoshimoto, T., T. Sakamoto, T. Watanabe, et al.: Experimental cerebral infarction. Part 3: Protective effect of mannitol in thalamic infarction in dogs. Stroke 9: 217–218, 1978
Youman, J. R., G. W. Kindt, O. C. Mitchell: Extended studies of direction of flow and pressure in the internal carotid artery following common carotid artery ligation. J. Neurosurg. 27: 250–254, 1967
Young, G., G. A. Fattal: Arteriosclerotic aneurysm of the middle cerebral artery. Canad. med. Ass. J. 89: 720–723, 1963

Chapter 7: Multiple Aneurysms

Af Björkesten, G., V. Halonen: Incidence of intracranial vascular lesions in patients with subarachnoid haemorrhage investigated by four-vessel angiography. J. Neurosurg. 23: 29–32, 1965
Af Björkesten, G., H. Troupp: Multiple intracranial arterial aneurysms. Acta chir. scand. 118: 387–391, 1959/60
Bassett, R. C., C. F. List, L. J. Lemmen: Surgical treatment of intra-cranial aneurysm. Surg. Gynec. Obstet. 95: 701–708, 1952
Bigelow, N. H.: Multiple intracranial arterial aneurysms. AMA Arch. Neurol. Psychiat. 73: 76–98, 1955
Crompton, M. R.: The pathology of ruptured middle cerebral aneurysms with special reference to the differences between the sexes. Lancet II: 421–425, 1962
Dandy, W. E.: Intracranial Arterial Aneurysms, Vol. VII. Comstock, Ithaca 1944 (147 pp)
Drake, C. G., J. P. Girvin: The surgical treatment of subarachnoid hemorrhage with multiple aneurysms. In Morley, T. P.: Current Controversies in Neurosurgery. Saunders, Philadelphia 1976 (pp. 274–278)
Hamby, W. B.: Intra-cranial Aneurysms, chapt. 11, Thomas, Springfield/Ill. 1952 (pp. 104, 106, 342–345)
Hamby, W. B.: Multiple intracranial aneurysms. J. Neurosurg. 16: 558–563, 1959

Heiskanen, O.: The identification of ruptured aneurysm in patients with multiple intracranial aneurysms. Neurochirurgia (Stuttg.) 8: 102–107, 1965
Heiskanen, O.: Risk of bleeding from unruptured aneurysms in cases with multiple intracranial aneurysms. J. Neurosurg. 55: 524–526, 1981
Heiskanen, O., I. Marttila: Risk of rupture of a second aneurysm in patients with multiple aneurysms. J. Neurosurg. 32: 295–299, 1970
Karasawa, J., H. Kikuchi, S. Furuse, T. Manabe, T. Sakai: Surgery of multiple intracranial aneurysms. Neurol. Surg. 2: 763–769, 1974
King, G., H. W. Slade, F. Campoy: Bilateral intracranial aneurysms. Arch. Neurol. Psychiat. (Chic.) 71: 326–336, 1954
Locksley, H. B.: Report on the Cooperative Study of Intracranial Aneurysms and Subarachnoid Hemorrhage. Section V. Part I. Natural history of subarachnoid hemorrhage, intracranial aneurysms and arteriovenous malformations. Based on 6368 cases in the Cooperative Study. J. Neurosurg. 25: 219–239, 1966
McKissock, W., A. Richardson, L. Walsh, et al.: Multiple intracranial aneurysms. Lancet I: 623–626, 1964
McKissock, W., I. Walsh: Subarachnoid haemorrhage due to intracranial aneurysms. Results of treatment of 249 verified cases. Brit. med. J. II: 559–565, 1956
Magee, C. G.: Spontaneous subarachnoid hemorhage. Lancet 2: 497–500, 1943
Mount, L. A., R. Brisman: Treatment of multiple intracranial aneurysms. J. Neurosurg. 35: 728–730, 1971
Mount, L. A., R. Brisman: Treatment of multiple aneurysms – symptomatic and asymptomatic. Clin. Neurosurg. 21: 166–170, 1974
Moyes, P. D.: Surgical treatment of multiple aneurysms and of incidentally discovered unruptured aneurysms. J. Neurosurg. 35: 291–295, 1971
Nagamine, Y., S. Takahashi, M. Sonobe: Multiple intracranial aneurysms associated with moya moya disease. J. Neurosurg. 54: 673–676, 1981
Norlén, G., H. Olivecrona: The treatment of aneurysms of the circle of Willis. J. Neurosurg. 10: 404–415, 1953
Paterson, A., M. R. Bond: Treatment of multiple intracranial arterial aneurysms. Lancet I: 1302–1304, 1973
Pool, J. L., D. G. Potts: Aneurysms and Arteriovenous Anamolies of the Brain. Diagnosis and Treatment. Harper & Row, New York 1965
Poppen, J. L., C. A. Fager: Multiple intracranial aneurysms. J. Neurosurg. 16: 581–589, 1959
Pouyanne, H., A. Banayan, J. Guerin, V. Riemens: Les anévrysmes sacculaires multiples du système carotidien supra-clinoîdien. Etude anatomo-clinique et thérapeutique. Neuro-chirurgie 19, Suppl. 1: 96, 1973
Richardson, J. C., H. H. Hyland: Intracranial aneurysms. A clinical and pathological study of subarachnoid and intracerebral hemorrhage caused by berry aneurysms. Medicine (Baltimore) 20: 1–83, 1941
Riggs, H., C. Rupp: Miliary aneurysms: relations of anomalies of the circle of Willis to formation of aneurysms. Arch. Neurol. Psychiat. (Chic.) 49: 615–616, 1943
Sengupta, R. P., J. Hankinson: An unusual case of multiple intracranial aneurysms. Acta neurochir. (Wien) 45: 259–275, 1975
Sengupta, R. P., L. P. Lassen: Identification of the source of bleeding in multiple intracranial aneurysms. Vasc. Surg. 8: 177–183, 1974
Suzuki, J., Y. Sakurai: The treatment of intracranial multiple aneurysms. In Suzuki, J.: Cerebral Aneurysms. Neuron, Tokyo 1979 (pp. 293–307)
Suzuki, J., Shigeaki, Y. Sakurai: Intracranial aneurysms in the neurosurgical clinics in Japan. J. Neurosurg. 35: 34–39, 1971
Taveras, J. M., E. H. Wood: Diagnostic Neuroradiology. Williams & Wilkins, Baltimore 1963
Walton, J. N.: Subarachnoid Haemorrhage. Livingstone, Edinburgh 1956
Williams, R. R., R. C. Bahn, G. P. Sayre: Congenital cerebral aneurysms. Proc. Mayo Clin. 30: 161–168, 1955
Wilson, G., H. E. Riggs, C. Rupp: The pathologic anatomy of ruptured cerebral aneurysms. J. Neurosurg. 11: 128–134, 1954

Wood, E. H.: Angiographic identification of the ruptured lesion in patients with multiple cerebral aneurysms. J. Neurosurg. 21: 182–198, 1964

Kassel, N. F., C. G. Drake: Review of the management of saccular aneurysms. Neurol. Clin. North America Vol. 1, No. 1, 1983

Chapter 11: Final Comments

Bucy, P. C.: Intracranial aneurysms – some important statistics. Surg. Neurol. 19: 390–391, 1983

Index

A

Addendum (second series of cases 1979–1983) 340ff
Age
– and sex 48, 68, 89, 103, 119, 160f, 206, 252
– related incidence of SAH, 29ff, 340
– – to surgical results 206
Aneurysms
– alternative treatments 254
– arterial relationships 99, 109ff, 126, 178f
– asymptomatic 2ff, 28f
– enlargement: Vol. I 295
– giant 296ff
– multiple 305ff
– ruptured (clinical presentation) 1f
– suprachiasmatic, elevation of 46
– unclipped 47
– unoperated 329f
– unruptured 28f
– – asymptomatic 28f
– – symptomatic 2
Angiography and vasospasm 17ff
Anterior clinoid process, relationship to 44
Antifibrinolysis 27f
Approach, initial 44f, 167, 185, 226, 237f, 254
Arteries
– anterior cerebral 165ff
– – – contralateral, relationship to 185
– – – distal 224ff
– – – ipsilateral, relationship to 185
– – – proximal 165ff
– – choroidal 99ff
– – – identification of 82
– – – relationship to 77, 99
– – communicating 169ff
– – – complex and exposure 185f
– basilar bifurcation 233ff
– – – alternative treatments 254
– – lower trunk, fusiform 272ff
– – – – saccular 270f
– – upper trunk 257ff
– – internal carotid 33ff
– – – bifurcation 109ff
– – – cervical 33ff
– – – distal (medial wall) 58f
– – – inferior wall 60ff
– – – intracavernous 37ff
– – – petrous portion 37
– – – summary of ICA aneurysms 122f

– – – superior wall 59
– middle cerebral 124ff
– – – bifurcation 129ff
– – – – secondary 131
– – – distal branches 132
– – – proximal, lateral wall 127
– – – – medial wall 128
– – – relationship to 126
– ophthalmic 43ff
– – exposure 45
– – relationship to 44
– pericallosal 224ff
– posterior cerebral, dissection of 240
– – – (P1/2 junction) 265ff
– – – (P1 segment) 260ff
– – – (P2 segment) 266f
– – – (P3 segment) 268f
– – – relationships to 236
– – communicating 71ff
– – – dissection of 240
– – – identification of 78ff
– – – relationship to 76, 236
– – inferior cerebellar (distal) 290ff
– – superior cerebellar (distal) 279f
– – vertebral, fusiform 286ff
– – – saccular 281ff
– – vertebrobasilar 232ff

B

Bilateral 46f, 85ff, 100ff, 116ff, 140ff
Botterell grading 7

C

Cerebral blood flow and timing of operation 26
– ischemia and infarction 212f
Cerebrospinal fluid circulation after aneurysm surgery 332, 336f
Cervical carotid ligation 38f
Children, aneurysms in 30ff
Circle of Willis, dividing of 240f, 255
Cisternal exposure 46
Cisterns
– carotid 102
– dissection 102, 113, 167
– hematoma 228, 345
– interpeduncular, entering 237ff
– lamina terminalis, dissection 113
– relationship to 74ff, 109, 125f, 184
Clinical condition, relationship to 7ff
– considerations 1ff
– presentation of SAH 1f, 340

Clinoid process, relationship to 44, 78, 242
Clipping 46, 85, 102f, 114f, 136ff, 167, 193ff, 228, 242ff
– temporary 163, 219
Closure 85, 115, 139, 199, 246
Coagulation of aneurysm neck 84, 255
Complications, surgical 159, 220f, 331ff, 343ff
– – alterations in CSF circulation 336f
– – classification 331f
– – conclusions 338f
– – epilepsy 335
– – general medical problems 338
– – infection 333
– – intracranial hematoma 333
– – introduction 331
– – ischemia 333f
– – personality and mental changes 335
Control, distal 45
– proximal 44f
Cranial nerve deficit as complications of aneurysm surgery 332
Craniotomy and approach 254
CT scan findings in aneurysm patients 340f
– in giant intracranial aneurysms 297ff

D

Diagnosis of SAH 1f, 340
Differentialdiagnosis of SAH 1f, 340
Dissection of
– aneurysms 134f, 167, 186ff, 228
– – neck 83, 102, 242
– bifurcation 114
– cisterns 102, 167
– lamina terminalis cistern 113
– posterior cerebral arteries 240
– – communicating arteries 240
– Sylvian fissure 113
Distal control 45
Dorsum sellae, relationship to 236

E

Early surgery 9ff, 23, 345
Electrolyte disturbances associated with surgery 214
Epidural extension 78
Epilepsy after aneurysm surgery 159, 215, 332, 335
Exploration, initial 102

Index

Exposure, cisternal 46
– initial 113, 132ff

F

Final comments 346f
Fits following rupture 95
– – surgery 95, 215
Frequency and location of vertebrobasilar aneurysms 232
Fundus
– direction 72f, 109, 180ff, 253
– dissection 186ff
– projection 44, 233ff, 236
– resection 85, 115, 199, 228
– size 109, 236, 253

G

General medical care in SAH 26
– condition related to timing of surgery 16f, 345
Giant aneurysms 146ff, 296ff
Grading, clinical 7ff
– – Botterell 7
– – Hunt and Hess 7
– – Lougheed 7

H

Hematoma, cisternal 228
– – removal of (in early surgery) 345
– intracranial 92f, 162, 210f
– – (as complication of aneurysm surgery) 333
Hemostasis and closure 199
Historical aspects 88, 103, 118, 149, 169, 232
Hydrocephalus 94, 159, 209f, 252
Hypertension 92
Hypotension in present recurrent hemorrhage 27

I

Infection after aneurysm surgery 333
Intracranial pressure and timing of surgery 25f
Intraoperative rupture 85, 218f, 255
Investigations in SAH 346f
Ischemia and infarction, cerebral 212f
– after aneurysm surgery 333f

J

Juvenile aneurysms 30ff

L

Laterality of aneurysms 32, 43, 71, 109, 124, 173ff

Ligation of aneurysm 85, 114f
– – internal carotid artery 38f, 114f
Location 173ff, 232
Lougheed grading 7

M

Meningeal irritation and meningitis, differential diagnosis in SAH 1f
Morbidity 92ff, 95ff, 163f, 218ff
Morphology and size 125
Mortality 92ff
Multiple aneurysms 46f, 116ff, 140ff, 305ff
– – bilateral 46f, 100ff, 116ff, 140ff
– – incidence and epidemiology 305
– – operative results 327
Multiplicity 43, 60, 71, 124, 170ff, 225, 233

O

Oculomotor nerve
– – identification 82
– – palsy 82
– – – outcome 90, 252
– – – relationship to 77
Operative complications 159, 220f
– morbidity related to outcome 95ff, 163f, 218ff
– problems 254f

P

Parent arteries identification 228
Partial cervical carotid artery occlusion 28
Posterior clinoid process, removal 242
Pregnancy and subarachnoid hemorrhage 29
Preoperative condition related to results 92, 160, 206ff
– rebleed, prevention of 26ff
Proximal control 44f
Psycho-organic syndrome 215

R

Recurrent hemorrhage, preoperative (prevention of) 26ff, 345
– – – – antifibrinolysis 27f
– – – – general medical measures 26
– – – – hypotension 27
– – – – partial cervical carotid artery occlusion 28
Relationship
– arterial 76f, 109ff, 126, 178f, 185, 236
– cisternal 74ff, 109, 125f, 184
– uncus and tentorium 100
Risk of hemorrhage in unruptured aneurysms 28f

Rupture, intraoperative 95, 218f, 255
Ruptured cerebral aneurysms, clinical presentation 1f, 340f

S

Sites of aneurysm formation 328, 343
Size 163, 236
– and morphology 125
Special clinical presentations 28ff, 340ff
– – – age 29f, 340
– – – children 30ff
– – – laterality 32
– – – pregnancy 29
– – – unruptured, asymptomatic aneurysms 28f
Subarachnoid hemorrhage, number of 93f, 162, 206ff
Sylvian fissure, dissection 113

T

Temporal lobe, relationship to 78
Temporary clipping 163, 219
Tentorium cerebelli, relationship to 78
Thrombosis of aneurysm 254
Timing of surgery 7ff, 54, 70, 95, 106, 120ff, 161, 216ff, 229f, 252f, 341ff
– – cerebral blood flow, relationship to 26
– – intracranial pressure, relationship to 25f
– – preoperative condition, relationship to 7ff
– – – vasospasm, relationship to 17ff

U

Unclipped aneurysms 47
Uncus and tentorium, relationship to 100
Unoperated aneurysms 329f
– – asymptomatic 2ff, 28f
– – symptomatic 2
Unruptured aneurysms 28f

V

Vasospasm, cerebral, angiography and 17ff
– – preoperative 17ff
– – postoperative 23f
Veins, Sylvian in middle cerebral artery aneurysms 133
Venous relationships 113, 184
– thrombosis, pulmonary embolism 345

W

Warning hemorrhage 1, 31, 347